ORTHOPEDIC PHYSICAL ASSESSMENT

ORTHOPEDIC PHYSICAL ASSESSMENT

DAVID J. MAGEE, Ph.D., B.P.T.

Professor
Department of Physical Therapy
Faculty of Rehabilitation Medicine
University of Alberta
Edmonton, Alberta, Canada

W. B. SAUNDERS COMPANY
Harcourt Brace Jovanovich, Inc.
Philadelphia London Toronto Montreal Sydney Tokyo

W. B. SAUNDERS COMPANY
Harcourt Brace Jovanovich, Inc.

The Curtis Center
Independence Square West
Philadelphia, Pennsylvania 19106

Library of Congress Cataloging-in-Publication Data

Magee, David J.
    Orthopedic physical assessment / David J. Magee.—2nd ed.

        p. cm.

    Includes bibliographical references and index.

    ISBN 0–7216–4344–2

    1. Orthopedics—Diagnosis.   2. Physical diagnosis.
        3. Physical orthopedic tests.   I. Title.

    [DNLM: 1. Bone diseases—diagnosis.   2. Joint Diseases—
    diagnosis.   3. Orthopedics.   WE 168 M191o]

    RD734.M34   1992

    617.3—dc20

    DNLM/DLC   91-36021

Listed here are the latest translated editions of this book together with the language of the translation and the publisher.

French (1st Edition)—EDISEM, Inc., St. Hyacinthe, Quebec, Canada
Japanese (1st Edition)—Ishiyaku Publishers, Inc., Tokyo, Japan

Editor: Margaret M. Biblis
Designer: Susan Hess Blaker
Cover Designer: Karen O'Keefe
Cover Artist: Phillip Ashley
Production Manager: Linda R. Garber
Manuscript Editors: Allison Esposito and Amy Norwitz
Illustration Specialist: Peg Shaw
Page Layout Artist: B. J. Crim

Orthopedic Physical Assessment, 2nd edition   ISBN 0–7216–4344–2

Last digit is the print number: 9   8   7   6   5   4   3   2   1

To my parents,
who taught me to pick a goal in life
and to take it seriously

Preface
to the First Edition

This manuscript was originally developed as part of a manual for physical therapy students at the University of Alberta. That original manual covered conditions and treatment as well as assessment.

The text is the result of my interpretation of the teachings of recognized experts in the field of orthopedic assessment: James Cyriax, Hans Debrunner, Stanley Hoppenfeld, Freddy Kaltenborn, Geoff Maitland, Robin McKenzie, John Mennell, and Alan Stoddard, to name a few. It is my belief that a book such as this will be of benefit to paramedical and medical students throughout their training and into their practice as well as to other health professionals.

The aim of the book is to provide the reader with a systematic approach to carry out an orthopedic assessment and an understanding of the reason for the various aspects of the assessment. Initially, in each chapter, pertinent arthrology is reviewed. The reader is then taken through history, observation, and examination of each joint of the body. The examination is organized in a consistent fashion beginning with active, passive, and resisted isometric movements. The movements are followed by tests designed by different individuals to evaluate specific structures, and a quick assessment of sensory distribution and reflexes to differentiate between peripheral nerves and nerve root problems. Palpation is discussed next to help the examiner pinpoint the problem. The assessment is concluded by a review of different roentgenographic views and the possible findings that the examiner might see in these views.

At the end of each chapter is a précis for quick review prior to beginning an assessment and a list of references should the examiner wish to do further in-depth reading.

The text is liberally provided with artistic renderings and photos to illustrate different points and to provide visual examples of the conditions and anatomic variations referred to in the manuscript.

This book is my first attempt at a project of this magnitude. Any feedback from readers with constructive ideas of how to improve the text would be greatly appreciated.

DAVID J. MAGEE
1987

Preface
to the Second Edition

The second edition of *Orthopedic Physical Assessment* is an update and rearrangement of information provided in the first edition. In most chapters, several different ways of testing structures are given. This is done not to confuse the reader but to give the reader a choice. The examiner should use the technique that he or she finds works the best and that gives the best results. By providing several tests for the same structures, the book acts as a reference source. I have added new sections dealing with functional assessment and new radiographic techniques to each chapter. Case studies included at the end of most chapters provide the reader with assessment exercises. Two new chapters, "Head and Face" and "Emergency Sports Assessment," have been added at the suggestion of some readers of the first edition.

I am grateful to all those who spoke to me or wrote offering suggestions and corrections to the first edition, especially the late Gail Gilewich. Their help was very much appreciated and many of their suggestions have been incorporated into the second edition. I hope readers will provide feedback to this edition as well.

DAVID J. MAGEE
1992

Acknowledgments

The writing of a book such as this, although a task undertaken by one person, is in reality a bringing together of ideas of colleagues, friends, and experts in the field of orthopedic assessment. In particular, I would like to thank:

Dr. David C. Reid, F.R.C.S.(C), for his teachings, contributions, and ideas in the preparation of this manuscript.

The physical therapy staffs of the Royal Alexandra Hospital, the Glenrose Provincial Hospital, and the Workers' Compensation Board Clinic in Edmonton, Alberta, for their valued suggestions.

My graduate and undergraduate students, who helped collect many of the articles used as references in this book.

The many authors and publishers who have agreed to have some of their photographs, drawings, and tables appear in the text so that explanations can be clearer and more easily understood. Without these additions, the book would not be what I hoped.

Paul Wodehouse, for the new photographs in the second edition.

Alan Garard, Georgina Gray, Marney Dickey, Doug Gilroy, and Martin Parfitt, for being models for many of the photographs in the first edition. For modeling in the second edition, I would like to thank Bev Aindow, Trent Brown, Ian Halworth, Dwayne Man-drusiak, Leslie Ann Marcuk, Jim Meadows, Kevin Wagner, my children, Shawn and Wendy, and my wife, Bernice.

Dorothy Tomniuk, for her untiring and uncomplaining efforts of typing and retyping the first edition.

Dr. Parkinson, Mrs. Kehoe, and the staff of Associated Radiologists, for providing x-ray film to be photographed to illustrate many of the physical conditions discussed in this book.

Martin Parfitt and Donna Ford, for taking the time and effort to review the manuscript.

Baxter Venable, Carol Robins Wolf, and the staff of W. B. Saunders Company, for their suggestions in writing the first edition. For the second edition, I would like to thank Margaret Biblis, Charlie Keenan, and the W. B. Saunders staff for their assistance and patience.

My teachers and colleagues, who encouraged me to pursue my chosen career.

Finally, I must extend a word of appreciation to my irreplaceable secretary, Bev Aindow. Without her help and persistence, this second edition would never have been completed.

To these people, and many others, I say thank you. Without your help and encouragement, this book would never have been written or revised.

Contents

McGill-Melzack
PAIN QUESTIONNAIRE

Patient's name _____ Age _____
File No. _____ Date _____
Clinical category (eg. cardiac, neurological, etc.):

Diagnosis : _____

_____

Analgesic (if already administered):
1. Type _____
2. Dosage _____
3. Time given in relation to this test _____

Patient's intelligence: circle number that represents best estimate

1 (low)   2   3   4   5 (high)

****

This questionnaire has been designed to tell us more about your pain. Four major questions we ask are:

1. Where is your pain?
2. What does it feel like?
3. How does it change with time?
4. How strong is it?

It is important that you tell us how your pain feels now. Please follow the instructions at the beginning of each part.

© R. Melzack, Oct. 1970

Part 1.   Where is your Pain?

Please mark, on the drawings below, the areas where you feel pain. Put E if external, or I if internal, near the areas which you mark. Put EI if both external and internal.

Part 2.   What Does Your Pain Feel Like?

Some of the words below describe your present pain. Circle ONLY those words that best describe it. Leave out any category that is not suitable. Use only a single word in each appropriate category—the one that applies best.

1	2	3	4
Flickering	Jumping	Pricking	Sharp
Quivering	Flashing	Boring	Cutting
Pulsing	Shooting	Drilling	Lacerating
Throbbing		Stabbing	
Beating		Lancinating	
Pounding			

5	6	7	8
Pinching	Tugging	Hot	Tingling
Pressing	Pulling	Burning	Itchy
Gnawing	Wrenching	Scalding	Smarting
Cramping		Searing	Stinging
Crushing			

9	10	11	12
Dull	Tender	Tiring	Sickening
Sore	Taut	Exhausting	Suffocating
Hurting	Rasping		
Aching	Splitting		
Heavy			

13	14	15	16
Fearful	Punishing	Wretched	Annoying
Frightful	Gruelling	Blinding	Troublesome
Terrifying	Cruel		Miserable
	Vicious		Intense
	Killing		Unbearable

17	18	19	20
Spreading	Tight	Cool	Nagging
Radiating	Numb	Cold	Nauseating
Penetrating	Drawing	Freezing	Agonizing
Piercing	Squeezing		Dreadful
	Tearing		Torturing

Part 3.   How Does Your Pain Change With Time?

1. Which word or words would you use to describe the pattern of your pain?

1	2	3
Continuous	Rhythmic	Brief
Steady	Periodic	Momentary
Constant	Intermittent	Transient

2. What kind of things relieve your pain?

3. What kind of things increase your pain?

Part 4.   How Strong Is Your Pain?

People agree that the following 5 words represent pain of increasing intensity. They are:

1	2	3	4	5
Mild	Discomforting	Distressing	Horrible	Excruciating

To answer each question below, write the number of the most appropriate word in the space beside the question.

1. Which word describes your pain right now? _____
2. Which word describes it at its worst? _____
3. Which word describes it when it is least? _____
4. Which word describes the worst toothache you ever had? _____
5. Which word describes the worst headache you ever had? _____
6. Which word describes the worst stomach-ache you ever had? _____

FIGURE 1–1. McGill Melzack Pain Questionnaire. (From Melzack, R.: Pain 1:280–281, 1975.)

---

areas. Repetition helps the examiner to become familiar with the characteristic history of the patient's complaints so that unusual deviation, which often indicates problems, can be noticed immediately. Even if the diagnosis is obvious, the history will give valuable information about the disorder, its prognosis, and the appropriate treatment desired. The history also enables the examiner to determine the type of person the patient is, the treatment the patient has received, and the behavior of the injury. In addition to the history of the present illness or injury, relevant past history, treatment, and results should also be noted. Past medical history should include any major illnesses or surgery, accidents, or allergies. In some cases, it may be necessary to delve into the social and family histories of the patient when they appear relevant. Lifestyle habit patterns, including sleep patterns, stress, work load, and recreational pursuits, should also be noted.

It is important that the examiner help to keep the patient to the point and discourage irrelevant information; this should be done politely but firmly. At the same time, however, to obtain optimum results in the assessment, it is important to establish a good rapport with the patient.

The history is usually taken in an orderly sequence. It offers the patient an opportunity to describe the problem and the limitations caused by the problem as perceived by the patient. The questions asked should be easy to understand and should not "lead" the patient. For example, the examiner should not say, "Does this increase your pain?" It would be better to say, "Does this alter your pain in any way?" The examiner should ask one question at a time and receive an answer to each question before proceeding with another question. The examiner should pose the following pertinent questions:

1. What is the patient's age? Many conditions occur within certain age ranges. For example, various growth disorders, such as Legg-Perthes disease or Scheuermann's disease, are seen in adolescents or teenagers. Degenerative conditions, such as osteoarthritis and osteoporosis, are more likely to be seen in an older population.

2. What is the patient's occupation? As an example, one would expect a laborer to have stronger muscles than a sedentary worker and possibly be less likely to suffer a muscle strain. In contrast, laborers would be more susceptible to injury because of the type of job they have. Although sedentary workers usually have no need for immediate muscle strength, they may find that on weekends, for example, their muscles or joints become overstressed. It is important to remember that habitual postures caused by some occupations may give an indication as to the location of the problem.

3. Was the onset of the problem slow or sudden? Did the condition start as an insidious mild ache and then progress to continuous pain? Does the pain get worse as the day progresses? Was it a sudden onset due to trauma, or was it sudden with locking? Knowledge of these facts helps the examiner determine the cause of the problem.

4. Has the condition occurred before? If so, what was the onset like? Where was the site of the original condition, and has there been any radiation (spread of pain)? If the person is feeling better, how long did it take to recover? Did any treatment help to relieve symptoms? Does the current problem appear to be the same as the previous problem, or is it different? Answers to these questions help the examiner to determine the location and severity of the injury.

5. Was there any inciting trauma? What was the mechanism of injury? Does the patient remember a specific episode in which the body part was injured, or did the problem slowly develop over a period of

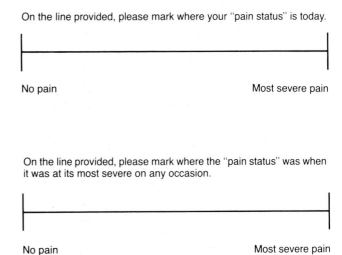

On the line provided, please mark where your "pain status" is today.

|————————————————————————|

No pain   Most severe pain

On the line provided, please mark where the "pain status" was when it was at its most severe on any occasion.

|————————————————————————|

No pain   Most severe pain

FIGURE 1–2. *Visual-analog scales for pain.*

time? If there has been inciting trauma, it is often easier to determine the location of the problem.

6. How long has the patient had the problem? What are the duration and frequency of the symptoms? Answers to these questions help the examiner to determine whether the condition is acute or chronic and to get an idea of the patient's tolerance to pain. When discussing pain, it is often worthwhile to provide the patient with a pain questionnaire or a visual-analog scale (VAS) that can be completed while the patient is waiting to be assessed. An example of such a questionnaire is the McGill-Melzack pain questionnaire (Fig. 1–1).[3] Examples of VASs, or pain-rating scales in which the patient "gauges" the amount of pain, are also illustrated (Fig. 1–2 and 1–3).[4] Once the patient has completed the questionnaire or scale, the examiner can use it to indicate the perception of the pain as described or perceived by the patient.

7. Is the intensity, duration, and/or frequency of pain increasing? These changes usually mean the condition is getting worse. Is the pain decreasing? This change usually means the condition is improving. Is the pain static? If so, how long has it been that way? This question may help the examiner to learn whether the condition is acute or chronic or how long it has been chronic. These factors may become important in treatment. Is the pain associated with other physiological functions? For example, is the pain worse with menstruation? If so, when did the patient last have a pelvic examination? Questions such as these may give the examiner an indication of what is causing the problem or what factors affect the problem.

8. Is the pain constant, periodic, or occasional? Does the condition bother the patient at that exact moment? If the patient is not bothered, the pain is

Pain Rating Scale

Instructions:

Below is a thermometer with various grades of pain on it from "No Pain at all" to "The pain is almost unbearable." Put a × by the words that describe your pain best. Mark how bad your pain is AT THIS MOMENT IN TIME.

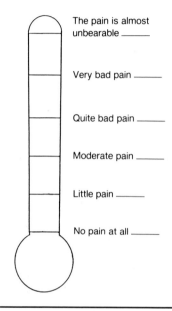

The pain is almost unbearable _____

Very bad pain _____

Quite bad pain _____

Moderate pain _____

Little pain _____

No pain at all _____

FIGURE 1–3. "Thermometer" pain rating scale. (From Brodie, et al.: Evaluation of low back pain by patient questionnaires and therapist assessment. J.O.S.P.T. 11:528, 1990.)

not constant. If the pain is periodic or occasional, the examiner should try to determine the patient's activity, position, or posture that irritates the problem. The examiner should be observing the patient at the same time. Does there appear to be constant pain? Does the patient appear to be lacking sleep because of pain? Does the patient move around a great deal in an attempt to find a comfortable position?

9. Where was the pain when the individual first had the complaint? Has the pain moved or spread? Ask the patient to point to exactly where the pain was and where it is now. In general, the area of pain enlarges or becomes more distal as the lesion worsens and vice versa. The more distal and superficial the problem, the more accurately the patient can determine the location of the pain. In the case of referred pain, the patient will usually point out a general area; with a localized lesion, the patient will point to a specific location. Pain also may shift as the lesion shifts. For example, with an internal derangement of the knee, pain may occur in flexion one time and in extension another time if it is due to a loose body within the joint. What are the exact movements that cause pain? At this stage, the patient should not be asked to do the movements because

they will be done in the examination. However, the examiner should remember which movements the patient says are painful so that when the examination is carried out these movements can be done last to avoid overflow of painful symptoms. Are there any other factors that aggravate or help to relieve the pain? Is there any alteration in intensity of the pain?

10. Is the pain associated with rest? Activity? Certain postures? Visceral function? Time of day? For example, pain on activity that decreases with rest usually indicates a mechanical obstruction to movement, such as adhesions. Morning pain with stiffness that improves with activity usually indicates chronic inflammation and edema. Pain or aching as the day progresses usually indicates increased congestion in a joint. Peripheral nerve entrapments and thoracic outlet syndromes tend to be worse at night. Pain that is not affected by rest or activity usually indicates bone pain. Chronic pain is often associated with multiple factors such as fatigue, posture, or activity. If the pain occurs at night, how does the patient lie in bed—supine, on the side, or prone? Does sleeping alter the pain, or does it wake the patient when changing position? Pain and cramping with prolonged walking may indicate lumbar spinal stenosis (neurogenic intermittent claudication). Disc pain is aggravated by sitting and bending forward. Facet joint pain is often relieved by sitting and bending forward. What types of mattress and pillow are used? Foam pillows will often cause more problems for persons with cervical problems because these pillows have more "bounce" to them than do feather pillows. Too many pillows, pillows improperly positioned, or too soft a mattress may also cause problems.

11. What type of pain is exhibited? Nerve pain tends to be sharp, bright, and burning in quality and also tends to run in the distribution of specific nerves. Bone pain tends to be deep, boring, and very localized. Vascular pain tends to be diffuse, aching, and poorly localized and may be referred to other areas of the body. Muscle pain is usually hard to localize, is dull and aching, is often aggravated by injury, and may be referred to other areas (Table 1–1).

TABLE 1–1. Pain Descriptions and Related Structures

Type of Pain	Structure
Cramping, dull, aching	Muscle
Sharp, shooting	Nerve root
Sharp, bright, lightninglike	Nerve
Burning, pressurelike, stinging, aching	Sympathetic nerve
Deep, nagging, dull	Bone
Sharp, severe, intolerable	Fracture
Throbbing, diffuse	Vasculature

12. What types of sensations does the patient feel? If the problem is in bone, there usually is very little radiation of pain. If pressure is applied to a nerve root, there will be pain caused by pressure on the dura mater, which is the outermost covering of the spinal cord. If there is pressure on the nerve trunk, no pain occurs but there is paresthesia or an abnormal sensation such as a "pins and needles" feeling or a tingling. If the nerve itself is affected, regardless of where the irritation occurs along the nerve, the pain is perceived by the brain as coming from the periphery. This is an example of referred pain. Muscular, ligamentous, and bursal types of pain are indistinguishable.

13. Does a joint exhibit locking, unlocking, twinges, instability, or giving way? Locking may just mean that the joint will not fully extend, as is the case with a meniscal tear, or it may mean that it will not extend one time or flex the next time in the case of a loose body moving around within the joint. Giving way is often due to reflex inhibition of the muscles so that the patient feels that the limb will buckle if weight is placed on it. The inhibition may be due to anticipated pain or instability.

14. Are there any changes in color of the limb? Ischemic changes resulting from circulatory problems may include white, brittle skin; loss of hair; and abnormal nails on the foot or hand.

15. Has the patient been experiencing any life or economic stresses? Divorce, marital problems, financial problems, or job insecurity can all contribute to increasing the pain because of psychological stress.

When taking the history, the examiner should determine the following:

1. Has the patient had an x-ray examination? If so, x-ray overexposure has to be considered; if not, an x-ray examination may help yield a diagnosis.

2. Has the patient been receiving steroids or any other medication? If so, for how long? High dosages of steroids for long periods of time may, for example, lead to osteoporosis.

3. Has the patient been taking any other medication that is pertinent? Patients do not always regard every drug as "medication." An example is the birth control pill; if a person takes such medication over a long period of time, it may not seem as pertinent to her.

4. Does the patient have any bilateral cord symptoms, fainting, or "drop attacks"? Is bladder function normal? Is there any "saddle" involvement or vertigo? Vertigo and dizziness are often used synonymously although vertigo usually indicates more severe symptoms. The terms describe a swaying, spinning sensation accompanied by feelings of unsteadiness and loss of balance. These last questions are important to ask because these symptoms indicate severe neurological problems that must be dealt with carefully.

5. Does the patient have a history of surgery? If so, when was the surgery performed, what was the site of operation, and what condition was being treated? Sometimes the condition the examiner will be asked to treat is the result of the surgery.

It is evident that the taking of an accurate, detailed history is very important. With experience, one is often able to make a "preliminary" diagnosis from the history alone.

OBSERVATION

In an assessment, observation is the "looking" phase. The examiner should note the patient's way of moving as well as the general posture, manner, and attitude and willingness to cooperate. The patient must be undressed adequately to be observed properly. Males should wear only shorts, and females should wear bra and shorts. Because the patient is in a state of undress, it is important for the examiner to explain to the patient that observation and detailed looking are an integral part of the assessment. This explanation may prevent a potentially embarrassing situation. On entering the assessment area, the patient's gait should be observed. This initial gait assessment is only a cursory one. (If there appears to be a gait abnormality, the gait may be checked in greater detail once the patient is suitably undressed.) Problems such as a Trendelenburg sign or drop foot are easily noticed even if the patient is dressed.

Once the patient is in the examining room and suitably undressed, the examiner should observe the posture, noting the following:

1. Is there any obvious deformity? Deformities may take the form of restricted range of motion (e.g., flexion deformity), malalignment (e.g., genu varum), alteration in the shape of a bone (e.g., fracture), or alteration in the relation of two articulating structures (e.g., subluxation, dislocation). Structural deformities are present even at rest. Dynamic deformities are caused by muscle action and therefore are not usually evident when the muscles are relaxed. Examples of deformities include torticollis, fractures, scoliosis, or kyphosis.

2. Are the bony contours of the body normal and symmetric, or is there an obvious deviation? The examiner must remember that the body is not perfectly symmetric and deviation may mean nothing. For example, individuals will often have a lower shoulder on the dominant side or they may demonstrate a slight scoliosis of the spine adjacent to

the heart. However, any deviation should be noted because it may contribute to a more accurate diagnosis.

3. Are the soft-tissue (e.g., muscle, skin) contours normal and symmetric? Is there any obvious muscle wasting?

4. Are the limb positions equal or symmetric? Compare limb size, shape, any atrophy, color, and temperature.

5. Are the color and texture of the skin normal? Does the appearance of the skin differ in the area of pain from other areas of the body, or are other areas of the body different in skin texture? For example, trophic changes in the skin resulting from peripheral nerve lesions include loss of skin elasticity, skin becoming shiny, hair loss on the skin, and skin breaking down easily and healing slowly. The nails may become brittle and ridged. Cyanosis, or a bluish color to the skin, is usually an indication of poor blood perfusion. Redness indicates increased blood flow and/or inflammation.

6. Are there any scars that may indicate recent injury or surgery? Recent scars will be red because they are still healing and contain capillaries; older scars are white and primarily avascular. Are there any callosities, blisters, or inflamed bursae, which are indicative of excessive pressure or friction to the skin? Are there any sinuses that may indicate infection? If so, are the sinuses draining or dry?

7. Is there any crepitus or abnormal sound in the joints when the patient moves them?

8. Is there any heat, swelling, or redness in the area being observed? All of these signs are indications of inflammation or an active inflammatory condition.

9. What attitude does the patient appear to have toward the condition or you as an examiner? Is the patient apprehensive, restless, resentful, or depressed? These questions will give the examiner some indication of the patient's psychological state and how the patient will respond to treatment.

10. What is the patient's facial expression? Is it evident that the patient appears to be in discomfort or is lacking sleep?

11. Is the patient willing to move? Are patterns of movement normal? If not, how are they abnormal? Any alteration should be noted and included in the observation portion of the assessment.

The examiner should be positioned so that the dominant eye is used and both sides of the patient are compared simultaneously. During the observation stage, the examiner is only looking at the patient and does not ask the patient to move; the examiner does not palpate, except possibly to learn whether an area is warm or hot.

EXAMINATION

Principles

In the examination portion of the assessment, a number of principles must be followed:

1. Unless bilateral movement is required, the normal side is tested first. Testing the normal side first allows the examiner to establish a baseline for normal movement and shows the patient what to expect, resulting in increased patient confidence.

2. *Active* movements are done before *passive* movements. Passive movements are followed by *resisted isometric* movements. (These movements are detailed later in this section.)

3. Any movements that are painful are done last if possible to prevent an overflow of painful symptoms to the next movement.

4. If active range of motion is not full, overpressure is applied only with extreme care.

5. When the patient is doing active movements, if the range of motion is full, overpressure may be applied to determine the end feel of the joint. This often negates the need to do passive movements.

6. Each active, passive, or resisted isometric movement is repeated several times to see whether symptoms increase or decrease, whether a different pattern of movement results, whether there is increased weakness, and whether there is possible vascular insufficiency.

7. Resisted isometric movements are done with the patient in a neutral or resting position.

8. When the examiner is doing passive range of motion or ligamentous tests, it is not only the degree of the opening but also the quality (i.e., end feel) of the opening that is important.

9. When the examiner is doing ligamentous tests, the appropriate stress is applied gently and repeated several times; the stress is increased up to but not beyond the point of pain. By doing the test this way, maximum instability can be demonstrated without causing muscle spasm.

10. When *myotomes* (a group of muscles supplied by a single nerve root) are being tested, each contraction is held for a minimum of 5 seconds to see if weakness becomes evident. Myotomal weakness takes time to develop.

11. At the completion of an assessment, the examiner must warn the patient that the movements may exacerbate symptoms.

The examination described in this chapter emphasizes the joints of the body. It is necessary to examine all appropriate tissues to delineate the affected area, which can then be examined in detail.

Applying tension, stretch, or isometric contraction to specific tissues in turn produces either a normal or an appropriate abnormal response. This action enables the examiner to determine the nature and site of the present symptoms as well as the patient's response to these symptoms. The examination shows whether these activities provoke or change the patient's pain and, in this way, gives subjective information. Thus, the examiner focuses on the patient's feelings or opinions as well as objective observation. The patient must be clear about the patient's (the subjective) side of the examination. For instance, when responding to the question "Does the movement make any difference to the pain?" or "Does the movement bring on or change the pain," the patient must not confuse movement-associated pain with a query about already existing pain. In addition, the examiner is attempting to see whether patient responses are measurably abnormal. Do the movements cause any abnormalities in function? For example, a loss of movement or weakness in muscles can be measured and therefore is an objective response. Thus, the examiner looks for two sets of data: (1) what the patient feels (subjective) and (2) responses that can be measured or are found by the examiner (objective).

The examination is therefore very extensive. In the upper part of the body, the examination begins with the cervical spine and includes the temporomandibular joints, the entire scapular area, the shoulder region, and the upper limb to the fingers. In the lower part of the body, the examination begins at the lumbar spine and continues to the toes. This phase, often called a *scanning* or *screening examination*, may not be essential if there is a definite history of trauma to a specific joint. However, if one has any doubt as to where the injury is located, it is necessary to perform this scanning examination. The goal of the scanning examination is to rule out problems in the upper or lower extremity and to note areas needing more specific testing. The "scan" should add no more than 5 or 10 minutes to the assessment.

As with all assessments, when doing the scanning examination, the examiner begins with the history and observation. The scanning examination is a modification of the cervical or lumbar spinal assessment. Following the active, passive, and resisted isometric movements of the cervical or lumbar spine, the peripheral joints are scanned with the patient doing only a few movements. The examiner then tests the upper or lower limb myotomes. After these tests, the appropriate reflexes and cutaneous distribution can be checked or left until later. At this point, the examiner makes a decision or an educated guess regarding whether the problem is in

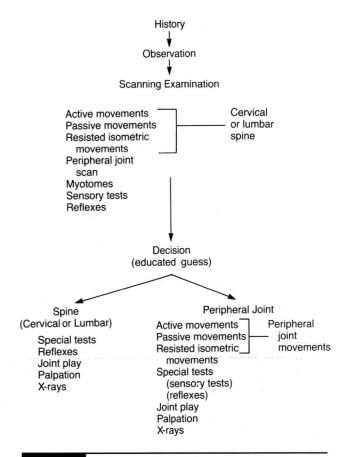

FIGURE 1–4. *The scanning examination.*

the cervical or lumbar spine or one of the peripheral joints. Once the decision is made, the examiner either continues with the spinal assessment or changes to the appropriate peripheral joint (Fig. 1–4).

The idea of the scanning examination was developed by James Cyriax,[1] who, more than any other author, also originated the concepts of "contractile" and "inert" tissue, "end feel," and "capsular patterns." The medical and paramedical professions owe a great deal to this man for his development of a comprehensive and systematic physical examination of the moving parts of the body.

In the examination, there should be an unchanging pattern that varies only slightly to elaborate certain clues given by the history. For example, if the history is characteristic of a disc lesion, the examination should be a detailed one of all the tissues that might be affected by the disc and a brief one of all the other joints to exclude contradictory signs. If the history suggests arthritis of the hip, the examination should be a detailed one of the hip and a brief one of the other joints—again, to exclude contradictory signs. As the movements are tested, the examiner is looking sometimes for the patient's subjective responses and sometimes for objective findings. For

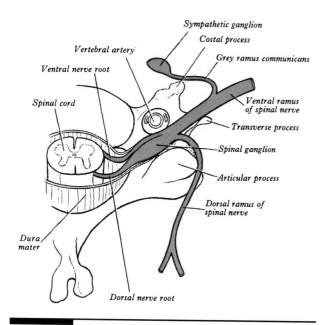

FIGURE 1–5. *Scheme showing spinal cord, nerve root portions, and spinal nerve. (From Williams, P., and R. Warwick (eds.): Gray's Anatomy, 37th ed. Edinburgh, Churchill Livingstone, 1989, p. 1125.)*

example, if examination of the cervical spine shows clear signs of a disc problem, as the examination is continued down the arm, the examiner will be looking more for muscle weakness (objective) rather than expecting to elicit pain (subjective). In contrast, if the history suggests a muscle lesion, pain will probably be provoked when the arm is examined. In either case, the structures expected to be normal are not omitted from examination.

Nerve Root System

To further comprehend the value of the scanning examination, the examiner must understand peripheral nerve distribution and the nerve root system of the body (Fig. 1–5). A nerve root is the portion of the nerve that connects it to the spinal cord. Nerve roots are made up of anterior (ventral) and posterior (dorsal) parts that unite near or in the intervertebral foramen to form a single nerve root or *spinal nerve*. They are the most proximal parts of the peripheral nervous system.

Within the human body, there are 31 nerve roots: eight cervical, 12 thoracic, five lumbar, five sacral, and one coccygeal. Each nerve root has two components: (1) a *somatic* portion that innervates the skeletal muscles and provides sensory input from the skin, fascia, muscles, and joints; and (2) a *visceral* component that is part of the autonomic nervous system.[4] The autonomic system supplies the blood vessels, dura mater, periosteum, ligaments, and intervertebral discs, among many other struc-

tures. The spinal nerve roots may combine to form a plexus, such as the *brachial plexus*. Thus, the nerve roots, by intermingling, form the peripheral nerves, such as the *median nerve*. For this reason, if pressure is applied to the nerve root, the distribution of the sensation or motor function will often be felt or exhibited in more than one peripheral nerve and will not demonstrate the same sensory distribution or altered motor function as the peripheral nerve (Table 1–2). In addition, neurological signs and symptoms such as paresthesia and altered deep tendon reflexes may result from irritation of tissues such as facet joints and interspinous ligaments. This irritation can contribute to the referred pain discussed below.

Dermatomes

The sensory distribution of each nerve root, or dermatome, varies from person to person, and there is often a great deal of overlap. A dermatome is defined as the area skin supplied by a single nerve root. One must be aware of the general distribution of these dermatomes and realize that there is a great deal of variability and overlap. Thus, when dermatomes are described in the following chapters, they should be considered as examples only, since slight differences may occur. The variability in dermatomes was aptly demonstrated by Keegan and Garrett in 1948[5] (Fig. 1–6).

Peripheral Nerves

The examiner must also be aware of the sensory, motor, and sympathetic distributions of peripheral nerves to be able to differentiate between lesions of nerve roots and lesions of peripheral nerves. The effects of a mixed (motor, sensory, and sympathetic) peripheral nerve lesion include:

1. Flaccid paralysis (motor).
2. Loss of reflexes (motor).
3. Muscle wasting and atrophy (motor).
4. Loss of sensation (sensory).
5. Trophic changes in the skin (sensory).
6. Loss of secretions from sweat glands (sympathetic).
7. Loss of pilomotor response (sympathetic).

Pressure on a peripheral nerve resulting in a neuropraxia leads to temporary nonfunction of the nerve. With this type of injury, there is primarily motor involvement with little sensory or autonomic involvement. Pressure on a nerve root leads to loss of tone and muscle mass. Spinal nerve roots have a poorly developed *epineurium* and lack a *perineurium*. This development makes the nerve root more susceptible to compressive forces, tensile deforma-

TABLE 1–2. Nerve Root Dermatomes, Myotomes, Reflexes, and Paresthetic Areas

Nerve Root	Dermatome*	Muscle Weakness (Myotome)	Reflexes Affected	Paresthesias
C1	Vertex of skull			
C2	Temple, forehead, occiput			
C3	Entire neck, posterior cheek, temporal area, prolongation forward under mandible			Cheek, side of neck
C4	Shoulder area, clavicular area, upper scapular area			Horizontal band along clavicle and upper scapula
C5	Deltoid area, anterior aspect of entire arm to base of thumb	Supraspinatus, intraspinatus, deltoid, biceps	Biceps, brachioradialis	
C6	Anterior arm, radial side of hand to thumb and index finger	Biceps, supinator, wrist extensors	Biceps, brachioradialis	Thumb and index finger
C7	Lateral arm and forearm to index, long, and ring fingers	Triceps, wrist flexors (rarely, wrist extensors)	Triceps	Index, long, and ring fingers
C8	Medial arm and forearm to long, ring, and little fingers	Ulnar deviators, thumb extensors, thumb adductors (rarely, triceps)	Triceps	Little finger alone or with two adjacent fingers; *not* ring or long fingers, alone or together (C7)
T1	Medial side of forearm to base of little finger	Disc lesions at upper two thoracic levels do not appear to give rise to root weakness. Weakness of intrinsic muscles of the hand is due to other pathology (e.g., thoracic outlet pressure, neoplasm of lung, and ulnar nerve lesion). Dural and nerve root stress has T1 elbow flexion with arm horizontal. T1 and T2 scapulae forward and backward on chest wall. Neck flexion at any thoracic level.		
T2	Medial side of upper arm to medial elbow, pectoral and midscapular areas			
T3–T12	T3–T6, upper thorax; T5–T7, costal margin; T8–T12, abdomen and lumbar region	Articular and dural signs and root pain are common. Root signs (cutaneous analgesia) are rare and have such indefinite area that they have little localizing value. Weakness is not detectable.		
L1	Back, over trochanter and groin	None	None	Groin; after holding posture, which causes pain
L2	Back, front of thigh to knee	Psoas, hip adductors	None	Occasionally anterior thigh
L3	Back, upper buttock, anterior thigh and knee, medial lower leg	Psoas, quadriceps, thigh atrophy	Knee jerk sluggish, PKB positive, pain on full SLR	Medial knee, anterior lower leg
L4	Medial buttock, lateral thigh, medial leg, dorsum of foot, big toe	Tibialis anterior, extensor hallucis	SLR limited neck flexion pain, weak or absent knee jerk, side flexion limited	Medial aspect of calf and ankle
L5	Buttock, posterior and lateral thigh, lateral aspect of leg, dorsum of foot, medial half of sole, first, second, and third toes	Extensor hallucis, peroneals, gluteus medius, dorsiflexor, hamstring and calf atrophy	SLR limited one side, neck flexion painful, ankle decreased, crossed-leg raising—pain	Lateral aspect of leg, medial three toes
S1	Buttock, thigh, and leg posterior	Calf and hamstring, wasting of gluteals, peroneals, plantar flexors	SLR limited, Achilles reflex weak or absent	Lateral two toes, lateral foot, lateral leg to knee, plantar aspect of foot
S2	Same as S1	Same as S1 except peroneals	Same as S1	Lateral leg, knee, and heel
S3	Groin, medial thigh to knee	None	None	None
S4	Perineum, genitals, lower sacrum	Bladder, rectum	None	Saddle area, genitals, anus, impotence, massive posterior

*In any part of which pain may be felt.
Abbreviations: PKB = prone knee bending; SLR = straight leg raising.

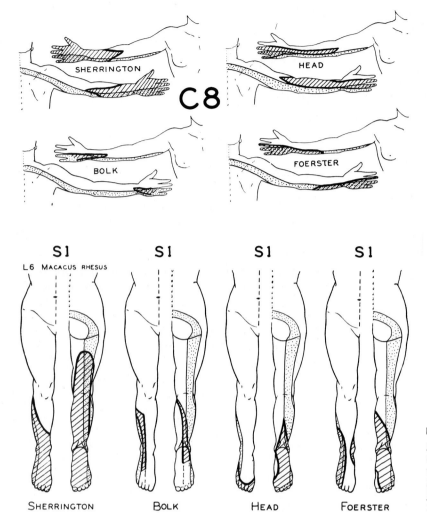

FIGURE 1–6. The variability of dermatomes at C8 and S1 as found by researchers. Similar variability is demonstrated in most cervical, lumbar, and sacral vertebrae. (From Keegan, J. J., and F. D. Garrett: Anat. Rec. 102:430, 433, 1948.)

tion, chemical irritants (e.g., alcohol, lead, or arsenic), or metabolic abnormalities. For example, diabetes may cause a metabolic peripheral neuropathy of one or more nerves.

In peripheral nerves, the epineurium consists of a loose areolar connective tissue matrix surrounding the nerve fiber and allows changes in growth length of the bundled nerve fibers (funiculi) without allowing the bundles to be strained. The perineurium protects the nerve bundles by acting as a diffusion barrier to irritants and provides tensile strength and elasticity to the nerve.

Myotomes

As defined earlier, *myotomes* are groups of muscles supplied by a single nerve root. A lesion of a single nerve root is usually associated with *paresis* (incomplete paralysis) of the muscle (myotome) supplied by that nerve root. On the other hand, a lesion of a peripheral nerve leads to complete paralysis of the muscles supplied by that nerve, especially if the injury results in *axonotmesis* or *neurotmesis*. The

difference in the amount of resulting paralysis results from the fact that more than one myotome contributes to the formation of a muscle embryologically.

Sclerotomes

A *sclerotome* is an area of bone or fascia supplied by a single nerve root (Fig. 1–7). As with dermatomes, sclerotomes can show a great deal of variability among individuals.

Referred Pain

It is the nature of this makeup of dermatomes, myotomes, and sclerotomes that can lead to referred pain, which is felt in a part of the body that is usually a considerable distance from the tissues that have caused the pain and is explained as an error in perception on the part of the brain. Many theories of the mechanism of referred pain have been developed, but none has been proved conclusively. Gen-

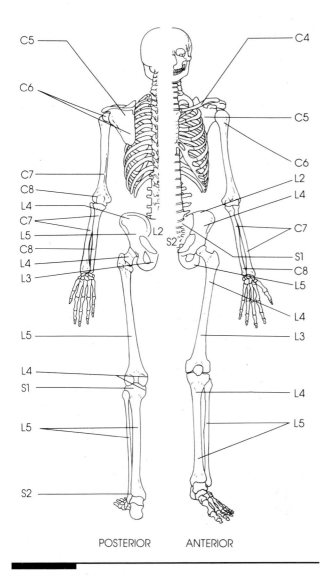

FIGURE 1–7. Sclerotomes of the body. Lines from nerve roots show area supplied by sclerotomes.

POSTERIOR   ANTERIOR

erally, referred pain may involve one or more of the following mechanisms:

1. Misinterpretation by the brain as to the source of the painful impulses.
2. Inability of the brain to interpret a summation of noxious stimuli from various sources.
3. Disturbance of the internuncial pool by afferent nerve impulses.

Referral of pain is a common occurrence in problems associated with the musculoskeletal system. Pain is often felt at points remote from the site of the lesion. The reference of pain is an indicator of the segment that is at fault. For example, pain in the L5 dermatome could arise from irritation around the L5 nerve root, from an L5 disc, from facet involvement of L4–L5, from any muscle supplied by the L5 nerve root, or from any visceral structures having L5 innervation.

Movements

Because the assessment is an examination of the moving parts of the body, testing of the active, passive, and resisted isometric movements can yield information concerning the tissues that could be at fault.

Active Movements

Active movements can be "actively" performed by voluntary muscles and have their own special value (i.e., they combine tests of a patient's willingness to perform the movement, joint range, control, and muscle power). Both contractile and inert tissues are involved or moved during active movements. When active movements occur, one or more rigid structures (bones) move, and such movement results in all structures that attach to that bone also moving. The examiner should note which movements, if any, cause pain and the amount and quality of pain that results. For example, small, unguarded movements causing intense pain indicate an irritable joint.

Contractile tissues may have tension placed on them by stretching or contracting.[1] These structures include the muscles, their tendons, and their attachments into the bone. *Inert tissues* have tension put on them by stretching or pinching.[1] They include all structures that would not be considered contractile, such as joint capsules, ligaments, bursae, blood vessels, nerves and their sheaths, cartilage, dura mater, and so on.

If there is an organic lesion, some movements will be found to be abnormal or painful and others will not. Negative findings must balance positive ones, and the examination must be extensive enough to allow characteristic patterns to emerge. Determination of the problem is not made on the strength of the first positive finding; it is made only when it is clear that there are no other contradictory signs. Movements should be repeated several times quickly to rule out any problem such as vascular insufficiency. The active component is a functional test of the anatomic and dynamic aspects of the body and joints. When testing active movements, the examiner should note:

1. When and where during the movement the onset of pain occurs.
2. Whether the movement increases the intensity and quality of the pain.
3. The reaction of the patient to pain.
4. The amount of observable restriction.
5. The pattern of movement.
6. The movement of associated joints.
7. The willingness of the patient to move the part.
8. The quality of the movement.
9. Any limitation and its nature.

Passive Movements

In passive movement, the joint is put through a range of motion by the examiner while the patient is relaxed. The movement must proceed through as full a range of movement as possible. Although the movement must be gentle, the examiner must find out whether there is any limitation of range (hypomobility) or excess of range (hypermobility) and, if so, whether it is painful. Hypermobile joints tend to be more susceptible to ligament sprains, joint effusion, chronic pain, recurrent injury, tendinitis resulting from lack of control, and early osteoarthritis. Hypomobile joints are more susceptible to muscle strains, pinched nerve syndromes, and tendinitis resulting from overstress.[6, 7] Although there are tests to demonstrate general hypermobility in an individual, these tests should be interpreted with caution because individuals demonstrate a wide range of variability between joints. It must also be remembered that for the individual being assessed, evidence of hypomobility or hypermobility does not necessarily indicate a pathological state. The examiner should also attempt to determine the cause of the limitation (e.g., pain, spasm, adhesions, or compression) and the quality of the movement (e.g., lead pipe, cogwheel).

END FEEL[1]

The examiner should determine the quality of end feel (the sensation the examiner "feels" in the joint as it reaches the end of the range of motion) of each passive movement. A proper evaluation of end feel can help the examiner to assess the type of pathology present to determine a prognosis for the condition and learn the severity or stage of the problem.

There are three classic *normal* end feels:

Bone to Bone. This is a "hard," unyielding sensation that is painless. An example of normal bone-to-bone end feel would be elbow extension.

Soft-Tissue Approximation. With this type of end feel, there is a yielding compression that stops further movement. Examples are elbow and knee flexion in which movement is stopped by the muscles. In a particularly slim individual with little muscle bulk, the end feel of the elbow flexion might be a bone-to-bone type.

Tissue Stretch. There is a hard or firm (springy) type of movement with a slight give. Toward the end of range of motion, there is a feeling of "springy" or elastic resistance. Thus, the normal tissue stretch end feel has a feeling of "rising tension." This elastic feeling depends on the thickness of the tissue and may be very elastic, as in the Achilles tendon stretch, or slightly elastic, as in wrist flexion. Major injury to ligaments often causes a softer end feel until the tension is taken up by other structures.[8] Tissue stretch is the most common type of normal end feel. Examples are lateral rotation of the shoulder and knee and metacarpophalangeal joint extension.

There are five classic *abnormal* end feels[1]:

Muscle Spasm. Invoked by movement, with a sudden dramatic arrest of movement often accompanied by pain, the end feel is sudden and hard. Cyriax calls this a "vibrant twang."[1] Some examiners divide muscle spasm into two parts. *Early* muscle spasm occurs early in the range of motion, almost as soon as movement starts; this type of muscle spasm is associated with inflammation. The second, or *late,* muscle spasm occurs at or near the end of the range of motion. It is due to instability and the resulting irritability caused by movement.

Capsular. Although this end feel is very similar to tissue stretch, it does not occur where one would expect. The range of movement is obviously reduced, and the capsule can be postulated to be at fault. Muscle spasm usually does not occur in conjunction with the capsular type of end feel. Some examiners divide this capsular end feel into *hard capsular* when the end feel has a "thick" quality to it and *soft capsular* when it is similar to normal but has a restricted range of motion. The hard capsular end feel is seen in more chronic conditions; the limitation comes on rather abruptly following a smooth friction-free movement. The soft capsular end feel is more often seen in more acute conditions, with stiffness occurring early in the range and increasing until the end of range is reached. Maitland[9] calls this "resistance through range." Some authors[10] add a modification to this end feel, calling it soft. They interpret this soft and boggy end feel as being the result of synovitis or soft-tissue edema.

Bone to Bone. This abnormal end feel is similar to the normal bone-to-bone type, but the restriction or sensation of restriction occurs before the normal end of range of movement would normally occur or where one would not expect to have a bone-to-bone end feel.

Empty. The empty end feel is detected when considerable pain is produced by movement. The movement is obviously impossible because of the pain, although no real mechanical resistance is being detected. Examples might include an acute subacromial bursitis or a neoplasm. Patients often have difficulty describing the empty end feel, and there is no muscle spasm involved.

Springy Block. Similar to a tissue stretch, this occurs where one would not expect it to occur; it tends to be found in joints with menisci. There is a rebound effect, and it usually indicates an internal derangement within the joint. One might find a springy block end feel with a torn meniscus of a knee when it is locked or unable to go into full extension.

TABLE 1–3. Common Capsular Patterns of Joints

Joint(s)	Restriction*
Temporomandibular	Limitation of mouth opening
Occipitoatlanto	Extension, side flexion equally limited
Cervical spine	Side flexion and rotation equally limited, extension
Glenohumeral	Lateral rotation, abduction, medial rotation
Sternoclavicular	Pain at extreme of range of movement
Acromioclavicular	Pain at extreme of range of movement
Humeroulnar	Flexion, extension
Radiohumeral	Flexion, extension supination, pronation
Proximal radioulnar	Supination, pronation
Distal radioulnar	Full range of movement, pain at extremes of rotation
Wrist	Flexion and extension equally limited
Trapeziometacarpal	Abduction, extension
Metacarpophalangeal and interphalangeal	Flexion, extension
Thoracic spine	Side flexion and rotation equally limited, extension
Lumbar spine	Side flexion and rotation equally limited, extension
Sacroiliac, symphysis pubis, and sacro-coccygeal	Pain when joints are stressed
Hip†	Flexion, abduction, medial rotation (but in some cases medial rotation is most limited)
Knee	Flexion, extension
Tibiofibular	Pain when joint stressed
Talocrural	Plantar flexion, dorsiflexion
Talocalcaneal (subtalar)	Limitation of varus range of movement
Midtarsal	Dorsiflexion, plantar flexion, adduction, medial rotation
First metatarsophalangeal	Extension, flexion
Second to fifth metatarso-phalangeal	Variable
Interphalangeal	Flexion, extension

*Movements are listed in order of restriction.
†For the hip, flexion, abduction, and medial rotation will always be the movements most limited in a capsular pattern. However, the order of restriction may vary.

CAPSULAR PATTERN[1]

With passive movement, it must be remembered that a full range of motion must be carried out. A short, too-soft movement in the midrange does not achieve the proper results. In addition to looking at the end feel, the examiner must look at the *pattern of limitation*. If the capsule of the joint is affected, it will be found that a pattern of proportional limitation is the feature that indicates the presence of a capsular pattern in the joint. It is the result of a total joint reaction, with muscle spasm, capsular contraction, and generalized osteophyte formation being possible mechanisms at fault. Each joint has a characteristic pattern of proportional limitation. The presence of this capsular pattern does not indicate the type of joint involvement present; only an analysis of the

end feel can do this. Only joints that are controlled by muscles have a capsular pattern. Thus, joints such as the sacroiliac and distal tibiofibular joints do not exhibit a capsular pattern. Table 1–3 illustrates some of the common capsular patterns seen in joints.

NONCAPSULAR PATTERN[1]

The examiner must also be aware of *noncapsular patterns*, which suggest a limitation of movement that exists but does not correspond to the classic capsular pattern for that joint. In the shoulder, abduction might be restricted but there might be very little rotational restriction. Thus, a total capsular reaction is absent, but there are other possibilities, such as ligamentous adhesions, in which only part of a capsule or the accessory ligaments are involved. Thus, a local restriction in one direction, often accompanied by pain, is produced, and full pain-free range of movement in all other directions is obvious. A second possibility is *internal derangement of a joint*. Only certain joints, such as the knee and elbow, are commonly affected in this case. Intercapsular fragments may interfere with the normal sequence of motion. Movements causing impingement with the fragments will be limited, whereas other motions will be free. In the knee, for example, a torn meniscus may cause a blocking of extension, but flexion is usually free. Loose bodies cause limitation when they are caught between articular surfaces. A third possibility is *extra-articular lesions*. These lesions are revealed by disproportionate limitation, extra-articular adhesions, or an acutely inflamed structure limiting movement in a particular direction. For example, limited straight leg raising in the lumbar disc syndrome is referred to as a *constant length phenomenon*. This phenomenon results when the limitation of movement in one joint is dependent on the position in which another joint is held. Thus, the restricted tissue (in this case, the sciatic nerve) must lie outside the joint or joints (in this case, hip and knee) being tested. Muscle adhesion causing restriction of motion is a further example of this phenomenon.

Inert Tissue[1]

Once the active and passive movements are completed, the examiner should be able to determine whether there are problems with any of the *inert tissues*. The examiner makes such a determination by judging the degree of pain and the limitation of movement within the joint. For lesions of inert tissue, the examiner may find that active and passive movements are painful in the same direction. Usually pain occurs as the limitation of motion approaches. Resisted isometric movements, which will be discussed shortly, are not usually painful unless there is some compression occurring.

Inert tissue refers to all tissue that is not considered contractile. Four classic patterns may be seen in lesions of inert tissue:

1. The first pattern is one of **pain and limitation of movement in every direction.** In this pattern, the entire joint is affected, indicating arthritis or capsulitis. As previously stated, each joint has its own capsular pattern, and the amount of limitation is not usually the same in each direction. With capsular patterns, although there is a set "pattern" for each joint, other directions may also be affected. All movements of the joint may be affected, but it will be found that the motions described for capsular pattern are always in that particular order. In early capsular patterns, only one movement may be restricted; this movement is usually the one that has the potential for the greatest restriction. For example, in an early capsular pattern of the shoulder, only lateral rotation may be limited and the limitation may be slight.

2. A patient with a lesion of inert tissue may experience **pain and limitation or excessive movement in some directions but not in others,** such as in a ligament sprain or local capsular adhesion. The movements that stretch or move the affected structure cause the pain. Internal derangement that results in the blocking of a joint may also be an example of a lesion of inert tissue where a variable pattern exists. Extra-articular limitation occurs when a lesion outside the joint affects the movement of that joint. Because these movements pinch or stretch the involved structure (e.g., bursitis in the buttock or acute subacromial bursitis), there will be pain and limitation of movement on stretch or compression of these structures. If a structure such as a ligament has been torn, the range of motion may increase if swelling is minimal, indicating instability of the joint. Swelling often masks this instability because it stretches the tissues.

3. There may be **limited movement that is pain-free.** The end feel for this type of condition is often the abnormal bone-to-bone type, and it usually indicates a symptomless osteoarthritis. If this situation is encountered, it should be left alone because it is not causing the patient any problem other than restricted range of motion and to deal with it could lead to further problems.

4. If the **range of movement is full and there is no pain,** there is no lesion of the inert tissues being tested by that movement; however, there may be lesions of inert tissue in other directions or around the other joints.

Resisted Isometric Movements

Resisted isometric movements are tested last in the examination of the joints. This type of movement consists of a strong, static (isometric) voluntary muscle contraction. If movement is allowed to occur at the joint, inert tissue around the joint will also move, and if pain is felt, it will not be clear whether it arises from contractile or inert tissues. The joint, therefore, is put in a neutral or resting position so that minimal tension is placed on the inert tissue. The patient is asked to contract the muscle strongly while the examiner resists to prevent any movement from occurring and to ensure that the patient is using maximum effort. There is no question that movement cannot be completely eliminated, but by doing it in this fashion movement will be minimized. Some compression of the inert tissues (cartilage and so on) will occur with the contraction; there may be some joint shear as well, but it will be minimal if done as just described. To do the test properly, the examiner positions the joint in the resting position, asks the patient to hold the limb in that position, and applies resistance. In this way, the examiner can ensure the contraction is isometric. Muscle weakness, if elicited, may be due to an upper motor neuron lesion, injury to a peripheral nerve, pathology at the neuromuscular junction, or the muscles themselves. For the first three causes above, a grade system of testing (Table 1–4) may be used. However, because this grading system involves moving through a range of motion, when testing for muscle lesions it is more appropriate to test the resisted movements isometrically to determine which movements are painful, then to perform individual muscle tests[11] to determine exactly which muscle is at fault.

TABLE 1–4. Muscle Test Grading

Grade	Value	Movement
5	Normal	Complete range of motion against gravity with maximal resistance
4	Good	Complete range of motion against gravity with some (moderate) resistance
3 +	Fair +	Complete range of motion against gravity with minimal resistance
3	Fair	Complete range of motion against gravity
3 −	Fair −	Some but no complete range of motion against gravity
2 +	Poor +	Initiates motion against gravity
2	Poor	Complete range of motion with gravity eliminated
2 −	Poor −	Initiates motion if gravity is eliminated
1	Trace	Evidence of slight contractility but no joint motion
0	Zero	No contraction palpated

If the contraction appears weak, the examiner must make sure that the weakness is not due to pain or the patient's fear or unwillingness. Weakness that is not associated with pain or disuse is a positive neurological sign. The examiner can often resolve such a finding by having the patient make a contraction on the good side first so that the movement normally will not cause pain. The movement must be as pure as possible. Although some inert tissue may be compressed during this action, compression will be minimal and a clear pattern of the problem will usually emerge.

CONTRACTILE TISSUE[1]

With resisted isometric testing, the examiner checks for problems of *contractile tissue*, which consists of muscles, tendons, and their attachments. One would find both active movements and resisted isometric testing to be affected. Usually, passive movements are normal; in other words, passive movements are full and pain free, although pain may be exhibited at the end of the range of motion when the muscle is stretched. If the muscles are tested as described, the examiner will find that not all movements are affected except in patients with psychogenic pain and sometimes in patients with an acute joint lesion, when even a small amount of tension on the muscles around the joints provokes pain. However, if the joint lesion is severe, passive movements, when tested, will be markedly affected so that no confusion arises as to where the lesion lies. As with testing lesions of inert tissue, there are four classic patterns that may be seen with lesions of contractile tissue.[1] (In this case, however, we are dealing with pain and strength rather than pain and limited or excessive range of motion.)

1. Movement that is **strong and pain free** indicates that there is no lesion of the muscles being tested, regardless of how tender the muscles may be when touched. The muscles function painlessly and are not the source of the patient's discomfort.

2. Movement that is **strong and painful** indicates a local lesion of the muscle or tendon. Such a lesion could be a first- or second-degree muscle strain. Typically, there is no primary limitation of passive movement, except, for example, in a gross muscle tear with hematoma and muscle spasm. In this case, the patient may develop secondary joint stiffness caused by disuse superimposed on the muscle lesion. This stiffness then takes precedence in the treatment.

3. Movement that is **weak and painful** indicates a severe lesion around that joint, such as a fracture. The weakness that results is usually due to reflex inhibition of the muscles around the joint.

4. Movement that is **weak and pain free** indicates a rupture of a muscle (third-degree strain) or involvement of the nerve supplying that muscle.

If all movements appear painful, pain is often due to fatigue, emotional hypersensitivity, or emotional problems. It must be remembered that patients may equate effort with discomfort, and they must be told that this is not necessarily the case. Janda[12] put forth an interesting concept by dividing muscles into two groups—postural and phasic. He believed that postural or tonic muscles, which were the muscles responsible for maintaining upright posture, had a tendency to become tight with pathology and develop contractures, whereas phasic muscles, which included almost all other muscles, tended to become weak and inhibited with pathology. Thus, the examiner must be careful to note the range of motion available (active movements) as well as strength (resisted isometric movements) when testing the muscles. Janda described the primary postural muscles as triceps, rectus femoris, thigh adductors, hamstrings, iliopsoas, tensor fasciae latae, trunk erectors, quadratus lumborum, pectoralis major (sternal portion), upper trapezius, levator scapulae, and upper limb flexors. The phasic muscles included tibialis anterior, the vasti, gluteal muscles, abdominal muscles, lower stabilizers of the scapula, and deep flexors of the neck. All other muscles were described by Janda as neutral.

Other Findings

When carrying out the examination of the joints, the examiner must be aware of other findings that may become evident and will help to determine the nature and location of the problem. For example, it should be noted whether there is excessive range of motion or *hypermobility* within the joints. When doing any examination, the examiner should compare both the normal and involved sides of the body. This comparison will give some idea as to whether the findings on the affected side would be considered normal. For example, the excessive range may just be a normal range of motion for that individual. It must also be remembered that joints on the nondominant side tend to be more flexible than those on the dominant side.

It is also important to note whether a *painful arc* is present; this finding indicates that an internal structure is being squeezed. *Sounds* such as crepitus, clicking, or snapping should be noted because they are often due to structures slipping over one another (e.g., tendons slipping over bone). *Pain at the extreme of range of motion* may be due to squeezing or stretching in which a particular joint may be affected.

Functional Assessment

Some aspect of functional assessment should always be performed on the joint during the examination. This procedure may involve task analysis or simply observation of certain patient activities. The functional assessment is important to determine the effect of the condition or injury on the patient's daily life, including the sex life.[10] Functional impairment may be just annoying or completely disabling. Functional activities that should be tested, if appropriate, include self-care activities such as walking, dressing, daily hygiene (e.g., washing, bathing, shaving, combing hair), eating, and going to the bathroom; recreational activities such as reading, sewing, watching television, gardening, and playing a musical instrument; and instrumental activities such as driving, dialing a telephone, getting grocer-

ies, preparing meals, and hanging clothes. Table 1–5 shows some of the daily living skills and mobility questions with which the examiner may be concerned. Part of this assessment will occur during the history when the examiner asks the patient which activities can be done easily, which with some difficulty, or which not at all. During the observation, the examiner will note what the patient can and cannot do within the confines of the assessment area. Finally, during the examination, function testing may be carried out. For example, when examining the hand, it is important to note power and dexterity when performing fundamental maneuvers such as gripping and pinching. Regardless of which functional test is used, it is important for the examiner to understand the purpose of the test. A functional test should not be done just because it is available. It should also not be used in isolation but

TABLE 1–5. Daily Living Skill and Mobility Questions for Functional Assessment*

Daily Living Skills	Mobility
Feeding	**Supine to Sit**
(7) Are you able to feed yourself from a tray or table using ordinary utensils? Can you cut meat? Can you pour liquids from open containers?	(7) When you are lying on your back, can you sit up without using your arms or without rolling to the side? Can you do this smoothly and easily?
(4) If you use a spork or rocker knife or other helpful aid, are you able to feed yourself in a reasonable length of time?	(4) Do you use your arms to help you sit up, or do you roll to the side before sitting up? Do you have to try several times before sitting up?
(2) Are you able to feed yourself with some help from another person, for example, to help you raise a cup to your mouth or to cut meat?	(2) Does someone help you to sit up?
(0) Do you depend on another person to feed you?	(0) Are you unable to sit up?
	Sitting to Standing
	(7) Are you able to stand up from a regular chair without using your arms?
Dress Upper Body	(4) Do you need to use your arms to help you stand up, or do you need to try several times?
(7) Are you able to get clothes out of your closets and drawers and put them on and remove them from your upper body by yourself, including bra, slip, pullovers, and front opening shirts and blouses, as well as managing zippers, buttons, and snaps?	(2) Does someone need to help you stand up out of a chair?
	(0) Do you depend on someone else entirely to get you out of a chair?
(4) If someone lays your clothes out for you or hands them to you, are you able to dress your upper body by yourself even if it takes a little more time, or do you need some help with closures, such as buttons, zippers, snaps, or hooks? Do you use aids such as reachers, dressing hooks, button hooks, or zipper pulls?	**Transfer—Toilet**
	(7) Are you able to get on and off the toilet easily and without using your hands?
	(4) Do you need to use your arms to help you get on and off the toilet, or do you require assistive devices such as elevated toilet seats or grab bars?
(2) Does someone help you put on your blouse or shirt or sweater because you are limited by pain, lack of strength, or limited range of motion?	(2) Does someone need to help you get on and off the toilet?
(0) Do you depend on another person to dress your upper body?	(0) Are you unable to use the toilet?
	Transfer—Tub or Shower
	(7) Are you able to get in and out of a tub or shower safely?
	(4) Can you get in and out of a tub or shower using aids such as grab bars or special seat or lift?
Dress Lower Body	(2) Does someone need to help you to get in and out of the tub or shower?
(7) Are you able to put on undergarments, slacks, socks, nylons, and shoes by yourself? Can you tie shoelaces?	(0) Are you unable to get in and out of the tub or shower?
(4) Are you able to put on undergarments, slacks, socks, nylons, and shoes by yourself if they are laid out for you or handed to you? Do you use dressing aids such as long handled reachers? Do you avoid shoes that have laces or buckles, or do you use elastic laces or velcro shoe closures by yourself?	**Transfer—Automobile**
	(7) Can you get in and out of a car easily, including opening and closing the door?
	(4) Can you get in and out of a car by yourself if you use aids such as grab bars or if someone opens the door for you?
(2) Does someone help you to put on undergarments, slacks, nylons, or shoes?	(2) Does someone help you get in and out of a car?
(0) Do you depend on another person to dress your lower body?	(0) Are you unable to get in and out of a car even with assistance?

TABLE 1–5. Daily Living Skill and Mobility Questions for Functional Assessment* *Continued*

Daily Living Skills	Mobility
Grooming	*Walk on Level*
(7) Are you able to comb and brush and shampoo your hair, shave, apply makeup, clean your teeth or dentures, and manage nail care by yourself without adaptations or modifications?	(7) Are you able to walk two blocks at an even pace without using a cane, crutches, walker, or adapted shoes?
(4) Do you use assistive devices or adapted methods for grooming: If someone places what you need within reach, are you then able to complete grooming activities unaided? Do you use long handled combs or brushes, suction brushes for cleaning nails or dentures, adapted shaving equipment or adapted key for rolling toothpaste tubes?	(4) Do you need a cane, crutches, or walker to walk two blocks?
	(2) Can you walk one block with assistance?
	(0) Are you unable to walk one block even with assistance?
	Walk Outdoors
(2) Does someone actually help you shampoo or brush your hair, shave, apply makeup, clean your teeth or dentures, or manicure your nails?	(7) Are you able to walk outdoors at least two blocks without avoiding rough terrain such as grass, sand, gravel, curbs, ramps, or hills?
(0) Do you depend on someone else entirely for your grooming needs?	(4) Do you try to avoid uneven terrain? Do you use a crutch or cane for safety or balance purposes only when outside?
Care of Perineum/Clothing at Toilet	(2) Must you use a cane or crutches to walk at least two blocks on uneven terrain?
(7) Are you able to go to the bathroom by yourself including managing your clothes, wiping yourself (and placing sanitary napkins or tampons)?	(0) Are you unable to walk on uneven terrain?
(4) Are you able to manage your clothing at the toilet and wipe yourself independently although it may be difficult, or do you use aids such as an extended reacher for wiping yourself or clothing aids?	*Up and Down Stairs*
	(7) Can you go up and down at least five steps safely, step over step without using the hand rail or other support?
(2) Does someone help you with your clothing at the toilet or assist you with wiping yourself (or in placement of sanitary napkins or tampons)?	(4) Are you able to go up and down at least five steps if you use a hand rail, cane, or crutches or if you go one step at a time?
(0) Do you depend on someone else to manage your clothes at the toilet for you or to wipe you (or to place sanitary napkins or tampons)?	(2) Do you need someone to help you go up and down at least five steps?
	(0) Are you unable to go up and down at least five steps even with help?
Wash or Bathe	*Wheelchair/10 Yards*
(7) Are you able to wash and dry your entire body by yourself, including your back and feet? Are you able to turn water faucets?	(7) Are you able to push your wheelchair without help for 10 yards? Can you turn corners and get close to bed, table, and toilet?
(4) Do you use bathing aids such as long handled bath brushes or sponges? Are you unable to reach some parts of your body for bathing or drying thoroughly but can still manage without help?	(4) Do you use a motorized wheelchair?
	(2) Do you need someone to help you maneuver your wheelchair around corners or to help you position it?
(2) Are you able to bathe and dry most parts of your body and have someone help you with the rest?	(0) Are you unable to push your wheelchair 10 yards?
(0) Does someone else bathe you?	
Vocational	
(2) Are you employed full-time in your usual occupation? Are you a full-time homemaker and require no assistance? Are you retired for other than medical reasons?	
(0) Not able to do the above	

*Modified from Convery, F. R., et. al. Polyarticular disability: A functional assessment. Arch. Phys. Med. Rehab. 58:498, 1977.

rather in conjunction with the overall assessment so that a complete assessment picture of the patient can be developed. Table 1–6 demonstrates an assessment form for the shoulder[13] in which a functional assessment plays an integral part. Table 1–7 shows a functional assessment involving the entire upper limb.[14] Table 1–8 demonstrates tests that could be used in a simulated activities of daily living examination.[15] Similar charts can and have been developed for almost all joints of the body.

Special Tests

Once the examiner has completed the history, observation, and evaluation of movement, special tests may be performed for the involved joint. Many special tests can be used for each joint to determine whether a particular type of disease, condition, or injury is present. These tests are strongly suggestive of a particular problem and must be viewed as such.

TABLE 1–8. Summary Description of Tests in Simulated Activities of Daily Living Examination (SADLE)*

Test	Measure	Units	Instrumentation
Two leg standing, eyes open	Maximum time of three 30-second trials	Seconds	Stopwatch
One leg standing, eyes open	Maximum time of three 30-second trials	Seconds	Stopwatch
Two leg standing, eyes closed	Maximum time of three 30-second trials	Seconds	Stopwatch
One leg standing, eyes closed	Maximum time of three 30-second trials	Seconds	Stopwatch
Tandem walking with supports	Time to take 10 heel-to-toe steps	Steps/sec	Stopwatch and parallel bars
Tandem walking without supports	Time to take 10 heel-to-toe steps	Steps/sec	Stopwatch and parallel bars
Putting on a shirt	Average time of two trials	Seconds	Stopwatch and shirt
Managing three visible buttons	Average time of two trials	Seconds	Stopwatch and cloth with three buttons mounted on a board
Zipping a garment	Average time of two trials	Seconds	Stopwatch and cloth with zipper mounted on a board
Putting on gloves	Average time of two trials	Seconds	Stopwatch and two garden gloves
Dialing a telephone	Average time of two trials	Seconds	Stopwatch and telephone
Tying a bow	Average time of two trials	Seconds	Stopwatch and large shoelaces mounted on a board
Manipulating safety pins	Average time of two trials	Seconds	Stopwatch and two safety pins
Picking up coins	Average time of two trials	Seconds	Stopwatch and four coins placed on a plastic sheet
Threading a needle	Average time of two trials	Seconds	Stopwatch, thread, and large-eyed needle
Unwrapping a Band-Aid	Time for one trial	Seconds	Stopwatch and one Band-Aid
Squeezing toothpaste	Average time of two trials	Seconds	Stopwatch, tube of toothpaste, and a board
Cutting with a knife	Average time of two trials	Seconds	Stopwatch, plate, fork, knife, and permoplast
Using a fork	Average time of two trials	Seconds	Stopwatch, plate, fork, and permoplast

*Modified from Potvin, A. R., et. al.: Simulated activities of daily living examination. Arch. Phys. Med. Rehab. 53:478, 1972.

In addition, these tests, while strongly suggestive of disease when they yield positive results, do not necessarily rule out the disease when they yield negative results. For each joint examination described herein, specific tests are mentioned for specific conditions. Whether to do these special tests is up to the individual examiner. Often, many tests will show the same results. These different methods will be shown, and the examiner should pick the ones that give the best results.

For example, for years, the *anterior drawer sign* had been the test to determine whether there was a problem with the anterior cruciate ligament of the knee. However, literature from the past few years has indicated that the *Lachman test* is much more effective.

In addition to physical tests, the examiner may also make use of *laboratory tests* for specific conditions. With osteomyelitis, for example, a positive blood culture is likely to be obtained, the white blood cell (WBC) count will be elevated, and the erythrocyte sedimentation rate (ESR) will be increased. The examiner, if a physician, may decide to draw fluid out of a joint with a hypodermic needle to view the synovial fluid. Tables 1–9 and 1–10 present laboratory findings in bone disease and a classification of synovial fluid as examples of laboratory tests.

TABLE 1–9. Laboratory Findings in Bone Disease*

Condition	Calcium	Inorganic Phosphorus	Alkaline Phosphatase	Calcium	Phosphorus
Hyperparathyroidism, primary	↑	↓	↑	↑	↑
Hyperparathyroidism, secondary	N-↓	↑	R↑	↑	↑
Hyperthyroidism, marked	N	N	↑	↑	↑
Hypothyroidism	N	N	N	N	N
Senile osteoporosis	N	N-O↓	N	N	N
Rickets (child)	↓	↓	↑	N	N
Osteomalacia (adult)	N-↓	↓	↑	N	N
Paget's disease	R↑	R↓	↑	N	N
Multiple myeloma	↑	N-↑	R↑.	↑	↑

*Adapted from Quinn, J.: In Meschan, I.: Synopsis of Roentgen Signs in General Radiology. Philadelphia, W. B. Saunders Co., 1976, p. 27.
Key: N = normal; O = occasionally; R = rarely; ↑ = increased; ↓ = decreased.

TABLE 1–10. Classification of Synovial Fluid*

Type	Appearance	Significance
Group 1	Clear yellow	Noninflammatory states, trauma
Group 2†	Cloudy	Inflammatory arthritis; excludes most patients with osteoarthritis
Group 3	Thick exudate, brownish	Septic arthritis; occasionally seen in gout
Group 4	Hemorrhagic	Trauma, bleeding disorders, tumors, fractures

*From Curran, J. F., et al.: Rheumatologic aspects of painful conditions affecting the shoulder. Clin. Orthop. Relat. Res. 173:28, 1983.

†Inflammatory fluids will clot and should be collected in heparin-containing tubes. All group 2 or 3 fluids should be cultured when the diagnosis is uncertain.

Reflexes and Cutaneous Distribution

After the special tests, the examiner can test the superficial, deep, and/or pathological reflexes to obtain an indication of the state of the nerve or nerve roots supplying the reflex. Most often, the deep tendon reflexes are tested. It should be remembered that a deep tendon reflex can be elicited from almost any tendon with practice. The more common deep tendon reflexes tested are shown in Table 1–11. Tables 1–12 and 1–13 demonstrate superficial and pathological reflexes.

With a loss or abnormality of conduction, there will be a diminution (hyporeflexia) or loss (areflexia) of the stretch reflex. Upper motor neuron lesions produce findings of spasticity, hyperreflexia, hypertonicity, extensor plantar responses, reduced or absent superficial reflexes, and weakness of muscles distal to the lesion. Lower motor neuron lesions involving nerve roots or peripheral nerves produce findings of flaccidity, hyporeflexia or areflexia, hy-

potonicity, fasciculations, fibrillations, and weakness and atrophy of the involved muscles.[16] To test a deep tendon reflex properly, the examiner should tap the tendon five or six times to uncover any fading reflex response indicative of developing root signs. If the deep tendon reflexes are difficult to elicit, the reflexes can often be enhanced by having the patient clench the teeth or squeeze the hands together (Jendrassik maneuver) when testing the lower limb or squeeze the legs together when testing the upper limb. These activities increase the facilitative activity of the spinal cord and thus accentuate minimally active reflexes. The reflexes may be graded as follows:

0—Absent
1—Diminished
2—Average
3—Exaggerated
4—Clonus

Superficial reflexes are tested by stroking the skin with a moderately sharp object that does not break the skin. The response expected when testing these superficial reflexes is shown in Table 1–12. A great deal of practice is needed to become proficient when testing the superficial reflexes.

Pathological reflexes (Table 1–13) may indicate upper motor neuron lesions if absent on both sides or lower motor neuron lesions if absent on only one side. Improper stimulation (e.g., too much pressure) may lead to voluntary withdrawal in normal subjects, and the examiner must take care not to confuse this reaction with the pathological response.

To be of clinical significance, findings must show asymmetry between bilateral reflexes unless it is a central lesion. The examiner should not be overly concerned if the reflexes are absent, diminished, or

TABLE 1–11. Deep Tendon Reflexes

Reflex	Site of Stimulus	Normal Response	Pertinent Central Nervous System Segment
Jaw	Mandible	Mouth closes	Cranial nerve V
Biceps	Biceps tendon	Biceps contraction	C5–C6
Brachioradialis	Brachioradialis tendon or just distal to the musculotendinous junction	Flexion of elbow and/or pronation of forearm	C5–C6
Triceps	Distal triceps tendon above the olecranon process	Elbow extension	C7–C8
Patellar	Patellar tendon	Leg extension	L3–L4
Medial hamstrings	Semimembranosus tendon	Knee flexion	L5, S1
Lateral hamstrings	Biceps femoris tendon	Knee flexion	S1–S2
Tibialis posterior	Tibialis posterior tendon behind medial malleolus	Plantar flexion of foot with inversion	L4–L5
Achilles	Achilles tendon	Plantar flexion of foot	S1–S2

TABLE 1–12. Superficial Reflexes

Reflex	Normal Response	Pertinent Central Nervous System Segment
Upper abdominal	Umbilicus moves up and toward area being stroked	T7–T9
Lower abdominal	Umbilicus moves down and toward area being stroked	T11–T12
Cremasteric	Scrotum elevates	T12, L1
Plantar	Flexion of toes	S1–S2
Gluteal	Skin tenses in gluteal area	L4–L5, S1–S3
Anal	Contraction of anal sphincter muscles	S2–S4

excessive on both sides when tested unless there is a suspected central lesion. This difference is especially true in young people. Decreased (hyporeflexia) or absence of reflexes (areflexia) are indicative of injury to a peripheral nerve or spinal nerve root due to impingement, entrapment, or injury. Hyperactive or exaggerated reflexes (hyperreflexia) indicate upper motor neuron lesions. In the cervical spine, if a disc herniation and compression occur above the cervical enlargement, the reflexes of the upper extremity are exaggerated. If the cervical enlargement is involved (more common), then some reflexes are exaggerated and some are decreased.[17]

At the same time, the examiner should check the cutaneous distribution of the various peripheral nerves and the dermatomes around the joint being examined. One must remember that the dermatomes will vary from person to person, and there is considerable overlap.[5, 18] Although the sensory distribution of peripheral nerves may vary from person to person, they tend to be much more consistent than dermatomes. The examiner must be able to differentiate between sensory loss due to a nerve root (dermatome) and that due to a peripheral nerve. The same is true for muscle innervation. The examiner must be able to differentiate between the muscle innervation of a nerve root (myotome) and the muscle innervation of a peripheral nerve.

Throughout the sensory examination, the examiner should note the patient's ability to perceive the sensation being tested and the difference, if any, between the two sides of the body. In addition, distal and proximal sensitivities should be compared for each form of sensation tested. During the sensory tests, the patient should keep the eyes closed so that the results will indicate the patient's perception and interpretation of the stimuli, not what the patient sees happening.

The examiner should test for altered sensation by relaxing the hands and fingers and running them while relaxed over the area to be tested. After this quick sensory "scanning" examination, if the patient feels a difference in sensation between the two sides of the body, the examiner should note where the difference is so that the area can be "mapped out" in greater detail. Superficial tactile sensation can be tested with a wisp of cotton or a soft hair brush, whereas superficial pain can be tested with a pin, pinwheel, or other sharp object. The examiner then has to determine if the pattern mapped out follows a peripheral nerve or dermatome distribution. When looking at dermatome or peripheral nerve distribution, one must keep in mind that the sensation felt does not necessarily come from the indicated nerve root or peripheral nerve. Because of referred pain, it may come from any structure supplied by that nerve root. In some cases, the paresthesia may involve no specific pattern, or it may involve the entire circumference of the limb. In this case, the "opera glove" or "stocking" paresthesia or anesthesia may result from vascular insufficiency.

If desired, the examiner may also test other sensibilities. Sensitivity to temperature is tested by using two test tubes, one containing hot water and one containing cold water, whereas sensitivity to vibration (i.e., how long until vibration stops) may be tested by holding a tuning fork (usually 30- or 256-cps tuning forks are used) against bony prominences. Deep pressure pain can be tested by squeezing the Achilles tendon, the trapezius muscle, or the web space between the thumb and index finger or by applying a knuckle to the sternum. To test proprioception and motion, the patient's fingers or toes can be passively moved, and the patient is asked to indicate the direction of movement and final position while keeping the eyes closed. Care must be taken to ensure that pressure on the patient's skin cannot be used as a clue to direction of movement. Thus, the test digit should be grasped between the thumb and index finger of the examiner.

Cortical and discriminatory sensations may be tested by two-point discrimination, point localization, texture discrimination, stereognostic function (i.e., identification of familiar objects held in the

TABLE 1–13. Pathological Reflexes

Reflex	How to Elicit	Positive Response
Babinski	Stroke lateral aspect of sole of foot	Extension of big toe and fanning of four small toes
Chaddock	Stroke lateral aspect of foot beneath lateral malleolus	Same response as above
Oppenheim	Stroke anteromedial tibial surface	Same response as above
Gordon	Squeeze calf muscles firmly	Same response as above

hand), and graphesthesia (i.e., recognition of letters or numbers written with a blunt object on patient's palms or other body parts).

The examiner should look for possibilities of referred pain, try to remember which structure could refer pain to the joint being assessed, and ensure that these structures are normal and are not, in fact, referring pain to the joint. If a patient complains of low back pain but the lumbar spine is found to be normal, the examiner may want to look at the hip or sacroiliac joints because they may refer pain to the lumbar spine.

Joint Play (Accessory) Movements

All synovial and secondary cartilaginous joints, to some extent, are capable of an active range of motion, termed *voluntary movement*. In addition, there is a small range of movement that can be obtained only passively by the examiner; this movement is called *joint play*, or *accessory*, *movement*. These accessory movements are not under voluntary control; they are necessary, however, for full painless function of the joint and full range of motion of the joint. Joint dysfunction signifies a loss of joint play movement.

TABLE 1–14. Resting (Loose Packed) Positions of Joints

Joint(s)	Position
Facet (spine)	Midway between flexion and extension
Temporomandibular	Mouth slightly open (freeway space)
Glenohumeral	55° abduction, 30° horizontal adduction
Acromioclavicular	Arm resting by side in normal physiological position
Sternoclavicular	Arm resting by side in normal physiological position
Ulnohumeral (elbow)	70° flexion, 10° supination
Radiohumeral	Full extension, full supination
Proximal radioulnar	70° flexion, 35° supination
Distal radioulnar	10° supination
Radiocarpal (wrist)	Neutral with slight ulnar deviation
Carpometacarpal	Midway between abduction-adduction and flexion-extension
Metacarpophalangeal	Slight flexion
Interphalangeal	Slight flexion
Hip	30° flexion, 30° abduction, slight lateral rotation
Knee	25° flexion
Talocrural (ankle)	10° plantar flexion, midway between maximum inversion and eversion
Subtalar	Midway between extremes of range of movement
Midtarsal	Midway between extremes of range of movement
Tarsometatarsal	Midway between extremes of range of movement
Metatarsophalangeal	Neutral
Interphalangeal	Slight flexion

The existence of joint play movement is necessary for full pain-free voluntary movement to occur. An essential part of the detailed assessment of any joint includes an examination of its joint play movements. If any joint play movement is found to be absent, this movement must be freed before functional voluntary movement can be fully restored. In most joints, this movement is less than 4 mm in any one direction.

Mennell[19] stated that the following rules should be followed when testing joint play or accessory movements:

1. The patient should be relaxed and fully supported.
2. The examiner should be relaxed and use a firm but comfortable grasp.
3. One joint should be examined at a time.
4. One movement should be examined at a time.
5. The unaffected side should be tested first.
6. One articular surface is stabilized while the other surface is moved.
7. Movements must be normal and not forced.
8. Movements should not cause undue discomfort.

Loose Packed (Resting) Position

To test joint play movement, the examiner places the joint in a resting position, which is the position of a joint in its range of motion where the joint is under the least amount of stress; it is also the position in which the joint capsule has its greatest capacity.[20] The resting position (sometimes called the loose packed position) is one of minimal congruency between the articular surfaces and the joint capsule, with the ligaments being in the position of greatest laxity and passive separation of the joint surfaces being the greatest. This position may be the anatomic resting position that is usually considered in the midrange, or it may be just outside the range of pain and spasm. The advantage of the loose packed position is that the joint surface contact areas are reduced and always changing to decrease friction and erosion in the joints. The position also provides proper joint lubrication and allows the movements of spin, slide, and roll in a joint; thus, this is the ideal position for joint play mobilizations. Examples of resting positions are shown in Table 1–14.

Close Packed (Synarthrodial) Position

The close packed position should be avoided as much as possible during an assessment. In this position, the two joint surfaces fit together precisely;

TABLE 1–15. Close Packed Positions of Joints

Joint(s)	Position
Facet (spine)	Extension
Temporomandibular	Clenched teeth
Glenohumeral	Abduction and lateral rotation
Acromioclavicular	Arm abducted to 90°
Sternoclavicular	Maximum shoulder elevation
Ulnohumeral (elbow)	Extension
Radiohumeral	Elbow flexed 90°, forearm supinated 5°
Proximal radioulnar	5° supination
Distal radioulnar	5° supination
Radiocarpal (wrist)	Extension with radial deviation
Metacarpophalangeal (fingers)	Full flexion
Metacarpophalangeal (thumb)	Full opposition
Interphalangeal	Full extension
Hip	Full extension, medial rotation*
Knee	Full extension, lateral rotation of tibia
Talocrural (ankle)	Maximum dorsiflexion
Subtalar	Supination
Midtarsal	Supination
Tarsometatarsal	Supination
Metatarsophalangeal	Full extension
Interphalangeal	Full extension

*Some authors include abduction, e.g., Kaltenborn.[20]

that is, they are fully congruent. The joint surfaces are tightly compressed; the ligaments and capsule of the joint are maximally tight; and the joint surfaces cannot be separated by distractive forces. The majority of joint structures are under maximum tension. Thus, ligaments or bone, if injured, will become more painful as the close packed position is approached. If a joint is swollen, the close packed position cannot be achieved.[8] In the close packed position, no accessory movement is possible. Examples of the close packed positions of most joints are shown in Table 1–15.

Palpation

Initially, palpation for tenderness plays no part in the assessment, since "referred" tenderness is very real and can be misleading. Only when the tissue at fault has been identified is palpation for tenderness used to determine the exact extent of the lesion within that tissue, and then palpation is done only if the tissue lies superficially and within easy reach of the fingers. Tenderness often does enable the examiner to name the affected ligament or the specific section or exact point of the tearing or bruising.

To palpate properly, the examiner must ensure that the area to be palpated is as relaxed as possible. For this to be done, the body part must be supported as much as possible. As the ability to develop palpation develops, the examiner should be able to:

1. Discriminate differences in tissue tension (e.g., effusion and spasm) and muscle tone (i.e., spasticity, rigidity, and flaccidity). Spasticity refers to muscle tonus in which there may be a collapse of muscle tone during testing. Rigidity refers to involuntary resistance being maintained during passive movement and without collapse of the muscle. Flaccidity means there is no muscle tone.
2. Distinguish differences in tissue texture.
3. Identify shapes, structures, and tissue type and thus detect abnormalities.
4. Determine tissue thickness and texture and thus determine whether it is pliable, soft, and resilient. Is there any obvious swelling? Edema is an abnormal accumulation of fluid in the intercellular spaces. Swelling is the abnormal enlargement of a body part. It may be intracellular or extracellular and intracapsular or extracapsular. Swelling that develops immediately in response to injury or within 2 to 4 hours of the injury is most likely due to blood extravasation into the tissues or joint. Swelling becoming evident after 12 to 24 hours is due to inflammation and, in a joint, is synovial swelling. Bony or hard swelling may be due to osteophytes or new bone formation. Soft-tissue swelling such as edematous synovium produces a boggy feeling, whereas fluid swelling is softer and more mobile. Older, long-standing soft-tissue swelling, such as a skin callus, feels like tough, dry leather. The more leathery the thickening feels, the more likely it is to be causing local symptoms. Softer thickenings tend to be more acute and associated with recent symptoms.[9] Pitting edema is thick and slow moving, leaving an indentation after pressure is applied and removed. The swelling may be localized or encapsulated. This finding may indicate intra-articular swelling, a cyst, or swollen bursa. Long-lasting swelling may cause reflex inhibition of the muscles around the joint leading to atrophy and weakness.
5. Determine joint tenderness by applying firm pressure to the joint. The pressure should always be applied with care. The degree of tenderness can be graded as follows:

Grade I: Patient complains of pain.
Grade II: Patient complains of pain and winces.
Grade III: Patient winces and withdraws the joint.
Grade IV: Patient will not allow palpation of the joint.

6. Feel variations in temperature. This determination is usually best done by using the back of the examiner's hand or fingers and comparing both sides.

7. Feel pulses, tremors, and fasciculations. Fasciculations are the result of a number of muscle cells innervated by the contraction of a single motor axon. Tremors are involuntary movements in which agonist/antagonist muscle groups contract to cause rhythmic movements of a joint. Pulses are an indication of circulatory sufficiency and should be tested for rhythm and strength if circulatory problems are suspected. Table 1–16 indicates the more common pulses that may be used to determine circulatory sufficiency and location.

8. Determine the state of the periarticular tissues.

9. Feel dryness or excessive moisture of the skin. For example, acute gouty joints tend to be dry, whereas septic joints tend to be moist.

10. Note any abnormal sensation (e.g., dysesthesia, diminished sensation; hyperesthesia, increased sensation; and anesthesia, absence of sensation) or crepitus. Soft, fine crepitus may indicate roughening of the articular cartilage, whereas coarse grating may indicate badly damaged articular cartilage. A creaking, leathery (snowball crepitation) crepitus is sometimes seen in tendons, indicating pathology. Tendons may "snap" over one another or over a bony prominence. Loud, snapping, pain-free noises in joints are usually due to cavitation in which gas bubbles form suddenly and transiently due to a negative pressure in the joint.

Palpation of a joint and surrounding area must be carried out in a systematic fashion to ensure that all structures are examined. This procedure involves having a starting point and working from that point to surrounding tissues to ensure their normality or the possibility of pathological involvement. The examiner must work slowly and carefully, applying light pressure initially and working into a deeper pressure of palpation, "feeling" for pathological conditions. The uninvolved side should be palpated first so that the patient has some idea of what to expect. Any differences or abnormalities should be noted.

Radiographic Examination

The examiner may view the x-ray films.[21, 22] However, it should be remembered that although impor-

TABLE 1–16. Common Circulatory Pulse Locations

Artery	Location
Carotid	Anterior to sternocleidomastoid muscle
Brachial	Medial aspect of arm midway between shoulder and elbow
Radial	At wrist, lateral to flexor carpi radialis tendon
Ulnar	At wrist, between flexor digitorum superficialis and flexor carpi ulnaris tendons
Femoral	In femoral triangle (sartorius, adductor longus, and inguinal ligament)
Popliteal	Posterior aspect of knee (deep and hard to palpate)
Posterior tibial	Posterior aspect of medial malleolus
Dorsalis pedis	Between first and second metatarsal bones on superior aspect

tant, radiographic examination is usually used only to confirm a clinical opinion. X-rays are part of the electromagnetic spectrum and have the ability to penetrate tissue to varying degrees. The x-ray plates that are developed after exposure to the roentgen rays enable the examiner to see any fractures, dislocations, foreign bodies, or radiopaque substances that may be present. The main function of x-ray examination is to rule out or exclude serious disease, such as infection (osteomyelitis), ankylosing spondylitis, or neoplasm. In soft-tissue injuries, clinical findings should take precedence over x-ray findings. It is desirable to know whether an x-ray has been taken so the examiner can obtain this information if necessary. The examiner should be aware of obvious unusual x-ray findings that distract attention from other tissue that is actually the cause of the pain. Such x-ray abnormalities are significant only if clinical examination bears out their relevance. With experience, the examiner becomes able to detect on x-ray examination many important soft-tissue changes, such as effusion in joints, tendinous calcifications, ectopic bone in muscle, tissue displaced by tumor, and presence of air or foreign body material in the tissues. Roentgenograms may also be used to give an indication of bone loss. For osteoporosis to be evident on film, approximately 30 to 35 per cent of the bone must be lost.

When viewing bone films, the examiner should note whether the following features vary from normal:

1. Overall size and shape of bone.
2. Local size and shape of bone.
3. Thickness of the cortex.
4. Trabecular pattern of the bone.
5. General density of the entire bone.
6. Local density change.
7. Margins of local lesions.
8. Any break in continuity of the bone.
9. Any periosteal change.

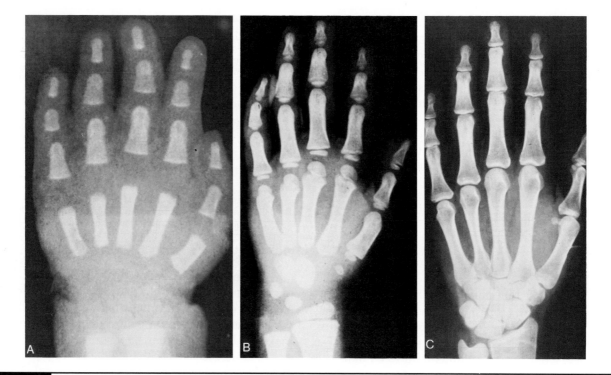

FIGURE 1–8. X-ray films showing skeletal maturity. (A) Male, newborn. (B) Male, 5 years old. (C) Female, 17 years old.

10. Any soft-tissue change.
11. Relation among bones.
12. Thickness of the cartilage (cartilage space within joints).

The examiner should keep in mind the maturity of the individual when viewing films. Skeletal changes occur with age,[23] and the appearance and fusion of epiphysis, for example, may be important in interpreting the pathology of the condition seen. Soft-tissue structures can be seen as well as bone, provided there is something to outline them (i.e., the joint capsule may be silhouetted by the pericapsular fat, or a cardiac shadow may be silhouetted by air in the lungs). Anatomic variations and anomalies must all be ruled out before pathology can be ruled in (i.e., accessory navicular, bipartite patella, or os trigonum may all be confused with fractures by the unsuspecting examiner). The fabella is often confused with a loose body in the knee in the anteroposterior projection x-ray film.

The basic principle of roentgen ray use is as follows. The greater the density of the tissue, the less penetration by x-rays; thus, the greater the density of the tissue, the whiter it will appear on the film. This fact is illustrated by varying degrees of white, gray, and black on the film. In order of descending degree of density are the following structures: metal, bone, soft tissue, water, fat, and air.

This difference gives the six basic densities on the x-ray plate. When viewing the x-rays, the examiner must identify the film, noting the name, age, date, and sex of the individual, and must identify the type of projection taken. For example, it should be noted if the view is an anteroposterior, lateral, tunnel, skyline, weight-bearing, or stress type.

Roentgenograms may also be used to determine the maturity index of an individual. A special film of the wrist is taken to assess skeletal maturity (Fig. 1–8). These films can be compared with established films in a bone atlas compiled by Gruelich and Pyle.[23] This technique is often done before epiphysiodesis and leg-lengthening procedures to ensure that the child is of a suitable skeletal age to do the procedure.

In addition to basic x-ray films, there are special techniques that may often be used in orthopedics. For example, *arthrograms* are used to outline structures within a joint (Fig. 1–9), most often the knee. There are three types of arthrograms:

Air. Air is used to outline the joint structures.

Dye or Contrast. A radiopaque dye is used to outline the joint structures.

Double-Contrast. Air and radiopaque dye are used to outline the joint structures.

Another specialized technique is a *myelogram* (Figs. 1–10 and 1–11). A radiopaque dye is placed within the epidural space and allowed to flow to

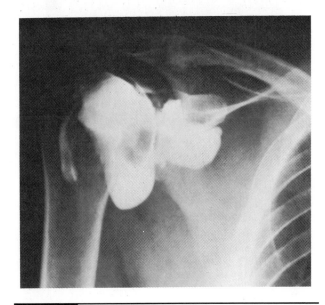

FIGURE 1–9. Normal arthrogram, shoulder in external rotation. Note the good dependent fold and the outline of the bicipital tendon. (From Neviaser, T. J.: Orthop. Clin. North Am. 11:209, 1980.)

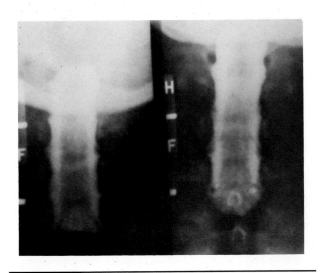

FIGURE 1–10. Myelogram of cervical spine. Note how radiopaque dye fills root sheaths.

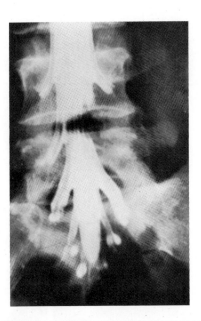

FIGURE 1–11. Myelogram of lumbar spine showing extrusion of nucleus pulposus of L4–L5. Note how radiopaque dye fills dural recesses. (From Selby, D. K., et al.: Orthop. Clin. North Am. 8:82, 1977.)

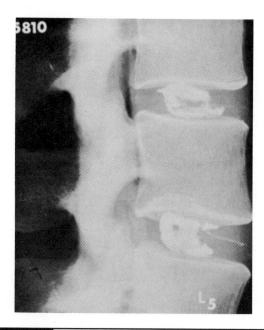

FIGURE 1–12. *Normal discogram shown with barium paste. (From Farfan, H. F.: Mechanical Disorders of the Low Back. Philadelphia, Lea & Febiger, 1973, p. 96.)*

different levels of the spinal cord. This technique is used to detect disc disease, nerve root entrapment, spinal stenosis, and tumors of the spinal cord. Extradural techniques can also be used. In epidural venography, radiopaque dye is allowed to flow through the epidural veins. This technique can yield supplementary information regarding the state of the disc.

Discography involves injecting a radiopaque dye into the disc to reproduce signs of disc disease and localize the level of impingement (Fig. 1–12).

With a *venogram* and an *arteriogram*, radiopaque dye is injected into specific vessels to outline abnormal conditions (Fig. 1–13). This technique may be used to diagnose arteriosclerosis, investigate tumors, or demonstrate blockage after trauma.

Increasing use is being made of *bone scans* (Fig. 1–14). With this technique, chemicals labeled with isotopes, such as technetium-99m–labeled phosphorus complexes, may be intravenously injected and used to localize specific organs that concentrate the particular chemical. The isotope may be localized where there is a high level of activity relative to the rest of a bone. Thus, the bone scan can be used to detect stress fractures and tumors. The bone scan images are usually taken 2 to 3 hours after the injection to allow clearance of the isotope from the blood. Because the isotope is excreted by the kidneys, the kidneys and bladder are often visible in bone scans.

Tomography has also become a common technique. Cuts of film are taken at specific levels of the body. Tomograms may be plain (rather fuzzy) or

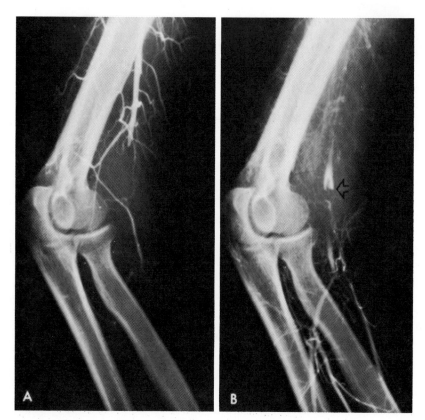

FIGURE 1–13. *Occlusion of brachial artery. (A) Arteriogram of a young man with a previously reduced elbow dislocation and an ischemic hand shows an occluded brachial artery. (B) A later film shows fresh clot (arrow) in the brachial artery and reconstituted radial and ulnar arteries. Primary repair and thrombectomy treated the ischemic symptoms. (From McLean, G., and D. B. Frieman: Orthop. Clin. North Am. 14:267, 1983.)*

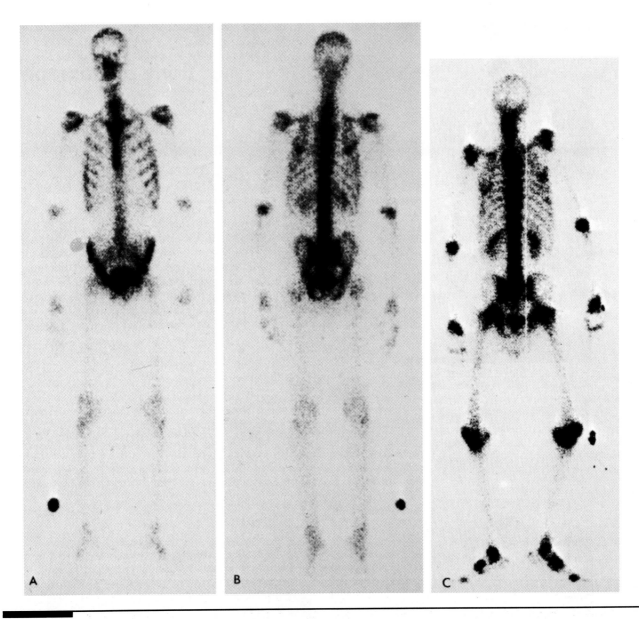

FIGURE 1–14. Whole body bone scans. (A) Normal adult anterior scan. (B) Normal adult posterior scan. (C) Posterior scan showing joint involvement of rheumatoid arthritis. (From Goldstein, H. A.: Orthop. Clin. North Am. 14:244, 250, 1983.)

computer enhanced. In the latter case, they are referred to as *CT scans* (computed tomography scans) or *CAT scans* (computer-assisted or -enhanced tomography scans). The CT scans can also be contrast enhanced (dye injected around the structure) to indicate tumor or bone or soft-tissue involvement. In this case, they may be called CTAs (computed tomoarthrograms). CT scans can be used to clearly define complicated fractures or outline structures deep within the body (Fig. 1–15).

Magnetic resonance imaging (MRI), or *nuclear magnetic resonance* (NMR), is a noninvasive, painless imaging technique that uses magnetic fields to obtain an image of bone and soft tissue. The two terms mean the same thing. MRI is the more often used term because patients frequently become uncomfortable when the word "nuclear" is mentioned. This technique uses no ionizing radiation to visualize the structures being evaluated and can be used to visualize soft-tissue detail (Fig. 1–16). However, MRIs should be interpreted only with the full knowledge of other findings such as plain x-rays.

Xeroradiography is a technique in which a xeroradiographic plate replaces the normal x-ray film. On the plate, there is a thin layer of a photoconductor to enhance the picture (Fig. 1–17). This tech-

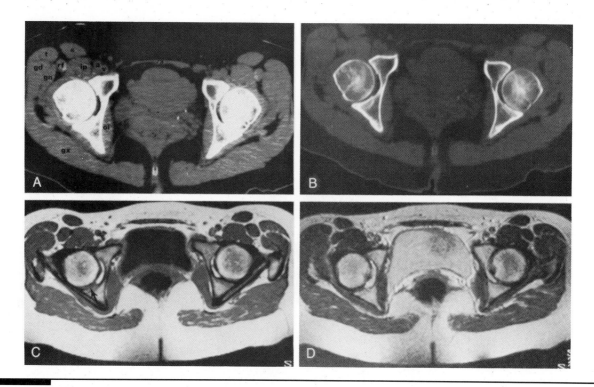

FIGURE 1–15. (A) Normal CT image at the level of the midacetabulum obtained with soft-tissue window settings shows the homogeneous, intermediate signal of musculature. a = common femoral artery; gd = gluteus medius; gn = gluteus minimum; gx = gluteus maximum; ip = iliopsoas; oi = obturator internus; ra = rectus abdominis; rf = rectus femoris; s = sartorius; t = tensor fascia lata; v = common femoral vein. (B) Axial CT at bone window settings reveals improved delineation of cortical and medullary osseous detail. Note anterior and posterior semilunar acetabular articular surfaces and the central nonarticular acetabular fossa. (C) Normal midacetabular T1-weighted axial 0.4-T MRI (TR, 600 msec; TE, 20 msec) of a different patient shows normal, high signal intensity image of fatty marrow (adult pattern) and subcutaneous tissue, low-signal intensity image of muscle, and absence of signal in the cortical bone. The thin articular hyaline cartilage is of intermediate signal (arrow). (D) T2-weighted MRI (TR, 2,000 msec; TE, 80 msec) shows decreasing high-signal intensity in fatty marrow and subcutaneous tissue with increased signal intensity in the fluid-filled urinary bladder. (From Pitt, M. J., et al.: Orthop. Clin. North Am. 21:553, 1990.)

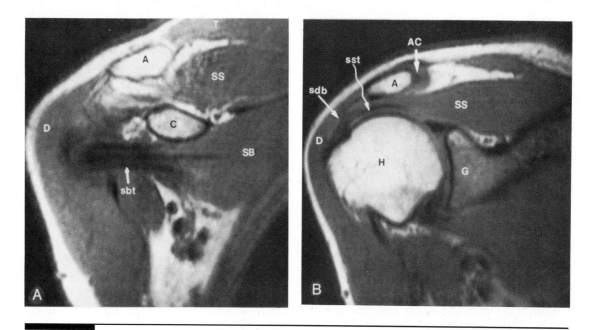

FIGURE 1–16. MRI T1-weighted coronal oblique images from anterior (A) to posterior (C). T = trapezius muscle, A = acromion, SS = supraspinatus muscle, D = deltoid muscle, C = coracoid, SB = subscapularis muscle, sbt = subscapularis tendon, AC = acromioclavicular joint, sst = supraspinatus tendon, SDB = subdeltoid-subacromial bursa, H = humerus, G = glenoid of scapula, ist = infraspinatus tendon, IS = infraspinatus muscle. (From Mayer, S. J., and M. K. Dalinka: Orthop. Clin. North Am. 21:500, 1990.)

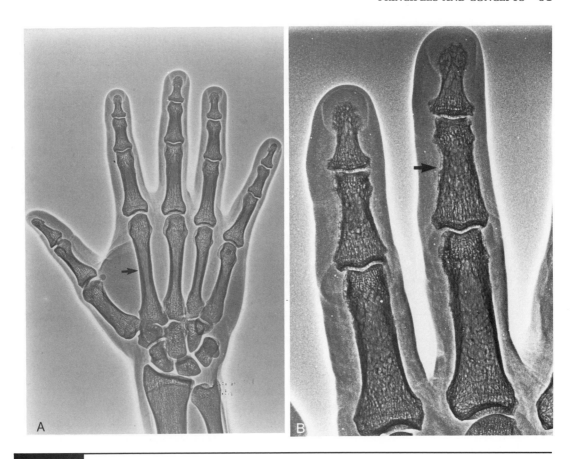

FIGURE 1–17. Xeroradiography. (A) Normal examination. Note the ability to demonstrate both soft tissues and bony structures on a single examination. The halo effect (arrow) around the bony cortices is an example of edge enhancement. (B) Hyperparathyroid bone changes shown on xeroradiography. The subperiosteal bone resorption (arrow) and distal tuft erosion are well seen. (A, from Weissman, B. N. W., and C. B. Sledge: Orthopedic Radiology. Philadelphia, W. B. Saunders Co., 1986, p. 11; B, from Seltzer, S. E., et al.: Semin. Arthritis Rheum. 11:315, 1982.)

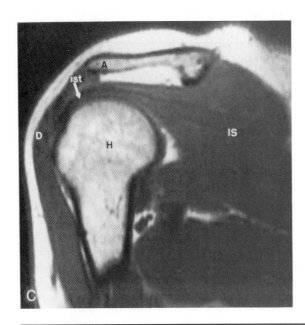

FIGURE 1–16C See legend on opposite page.

TABLE 1–17. Symptoms and Differentiation of Claudication*

Vascular Claudication	Neurogenic Claudication	Spinal Stenosis
Pain† is usually bilateral	Pain is usually bilateral but may be unilateral	Usually bilateral pain
Occurs in the calf (foot, thigh, hip, or buttocks)	Occurs in back, buttocks, thighs, calves, feet	Occurs in back, buttocks, thighs, calves, and feet
Pain consistent in all spinal positions	Pain decreased in spinal flexion	Pain decreased in spinal flexion
	Pain increased in spinal extension	Pain increased in spinal extension
Pain brought on by physical exertion (e.g., walking)	Pain increased with walking	Pain increased with walking
Pain relieved promptly by rest (1 to 5 minutes)	Pain decreased by recumbency	Pain relieved with prolonged rest (may persist hours after resting)
Pain increased by walking uphill		Pain decreased when walking uphill
No burning or dysesthesia	Burning and dysesthesia from the back to buttocks and leg(s)	Burning and numbness present in lower extremities
Decreased or absent pulses in lower extremities	Normal pulses	Normal pulses
Color and skin changes in feet—cold, numb, dry, or scaly skin, poor nail and hair growth	Good skin nutrition	Good skin nutrition
Affects ages from 40 to over 60	Affects ages from 40 to over 60	Peaks in seventh decade of life; affects men primarily

*Modified from Goodman, C. C., and T. E. Kelly Snyder: Differential Diagnosis in Physical Therapy. Philadelphia, W. B. Saunders Co., 1990, p. 339.
†"Pain" associated with vascular claudication may also be described as an "aching," "cramping," or "tired" feeling.

nique is used when the margins between areas of different densities need to be exaggerated.[24]

PRÉCIS

At the end of each chapter, the reader will find a précis of the assessment for that joint as a quick reference. The précis does not follow the text description exactly but is laid out so that each assessment involves minimal movement of the patient, which hopefully will decrease patient discomfort. Thus, all of the examination is performed with the patient standing, followed by sitting and so on.

CASE STUDIES

Case studies are provided for the reader as written exercises to help the examiner develop skills in assessment. Based on the presented case study, the reader should develop a list of appropriate questions to ask in the history, what things should be especially noted in observation, and what part of the examination is essential to make a definitive diagnosis. Where appropriate, example diagnoses are given in parentheses at the end of each question. At the end of the case study, the reader can develop a table showing the differential diagnosis for the case described. Table 1–17 illustrates just such a differential diagnosis chart for intermittent claudication and spinal stenosis.

CONCLUSION

Having completed all parts of the assessment, the examiner can look at the pertinent objective and subjective facts, note the significant signs and symptoms to determine what is causing the patient's problems, and design a proper treatment regimen based on the findings. If the assessment is not followed through completely, the treatment regimen may not be implemented properly, and this may lead to unwarranted extended care of the patient and increase health care costs.

Occasionally, patients present with a mixture of signs and symptoms that indicates two or more possible problem areas. Only by adding the positive findings and subtracting the negative findings can the examiner determine the probable cause of the problem. In many cases, the decision may be an educated guess because very few problems are "textbook perfect." Only the examiner's knowledge, clinical experience, and diagnosis followed by trial treatment can conclusively delineate the problem.

REFERENCES

CITED REFERENCES

1. Cyriax, J.: Textbook of Orthopaedic Medicine, vol. 1: Diagnosis of Soft Tissue Lesions, 8th ed. London, Bailliere Tindall, 1982.
2. Weed, L.: Medical records that guide and teach, Part I. New Engl. J. Med. 278:593–600, 1968.
3. Melzack, R.: The McGill pain questionnaire: Major properties and scoring methods. Pain 1:277–299, 1975.

4. Williams, P., and R. Warwick (eds.): Gray's Anatomy, 36th British ed. Philadelphia, W. B. Saunders Co., 1980.
5. Keegan, J. J., and E. D. Garrett: The segmental distribution of the cutaneous nerves in the limbs of man. Anat. Rec. 101:409, 1948.
6. Beighton, P., R. Grahame, and H. Borde: Hypermobility of Joints. Berlin, Springer-Verlag, 1983.
7. Wynne-Davies, R.: Hypermobility. Proc. Roy. Soc. Med. 64:689–693, 1971.
8. Evans, P.: Ligaments, joint surfaces, conjunct rotation and close pack. Physiother. 74:105–114, 1988.
9. Maitland, G. D.: Palpation examination of the posterior cervical spine: The ideal, average and abnormal. Aust. J. Physiother. 28:3–11, 1982.
10. Clarkson, H. M., and G. B. Gilewich: Musculoskeletal Assessment—Joint Range of Motion and Manual Muscle Strength. Baltimore, Williams & Wilkins, 1989.
11. Daniels, L., and C. Worthingham: Muscle Testing: Techniques of Manual Examination. Philadelphia, W. B. Saunders Co., 1980.
12. Janda, V.: On the concept of postural muscles and posture in man. Aust. J. Physiother. 29:83–85, 1983.
13. Rowe, C. R.: The Shoulder. Edinburgh, Churchill Livingstone, 1988.
14. Carroll, D.: A quantitative test of upper extremity function. J. Chron. Dis. 18:479–491, 1965.
15. Potvin, A. R., W. W. Tourtellotte, J. S. Dailey, J. W. Alberta, J. W. Walker, R. W. Pew, W. G. Henderson, and D. N. Snyder: Simulated activities of daily living examination. Arch. Phys. Med. Rehabil. 53:476–486, 1972.
16. Cervical Spine Research Society: The Cervical Spine. Philadelphia, J. B. Lippincott Co., 1989.
17. Bland, J. H.: Disorders of the Cervical Spine. Philadelphia, W. B. Saunders Co., 1987.
18. Hockaday, J. M., and C. W. M. Whitty: Patterns of referred pain in the normal subject. Brain 90:481, 1967.
19. Mennell, J. Mc. M.: Joint Pain. Boston, Little, Brown & Co., 1972.
20. Kaltenborn, F. M.: Mobilization of the Extremity Joints: Examination and Basic Treatment Techniques. Oslo, Olaf Norlis Bokhandel, 1980.
21. Jones, M. D.: Basic Diagnostic Radiology, St. Louis, C. V. Mosby Co., 1969.
22. Miller, W. T.: Introduction to Clinical Radiology. New York, MacMillan, 1982.
23. Greulich, W. W., and S. U. Pyle: Radiographic Atlas of Skeletal Development of the Wrist and Hand. Stanford, Calif., Stanford University Press, 1959.
24. Weissman, B. N. W., and C. B. Sledge: Orthopedic Radiology. Philadelphia, W. B. Saunders Co., 1986.

GENERAL REFERENCES

Bassett, L. W., R. H. Gold, and L. L. Seeger: MRI of the Musculoskeletal System. London, Martin Dunitz Ltd., 1989.
Bombardier, D., and P. Tugwell: Measuring disability: Guidelines for rheumatology studies. J. Rheum. Suppl. 10:68–73, 1983.
Bonica, J. J.: The Management of Pain. Philadelphia, Lea & Febiger, 1953.
Brodie, D. J., J. V. Burnett, J. M. Walker, and D. Lydes-Reid: Evaluation of low back pain by patient questionnaires and therapist assessment. J.O.S.P.T. 11:519–529, 1990.
Chafetz, N., and H. K. Genant: Computed tomography of the lumbar spine. Orthop. Clin. North Am. 14:147, 1983.
Cohen, J., M. Bonfiglio, and C. J. Campbell: Orthopedic Pathophysiology in Diagnosis and Treatment. Edinburgh, Churchill Livingstone, 1990.
Convery, F. R., M. A. Minteer, D. Amiel, and K. L. Connett: Polyarticular disability: A functional assessment. Arch. Phys. Med. Rehab. 58:494–499, 1977.
Curran, J. F., M. H. Ellman, and N. L. Brown: Rheumatologic aspects of painful conditions affecting the shoulder. Clin. Orthop. Rel. Res. 173:27, 1983.
Currey, H. L. F.: Clinical Examination of the Joints: An Introduction to Clinical Rheumatology. Toronto, Pitman Medical, 1975.
Cyriax, J.: Examination of the spinal column. Physiother. 56:2–6, 1970.

Farfan, H. F.: Mechanical Disorders of the Low Back. Philadelphia, Lea & Febiger, 1973.
Forrester, D. M., and J. C. Brown: The Radiology of Joint Disease. Philadelphia, W. B. Saunders Co., 1987.
French, S.: History taking in physiotherapy assessment. Physiother. 74:158–160, 1988.
Gartland, J. J.: Fundamentals of Orthopedics. Philadelphia, W. B. Saunders Co., 1979.
Goldstein, H. A.: Bone scintigraphy. Orthop. Clin. North Am. 14:243, 1983.
Goodman, C. C., and T. E. Kelly Snyder: Differential Diagnosis in Physical Therapy—Musculoskeletal and Systemic Conditions. Philadelphia, W. B. Saunders Co., 1990.
Grieve, G. P.: Common Vertebral Joint Problems. London, Churchill Livingstone, 1981.
Grieve, G. P.: Modern Manual Therapy of the Vertebral Column. London, Churchill Livingstone, 1986.
Hammond, M. J.: Clinical examination and the physiotherapist. Aust. J. Physiother. 15:47, 1969.
Health, J. R.: Problem oriented medical systems. Physiother. 64:269–270, 1978.
Hoppenfeld, S.: Physical Examination of the Spine and Extremities. New York, Appleton-Century-Crofts, 1976.
Jackson, R.: Headaches associated with disorders of the cervical spine. Headache 6:175–179, 1967.
Janda, V.: Muscle Function Testing. London, Butterworths, 1983.
Judge, R. D., G. D. Zuidema, and F. T. Fitzgerald: Clinical Diagnosis: A Physiologic Approach. Boston, Little, Brown & Co., 1982.
Lee, P., M. K. Jasani, W. C. Dick, and W. W. Buchanan: Evaluation of a functional index in rheumatoid arthritis. Scand. J. Rheum. 2:71–77, 1973.
Little, H.: The Rheumatological Physical Examination. Orlando, Grune & Stratton, Inc., 1986.
MacConnaill, M. A., and J. V. Basmajian: Muscles and Movements: A Basis for Human Kinesiology. Baltimore, Williams & Wilkins, 1977.
Mayer, S. J., and M. K. Dalina: Magnetic resonance imaging of the shoulder. Orthop. Clin. North Am. 21:497–513, 1990.
McLean, G., and D. B. Freiman: Angiography of skeletal disease. Orthop. Clin. North Am. 14:257, 1983.
Melzack, R.: The McGill pain questionnaire: Major properties and scoring methods. Pain 1:277–299, 1975.
Neviaser, T. J.: Arthrography of the shoulder. Orthop. Clin. North Am. 11:205, 1980.
Novey, D. W.: Rapid Access Guide to the Physical Examination. Chicago, Year Book Medical Publishers, 1988.
Palmer, M. L., and M. Epler. Clinical Assessment Procedures in Physical Therapy. Philadelphia, J. B. Lippincott Co., 1990.
Pitt, M. J., P. J. Lund, and D. P. Speer: Imaging of the pelvis and hip. Orthop. Clin. North Am. 21:545–559, 1990.
Post, M.: Physical Examination of the Musculoskeletal System. Chicago, Year Book Medical Publishers, 1987.
Reading, A. E.: Testing pain mechanisms in persons in pain. In Wall, P. D., and R. Melzack (eds.): Textbook of Pain. Edinburgh, Churchill Livingstone, 1984, p 195–204.
Saunders, H. D.: Evaluation and Treatment of Musculoskeletal Disorders. Minneapolis, H. D. Saunders, 1982.
Saunders, H. D.: Evaluation of a musculoskeletal disorder. In Gould, J. A. (ed.): Orthopedics and Sports Physical Therapy. St. Louis, C. V. Mosby Co., 1990.
Seidal, H. M., J. W. Ball, J. E. Dains, and G. W. Benedict: Mosby's Guide to Physical Examination. St. Louis, C. V. Mosby Co., 1987.
Selby, D. K., A. J. Meril, K. J. Wagner, and R. R. G. Winans: Water-soluble myelography. Orthop. Clin. North Am. 8:79, 1977.
Singer, K. P.: A new musculoskeletal assessment in a student population. J.O.S.P.T. 8:34–41, 1986.
Smith, L. K.: Functional tests. Phys. Ther. Rev. 34:19–21, 1954.
Spengler, D. M.: Low Back Pain—Assessment and Management. Orlando, Grune & Stratton, Inc., 1982.
Squire, L. F., W. M. Colaiace, and N. Strutynsky: Exercises in Diagnostic Radiology, vol. III: Bone. Philadelphia, W. B. Saunders Co., 1972.
Wadsworth, C. T.: Manual Examination and Treatment of the Spine and Extremities. Baltimore, Williams & Wilkins, 1988.

CHAPTER 2

Cervical Spine

Examination of the cervical spine involves determining whether the injury or pathology occurs in the cervical spine or in a portion of the upper limb. Cyriax called this assessment the *scanning examination*.[1] In the initial assessment of a patient who complains of pain in the neck and/or upper limb, this procedure is always carried out unless the examiner is absolutely sure of where the lesion is localized. If the injury is in the neck, the scanning examination is definitely called for. Once the lesion site has been determined, a more detailed assessment of the affected area is performed if it is outside the cervical spine.

The cervical spine is a complicated area to assess properly, and adequate time must be allowed to ensure that as many causes or problems are examined as possible. Many conditions affecting the cervical spine can manifest in other parts of the body, and the examiner must be aware of this.

APPLIED ANATOMY

The cervical spine consists of several joints. It is an area in which stability has been sacrificed for mobility, making the cervical spine particularly vulnerable to injury. The *atlanto-occipital joints* (C0–C1) are the two uppermost joints. The principal motion at these two joints is flexion-extension (15 to 20°), or nodding of the head. In addition, side flexion is approximately 10° whereas rotation is negligible. The *atlas* (C1) has no vertebral body as such. During development, the vertebral body of C1 has evolved into the *odontoid process*, which is part of C2. The atlanto-occipital joints are ellipsoid and act in unison. Along with the atlantoaxial joints, these joints are the most complex articulation of the axial skeleton.

The *atlantoaxial joints* (C1–C2) constitute the most mobile articulation of the spine. Flexion-extension is approximately 10°, and side flexion is approximately 5°. Rotation, which is approximately

50°, is the primary movement of these joints. With rotation, there is a decrease in height of the cervical spine at this level as the vertebrae approximate because of the shape of the facet joints. The odontoid process of C2 acts as a pivot point for the rotation. This middle, or median, joint is classified as a *pivot (trochoidal)* type of joint. The lateral atlantoaxial, or facet, joints are classified as *plane* joints. Generally, if a person can talk and chew, there is probably some motion occurring at C1–C2.

It must be remembered that rotation past 50° in the cervical spine may lead to kinking of the contralateral vertebral artery; the ipsilateral vertebral artery may kink at 45° of rotation. This kinking may lead to vertigo, nausea, tinnitus, "drop attacks," visual disturbances, stroke, or death.

There are 14 *facet*, or *apophyseal*, joints in the cervical spine. The upper four facet joints in the two upper thoracic vertebrae are often included in the examination of the cervical spine. The superior facets of the cervical spine face upward, backward, and medially; the inferior facets face downward, forward, and laterally. This plane facilitates flexion and extension, but it prevents rotation and/or side flexion without both occurring to some degree together. These joints move primarily by gliding and are classified as a *synovial*, or *diarthrodial*, type of joints. The capsules are lax to allow for sufficient movement. At the same time, they provide support and a check-rein type of restriction. The greatest flexion-extension of the facet joints occurs between C5 and C6; however, there is almost as much movement between C4–C5 and C6–C7. The neutral or resting position of the cervical spine is slightly extended. The close packed position of the facet joints is complete extension. The facet joints are highly innervated by the recurrent *meningeal* or *sinuvertebral* nerve.

Some anatomists[2-5] refer to the *costal* or *uncovertebral processes* as *uncinate joints* or *joints of von Lushka*. These structures were described by von Lushka in 1858. The uncus gives a "saddle" form to the upper aspect of the cervical vertebra, which is more pronounced posterolaterally. It has the effect of limiting side flexion. Extending from the uncus is a "joint" that appears to form because of a weakness in the annulus fibrosus. The portion of the vertebra above, which "articulates" or conforms to the uncus, is called the *échancrure*, or notch. Notches are found from C3 to T1, but according to most of the authors,[2-5] they are not seen until the ages of 6 to 9 years and are fully developed by the age of 18 years. There is some controversy as to whether they should be classified as real joints because some authors believe they are the result of degeneration of the disc; degeneration tends to occur faster in the cervical spine than in any other parts of the spine.

The *intervertebral disc* makes up approximately 25 per cent of the height of the cervical spine. No disc is found between the atlas and the occiput (C0–C1) or between the atlas and the axis (C1–C2). It is the disc rather than the vertebrae that gives the cervical spine its lordotic shape. The *nucleus pulposus* functions as a buffer to axial compression in distributing compressive forces, while the annulus fibrosus acts to withstand tension within the disc. Although it is generally believed that the intervertebral disc has no innervation, research indicates there may be some innervation on the periphery of the annulus fibrosus.[6]

There are seven vertebrae in the cervical spine, with the body of each vertebra supporting the weight of those above it. The facet joints may bear some of the weight of the vertebrae above, but this weight is minimal. However, this slight amount of weight bearing can lead to spondylitic changes in these joints. The outer ring of the vertebral body is made of cortical bone, and the inner part is made of cancellous bone covered with the cartilaginous end plate. The vertebral arch protects the spinal cord; the spinous processes, the majority of which are bifid in the cervical spine, provide for attachment of muscles. The transverse processes have basically the same function. In the cervical spine, the spinous processes are at the level of the facet joints of the same vertebra. Generally, the spinous process is considered to be absent or at least rudimentary on C1. This is why the first palpable vertebra descending from the external occipital protuberance is the spinous process of C2.

PATIENT HISTORY

In addition to the questions listed under "Patient History" in Chapter 1, the examiner should ask the following:

1. What is the patient's usual activity or pastime? Do any particular activities or postures bother the patient? What type of work does the patient do? Are there any positions that the patient holds for long periods of time (e.g., when sewing, typing, or working at a desk)? Does the patient wear glasses? If so, are they bifocals or trifocals? Cervicothoracic joint problems are painful when activities that require push-and-pull motion, like lawnmowing, sawing, and cleaning windows, are performed.

2. What are the sites and boundaries of the pain? Have the patient point to the location(s). Symptoms do not go down the arm for a C4 nerve root injury or for nerve roots above that level.

3. Did the head strike anything, or did the patient lose consciousness? If the injury was due to a motor vehicle accident, it is important to know if the patient was wearing a seat belt, the type of seat belt (lap or shoulder), and whether the patient saw the accident coming. These questions will give some idea of the severity of the injury as well as the mechanisms of injury. If the patient was unconscious or unsteady, the character of each episode of altered consciousness should be noted.

4. Did the symptoms come on right away? For example, bone pain usually occurs immediately, whereas muscle or ligamentous pain may come on immediately (e.g., a tear) or occur several hours or days later (e.g., stretching as can occur from a motor vehicle accident).

5. Is there any radiation of pain? It is helpful to remember this and correlate it with dermatome findings when doing palpation. Is the pain deep? Superficial? Shooting? Burning? Aching?

6. Is there paresthesia ("pins and needles")? This sensation is present if pressure is applied to the nerve root. It may become evident if pressure is relieved from a nerve trunk.

7. Which activities aggravate the problem? Which activities ease the problem? Are there any head or neck positions that the patient finds particularly bothersome? These positions should be noted. For example, does reading (flexed cervical spine) bother the patient? If symptoms are not varied by a change in position, the problem is not likely to be mechanical in origin. Lesions of C3, C4, and C5 may affect the diaphragm and, thus, breathing.

8. Is the condition improving? Worsening? Staying the same?

9. What can be learned about the patient's sleeping position? Is there any problem sleeping? How many pillows does the patient use, and what type are they (e.g., feather, foam)? Foam pillows tend to retain their shape and have more "bounce" and do not offer as much support as a good feather pillow. What type of mattress does the patient use (e.g., hard, soft)? Does the patient "hug" the pillow or abduct the arms when sleeping? These positions can increase the stress on the lower cervical nerve roots.

TABLE 2–1. Type of Headache Pain and Usual Causes

Type of Pain	Usual Causes
Acute	Trauma, acute infection, impending cerebrovascular accident, subarachnoid hemorrhage
Chronic, recurrent	Migraine (definite pattern of irregular interval); eye strain; noise; excessive eating, drinking, or smoking; inadequate ventilation
Continuous, recurrent	Trauma
Severe, intense	Meningitis, aneurysm (ruptured), migraine, brain tumor
Intense, transient, shocklike	Neuralgia
Throbbing, pulsating (vascular)	Migraine, fever, hypertension, aortic insufficiency, neuralgia
Constant, tight (bandlike), bilateral	Muscle contraction

10. Does the patient have any headaches? If so, where? How frequently do they occur? How intense are they? How long do they last? Are there any precipitating factors (e.g., food, stress, posture)? Tables 2–1, 2–2, and 2–3 show the effect of time of day, body position, headache location, and type of pain on the type of headache the patient may have. Table 2–4 outlines the salient features of some of the more common headaches. For example, C1 headaches occur at the base and top of the head, whereas C2 headaches are referred to the temporal area.

11. Does a position change alter the headache or pain? If so, which position(s)? Sometimes, the patient may state that the pain and referred symptoms are decreased or relieved by placing the hand or arm on the affected side on top of the head. This is called *Bakody's sign* and is usually indicative of problems in the C4 or C5 area.[7]

12. Is the patient a mouth breather? Mouth breathing encourages forward head posture and increases activity of accessory respiratory muscles.

13. Does the patient experience dizziness, faintness, or seizures? Complete passing out is sometimes

TABLE 2–2. Location of Headache and Usual Causes

Location	Usual Causes
Forehead	Sinusitis, eye or nose disorder, muscle spasm of occipital or suboccipital region
Side of head	Migraine, eye or ear disorder, auriculotemporal neuralgia
Occipital	Myofascial problems, herniated disc, eye strain, hypertension, occipital neuralgia
Parietal	Hysteria (viselike), meningitis, constipation, tumor
Face	Maxillary sinusitis, trigeminal neuralgia, dental problems, tumor

TABLE 2–3. Effect of Position or Time of Day on Headache

Position or Time of Day When Headache Is Worst	Usual Causes
Morning	Sinusitis, migraine, hypertension, alcoholism, sleeping position
Afternoon	Eyestrain, muscle tension
Night	Intercranial disease, osteomyelitis, nephritis
Bending	Sinusitis
Lying horizontal	Migraine

called a *drop attack*. Did the patient experience any visual disturbances? Disturbances such as diplopia (double vision), loss of acuity, nystagmus ("dancing eyes"), scotomas (depressed visual field), and loss of acuity may indicate severity of injury, neurological injury, and sometimes increased intracranial pressure.[7]

14. Are there any lower limb symptoms? This finding may indicate a severe problem affecting the spinal cord.

15. Does the patient complain of any subjective restrictions when performing movements? If so, which movements are subjectively restricted?

16. Does the patient experience any tingling in the extremities? Are the symptoms bilateral? Bilateral symptoms usually indicate systemic disorders such as diabetes or alcohol abuse that are causing neuropathies or central space-occupying lesions.

17. Are symptoms improving or deteriorating?

18. Is there any difficulty in swallowing (dysphagia), or are there any voice changes? Such a change may be due to neurological problems, mechanical pressure, or muscle incoordination. Pain on swallowing may be indicative of soft-tissue swelling in the throat, vertebral subluxation, osteophyte projection, or disc protrusion into the esophagus or pharynx. One must remember that swallowing becomes more difficult and the voice becomes weaker as the neck is extended.

19. What is the patient's age? Spondylosis is often seen in persons 25 years old or older and is present in 60 per cent of those more than 45 years old and 85 per cent of those more than 65 years old. Symptoms of osteoarthritis do not usually appear until a person is 60 years old or older.

20. Is the pain affected by laughing? Coughing? Sneezing? Straining? If so, an increase in intrathoracic or intra-abdominal pressure may be causing the problem.

21. Does the patient exhibit or complain of any sympathetic symptoms? There may be injury to the cranial nerves or the sympathetic nervous system, which lies in the soft tissues of the neck anterior

TABLE 2–4. Headaches: A Differential Diagnosis*

Disorder	Sex/Age Pre-dominance	Nature of Pain	Frequency	Location	Duration	Prodromal Events	Precipitating Factors	Cause	Familial Pre-disposition	Other Possible Symptoms
Migraine	Female/20 to 40 years	Builds to throbbing and intense	Usually not more than twice a week May be nocturnal	Usually unilateral	Several hours to days	Visual disturbances can occur contralateral to pain site	Unknown, may be physical, emotional, hormonal, dietary	Vasomotor	Yes	Nausea, vomiting, pallor, photophobia, mood disturbances, fluid retention
Cluster (histamine) headache	Male/40 to 60 years	Excruciating, stabbing, burning, pulsating	1 to 4 episodes per 24 hours Nocturnal manifestation	Unilateral, eye, temple, forehead	Minutes to hours	Sleep disturbances or personality changes can occur	Unknown, may be serotonin, histamine, hormonal, blood flow	Vasomotor	Minor	Ipsilateral sweating of face, lacrimation, nasal congestion or discharge
Hypertension headache	None	Dull, throbbing, nonlocalized	Variable	Entire cranium, especially occipital region	Variable	None	Activity that increases blood pressure	High blood pressure; diastolic >120 mm Hg	Only as related to hypertension	
Trigeminal neuralgia (tic douloureux)	Female/40 to 60 years	Excruciating, spontaneous, lancinating, lightning	Can occur many (12 or more) times per day	Unilateral along trigeminal nerve area	30 seconds to 1 minute	Disagreeable tingling	Touch (cold) to affected area	Neurological	None	Reddened conjunctiva, lacrimation
Glossopharyngeal neuralgia	Male/40 to 60 years	Excruciating, spontaneous, lancinating, lightning	Can occur many (12 or more) times per day	Unilateral retrolingual area to ear	30 seconds to 1 minute	None	Movement or contact of the pharynx	Neurological	None	
Cervical neuralgia	None	Dull pain or pressure in head		Bilateral, occipital, frontal, or facial		None	Posture or head movement	Neurological, pressure on roots of spinal nerves	None	Dizziness, auditory disturbances
Eye disorders	None	Generalized discomfort in or around the eyes	Intensify with sustained visual effort	Entire cranium	During and after visual effort	None	Impairment of eye function	Cornea, iris, or intraocular pain	Possible	Diminished vision, sensitivity to light, tearing
Sinus, ear, and nasal disorders	None	Dull, persistent	Variable	Frontal, temporal, ear, nose, occipital	Variable	None	Infection, allergy, chemical, bending, straining	Blockage, inflammation, infection	None	

*Modified from Esposito, C. J., et al.: Headaches: A differential diagnosis. J. Craniomand. Pract. 4:318–322, 1986, p. 320–321.

and lateral to the cervical vertebrae. The cranial nerves and their functions are shown in Table 2–5. Some of the sympathetic symptoms the examiner may see are "ringing" in the ears, dizziness, blurred vision, photophobia, rhinorrhea, sweating, lacrimation, and hypothemia (loss of strength).

OBSERVATION

For a proper observation, the patient must be suitably undressed. However, the examiner should watch the patient before or while the patient undresses. These spontaneous movements can be very helpful in determining the patient's problems. For example, can the patient easily move the head when undressing? A male should wear only shorts, and a female should wear a bra and shorts. In some cases, the bra may have to be removed to determine whether there are any problems such as thoracic outlet syndrome, thoracic symptoms being referred to the cervical spine, or functional restriction of movement of the ribs. The examiner should note the willingness of the patient to move and the pattern of movement demonstrated. Facial expression of the patient will often give the examiner an indication of the amount of pain the patient is experiencing.

TABLE 2–5. Chief Functions and Distributions of the Cranial Nerves*

Nerve	Afferent	Efferent
I. Olfactory	Smell: nose	
II. Optic	Sight: eye	
III. Oculomotor		Vol. motor: levator of eyelid, sup., med., and inf. recti, inf. oblique of eyeball Autonomic: smooth muscle of eyeball
IV. Trochlear		Vol. motor: sup. oblique of eyeball
V. Trigeminal	Touch, pain: skin of face, mucous membranes of nose, sinuses, mouth, anterior tongue	Vol. motor: muscles of mastication
VI. Abducens		Vol. motor: lat. rectus of eyeball
VII. Facial	Taste: anterior tongue	Vol. motor: facial muscles Autonomic: lacrimal, submandibular, and sublingual glands
VIII. Vestibulocochlear	Hearing: ear Balance: ear	
IX. Glossopharyngeal	Touch, pain: posterior tongue, pharynx Taste: posterior tongue	Vol. motor: unimportant muscle of pharynx Autonomic: parotid gland
X. Vagus	Touch, pain: pharynx, larynx, bronchi Taste: tongue, epiglottis	Vol. motor: muscles of palate, pharynx, and larynx Autonomic: thoracic and abdominal viscera
XI. Accessory		Vol. motor: sternocleidomastoid and trapezius
XII. Hypoglossal		Vol. motor: muscles of tongue

*Modified from Hollinshead, W. H., and D. B. Jenkins: Functional Anatomy of the Limbs and Back. Philadelphia, W. B. Saunders Co., 1981, p. 358.

The patient may be seated or standing. The examiner should note the following:

Head and Neck Posture (Fig. 2–1). Is the head in the midline, or is there evidence of torticollis (Fig. 2–2), Klippel-Feil syndrome, or other neck deformity? Head and neck posture should be checked with the patient sitting and then standing, and any differences should be noted.

Shoulder Levels. Usually the dominant side will be slightly lower than the nondominant side.

Muscle Spasm or Any Asymmetry. Is there any atrophy of the deltoid muscle (circumflex or axillary nerve palsy) or torticollis (spasm, prominence, or tightness of the sternocleidomastoid muscle [Fig. 2–2])?

Facial Expression. The examiner should observe the patient's facial expression as the patient moves from position to position, makes different movements, and explains the problem. Such observation should give the examiner an idea of how much the patient is subjectively suffering.

Bony and Soft-Tissue Contours. If the cervical spine is injured, the head tends to be tilted and rotated away from the pain, and the face is tilted upward. If the patient is hysterical, the head tends to be tilted and rotated toward the pain, and the face is tilted down.

Evidence of Ischemia in Either Upper Limb.

Normal Sitting Posture. The nose should be in line with the manubrium and xiphoid process of the sternum. From the side, the ear lobe should be in line with the acromion process and the high point on the iliac crest for proper postural alignment. The examiner should remember that referred pain from conditions such as spondylosis tends to be in the shoulder and arm rather than the neck. It should also be remembered that the normal curve of the cervical spine is a lordotic type of curvature.

EXAMINATION

A complete examination of the cervical spine must be done, not only of the neck but also of the upper limbs. Many of the symptoms that occur in an upper limb can be originating from the neck. Unless there is a history of definite trauma to a peripheral joint, a screening examination must be done to rule out problems within the neck.

Active Movements

The first movements that are carried out are the active movements of the cervical spine, with the patient in the sitting position. The examiner is looking for differences in range of movement and the patient's willingness to do the movement. The range of motion taking place in this phase is the summation of all movements of the entire cervical

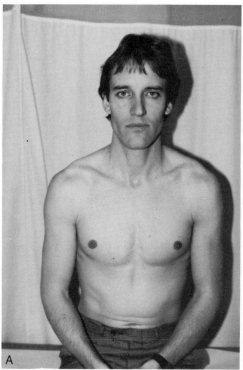

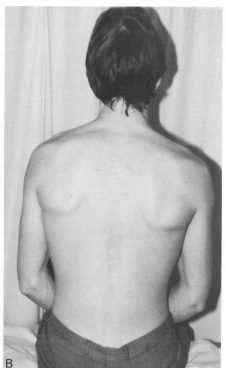

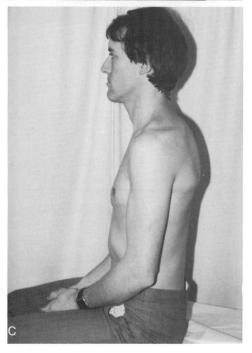

FIGURE 2–1. Observation views of head and neck. Note lower right shoulder and scapula; the ear is anterior to the shoulder.

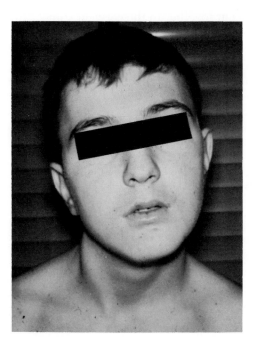

FIGURE 2–2. Example of torticollis showing prominent sternocleidomastoid muscle on the right. (From Gartland, J. J.: Fundamentals of Orthopedics. Philadelphia, W. B. Saunders Co., 1987, p. 279.)

spine, not just at one level. This combined movement allows for greater mobility in the cervical spine while still providing a firm support for the trunk and appendages. The range of motion available in the cervical spine is due to many factors, such as the flexibility of the intervertebral disc, the shape and inclination of the articular processes of the facet joints, and the slight laxity of the ligaments and joint capsules.

The movements should be done in a particular order so that the most painful movements are done last.[1] This is important so that there will be no residual pain carried over from the previous movement. When asking the individual to do the active movements, the examiner must remember to look for limitation of movement and possible reasons for pain, spasm, stiffness, or blocking. As the patient reaches the full range of active movement, passive overpressure may be applied very carefully—but only if the movement appears to be full and pain free. The overpressure will help to test the end feel of the movement. The examiner must be careful when applying overpressure to rotation.[8] In this position, the vertebral artery is often compressed; this can lead to a decrease in blood supply to the brain. Should this occur, the patient may complain of dizziness or feel faint. If the patient exhibits these symptoms, the examiner must use extreme care during these movements and during the following treatment.

The examiner can differentiate between movement in the upper and lower cervical spine. During flexion, "nodding" occurs in the upper cervical spine, whereas "flexion" occurs in the lower cervical spine. If this nodding movement does not occur, it indicates restriction of movement in the upper cervical spine; if flexion does not occur, it indicates restriction of motion in the lower cervical spine.

It must be remembered that movement can occur between C1 and C2 without affecting the other vertebrae but not between the other cervical vertebrae. That is, if one vertebra moves, the ones adjacent to it will also move.

The active movements that should be carried out in the cervical spine are as shown in Figure 2–3:

1. Flexion.
2. Extension.
3. Side flexion (left and right).
4. Rotation (left and right).

Flexion. For flexion, or forward bending, the maximum range of motion is 80 to 90°, and the extreme of range of motion is normally found when the chin is able to reach the chest with the mouth closed. However, up to two finger widths between the chin and chest is considered normal. In flexion, the intervertebral disc widens posteriorly and narrows anteriorly. The intervertebral foramen is 20 to 30 per cent larger on flexion than on extension. The vertebrae will shift forward in flexion and backward in extension. Also, the mastoid process will move away from the C1 transverse process on flexion and extension. As the patient forward flexes, the examiner should look for a posterior bulging of the spinous process of the axis. This bulging may be due to subluxation of the atlas forward, allowing the spinous process of the axis to become more prominent. If this sign appears, the examiner should exercise extreme caution during the remainder of the cervical assessment. If one has doubt about the subluxation, the Sharp-Purser test (see "Special Tests") may be performed but only with extreme care.

Extension. Extension, or backward bending, is normally limited to 70°. Because there is no anatomic block to stop movement going past this position, problems seen during whiplash or cervical strain often result. Normally, the plane of the nose and forehead is nearly horizontal. When the head is held in extension, the atlas tilts upward, resulting in posterior compression between the atlas and occiput.

Side Flexion. Side, or lateral, flexion is approximately 20 to 45° to the right and left. Most of the side flexion occurs between the occiput and C1 and between C1 and C2. When the patient does the movement, the examiner should ensure that the ear is taken to the shoulder and not the shoulder to the ear.

Rotation. Normally, rotation is 70 to 90° right and left, and the chin does not quite reach the plane of the shoulder. Remember that rotation and side flexion always occur together in the cervical spine. This combined movement may or may not be visible, depending on the movement involved. Rotation and side flexion occur together as a result of the shape of the articular surfaces of the facet joints; this shape is coronally oblique.

Figure 2–4 depicts active range of motion of the cervical spine.

Passive Movements

If the patient does not have full range of motion or the examiner has not applied overpressure to determine the end feel of the movement, the patient should be asked to lie down in a supine position. The examiner then passively tests flexion, extension, side flexion, and rotation, as in the active movements.

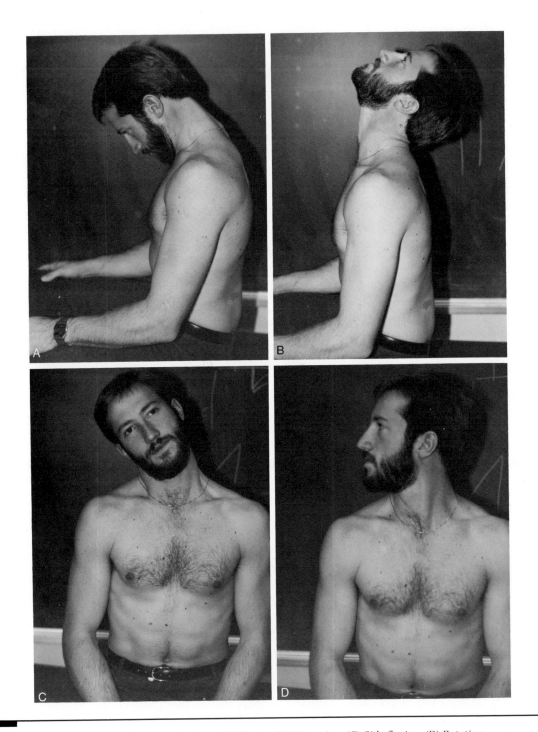

FIGURE 2–3. *Active movements of the cervical spine. (A) Flexion. (B) Extension. (C) Side flexion. (D) Rotation.*

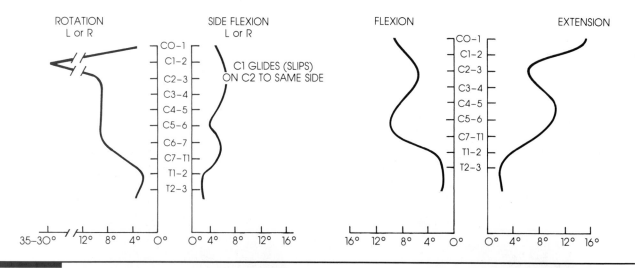

FIGURE 2–4. *Average active range of motion in the cervical spine. Individuals will vary widely, depending on age, body, type, and so on. (Adapted from Grieve, G. P.: Common Vertebral Joint Problems. Edinburgh, Churchill Livingstone, 1981, pp. 41, 42.)*

These movements are done to determine the end feel of each movement. This may give the examiner an idea of the pathology involved. The normal end feels of the cervical spine motions are tissue stretch for all four movements. As with active movements, the most painful movements are done last. The examiner should also note if a capsular pattern (side flexion and rotation equally limited; extension less limited) is present. Overpressure may be used to test the entire spine by testing it at the end of the range of motion, or proper positioning may be used to test different parts of the cervical spine.[9] For example, end feel for the lower cervical spine into extension is tested with minimal extension and the head pushed directly posterior (Fig. 2–5C), whereas the upper cervical spine is tested by "nodding" the head into extension and pushing posteriorly at an approximate 45° angle (Fig. 2–5B).[10]

Resisted Isometric Movements

The same movements that were done actively are done (flexion, extension, side flexion, and rotation), and there should be no movement. It is better for the examiner to say, "Don't let me move you," than to tell the patient to "contract the muscle as hard as possible." In this way, the examiner ensures that the movement is as isometric as possible and that a minimal amount of movement will occur (Fig. 2–6). The examiner should ensure that these movements are done with the cervical spine in the neutral position and that painful movements are done last. By using Table 2–6 and looking at the various combinations of muscles that cause the movement (Fig. 2–7), the examiner may be able to decide which muscle is at fault.

Peripheral Joints

Once the resisted isometric movements to the cervical spine have been completed, the peripheral joints should be quickly scanned to rule out obvious pathology in the extremities and to note areas that may need more detailed assessment.[1] The following joints are scanned bilaterally.

Temporomandibular Joint. The examiner checks the movement of the joint by placing the index or little fingers in the patient's ears (Fig. 2–8). The pulp aspect of the finger is placed forward to feel for equality of movement of the condyles of the temporomandibular joints and clicking or grinding as well as to ensure that the ears are clear. As the patient opens the mouth, the condyle will move forward. At the same time, the examiner should observe the patient open and close the mouth and should watch for any lateral deviation during the movement.

Shoulder Girdle. The examiner quickly scans this complex of joints by asking the patient to actively elevate the arm through abduction, followed by active elevation through forward flexion. In addition, the examiner quickly tests medial and lateral rotations of each shoulder. Any pattern of restriction should be noted. If the patient is able to reach full abduction without difficulty or pain, the examiner may decide that there is no problem with the shoulder complex.

Elbow Joints. The elbow joints are moved through flexion, extension, supination, and pronation. Any restriction of movement or abnormal sign and symptom should be noted because it may be indicative of pathology.

Wrist and Hand. The patient actively performs flexion, extension, and radial and ulnar deviations

Text continued on page 47

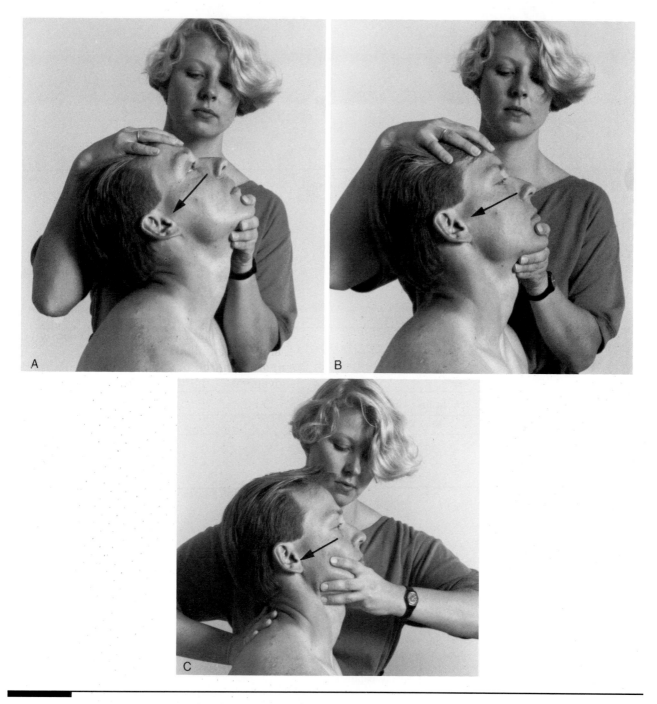

FIGURE 2–5. (A) *Overpressure to whole cervical spine.* (B) *Overpressure to upper cervical spine.* (C) *Overpressure to low cervical spine.*

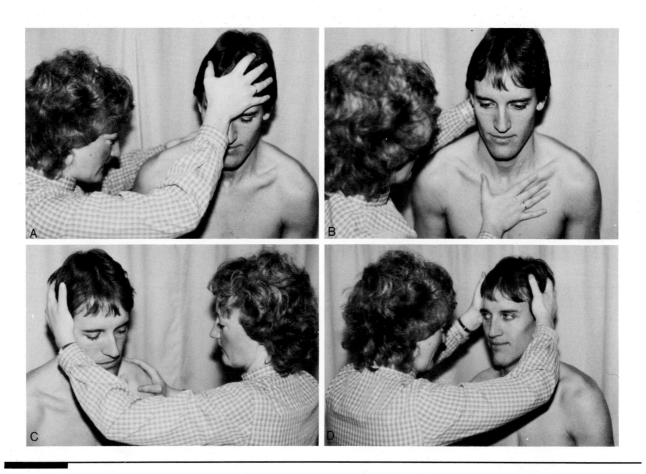

FIGURE 2–6. Positioning for resisted isometric movements. (A) Flexion. (B) Extension. (C) Side flexion. (D) Rotation.

TABLE 2–6. Muscles of the Cervical Spine: Their Actions and Nerve Supply

Action	Muscles Acting	Nerve Supply
Forward flexion of head	1. Rectus capitis anterior	C1–C2
	2. Rectus capitis lateralis	C1–C2
	3. Longus capitis	C1–C3
	4. Hyoid muscles	Inferior alveolar nerve
		Facial nerve
		Hypoglossal nerve
		Ansa cervicalis
	5. Obliquus capitis superior	C1
	6. Sternocleidomastoid (if head in neutral or flexion)	Accessory
		C2
Extension of head	1. Splenius capitis	C4–C6
	2. Semispinalis capitis	C1–C8
	3. Longissimus capitis	C6–C8
	4. Spinalis capitis	C6–C8
	5. Trapezius	Accessory
		C3–C4
	6. Rectus capitis posterior minor	C1
	7. Rectus capitis posterior major	C1
	8. Obliquus capitis superior	C1
	9. Obliquus capitis inferior	C1
	10. Sternocleidomastoid (if head in some extension)	Accessory
		C2
Rotation of head (muscles on one side contract)	1. Trapezius (face moves to opposite side)	Accessory
		C3, C4
	2. Splenius capitis (face moves to the same side)	C4–C6
	3. Longissimus capitis (face moves to same side)	C6–C8
	4. Semispinalis capitis (face moves to same side)	C1–C8
	5. Obliquus capitis inferior (face moves to same side)	C1
	6. Sternocleidomastoid (face moves to opposite side)	Accessory
		C2

TABLE 2–6. Muscles of the Cervical Spine: Their Actions and Nerve Supply *Continued*

Action	Muscles Acting	Nerve Supply
Side flexion of head	1. Trapezius	Accessory C3–C4
	2. Splenius capitis	C4–C6
	3. Longissimus capitis	C6–C8
	4. Semispinalis capitis	C1–C8
	5. Obliquus capitis inferior	C1
	6. Rectus capitis lateralis	C1–C2
	7. Longus capitis	C1–C3
	8. Sternocleidomastoid	Accessory C2
Flexion of neck	1. Longus coli	C2–C6
	2. Scalenus anterior	C4–C6
	3. Scalenus medius	C3–C8
	4. Scalenus posterior	C6–C8
Extension of neck	1. Splenius cervicis	C6–C8
	2. Semispinalis cervicis	C1–C8
	3. Longissimus cervicis	C6–C8
	4. Levator scapulae	C3–C4 Dorsal scapular
	5. Iliocostalis cervicis	C6–C8
	6. Spinalis cervicis	C6–C8
	7. Multifidus	C1–C8
	8. Interspinalis cervicis	C1–C8
	9. Trapezius	Accessory C3–C4
	10. Rectus capitus posterior major	C1
	11. Rotatores brevis	C1–C8
	12. Rotatores longi	C1–C8
Side flexion of neck	1. Levator scapulae	C3–C4 Dorsal scapular
	2. Splenius cervicis	C4–C6
	3. Iliocostalis cervicis	C6–C8
	4. Longissimus cervicis	C6–C8
	5. Semispinalis cervicis	C1–C8
	6. Multifidus	C1–C8
	7. Intertransversarii	C1–C8
	8. Scaleni	C3–C8
	9. Sternocleidomastoid	Accessory C2
	10. Obliquus capitis inferior	C1
	11. Rotatores breves	C1–C8
	12. Rotatores longi	C1–C8
	13. Longus coli	C2–C6
Rotation* of neck (muscles on one side contract)	1. Levator scapulae (face moves to same side)	C3–C4 Dorsal scapular
	2. Splenius cervicis (face moves to same side)	C4–C6
	3. Iliocostalis cervicis (face moves to same side)	C6–C8
	4. Longissimus cervicis (face moves to same side)	C6–C8
	5. Semispinalis cervicis (face moves to same side)	C1–C8
	6. Multifidus (face moves to opposite side)	C1–C8
	7. Intertransversarii (face moves to same side)	C1–C8
	8. Scaleni (face moves to opposite side)	C3–C8
	9. Sternocleidomastoid (face moves to opposite side)	Accessory C2
	10. Obliquus capitis inferior (face moves to same side)	C1
	11. Rotatores brevis (face moves to same side)	C1–C8
	12. Rotatores longi (face moves to same side)	C1–C8

*Occurs in conjunction with side flexion due to direction of facet joints.

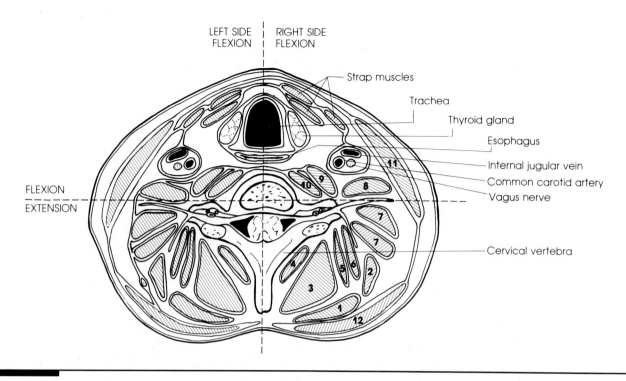

FIGURE 2–7. Anatomic relations of the lower cervical spine. (1) Splenius capitis. (2) Splenius cervicis. (3) Semispinalis cervicis and capitis. (4) Multifidus and rotatores. (5) Longissimus capitis. (6) Longissimus cervicis. (7) Levator scapulae. (8) Scalenus posterior. (9) Scalenus medius. (10) Scalenus anterior. (11) Sternocleidomastoid. (12) Trapezius.

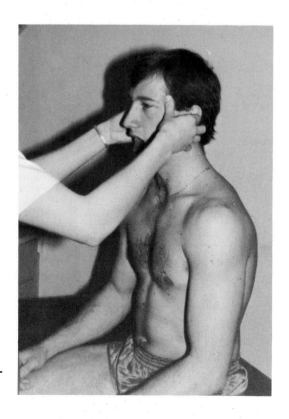

FIGURE 2–8. Testing temporomandibular joints.

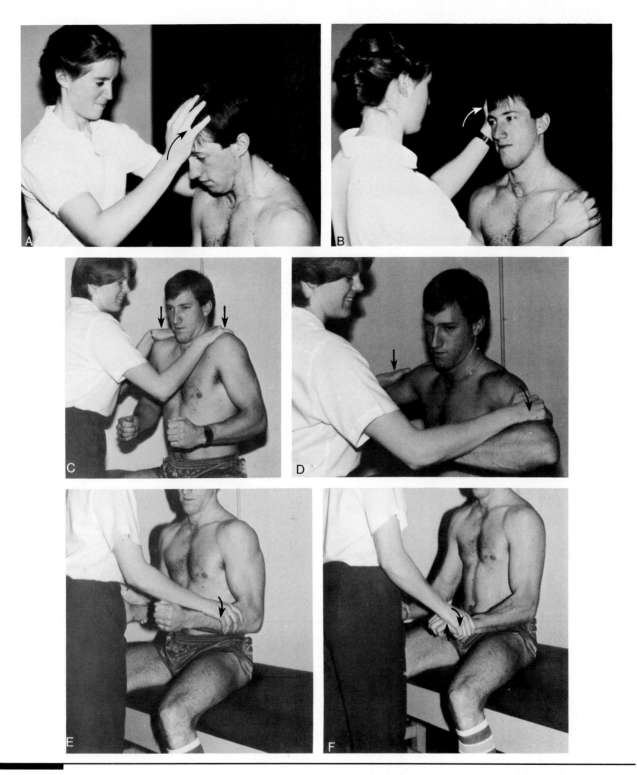

FIGURE 2–9. Positioning to test myotomes. (A) Neck flexion (C1, C2). (B) Neck side flexion (C3). (C) Shoulder elevation (C4). (D) Shoulder abduction (C5). (E) Elbow flexion (C6). (F) Wrist extension (C6).

Illustration continued on following page

of the wrist. Active movement (flexion, extension, abduction, adduction, and opposition) are done for the fingers and thumb. These actions can be accomplished by having the patient make a fist and then spread the fingers and thumb wide. Again, any alteration in sign and symptom or restriction of motion should be noted.

Myotomes

Having completed the scanning examination of the peripheral joints, the examiner should then determine muscle power and possible neurological weakness by testing the myotomes (Fig. 2–9). Myotomes

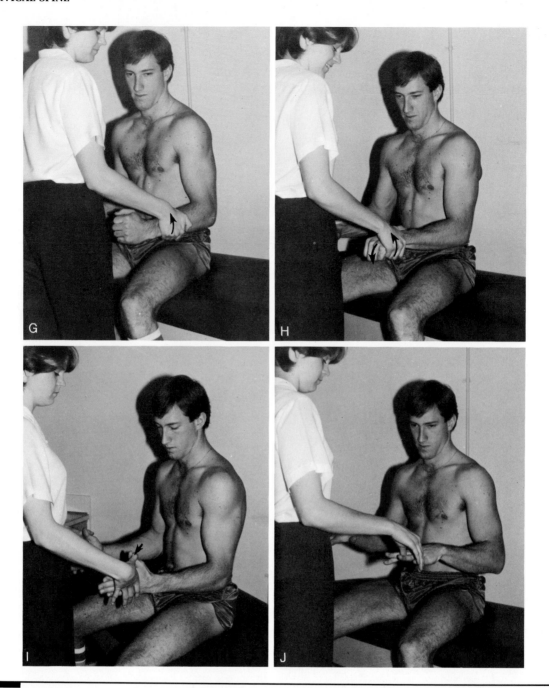

FIGURE 2–9 Continued (G) Elbow extension (C7). (H) Wrist flexion (C7). (I) Thumb extension (C8). (J) Finger abduction (T1).

are tested by the following isometric movements (Table 2–7):

1. Neck flexion, C1–C2.
2. Neck side flexion, C3.
3. Shoulder elevation, C4.
4. Shoulder abduction, C5.
5. Elbow flexion and/or wrist extension, C6.
6. Elbow extension and/or wrist flexion, C7.
7. Thumb extension and/or ulnar deviation, C8.
8. Abduction and/or adduction of hand intrinsics, T1.

With the patient in a sitting position, the examiner puts the test joint(s) in a neutral position and applies resisted isometric pressure. The contraction should be held for at least 5 seconds so that weakness, if any, can be noted. Where applicable, both sides are tested at the same time to provide a comparison. The examiner must not apply pressure over the joints because this action may mask symptoms or the true problem.

To test neck flexion, the patient's head should be slightly flexed. The examiner applies pressure to the

TABLE 2–7. Myotomes of the Upper Limb

Nerve Root	Test Action	Muscles*
C1–C2	Neck flexion	Rectus lateralis, rectus capitis anterior, rectus capitis, longus coli, longus cervicis, sternocleidomastoid
C3	Neck side flexion	Longus capitis, longus cervicis, trapezius, scalenus medius
C4	Shoulder elevation	Diaphragm, trapezius, levator scapulae, scalenus anterior, scalenus medius
C5	Shoulder abduction	Rhomboid major and minor, deltoid, supraspinatus, infraspinatus, teres minor, biceps, scalenus anterior and medius
C6	Elbow flexion and wrist extension	Serratus anterior, latissimus dorsi, subscapularis, teres major, pectoralis major (clavicular head), biceps, coracobrachialis, brachialis, brachioradialis, supinator, extensor carpi radialis longus, scalenus anterior, medius and posterior
C7	Elbow extension and wrist flexion	Serratus anterior, latissimus dorsi, pectoralis major (sternal head), pectoralis minor, triceps, pronator teres, flexor carpi radialis, flexor digitorum superficialis, extensor carpi radialis longus, extensor carpi radialis brevis, extensor digitorum, extensor digiti minimi, scalenus medius and posterior
C8	Thumb extension and ulnar deviation	Pectoralis major (sternal head), pectoralis minor, triceps, flexor digitorum superficialis, flexor digitorum profundus, flexor pollicis longus, pronator quadratus, flexor carpi ulnaris, abductor pollicis longus, extensor pollicis longus, extensor pollicis brevis, extensor indicis, abductor pollicis brevis, flexor pollicis brevis, opponens pollicis, scalenus medius and posterior
T1	Hand intrinsics	Flexor digitorum profundus, intrinsic muscles of the hand (except extensor pollicis brevis), flexor pollicis brevis, opponens pollicis

*Muscles listed may be supplied by additional nerve roots; only primary nerve root sources are listed.

forehead while stabilizing the trunk with a hand between the scapulae (Fig. 2–9A). To test neck side flexion, the examiner places one hand above the patient's ear and applies a side flexion force while stabilizing the trunk with the other hand on the opposite shoulder (Fig. 2–9B). Both right and left side flexion must be tested.

The examiner then asks the patient to elevate the shoulders to about one half of full elevation. The examiner applies a downward force on both of the patient's shoulders while the patient attempts to hold them in position.

For testing of shoulder abduction, the examiner asks the patient to abduct the arms to about 75 to 80° with the elbows flexed to 90° and the forearms pronated or in neutral. The examiner applies a downward force on the humerus while the patient attempts to hold the arms in position.

To test elbow flexion and extension, the examiner asks the patient to put the arms by the patient's side, with the elbows flexed to 90° and forearms in neutral. The examiner applies a downward isometric force to the forearms to test the elbow flexors (C6 myotome) and an upward isometric force to test the elbow extensors (C7 myotome).

For testing of wrist movements (flexion, extension, ulnar deviation) the patient's arms are by the side, elbows at 90°, forearms pronated, and wrists, hands, and fingers in neutral. The examiner applies a downward force to the hands to test wrist extension (C6 myotome), an upward force to test wrist flexion (C7 myotome), and a lateral force (radially deviated) to test ulnar deviation (C8 myotome) while the patient maintains the position.

In the test for thumb extension, the patient extends the thumb but not quite to full range of motion. The examiner applies an isometric force to the thumbs into flexion. For testing of hand intrinsics, the patient squeezes a piece of paper between the fingers while the examiner tries to pull it away; the patient may squeeze the examiner's fingers, or the patient may abduct the fingers slightly with the examiner isometrically adducting them.

Functional Assessment

If the patient has complained of functional difficulties or the examiner suspects some functional impairment, a series of functional tests or movements may be carried out to determine the patient's functional capacity, keeping in mind the patient's age and health. Some possible functional tests include:

Swallowing. This is a complex movement involving muscles of the lips, tongue, jaw, soft palate, pharynx, and larynx and the suprahyoid and infrahyoid muscles.

Looking Up at the Ceiling. At least 40 to 50° of neck extension is necessary. If this range is not available, the patient will bend the back and/or knees to obtain the desired range.

Looking Down at Belt Buckle or Shoe Laces. At least 60 to 70° of neck flexion is necessary. If this range is not available, the patient will flex the back to complete the task.

Shoulder Check. At least 60 to 70° of cervical rotation is necessary. If this range is not available, the patient will rotate the trunk to accomplish this task.

Tuck Chin In. This action produces upper cervical flexion with lower cervical extension.[10]

Poke Chin Out. This action produces upper cervical extension with lower cervical flexion.[10]

Neck Strength. In athletes, neck strength should be approximately 30% of body weight to decrease chance of injury.[11]

Paresthesia. Paresthesia may make cooking and handling utensils particularly difficult and, if severe, dangerous.

Table 2–8 lists functional strength tests that can give the examiner some indication of the patient's functional strength capacity.

Special Tests

There are several special tests that may be performed if the examiner feels they are relevant. Of these tests, some should always be done, and others should be done only if the examiner wants to use the tests as confirming tests. The foraminal compression test, distraction test, brachial plexus tension test, and vertebral artery test should always be done. The others should be done only as confirming tests.

Tests for Neurological Symptoms

Foraminal Compression (Spurling) Test. The patient bends or side flexes the head to one side (Fig. 2–10). The examiner carefully presses straight down on the head. A test result is classified as positive if pain radiates into the arm toward which the head is flexed during compression and indicates pressure on a nerve root. The distribution of the pain and

TABLE 2–8. Functional Strength Testing of the Cervical Spine†

Starting Position	Action	Functional Test*
Supine lying	Lift head keeping chin tucked in (neck flexion)	6 to 8 repetitions: functional 3 to 5 repetitions: functionally fair 1 to 2 repetitions: functionally poor 0 repetitions: nonfunctional
Prone lying	Lift head backward (neck extension)	Hold 20 to 25 seconds: functional Hold 10 to 19 seconds: functionally fair Hold 1 to 9 seconds: functionally poor Hold 0 seconds: nonfunctional
Side lying (pillows under head so head is not side flexed)	Lift head sideways away from pillow (neck side flexion) (must be repeated for other side)	Hold 20 to 25 seconds: functional Hold 10 to 19 seconds: functionally fair Hold 1 to 9 seconds: functionally poor Hold 0 seconds: nonfunctional
Supine lying	Lift head off bed and rotate to one side keeping head off bed or pillow (neck rotation) (must be repeated both ways)	Hold 20 to 25 seconds: functional Hold 10 to 19 seconds: functionally fair Hold 1 to 9 seconds: functionally poor Hold 0 seconds: nonfunctional

*Younger patients should be able to do the most repetitions and for the longest time. With age, time and repetitions decrease.

†Adapted from Palmer, M. L., and M. Epler: Clinical Assessment Procedures in Physical Therapy. Philadelphia, J. B. Lippincott, 1990, p. 181–182.

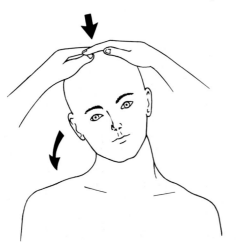

FIGURE 2–10. Foraminal compression test.

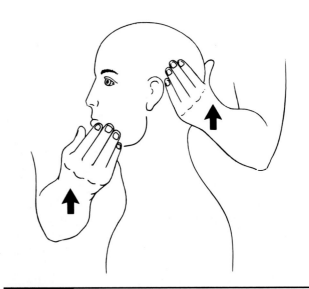

FIGURE 2–11. Distraction test.

altered sensation can give some indication as to which nerve root is involved.

Distraction Test. Placing one hand under the patient's chin and the other hand around the occiput, the examiner slowly lifts the patient's head (Fig. 2–11). The test would be classified as positive if the pain is relieved or decreased when the head is lifted or distracted. It is indicative of pressure on nerve roots that has been relieved. This test may also be used to check the shoulder. By the patient moving the arms while traction is applied, the symptoms are often relieved or lessened in the shoulder. In this case, the test would still be indicative of nerve root pressure in the cervical spine.

Brachial Plexus Tension (Upper Limb Tension) Test. The patient lies supine. The examiner passively abducts the patient's arm just behind the coronal plane to the point just short of pain. The

examiner then passively externally rotates the glenohumeral joint to a position just short of pain while the elbow is kept flexed. This shoulder position is held, and the forearm is supinated. While these positions are maintained, the elbow is passively extended. Reproduction of symptoms implies problems of cervical origin (C5–C7), primarily the C5 nerve root. In addition, if the cervical spine is then flexed, symptoms that include aching in the cubital fossa extending to the forearm (anterior and radial aspects) and into the radial side of the hand and tingling in the thumb and lateral three fingers will increase. Side flexion of the head to the test side will decrease the symptoms 70% of the time, whereas side flexion to the opposite side will increase the symptoms (Fig. 2–12).[9, 12]

Shoulder Depression Test. The examiner side flexes the patient's head while applying a downward

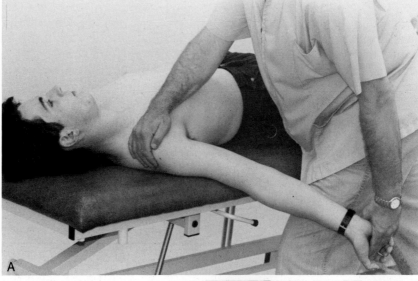

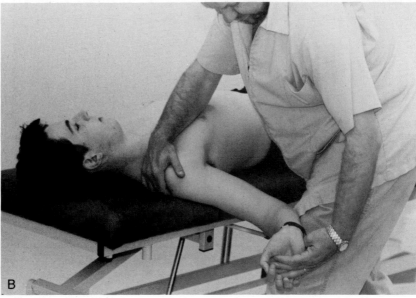

FIGURE 2–12. *Brachial plexus tension test (upper limb tension test). (A) The shoulder is fixed in depression with the glenohumeral joint in abduction and external rotation. The elbow is extended, the forearm supinated, and the wrist extended. (B) The elbow is then flexed.*

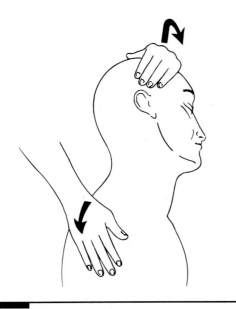

FIGURE 2–13. Shoulder depression test.

pressure on the opposite shoulder (Fig. 2–13). If the pain is increased, it indicates irritation or compression of the nerve roots, foraminal encroachments such as osteophytes in the area, or adhesions around the dural sleeves of the nerve and adjacent joint capsule on the side being stretched.

Lhermitte's Sign. The patient is in the long leg sitting position on the examining table. The examiner passively flexes the patient's head and hips (with legs straight) simultaneously. A positive test is indicated by a sharp pain down the spine and into the upper or lower limbs and is indicative of dural or meningeal irritation in the spine. The test is similar to a combination of the Brudzinski and double straight leg raise tests (described in Chapter 8, "Lumbar Spine"). If the patient actively flexes the head to the chest while in the supine lying position, the test is called the *Soto-Hall test.* If the hips are flexed to 45°, greater traction is placed on the spinal cord.[7]

Jackson's Compression Test. The patient rotates the head to one side. The examiner then carefully presses straight down on the head. The test is repeated with the head rotated to the other side. The test is positive if on testing, pain radiates into the arm, indicating pressure on a nerve root. The pain distribution can give some indication of which nerve root is affected (Fig. 2–14).[7]

Maximum Cervical Compression Test. The patient side flexes the head and then rotates it to the same side. The test is repeated to the other side. A positive test is indicated if pain radiates into the arm.[7] If the head is taken into extension, the intervertebral foramina close maximally and symptoms will be accentuated (Fig. 2–15).

Shoulder Abduction Test. The patient is sitting or lying down, and the examiner passively or the patient actively elevates the arm through abduction so that the hand or forearm rests on top of the head (Fig. 2–16).[13] A decrease in or relief of symptoms indicates a cervical extradural compression problem such as a herniated disc, epidural vein compression,

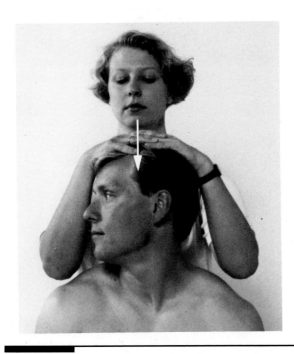

FIGURE 2–14. Jackson's compression test.

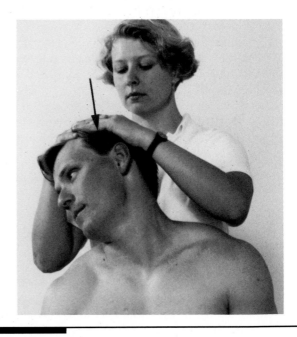

FIGURE 2–15. Maximum cervical compression test.

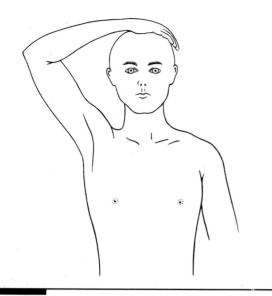

FIGURE 2–16. *Shoulder abduction test.*

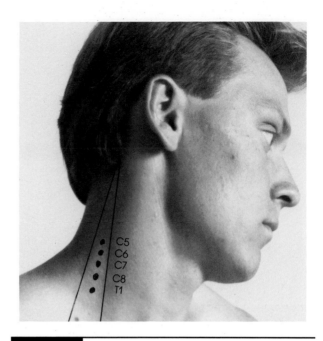

FIGURE 2–17. *Tinel's sign for brachial plexus lesions. Dots indicate percussion points.*

or nerve root compression, usually in the C5–C6 area.

Valsalva Test. The examiner asks the patient to take a deep breath and hold it while bearing down, as if moving the bowels. A positive test is indicated by increased pain, which may be due to increased intrathecal pressure. This increased pressure within the spinal cord is usually due to a space-occupying lesion, such as a herniated disc, a tumor, or osteophytes. Test results may be very subjective. The test should be done with care and caution because the patient may become dizzy and pass out while performing the test or shortly afterward as the procedure can block the blood supply to the brain.

Tinel's Sign for Brachial Plexus Lesions.[14] The patient sits with the neck slightly side flexed. The examiner taps the area of the brachial plexus (Fig. 2–17) with a finger along the nerve trunks in such a way that the different nerve roots are tested. Pure local pain implies there is an underlying cervical plexus lesion. A positive Tinel sign (tingling sensation in the distribution of a nerve) means the lesion is anatomically intact and some recovery is occurring. If pain is elicited in the distribution of a nerve, the sign is positive for a neuroma and indicates a disruption of the continuity of the nerve.

Tests for Vascular Signs

Vertebral Artery (Cervical Quadrant) Test. With the patient supine, the examiner passively takes the patient's head and neck into extension and side flexion.[15] When this movement is achieved, the examiner rotates the patient's neck to the same side and holds it for approximately 30 seconds. A positive test will provoke referring symptoms if the side

to which the head is taken is affected. This is a test for nerve root compression in the lower cervical spine (Fig. 2–18). To test the upper cervical spine, the examiner "pokes" the patient's chin and follows with extension, side flexion, and rotation. This test must be done with care. If dizziness or nystagmus occurs, it is an indication that the vertebral arteries are being compressed.

Static Vertebral Artery Tests. The examiner may test the following passive movements with the patient supine, watching for eye nystagmus and com-

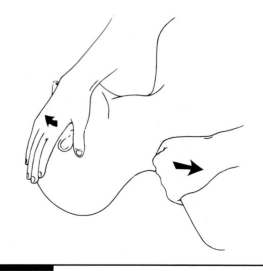

FIGURE 2–18. *Vertebral artery (cervical quadrant) test.*

TABLE 2–9. Aspinall's Progressive Clinical Tests for Vertebral Artery Pathology*

Vertebral Artery Area	Position		Test
	Sitting	*Lying*	
			Mid and Lower Cervical Spine
Area 1 (lower)	X		Active cervical rotation
Area 2 (middle)	X		Active cervical rotation
	X	X	Passive cervical rotation
	X		Active cervical extension
	X	X	Passive cervical extension
	X	X	Passive cervical extension with rotation
	X		Passive segmental extension with rotation
	X	X	Passive cervical flexion
	X	X	Cervical flexion with traction
		X	Accessory oscillatory anterior/posterior movement—transverse processes C2–C7 in combined extension and rotation
		X	Sustained manipulation position
			Upper Cervical Spine
Area 3 (upper)	X		Active cervical rotation
	X	X	Passive cervical rotation
	X		Active cervical extension
	X	X	Passive cervical extension
	X	X	Passive cervical rotation with extension
	X	X	Cervical rotation with extension and traction
	X		Cervical rotation with flexion
		X	Accessory oscillatory anterior/posterior movement—transverse processes C1–C2 in combined rotation and extension
		X	Sustained manipulation position

*From Aspinall, W.: Clinical testing for the craniovertebral hypermobility syndrome. J.O.S.P.T. 12:180–181, 1989.

plaints by the patient of dizziness, lightheadedness, or visual disturbances:

1. Full head and back extension.
2. Full head and neck rotation right and left.
3. Full head and neck rotation in extension, right and left.
4. Simulated mobilization position.

Each position should be held for at least 10 to 30 seconds unless symptoms are evoked. Ten seconds should elapse between each test to ensure that there are no latent symptoms. Extension is more likely to test the patency of the intervertebral foramen, whereas rotation and side flexion are more likely to test the vertebral artery. If symptoms are evoked,

care should be taken concerning any treatment to follow. These tests are often more effective if done with the patient sitting because the blood must flow against gravity and there is a restriction caused by the passive movement. However, the supine position allows greater passive movement.[16] Movements to the right tend to have more effect on the left vertebral artery, and movements to the left tend to have more effect on the right artery.

Aspinall[17] advocated the use of a progressive series of clinical tests to test the vertebral artery. With these tests, the examiner progressively moves from the lower cervical spine and, thus, lower vertebral artery to the upper cervical spine and upper vertebral artery. Table 2–9 demonstrates Aspinall's progressive clinical tests for the vertebral arteries.

Tests for Vertigo and Dizziness

Temperature (Caloric) Test. The examiner alternately applies hot and cold test tubes just behind the patient's ears on each side of the head; each side is done in turn. A positive test is associated with the inducement of vertigo, which indicates inner ear problems.

Dizziness Test. The examiner actively rotates the patient's head as far as possible to the right and then to the left. The patient's shoulders are then actively rotated as far to the right as possible and then to the left as far as possible while keeping the eyes looking straight ahead. If the patient experiences dizziness in both cases, the problem lies in the vertebral arteries. If the patient experiences dizziness only

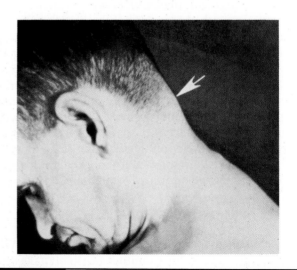

FIGURE 2–19. *Note the bulge in the posterior neck caused by the atlas subluxation forward, bringing the spinous process of the axis into prominence beneath the skin (arrow). (Courtesy of Harold S. Robinson, M.D., Vancouver, British Columbia.)*

when the head is rotated, the problem lies within the semicircular canals of the inner ear.

Tests for Instability

Sharp-Purser Test. This test should be performed with extreme caution. It is a test to determine subluxation of the atlas on the axis (Fig. 2–19). The examiner places one hand over the patient's forehead while the thumb of the other hand is placed over the spinous process of the axis to stabilize it (Fig. 2–20). The patient is asked to slowly flex the head; while this is occurring, the examiner presses backward with the palm. A positive test is indicated if the examiner feels the head slide backward during the movement. The slide backward indicates the subluxation of the atlas has been reduced and may be accompanied by a "clunk." Aspinall[18] advocates the use of an additional test if the Sharp-Purser test is negative. The examiner stabilizes the occiput on the atlas in flexion and holds the occiput in this flexed position. The examiner then applies an anteriorly directed force to the posterior aspect of the atlas (Fig. 2–21). Normally, no movement or symptoms are perceived by the patient. For the test to be positive, the patient should feel a lump in the throat as the atlas moves toward the esophagus; this is indicative of hypermobility at the atlantoaxial articulation.

Tests for Thoracic Outlet Syndrome

See Chapter 4, "Special Tests."

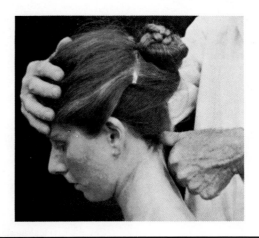

FIGURE 2–20. *The Sharp-Purser Test. The examiner's right hand is cupped over the forehead, and the left thumb is placed firmly over the spinous process of the axis. The head is gently pushed posteriorly. A sense of gliding movement or a sound or clunk is heard as the atlas and skull subluxate forward and backward. (From Bland, J. H.: Disorders of the Cervical Spine. Philadelphia, W. B. Saunders Co., 1987.)*

Reflexes and Cutaneous Distribution

The following reflexes should be checked for differences between the two sides, as in Figure 2–22: biceps (C5–C6), the brachioradialis (C5–C6), the triceps (C7–C8), and the jaw jerk (cranial nerve V). The reflexes are tested with a reflex hammer. The examiner tests the biceps and jaw jerk reflexes by placing the thumb over the patient's biceps tendon or midpoint of the chin and then tapping the thumb-

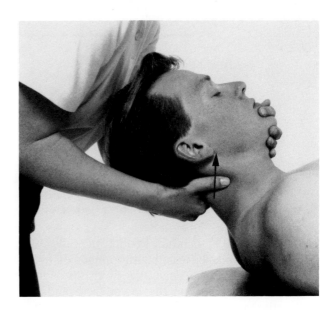

FIGURE 2–21. *Aspinall's transverse ligament test.*

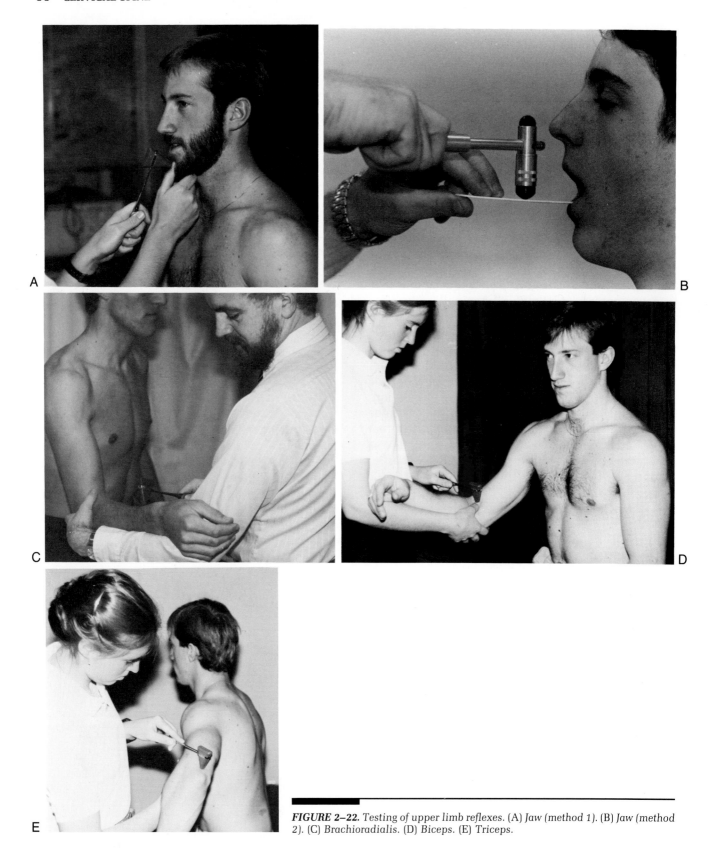

FIGURE 2–22. *Testing of upper limb reflexes. (A) Jaw (method 1). (B) Jaw (method 2). (C) Brachioradialis. (D) Biceps. (E) Triceps.*

nail with the reflex hammer to elicit the reflex. The jaw reflex may also be tested with a tongue depressor (see Fig. 2–22). The examiner holds the tongue depressor firmly against the lower teeth and then strikes the tongue depressor with the reflex hammer.

The brachioradialis and triceps reflexes are tested by directly tapping the tendon or muscle.

The examiner then checks the *dermatome pattern* of the various nerve roots as well as the distribution of the peripheral nerves (Figs. 2–23 and 2–24).

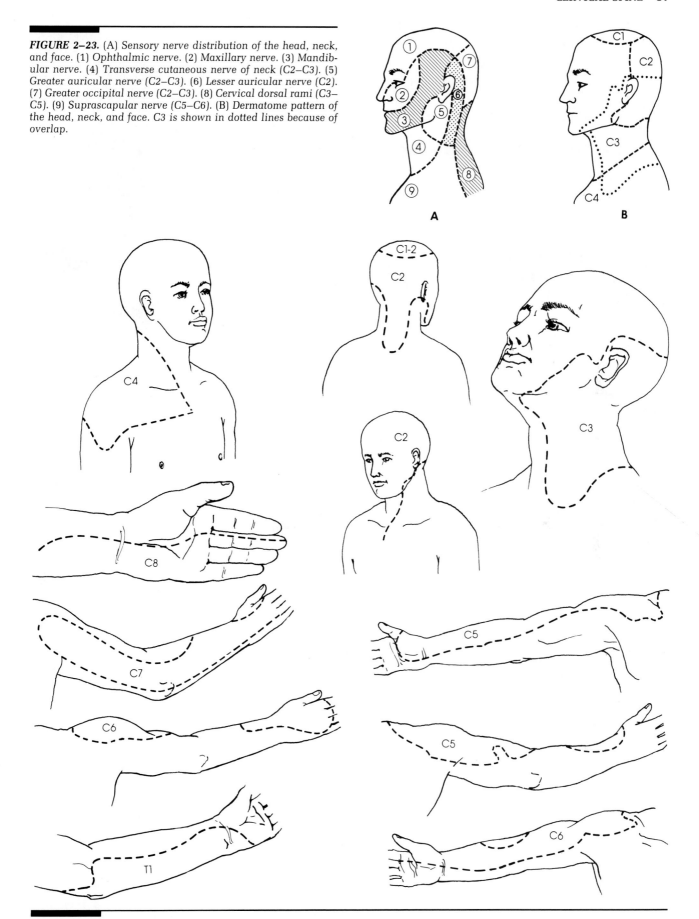

FIGURE 2–23. (A) Sensory nerve distribution of the head, neck, and face. (1) Ophthalmic nerve. (2) Maxillary nerve. (3) Mandibular nerve. (4) Transverse cutaneous nerve of neck (C2–C3). (5) Greater auricular nerve (C2–C3). (6) Lesser auricular nerve (C2). (7) Greater occipital nerve (C2–C3). (8) Cervical dorsal rami (C3–C5). (9) Suprascapular nerve (C5–C6). (B) Dermatome pattern of the head, neck, and face. C3 is shown in dotted lines because of overlap.

FIGURE 2–24. Dermatomes of the cervical spine.

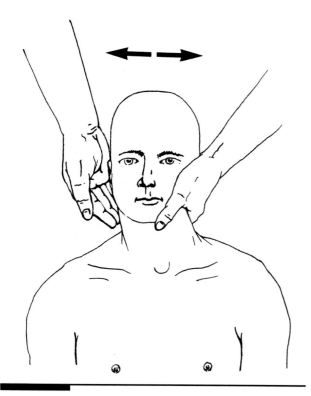

FIGURE 2–25. *Side glide of the cervical spine. Glide to the right is illustrated.*

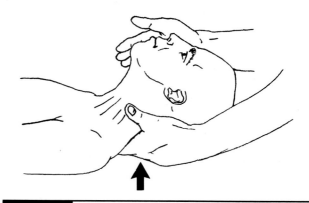

FIGURE 2–26. *Anterior glide of the cervical spine.*

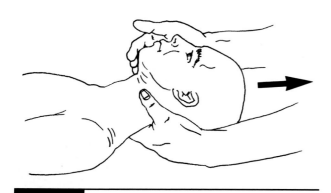

FIGURE 2–27. *Traction glide of the cervical spine.*

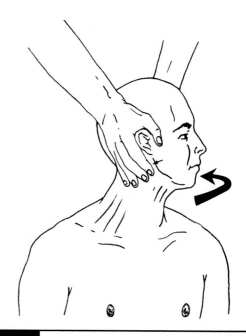

FIGURE 2–28. *Left rotation of the occiput on C1. Note the index finger (small arrow) palpating the right transverse process of C1.*

Dermatomes vary from person to person and overlap a great deal, and the accompanying diagrams are estimations only. For example, in the thoracic spine, one dermatome may be completely absent with no loss of sensation. The examiner tests sensation by running relaxed hands over the patient's head (sides and back); down over the shoulders, upper chest, and back; and down the arms, being sure to cover all aspects of the arm. If any difference is noted between the sides in this "sensation scan," the examiner may then use a pinwheel, pin, cotton batting, and/or brush to map out the exact area of sensory difference.

Joint Play Movements

The joint play movements that are carried out in the cervical spine are, for the most part, general movements involving the entire cervical spine and are not limited to one specific joint. The following joint play movements should be performed, and the examiner should note any decreased range of motion, pain, or difference in end feel:

1. Side glide of the cervical spine (general).
2. Anterior glide of the cervical spine (general).
3. Posterior glide of the cervical spine (general).
4. Traction glide of the cervical spine (general).
5. Rotation of the occiput on C1 (specific).
6. Posteroanterior central vertebral pressure (specific).
7. Posteroanterior unilateral vertebral pressure (specific).
8. Transverse vertebral pressure (specific).

Side Glide. The examiner holds the patient's head and moves it from side to side, keeping it in the same plane as the shoulder (Fig. 2–25).[19]

Anterior and Posterior Glide. The examiner holds the patient's head with one hand around the occiput and one hand around the chin, taking care to ensure the patient is not choked.[10] The examiner then draws the head forward for anterior glide (Fig. 2–26) and posteriorly for posterior glide. When doing these movements, the examiner must prevent flexion and extension of the head.

Traction Glide. The examiner places one hand around the patient's chin and the other hand on the occiput.[11] Traction is then applied in a straight longitudinal direction, with the majority of the pull being through the occiput (Fig. 2–27).

Rotation of the Occiput on C1. The examiner holds the patient's head and in this position palpates the transverse processes of C1 (Fig. 2–28). The examiner must first find the mastoid process on each side and then move the fingers inferiorly and anteriorly until a hard bump is palpated. (These bumps

are the transverse processes of C1.) Palpation in the area of C1 transverse process is generally painful so care must be taken. If the examiner then rotates the head while palpating the transverse processes, the transverse process on the side to which the head is rotated will normally disappear. If this disappearance does not occur, there is restriction of movement between C0 and C1 on that side.

Vertebral Pressures. For the last three joint play movements (Fig. 2–29), the patient lies prone with the forehead resting in the hands.[8] The examiner palpates the spinous processes of the cervical spine, starting at the C2 spinous process and working downward to the T2 spinous process. The positions of the examiner's hands, fingers, and thumbs in performing *posteroanterior central vertebral pressures* are shown in Figure 2–29A. Pressure is then applied through the examiner's thumbs, and the vertebra is pushed forward. The examiner must take care to apply pressure slowly with carefully controlled movements so as to "feel" the movement, which in reality is minimal. This "springing test" may be repeated several times to determine the quality of the movement.

For *posteroanterior unilateral vertebral pressure*, the examiner's fingers move laterally away from the tip of the spinous process so that the thumbs rest on the lamina or transverse process of the cervical or thoracic vertebrae (Fig. 2–29B). Anterior springing pressure is applied as in the central pressure technique. Both sides should be done and compared.

For *transverse vertebral pressure*, the examiner's thumbs are placed along the side of the spinous process of the cervical or thoracic spine (Fig. 2–29C). The examiner then applies a transverse springing pressure to the side of the spinous process, feeling for the quality of movement.

Palpation

If, after completing the scanning examination of the cervical spine, the examiner decides the problem is in another joint, palpation should be delayed until that joint is completely examined. However, during palpation of the cervical spine, the examiner should note any tenderness, muscle spasm, or other signs and symptoms that may indicate the source of the pathology. As with any palpation, the examiner should note the texture of the skin and surrounding bony and soft tissues on the posterior, lateral, and anterior aspects of the neck. Usually, the patient is palpated while supine so that maximum relaxation of the neck muscles is possible. However, the examiner may palpate the patient sitting (patient resting the head on forearms that are resting on something at shoulder height) or lying prone (on a table

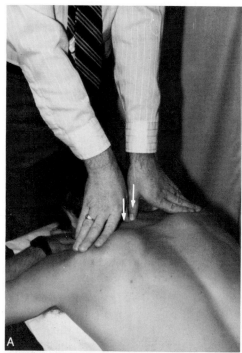

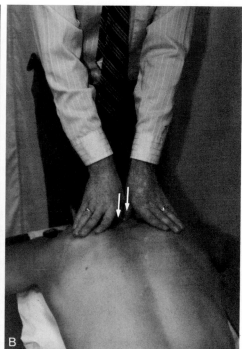

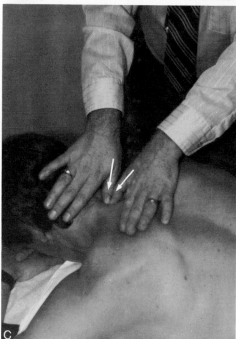

FIGURE 2–29. Vertebral pressures to the cervical spine. (A) Posteroanterior central vertebral pressure. (B) Posteroanterior unilateral vertebral pressure. (C) Transverse vertebral pressure.

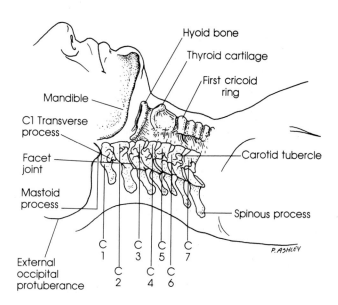

FIGURE 2–30. Palpation landmarks of the cervical spine.

with a face hole) if it is more comfortable for the patient. To palpate the posterior structures, the examiner stands behind the patient, and the patient's head is "cupped" in the examiner's hand while the examiner palpates with the fingers of both hands. For the lateral and anterior structures, the examiner stands at the patient's side. If the examiner suspects that the problem is in the cervical spine, palpation is done on the following structures (Fig. 2–30).

Posterior Aspect

External Occipital Protuberance. The protuberance may be found in posterior midline. The examiner palpates the posterior skull in midline and moves caudally until coming to a point where the fingers "dip" inward. The part of the bone just before the dip is the external occipital protuberance. The inion, or "bump of knowledge," is the most obvious point on the external occipital protuberance and lies in the midline of the occiput.

Spinous Processes and Facet Joints of Cervical Vertebrae. The spinous processes of C2, C6, and C7 are the most obvious. If the examiner palpates the occiput of the skull and descends in the midline, the C2 spinous process will be palpated as the first bump. The next spinous processes that are most obvious are C6 and C7. The examiner can differentiate between C6 and C7 by passively flexing and extending the neck. With this movement, the C6 spinous process will move in and out while the C7 spinous process remains stationary. The movement between the spinous processes of C2–C7 or T1 may be palpated by feeling between each set of spinous processes (e.g., C2 and C3, C3 and C4, and so on). While palpating between the spinous processes, the examiner flexes and extends the knees, causing the cervical spine to flex and extend around the palpating finger. Relative movement between the cervical vertebrae can then be determined (hypomobility versus normal versus hypermobility).[10] The facet joints may be palpated 1.5 to 3 cm lateral to the spinous process. The muscles in the adjacent area may be palpated for tenderness, swelling, and other signs of pathology. Careful palpation should also include the suboccipital structures.

Mastoid Processes (Below and Behind Ear Lobe). If the examiner palpates the skull following the posterior aspect of the ear, there will be a point on the skull where the finger again dips inward. The point just before the dip is the mastoid process.

Lateral Aspect

Transverse Processes of Cervical Vertebrae. The C1 transverse process is the easiest to palpate. The examiner first palpates the mastoid processes and then moves inferiorly and slightly anteriorly until a hard bump is felt. If the examiner applies slight pressure to the bump, the patient should say it feels uncomfortable. These bumps are the transverse processes of C1. The other transverse process may be palpated if the musculature is sufficiently relaxed. Once the C1 transverse process has been located, the examiner moves inferiorly, feeling for similar bumps. Normally, the bumps will not be directly inferior but rather will follow the lordotic path of the cervical vertebrae. These structures will be situated more anteriorly than one may suspect (see Fig. 2–30). If the examiner rotates the head while palpating the transverse processes of C1, the uppermost transverse process will protrude further and the lower one will disappear. During flexion, the space between the mastoid and the transverse processes will increase. On extension, it will decrease. On side flexion, the mastoid and transverse processes approach one another on the side to which the head is side flexed and separate on the other side.[10]

Lymph Nodes and Carotid Arteries. The lymph nodes are palpable only if they are swollen. The nodes lie along the line of the sternocleidomastoid muscle. The carotid pulse may be palpated in the midportion of the neck between the sternocleidomastoid muscle and the trachea. The examiner should determine whether the pulse is normal and equal on both sides.

Temporomandibular Joints, Mandible, and Parotid Glands. The temporomandibular joints may be palpated anterior to the external ear. The examiner may either palpate directly over the joint or place the little or index finger (pulp forward) in the external ear to feel for movement in the joint. The examiner can then move the fingers along the length of the mandible, feeling for any abnormalities. The angle of the mandible is at the level of C2 vertebra. Normally, the parotid gland is not palpable because it lies over the angle of the mandible. If it is swollen, however, it is palpable as a soft, boggy structure.

Anterior Aspect

Hyoid Bone, Thyroid Cartilage, and First Cricoid Ring. The hyoid bone may be palpated as part of the superior part of the trachea above the thyroid cartilage anterior to the C2–C3 vertebrae. The thyroid cartilage lies anterior to the C4–C5 vertebrae. With the neck in a neutral position, the thyroid cartilage can be easily moved. In extension, it is tight and crepitations may be felt. Adjacent to the cartilage is the thyroid gland, which the examiner should palpate. If the gland is abnormal, it will be tender and enlarged. The cricoid ring is the first part of the trachea and lies above the site for an emergency tracheostomy. The ring will move when the

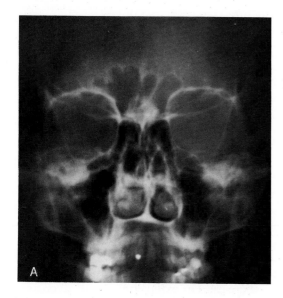

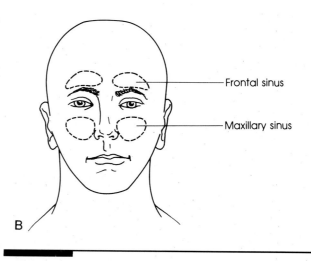

FIGURE 2–31. Paranasal sinuses. Radiograph (A) and illustration (B).

patient swallows. Rough palpation of the ring may cause the patient to gag. While palpating the hyoid bone, the examiner should ask the patient to swallow. Normally, the bone should move and cause no pain. The cricoid ring and thyroid cartilage also move when palpated as the patient swallows.

Paranasal Sinuses. Returning to the face, the examiner should palpate the paranasal sinuses (frontal and maxillary) for signs of tenderness and swelling (Fig. 2–31).

First Three Ribs. The examiner palpates the manubrium sternum and, moving the fingers laterally, follows the path of the first three ribs posteriorly. The examiner should palpate the ribs individually and with care, since it is difficult to palpate the ribs as they pass under the clavicle. The patient should be asked to breathe in and out deeply a few times so that the examiner can compare the movements of the ribs during breathing. Normally, there is equal mobility on both sides. The first rib is more prone to pathology than the second and third ribs and can refer pain to the neck and/or shoulder.

Supraclavicular Fossa. The examiner can palpate the supraclavicular fossa, which is superior to the clavicle. Normally, the fossa is a smooth indentation. The examiner should palpate for swelling after trauma (fractured clavicle?), abnormal soft tissue (swollen glands?), and abnormal bony tissue (cer-

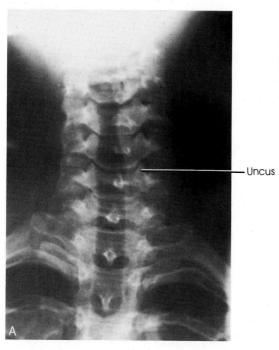

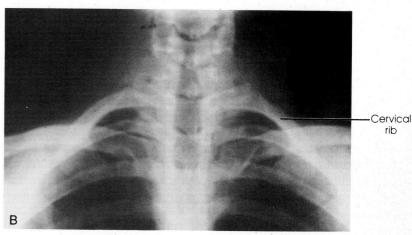

FIGURE 2–32. Anteroposterior films of the cervical spine. (A) Normal spine. (B) Cervical rib.

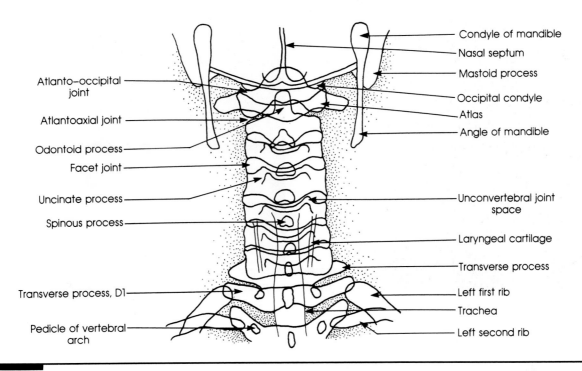

Condyle of mandible
Nasal septum
Mastoid process
Occipital condyle
Atlas
Angle of mandible

Atlanto–occipital joint
Atlantoaxial joint
Odontoid process
Facet joint
Uncinate process
Spinous process

Unconvertebral joint space
Laryngeal cartilage
Transverse process
Left first rib
Trachea
Left second rib

Transverse process, D1
Pedicle of vertebral arch

FIGURE 2–33. *Diagram of anteroposterior cervical spine film.*

vical rib?). In addition, the examiner should palpate the sternocleidomastoid muscle along its length for signs of pathology, especially in cases of torticollis.

Radiographic Examination

Anteroposterior View. The examiner should look for or note (Figs. 2–32 and 2–33):

1. The shape of the vertebra.
2. The presence of any lateral wedging.
3. The presence of a cervical rib.

Lateral View. The examiner should look for or note the following (Figs. 2–34, 2–35, and 2–36):

1. Normal or abnormal curvature. The curvature may be highly variable, since 20 per cent of "normal" spines have a straight or slightly kyphotic curve in neutral. Are the "lines" of the vertebra normal? For example, the line joining the anterior portion of the vertebral bodies (anterior vertebral line) should form a smooth, unbroken arc from C2 to C7 (see Fig. 2–35). Similar lines should be seen for the posterior vertebral bodies (posterior vertebral line) that form the anterior aspect of the spinal canal and the posterior aspect of the spinal canal (posterior canal line).

2. "Kinking" of the cervical spine. Kinking may

be indicative of a subluxation or dislocation in the cervical spine.

3. General shape of the vertebra. Is there any fusion, collapse, or wedging? The examiner should count the vertebrae because x-ray films do not always show C7 or T1.

4. Displacement.

5. Disc space. Is it normal? Narrow?

6. Lipping (see Fig. 2–34A).

7. Osteophytes.

8. Prevertebral soft-tissue width. Measured at the level of the anteroinferior border of the C3 vertebra, this is normally 2.6 to 4.8 mm in width. The retropharyngeal space lying between the anterior border of the vertebral body and the posterior border of the pharyngeal air shadow should be from 2 to 5 mm in width at C3. From C4 to C7, the space is called the retrotrachial space and should be 18 to 22 mm in width (see Fig. 2–35).

9. Subluxation of the facets.

10. Abnormal soft-tissue shadows.

11. Forward shifting of C1 on C2. This finding would indicate instability between C1 and C2. Normally, the joint space between the odontoid process and the anterior arch of the atlas (sometimes called the atlas dens index [ADI]) does not exceed 3 mm in the adult.

12. Instability. Instability is present when more than 3.5 mm of horizontal displacement of one vertebra occurs in relation to the adjacent vertebra.

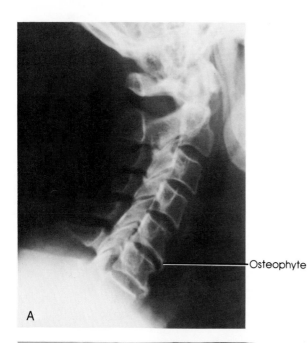

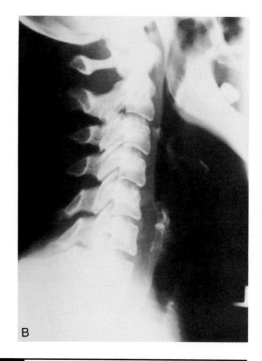

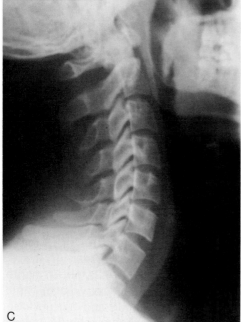

Osteophyte

FIGURE 2–34. Lateral radiograph of the cervical spine. (A) Normal curve showing osteophytic lipping. (B) Cervical spine in flexion. (C) Cervical spine in extension.

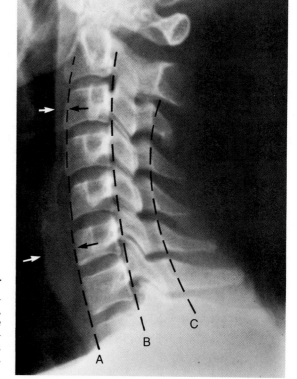

FIGURE 2–35. Normal cervical spine. Lateral projection. Note the alignment and appearance of the facet joints. A, Anterior vertebral line. B, Posterior vertebral line. C, Posterior canal line. Retropharyngeal space (between top arrows) should not exceed 5 mm. Retrotracheal space (between bottom arrows) should not exceed 22 mm. (Modified from Forrester, D. M., and J. C. Brown: The Radiology of Joint Disease. Philadelphia, W. B. Saunders Co., 1987, p. 408.)

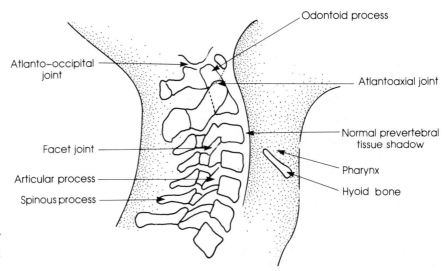

FIGURE 2-36. Diagram of structures seen in lateral film of the cervical spine.

Oblique Films. The examiner should look for or note the following (Figs. 2–37 and 2–38):

1. Lipping of the joints of von Lushka.
2. Overriding of the facet joints.
3. Facet joints and intervertebral foramen (Fig. 2–38). The oblique view is used primarily to evaluate these structures.

"Through-the-Mouth" View. With this view, the examiner is looking at the relation of the odontoid process to the adjacent bones (Fig. 2–39).

Pillar View. This view is used to evaluate the facet joints and their articular processes (Fig. 2–40).

CT Scan. CT helps to delineate the bone and soft-tissue anatomy of the cervical spine in cross section

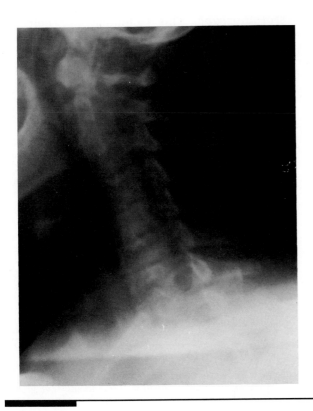

FIGURE 2–37. Abnormal x-ray findings on oblique view. Note loss of normal curve, narrowing at C4, C5, and C6; osteophytes and lipping of C4, C5, and C6; and encroachment on intervertebral foramen at C4–C5, C5–C6, and C6–C7.

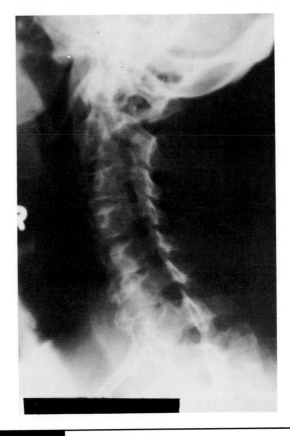

FIGURE 2–38. Oblique radiograph of the cervical spine showing intervertebral foramen and facet joints. Severe lipping in lower cervical spine and spondylosis are also evident.

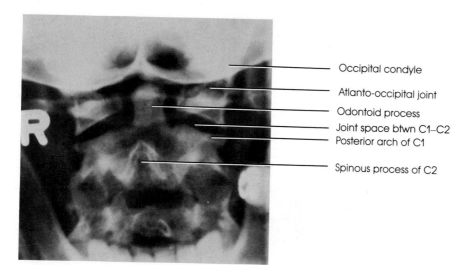

Occipital condyle

Atlanto-occipital joint

Odontoid process

Joint space btwn C1–C2

Posterior arch of C1

Spinous process of C2

FIGURE 2–39. Through-the-mouth radiograph.

showing, for example, a disc prolapse. It also shows the true size and extent of osteophytes better than do plain x-rays (Fig. 2–41). CT scans are used only after conventional radiographs have been taken and a need is shown for them.

MRI. This noninvasive technique can differentiate between various soft tissues and bone (Fig. 2–42).

Because it shows differences based on water content, it can differentiate between the nucleus pulposus and the annulus fibrosus.

Xeroradiograph. This technique also helps to delineate bone and soft tissue by enhancing the interfaces between tissues (Fig. 2–43).

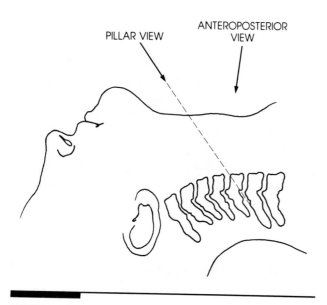

PILLAR VIEW ANTEROPOSTERIOR VIEW

FIGURE 2–40. Diagram of pillar view showing facet joints.

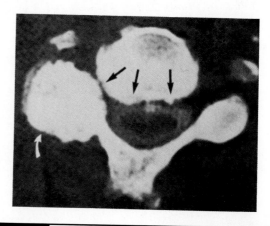

FIGURE 2–41. Foraminal stenosis by hypertrophic facet arthropathy and by spondylosis. Metrizamide-enhanced CT scan through C5–C6 foramina dramatically details the markedly overgrown facet (white arrow) and the bony "bar," or spondylotic spurring (black arrows). The right foramen is nearly occluded by abnormal bone. (From Dorwart, R. H., and D. L. LaMasters: Orthop. Clin. North Am. 16:386, 1985.)

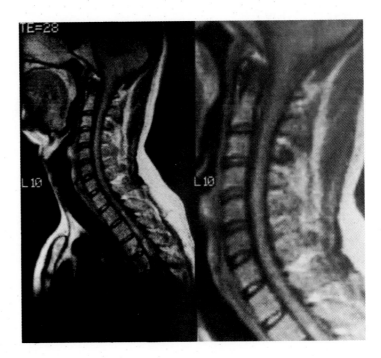

FIGURE 2–42. Magnetic resonance image of the cervical and upper thoracic spine. Sagittal view with close-up of cervical spine. (From Foreman, S. M., and A. C. Croft: Whiplash Injuries—The Cervical Acceleration/Deceleration Syndrome. Baltimore, Williams and Wilkins Co., 1988, p. 126.)

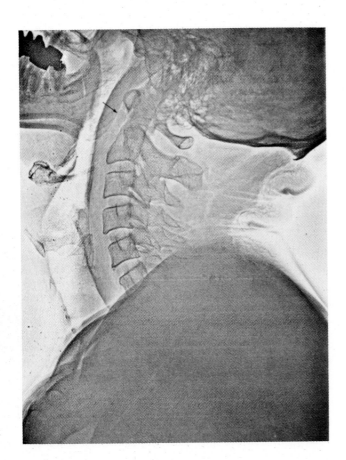

FIGURE 2–43. Xeroradiograph of cervical spine (lateral view). Arrow illustrates calcified mass. (From Forrester, D. M., and J. C. Brown: The Radiology of Joint Disease. Philadelphia, W. B. Saunders Co., 1987, p. 420.)

PRÉCIS OF THE CERVICAL SPINE ASSESSMENT*

History
Observation (standing or sitting)
Examination
  Active movements (sitting)
    Flexion
    Extension
    Side flexion (right and left)
    Rotation (right and left)
  Resisted isometric movements (sitting) (as in active movements)
  Peripheral joint scan (sitting)
    Temporomandibular joint (open and close mouth)
    Shoulder girdle (elevation through abduction, elevation through forward flexion, medial and lateral rotation)
    Elbow (flexion, extension, supination, pronation)
    Wrist (flexion, extension, radial and ulnar deviation)
    Fingers and thumb (flexion, extension, abduction, adduction, circumduction)
  Myotomes (sitting)
    Neck flexion (C1–C2)
    Neck side flexion (C3)
    Shoulder elevation (C4)
    Shoulder abduction (C5)
    Elbow flexion (C6) and/or extension (C7)
    Wrist flexion (C7) and/or extension (C6)
    Thumb extension (C8) and/or ulnar deviation (C8)
    Hand intrinsics (abduction or adduction [T1])
  Special tests (those in sitting)
  Reflexes and cutaneous distribution (sitting)
  Passive movements (supine lying) (as in active movements)
  Special tests (those in supine lying)
  Joint play movements (supine lying)
    Side glide of cervical spine
    Anterior glide of cervical spine
    Posterior glide of cervical spine
    Traction glide of cervical spine
    Rotation of occiput on C1
  Palpation (supine or prone lying)
  Joint play movements (prone lying)
    Posteroanterior central vertebral pressure
    Posteroanterior unilateral vertebral pressure
    Transverse vertebral pressure
  Radiographic examination

After any examination, the patient should always be warned of the possibility of exacerbation of symptoms as a result of the assessment.

---

*The précis is shown in an order that will limit the amount of moving that the patient has to do but ensure that all necessary structures are tested.

CASE STUDIES

When doing these case studies, the examiner should list the appropriate questions to be asked and why they are being asked, what to look for and why, and what things should be tested and why. Depending on the answer of the patient (and the examiner should consider different responses), several possible causes (two of which are given in parentheses) of the patient's problems may become evident. If so, a differential diagnosis chart should be made up. The examiner can then decide how different diagnoses may affect the treatment plan.

1. A 2-month-old baby is brought to you by a concerned parent. The child does not move the head properly, and the sternocleidomastoid muscle on the left side is prominent. Describe your assessment plan before beginning treatment (congenital torticollis versus Klippel-Feil syndrome).

2. A 54-year-old man comes to you complaining of neck stiffness, especially on rising; sometimes he has numbness into his left arm. Describe your assessment plan (cervical spondylosis versus subacromial bursitis).

3. An 18-year-old male football player comes to you complaining of a "dead arm" after a tackle he made 2 days ago. Although he can now move the left arm, it still does not feel right. Describe your assessment plan (brachial plexus lesion versus shoulder sprain).

4. A 23-year-old woman comes to you after a motor vehicle accident. She was "rear-ended" while stopped for a red light. She could tell the accident was going to occur because she could see in the rear-view mirror that the car behind her was not going to be able to stop. The car that hit her was going 50 kph (30 mph), and skid marks were visible for only 5 m from the location of her car. Describe your assessment plan (cervical sprain versus cervical facet syndrome).

5. A woman comes to you complaining of persistent headaches that last for days at a time. She is 35 years old and has recently lost her job. She complains that she sometimes sees flashing lights and cannot stand having anyone around her when the pain is very bad. Describe your assessment plan for this patient (migraine versus tension headache).

6. A 26-year-old man comes to you complaining of pain in his neck. The pain was evident yesterday when he got up and has not decreased significantly since then. He thinks that he may have "slept wrong." There is no previous history of trauma. Describe your assessment plan for this patient (acquired torticollis versus cervical disc lesion).

7. A 75-year-old woman comes to you complaining primarily of neck pain but also of stiffness. She exhibits a dowager's hump. There is no history of trauma. Describe your assessment plan for this patient (osteoporosis versus cervical spondylosis).

8. A 47-year-old man comes to you complaining of elbow and neck pain. There is no recent history of trauma, but he remembers being in a motor vehicle accident 19 years ago. He now works at a desk all day. Describe your assessment for this patient (cervical spondylosis versus tennis elbow).

9. A 16-year-old boy comes to you with a complaint of having hurt his neck. While "fooling" with some friends at the lake, he ran away from them and dove into the water to get away. The top of his head hit the bottom, and he felt a burning pain. The pain decreased as he came out of the water, but he still has a residual ache. Describe your plan for this patient (cervical fracture versus cervical sprain).

10. A 14-year-old girl comes to you complaining of neck pain. She has long hair. She states that when she "whipped" her hair out of her eyes, which she has done many times before, she felt a sudden pain in her neck.

Although the pain intensity has decreased, it is still there, and she cannot fully move her neck. Describe your assessment plan for this patient (cervical sprain versus acquired torticollis).

REFERENCES

CITED REFERENCES

1. Cyriax, J.: Testbook of Orthopaedic Medicine, vol. 1: Diagnosis of Soft Tissue Lesions. London, Bailliere Tindall, 1982.
2. Boreades, A. G., and J. Gershon-Cohen: Luschka joints of the cervical spine. Radiology 66:181, 1956.
3. Hall, M. C.: Luschka's Joint. Springfield, Ill., Charles C Thomas, 1965.
4. Silberstein, C. E.: The evolution of degenerative changes in the cervical spine and an investigation into the "joint of Luschka." Clin. Orthop. Relat. Res. 40:184, 1965.
5. Willis, T. A.: Luschka's joints. Clin. Orthop. Relat. Res. 46:121, 1966.
6. Ferlic, D.: The nerve supply of the cervical intervertebral disc in man. Johns Hopkins Hosp. Bull. 113:347, 1963.
7. Foreman, S. M., and A. C. Croft: Whiplash Injuries—The Cervical Acceleration/Deceleration Syndrome. Baltimore, Williams & Wilkins, 1988.
8. Toole, J., and S. H. Tucker: Influence of head position upon cervical circulation. Arch. Neurol. 2:616, 1960.
9. Elvey, R. L.: The investigation of arm pain. In Grieve, G. P. (ed.): Modern Manual Therapy of the Vertebral Column. Edinburgh, Churchill Livingstone, 1986.
10. Magarey, M. E.: Examination of the cervical spine. In Grieve, G. P. (ed.): Modern Manual Therapy of the Vertebral Column. Edinburgh, Churchill Livingstone, 1986.
11. Schneider, R., H. Gosch, H. Norrell, M. Jerva, L. Combs, and R. Smith: Vascular insufficiency and differential distortion of brain and cord caused by cervicomedullary football injuries. J. Neurosurg. 33:363–375, 1970.
12. Wells, P.: Cervical dysfunction and shoulder problems. Physiother. 68:66–73, 1982.
13. Davidson, R. I., E. J. Dunn, and J. N. Metzmaker: The shoulder abduction test in the diagnosis of radicular pain in cervical extradural compressive monoradiculopathies. Spine 6:441, 1981.
14. Landi, A., and S. Copeland: Value of the Tinel sign in brachial plexus lesions. Ann. Roy. Coll. Surg. Eng. 61:470–471, 1979.
15. Maitland, G. D.: Vertebral Manipulation. London, Butterworths, 1973.
16. Wadsworth, C. T.: Manual Examination and Treatment of the Spine and Extremities. Baltimore, Williams & Wilkins, 1988.
17. Aspinall, W.: Clinical testing for cervical mechanical disorders which produce ischemic vertigo. J.O.S.P.T. 11:176–182, 1989.
18. Aspinall, W.: Clinical testing for the craniovertebral hypermobility syndrome. J.O.S.P.T. 12:47–54, 1990.
19. Mennell, J. M.: Joint Pain. Boston, Little, Brown & Co., 1964.

GENERAL REFERENCES

Bassett, L. W., R. H. Gold, and L. L. Seeger: MRI Atlas of the Musculoskeletal System. London, Martin Dunitz Ltd., 1989.
Bateman, J. E.: The Shoulder and Neck. Philadelphia, W. B. Saunders Co., 1972.
Beggs, I.: Radiological assessment of degenerative diseases of the cervical spine. Semin. Orthoped. 2:63–73, 1987.
Bland, J. H.: Disorders of the Cervical Spine. Philadelphia, W. B. Saunders Co., 1987.
Bonica, J. J.: The Management of Pain. Philadelphia, Lea & Febiger, 1953.
Cailliet, R.: Neck and Arm Pain. Philadelphia, F. A. Davis Co., 1964.

Cervical Spine Research Society: The Cervical Spine. Philadelphia, J. B. Lippincott, 1989.
Crouch, J. E.: Functional Human Anatomy. Philadelphia, Lea & Febiger, 1973.
Darnell, M. W.: A proposed chronology of events for forward head posture. J. Craniomand. Pract. 1:50–54, 1983.
Dorwart, R. H., and D. L. LaMasters: Application of computed tomographic scanning of the cervical spine. Orthop. Clin. North Am. 16:381–393, 1985.
Dvorak, J., and V. Dvorak: Manual Medicine—Diagnostics. New York, Thieme-Stratton Inc., 1984.
Edwards, B. C.: Combined movements in the cervical spine (C2–7): Their value in examination and technique choice. Aust. J. Physiother. 26:165, 1980.
Esposito, C. J., G. A. Crim, and T. K. Binkley: Headaches: A differential diagnosis. J. Craniomand. Pract. 4:318–322, 1986.
Ferlic, D.: The range of motion of the 'normal' cervical spine. Johns Hopkins Hosp. Bull. 110:59, 1962.
Fielding, J. W.: Normal and selected abnormal motion of the cervical spine from the second cervical vertebra to the seventh cervical vertebra based on cineroentgenography. J. Bone Joint Surg. 46A:1799, 1964.
Fielding, J. W., G. V. B. Cochran, J. F. Lawsing, and M. Hohl: Tears of the transverse ligament of the atlas—a clinical and biomechanical study. J. Bone Joint Surg. 56A:1683, 1974.
Foreman, S. M., and A. C. Croft: Whiplash Injuries—The Cervical Acceleration/Deceleration Syndrome. Baltimore, Williams & Wilkins Co., 1988.
Forrester, D. M., and J. C. Brown: The Radiology of Joint Disease. Philadelphia, W. B. Saunders Co., 1987.
Franco, J. L., and A. Herzog: A comparative assessment of neck muscle strength and vertebral stability. J. Orthop. Sp. Phys. Ther. 8:351–356, 1987.
Frykholm, R.: Lower cervical vertebrae and intervertebral discs—surgical anatomy and pathology. Acta Chir. Scand. 101–102:345, 1951–1952.
Gould, G. A.: The Spine. In Gould, G. A. (ed.): Orthopedic and Sports Physical Therapy. St. Louis, C. V. Mosby Co., 1990.
Grieve, G. P.: Mobilisation of the Spine. New York, Churchill Livingstone, 1979.
Grieve, G. P.: Common Vertebral Joint Problems. New York, Churchill Livingstone, 1981.
Herrmann, D. B.: Validity study of head and neck flexion-extension motion comparing measurements of a pendulum goniometer and roentgenograms. J.O.S.P.T. 11:414–418, 1990.
Hohl, M.: Normal motions in the upper portion of the cervical spine. J. Bone Joint Surg. 46A:1777, 1964.
Hohl, M., and H. R. Baker: The atlanto-axial joint—roentgenographic and anatomic study of normal and abnormal motion. J. Bone Joint Surg. 46A:1739, 1964.
Hohl, M.: Soft-tissue injuries of the neck. Clin. Orthop. Relat. Res. 109:42, 1975.
Hollinshead, W. H., and D. B. Jenkins: Functional Anatomy of the Limbs and Back. Philadelphia, W. B. Saunders Co., 1981.
Hoppenfeld, S.: Physical Examination of the Spine and Extremities. New York, Appleton-Century-Crofts, 1976.
Jackson, R.: The Cervical Syndrome. Springfield, Ill., Charles C Thomas, 1976.
Judge, R. D., G. D. Zuidema, and F. T. Fitzgerald: Clinical Diagnosis—A Physiological Approach. Boston, Little, Brown & Co., 1982.
Kapandji, I. A.: The Physiology of Joints, vol. 3: The Trunk and the Vertebral Column. New York, Churchill Livingstone, 1974.
Kaye, J. J., and E. P. Nance: Cervical spine trauma. Orthop. Clin. North Am. 21:449–462, 1990.
Liebgott, B.: The Anatomical Basis of Dentistry. Philadelphia, W. B. Saunders Co., 1982.
Lysell, E.: Motion in the cervical spine. Acta Orthop. Scand. (Suppl.) 123:1–61, 1969.
Macnab, I.: Cervical spondylosis. Clin. Orthop. Relat. Res. 109:69, 1975.
Magarey, M. C.: Examination and assessment in spinal joint dysfunction. In Grieve, G. P. (ed.): Modern Manual Therapy of the Vertebral Column. Edinburgh, Churchill Livingstone, 1986.

Maigne, R.: Orthopaedic Medicine—A New Approach to Vertebral Manipulation. Springfield, Ill., Charles C Thomas, 1972.

Mathews, J. A., and J. Pemberton: Radiologic anatomy of the neck. Physiotherapy 65:77, 1979.

McRae, R.: Clinical Orthopaedic Examination. New York, Churchill Livingstone, 1976.

Palmer, M. L., and M. Epler: Clinical Assessment Procedures in Physical Therapy. Philadelphia, J. B. Lippincott Co., 1990.

Panjabi, M. M.: Cervical spine mechanics as a function of transection of components. J. Biomech. 8:327, 1975.

Patterson, R. H.: Cervical ribs and the scalenus muscle syndrome. Ann. Surg. 111:531, 1940.

Pedersen, H. E., C. F. J. Blunck, and E. Gardner: The anatomy of lumbosacral posterior rami and meningeal branches of spinal nerves (sinu-vertebral nerves). J. Bone Joint Surg. 38A:377, 1956.

Penning, L.: Functional pathology of the cervical spine. New York, Excerpta Medica Foundation, 1968.

Penning, L.: Normal movements of the cervical spine. Am. J. Roentgenol. 130:317–326, 1978.

Post, M.: Physical Examination of the Musculoskeletal System. Chicago, Year Book Medical Publishers, 1987.

Rothman, R. H.: The acute cervical disc. Clin. Orthop. Relat. Res. 109:59, 1975.

Rothman, R. H., and F. A. Simeone: The Spine. Philadelphia, W. B. Saunders Co., 1982.

Southwick, W. O. and K. Keggi: The normal cervical spine. J. Bone Joint Surg. 46A:1767, 1964.

Stratton, S. A., and J. M. Bryon: Dysfunction, evaluation and treatment of the cervical spine and thoracic inlet. In Donatelli, R. and M. J. Wooden (eds.): Orthopedic Physical Therapy. New York, Churchill Livingstone, 1989.

Sunderland, S.: Meningeal-neural relations in the intervertebral foramen. J. Neurosurg. 40:756, 1974.

Tatlow, W. F. T., and H. G. Bammer: Syndrome of vertebral artery compression. Neurology 7:331–340, 1957.

Travell, J. G., and D. G. Simons: Myofacial Pain and Dysfunction—The Trigger Point Manual. Baltimore, Williams & Wilkins, 1983.

Weir, D. C.: Roentgenographic signs of cervical injury. Clin. Orthop. Relat. Res. 109:9, 1975.

Wells, P.: Cervical dysfunction and shoulder problems. Physiotherapy 68:66, 1982.

White, A. A., R. M. Johnson, M. M. Panjabi, and W. O. Southwick: Biomechanical analysis of clinical stability in the cervical spine. Clin. Orthop. Relat. Res. 109:85, 1975.

White, A. A., and M. M. Panjabi: The clinical biomechanics of the occipito-atlantoaxial complex. Orthop. Clin. North Am. 9:867, 1978.

White, A. A., and M. M. Panjabi: Clinical Biomechanics of the Spine. Philadelphia, J. B. Lippincott Co., 1978.

Williams, P., and R. Warwick (eds.): Gray's Anatomy, 36th British ed. Philadelphia, W. B. Saunders Co., 1980.

Wyke, B.: Neurology of the cervical spine joints. Physiotherapy 65:72, 1979.

Temporoman- dibular Joints

The temporomandibular joint is one of the most frequently used joints in the body, but it probably receives the least amount of attention. In any examination of the head and neck, this joint should be included. Without these joints, we would be severely hindered when talking, eating, yawning, kissing, or sucking. Much of the work in this chapter has been developed from the teachings of Rocabado.[1]

APPLIED ANATOMY

The temporomandibular joint is a synovial, condylar, and hinge-type joint with fibrocartilaginous surfaces rather than hyaline cartilage and an articular disc; this disc completely divides each joint into two cavities (Fig. 3–1). There are two joints, one on either side of the jaw. Both joints must be considered together in any examination. Along with the teeth, these joints are considered to be a "trijoint complex."

Gliding or *sliding* movement occurs in the upper cavity of the joint, whereas *rotation* or *hinge* movement occurs in the lower cavity. Rotation occurs from the beginning to the midrange of movement. The upper head of the *lateral pterygoid muscles* draws the disc, or *meniscus*, anteriorly and prepares for condylar rotation during movement. The rotation occurs through the two condylar heads between the articular disc and the condyle. In addition, the disc provides congruent contours and lubrication for the joint. Gliding, which occurs as a second movement, is a translatory movement of the condyle and disc along the slope of the articular eminence. Both the gliding and the rotation are essential for opening and closing of the mouth (Fig. 3–2). The capsule of

the temporomandibular joints is thin and loose. In the resting position, the mouth is slightly opened so that the teeth are not in contact. In the close packed position, the teeth are tightly clenched and the heads of the condyles are in the posterior aspect of the joint. *Centric occlusion* occurs with maximum contact of the teeth, and it is the position assumed by the jaw in swallowing.

The temporomandibular joints will actively displace only anteriorly and slightly laterally. When the mouth is opening, the condyles of the joint rest on the articular eminences, and any sudden movement, such as a yawn, may displace one or both condyles forward.

The temporomandibular joints are innervated by branches of the auriculotemporal and masseteric branches of the mandibular nerve.

The *temporomandibular*, or *lateral*, *ligament* restrains movement of the lower jaw and prevents compression of the tissues behind the condyle. In reality, this collateral ligament is a thickness in the joint capsule.

The *sphenomandibular* and *stylomandibular ligaments* act as restraints to keep the condyle, disc, and temporal bone firmly opposed. The stylomandibular ligament is a specialized band of deep cerebral fascia with thickening of the parotid fascia.

In the human being, there are 20 deciduous, or temporary ("baby"), teeth and 32 permanent teeth (Fig. 3–3). There are no premolars. The temporary teeth are shed between the ages of 6 and 13 years. Missing teeth, abnormal eruption, malocclusion, or dental caries (decay) may lead to problems of the temporomandibular joint. By convention, the teeth are divided into four quadrants—the upper left, the upper right, the lower left, and the lower right quadrant (Fig. 3–4).

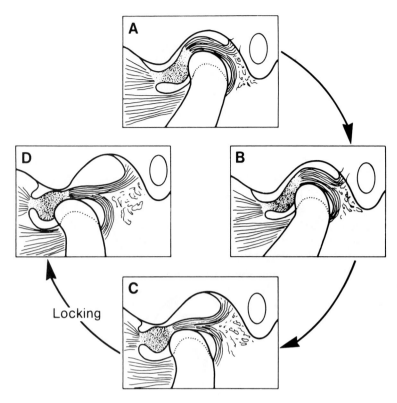

Locking

FIGURE 3–5. *Mechanism of blocking mandibular depression at one point caused by marked anterior displacement of the articular disc. (A) Rest position. (B) As the condyle translates forward, it impinges on the disc but is unable to ride over it. (C and D) This blocks full forward translation and thereby full jaw opening. (After D. D. Blaschke, reproduced with permission, from Solberg, W. K., and G. T. Clark: Temporomandibular Joint Problems: Biologic Diagnosis and Treatment. Chicago, Quintessence Publishing, 1980, p. 77.)*

PATIENT HISTORY

In addition to the questions listed under "Patient History" in Chapter 1, the examiner should ascertain the following information from the patient:

1. Is there pain on opening or closing the mouth? Pain in the fully opened position (e.g., associated with biting an apple, yawning) probably is due to an extra-articular problem, whereas pain associated with biting firm objects is probably due to an intra-articular problem.[2]

2. Is there pain on eating? Does the patient chew on the right? Left? Both sides equally? Loss of molars or worn dentures can lead to loss of vertical dimension, which can make chewing painful. Often, chewing on one side may be the result of malocclusion.[2]

3. What movements of the jaw cause pain?

4. Do any of these actions cause pain or discomfort? Yawning? Chewing? Swallowing? Speaking? Shouting? If so, where?

5. Does the patient breathe through the nose or the mouth? If the patient is a "mouth breather," the tongue does not sit in the proper position against the palate. In the young, if the tongue does not push against the palate, developmental abnormalities may occur because the tongue provides internal pressure to shape the mouth. The buccinator and orbicularis oris muscle complex provides external pressure to counterbalance the internal pressure of the tongue.

Loss of normal neck balance will often result in the individual's becoming a mouth breather and an upper respiratory breather, using the accessory muscles of respiration. Conditions such as adenoids, tonsils, and upper respiratory tract infections may cause the same problems.

6. Does the patient grind the teeth or hold them tightly? *Bruxism* is the forced clenching and grinding of the teeth, especially during sleep. If the front teeth are in contact and the back ones are not, facial and temporomandibular pain may develop as a result of malocclusion.

7. Are any teeth missing? If so, which ones and how many? The presence or absence of teeth and their relation to one another must be noted on a table similar to the one shown in Figure 3–4. Their presence or absence can have an effect on the temporomandibular joints and their muscles. If some teeth are missing, it may lead to deviation of the teeth to fill in the space, thus altering the vertical dimension. The examiner should watch the patient's jaw movement while the patient is talking.

8. Are any teeth painful or sensitive? This finding may be indicative of dental caries or abscess. Tooth pain may lead to incorrect biting when chewing, putting abnormal stresses on the temporomandibular joints.

9. Are there any ear problems such as hearing loss, ringing in the ears, blocking of the ears, earache, or dizziness? Any symptoms such as these may be due to inner ear, cervical spine, or temporomandibular joint problems.

10. Has the mouth or jaw ever locked? If the jaw has locked in the closed position, the locking is probably due to a disc, with the condyle being posterior to the disc. If locking occurs in the open position, it is probably due to subluxation of the joint (Fig. 3–5). Locking is usually preceded by reciprocal clicking (see below).

11. Does the patient smoke a pipe, use a cigarette holder, chew gum, bite the nails, chew hair, purse or chew lips, continually move the mouth, or have any other nervous habits? All these activities place additional stress on the temporomandibular joints.

12. Does the patient ever feel dizzy or faint?

13. Has the patient complained of any clicking? Normally, the condyles of the temporomandibular joint slide out of the concavity and onto the rim of the disc. Clicking may occur when the condyle slides back off the rim into the center (Fig. 3–6). There may be a partial anterior displacement (subluxation) of the disc, which the condyle must override to reach its normal position when the mouth is fully open. This override may also cause a click. If clicking occurs in both directions, it is called reciprocal clicking (Fig. 3–7). The opening click occurs somewhere during the opening or protrusive path, and the closing click occurs near the end of the closing or retrusive path. "Soft" or "popping" clicks that are sometimes heard in normal joints are due to ligament movement, articular surface separation, or sucking of loose tissue behind the condyle as it

moves forward. These clicks are usually due to muscle incoordination. "Hard" or "cracking" clicks are more likely to indicate joint pathology or joint surface defects. Soft crepitus (like rubbing knuckles together) is a sound that sometimes occurs in symptomless joints and is not an indication of pathology. Hard crepitus (like a footstep on gravel) is indicative of arthritic changes in the joints. The clicking may be due to uncoordinated muscle action of the lateral pterygoid muscles, a crack or perforation in the disc, osteoarthrosis, or occlusal imbalance. Normally, the upper head of the lateral pterygoid muscle pulls the disc forward. If the disc does not move first, the condyle will click over the disc as the condyles are pulled forward by the lower head of the lateral pterygoid muscle.

14. Has the patient noticed any voice changes? Changes may be due to muscle spasm.

15. Does the patient have any difficulty swallowing? Does the patient swallow normally or gulp? What happens to the tongue when the patient swallows? Does it move normally, anteriorly, or laterally? The normal resting position of the tongue is against the anterior palate (Fig. 3–8). It is the position in which one would place the tongue to make a "clicking" sound.

16. Does the patient have any habitual head postures? For example, holding the telephone between the ear and the shoulder compacts the temporomandibular joint on that side. Reading or listening to

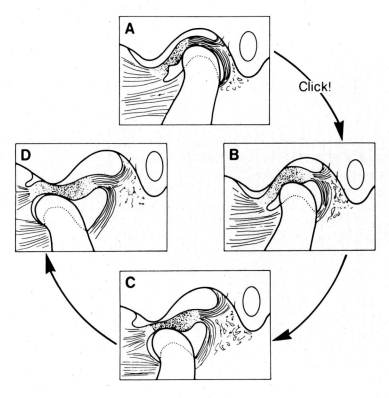

FIGURE 3–6. *Mechanism of early click caused by slight anterior displacement of the articular disc. (A) Rest position. (B) As the condyle begins to translate forward, it must override a thickness of posterior disc material, causing a click. This seats the condyle in the central, thin part of the disc. (C,D) After the click, mandibular opening and translation of the condyle proceed with apparently normal disc mechanics. (From Wilkes, C. H.: Arthrography of the temporomandibular joint. Minnesota Medicine 61:645–652, 1978.)*

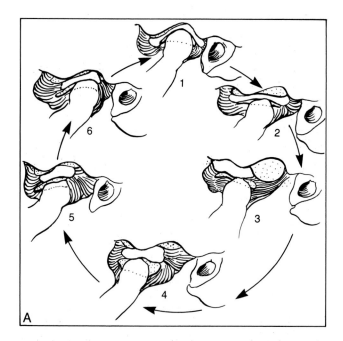
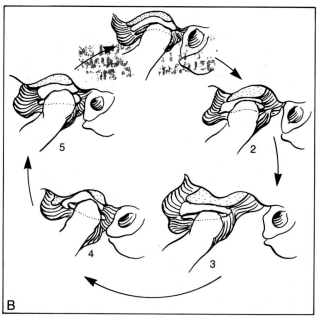

FIGURE 3–7. (A) In reciprocal clicking, the disc is displaced anteriorly in the closed position (1). As the condyle translates forward, the disc remains in front of the condyle until the opening click occurs (2 and 3). Coincident with the opening click, the condyle snaps downward beneath the thick posterior band of the disc, and condylar translation proceeds normally (4). During retrusion, the disc and condyle remain normally positioned until the last instant of retrusion (5). When the closing click occurs, the condyle is suddenly displaced posterosuperiorly, and the disc is displaced anteriorly (6). (B) In locking (a closed lock), the range of condylar translation is limited by the anteriorly dislocated disc. The disc thickens or becomes folded, and reciprocal clicking does not occur. (Redrawn from Farrar, W. B., and W. L. McCarty: The TMJ Dilemma. J. Alabama Dent. Assoc. 63:19–26, 1979.)

someone while leaning one hand against the jaw has the same effect.

17. Has the patient ever been seen by a dentist? A periodontist (a dentist who specializes in the study of tissues around the teeth and diseases of these tissues)? An orthodontist (a dentist who specializes in correction and prevention of irregularities of the teeth)? An endodontist (a dentist who specializes in the treatment of diseases of the tooth pulp, root canal, and periapical areas)? Or an ear, nose, and throat specialist? If the patient has been to one of the above, why did the patient see the specialist and what was done?

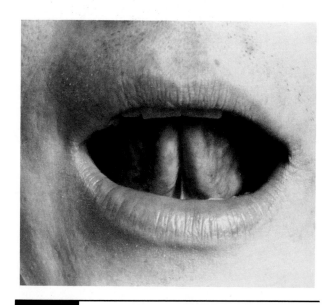

FIGURE 3–8. Resting position of the tongue.

OBSERVATION

When assessing a temporomandibular joint, the examiner must also assess the posture of the cervical spine and head. For example, it is necessary that the head be "balanced" on the cervical spine. The bipupital, otic, and occlusive lines should be parallel to each other (Fig. 3–9). The examiner should then determine whether the face is equally divided vertically between right and left (symmetric). If the head is normally developed vertically, in the adult it may be divided into three equal parts (Fig. 3–10). A quick way to measure the vertebral dimension is to measure from the lateral edge of the eye to the corner of the mouth and from the nose to the chin (Fig. 3–11). Normally, the two measurements are

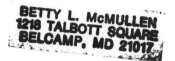

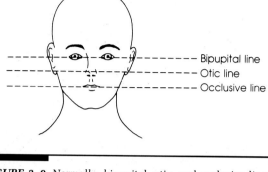

FIGURE 3–9. Normally, bipupital, otic, and occlusive lines are parallel.

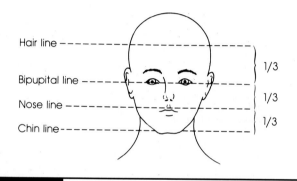

FIGURE 3–10. Divisions of the face (vertical dimension).

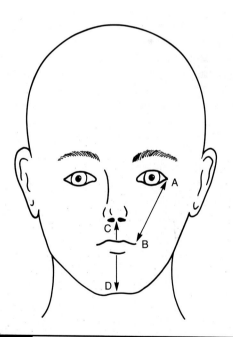

FIGURE 3–11. A quick measurement of vertical dimension showing lateral edge of eye to corner of mouth (A–B) and nose to point of chin (C–D). Normally, the two measurements are equal. (Redrawn from Trott, P. H.: Examination of the temporomandibular Joint. In Grieve, G. (ed.): Modern Manual Therapy of the Vertebral Column. Edinburgh, Churchill Livingstone, 1986.

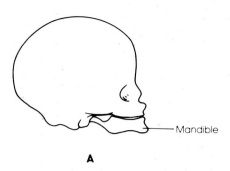

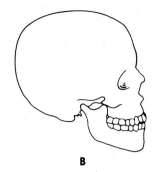

A

B

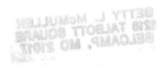

FIGURE 3–12. Human skull at birth (A) and in adult (B). Note the difference brought about by development of the teeth and the lower jaw in the adult.

equal. If the second measurement is smaller than the first measurement by 1 mm or more, there has been a loss of vertical dimension, which may have resulted from loss of teeth, overbite, or crossbite. In children, elderly persons, or those with massive tooth loss, the lower third is not well developed or it has recessed (Fig. 3–12). The examiner should notice whether there is any paralysis, which could be indicated by *ptosis* (drooping of an eyelid) or by drooping of the mouth on one side (Bell's palsy). The examiner should note whether there is any *malocclusion* that may result in a faulty bite. Malocclusion is a major factor in the development of disc problems of the temporomandibular joint.

The examiner should note whether there is any *crossbite* or *overbite* (Fig. 3–13).

In crossbite, the mandibular teeth are unilaterally, bilaterally, or in pairs in buccoversion (i.e., they lie anterior to the maxillary teeth). In overbite, the anterior maxillary teeth extend below the anterior mandibular teeth when the jaw is in centric occlusion. Any orthodontic appliances or false teeth present should also be noted for fit and possible sore spots. Is there any appearance of crossbite in which the mandible moves to the left or right as the patient's mouth is opened and closed?

The examiner should also notice whether there is normal *vertical dimension*. Vertical dimension is the distance between any two arbitrary points on the face, one of these points being above and the other point being below the mouth, usually in midline. Usually, the upper and lower teeth are used to measure vertical dimension. In the child, the lower third of the face is poorly developed because of lack of teeth. As the teeth grow, the lower third develops into its normal proportion.

The examiner should note whether the patient demonstrates normal bony and soft-tissue contours. If the patient bites down, do the masseter muscles bulge as they normally should? Is the patient able to move the tongue properly? Can the patient move the tongue up to and against the palate? Can the tongue be protruded? Is the patient able to "click" the tongue? All of these factors will give the examiner some idea of the mobility of the structures of the mouth and jaw and their neurological mechanisms. In addition, the examiner should be aware of any poor habits, such as biting the nails or chewing the hair, that may affect the temporomandibular joints.

EXAMINATION

The examiner must remember that many problems of the temporomandibular joints may be the result of or related to problems in the cervical spine or teeth.

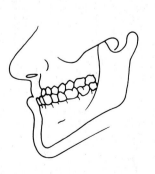

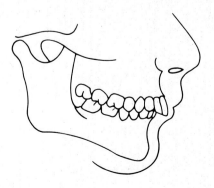

CROSSBITE   OVERBITE

FIGURE 3–13. Examples of crossbite and overbite.

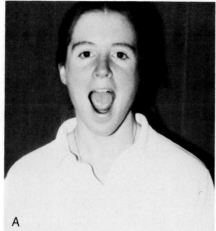 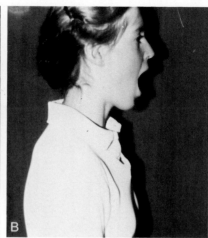

FIGURE 3–14. *Active opening of mouth.* (A) *Anteroposterior view. Note deviation to the left.* (B) *Side view.*

Active Movements

With the patient in the sitting position, the examiner watches the active movements occurring, noting whether they deviate from what would be considered normal range of motion and whether the patient is willing to do the movement.

The patient is first asked to carry out active movements of the neck. The most painful movements, if any, should be done last. These movements include:

1. Flexion.
2. Extension.
3. Side flexion (left and right).
4. Rotation (left and right).

During *flexion* of the neck, the mandible moves up and forward and the posterior structures of the neck become tight. During *extension*, the mandible moves down and back and the anterior structures of the neck become tight. The examiner should note whether the patient can flex and extend the neck while keeping the mouth closed or whether the patient must open the mouth to do these movements. The patient should be asked to place a fist under the chin and then open the mouth. If the mouth opens in this way, movement of the neck into extension is occurring. This test movement would be especially important if the patient subjectively feels that there is a loss of neck extension.

If *side flexion* of the neck occurs to the right, maximum occlusion will occur on the right and vice versa. Side flexion and *rotation* of the neck occur to the same side. Thus, if these movements occur to the right, maximum occlusion will occur to the right.

Having observed the neck movements, the examiner goes on to note the active movements of the temporomandibular joints. These movements include opening and closing of the mouth, protrusion of the mandible, and lateral deviation of the mandible.

Opening and Closing of Mouth

With opening and closing of the mouth, the normal arc of movement of the jaw is smooth and unbroken; that is, both temporomandibular joints are working in unison with no asymmetry or sideways movement. If deviation occurs to the left on opening (Fig. 3–14), the left temporomandibular joint is said to be hypomobile. If, on opening the mouth, the deviation is a "c"-type curve, hypomobility is evident toward the side of the deviation; if, on opening the mouth, the deviation is an "s"-type curve, the problem is probably muscular imbalance. The chin deviates toward the affected side and is usually the result of spasm of the pterygoid or masseter muscles or an obstruction in the joint. Early deviation on opening is usually due to muscle spasm, whereas late deviation on opening is usually due to capsulitis. The mandible should open and close in a straight line (Fig. 3–15). The examiner should then determine whether the patient's mouth can functionally be opened. The functional opening is determined by having the patient try to place two or three flexed proximal interphalangeal joints within the mouth opening (Fig. 3–16). This space should be approximately 35 to 50 mm. If the space is less than this, the temporomandibular joint is said to be hypomobile. As the mouth opens, the examiner should palpate the external auditory meatus with the finger (fleshy part anterior). The patient is then asked to close the mouth. When the examiner first feels the condyle touch the finger, the temporomandibular joints are in the resting position. This resting position of the temporomandibular joints is called the *freeway space*, or *interocclusal space*. Normally, the space between the front teeth at this point is 2

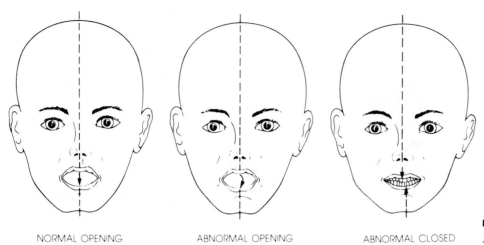

NORMAL OPENING   ABNORMAL OPENING   ABNORMAL CLOSED

FIGURE 3–15. Mandibular motion.

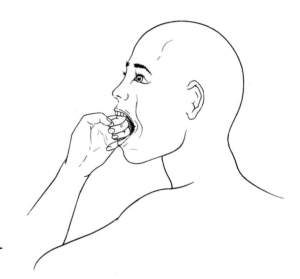

FIGURE 3–16. Functional opening "knuckle" test.

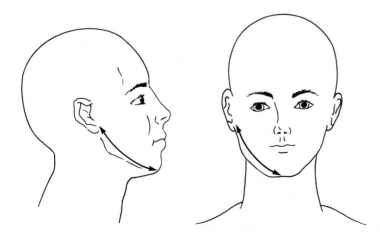

FIGURE 3–17. Measuring the mandible.

to 4 mm. If this space is greater than 4 mm, the temporomandibular joints are said to be hypermobile. Normally, when the mouth opens, the disc moves forward approximately 7 mm, and the condyle moves forward approximately 14 mm.[3]

If rotation does not occur at the temporomandibular joint, the mouth will not open. There may be gliding at the temporomandibular joint, but rotation has not occurred.

Protrusion of the Mandible

The examiner asks the patient to protrude or jut the lower jaw out past the upper teeth. The patient should be able to do this without difficulty. The normal movement is 5 mm.

The patient should then purse the lips in an attempt to whistle. If the patient is unable to do this or to wink or close an eye on one side, the symptoms may be indicative of Bell's palsy (paralysis of the facial nerve).

Retrusion of the Mandible

The examiner asks the patient to retrude or pull the lower jaw in as far as possible. In full retention or centric relation, the temporomandibular joint is in a close packed position. The normal movement is 3 to 4 mm.[2]

Lateral Deviation of the Mandible

Next, the examiner should measure the mandible from the posterior aspect of the temporomandibular joint to the notch of the chin (Fig. 3–17). Both sides are measured and compared for equality (normal is 10 to 12 mm). Any difference indicates a developmental problem or structural change so that the patient might not be able to obtain balancing in the midline. When doing lateral deviation, the opposite condyle moves forward, down, and toward the motion side. The condyle on the motion side (i.e., left condyle on left lateral deviation) remains relatively stationary and becomes more prominent.[2] When charting any changes, the examiner should note opening deviation as well as the functional opening and any lateral deviation (Fig. 3–18).

The movements of the mandible can be measured with a millimeter ruler or the depth gauge of a Vernier caliper. When using the ruler, the examiner should pick a midline point from which to measure opening and lateral deviation. This same ruler can be used to measure protrusion and retrusion. Any lateral deviation from the normal opening position or abnormal protrusion to one side indicates that

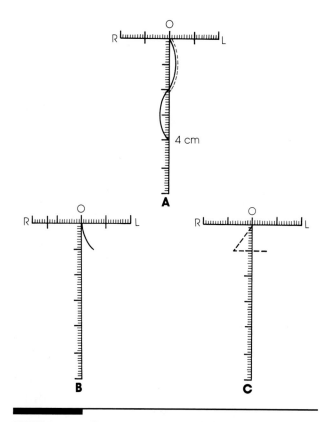

FIGURE 3–18. Charting temporomandibular motion. (A) Deviation R and L on opening; maximum opening, 4 cm; lateral deviation equal (1 cm each direction); protrusion on functional opening (dashed lines). (B) Capsule-ligamentous pattern; opening limited to 1 cm; lateral deviation greater to R than L; deviation to L on opening. (C) Protrusion is 1 cm; lateral deviation to R on protrusion (indicates weak lateral pterygoid on opposite side).

the lateral pterygoid, masseter, or temporalis muscle; the disc; or the lateral ligament on the opposite side is affected.

Passive Movements

Very seldom are passive movements carried out for the temporomandibular joints except when the examiner is attempting to determine the end feel of the joints. The normal end feel of these joints is tissue stretch on opening and teeth contact ("bone to bone") on closing. When the teeth are in maximum contact, the horizontal overjet is sometimes measured. The overjet is the horizontal distance from the edge of the upper central incisors to the lower central incisors (Fig. 3–19). This distance is the amount of the patient's protrusion. If the lower teeth extend over the upper teeth, this malocclusion condition is called a crossbite, and the horizontal distance between the two is the amount of crossbite. Overbite is the vertical overlap of the teeth.

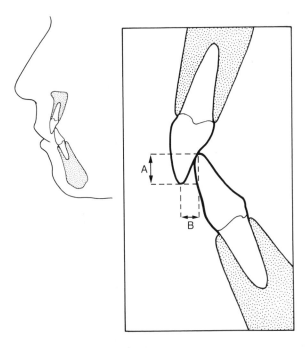

FIGURE 3–19. *Overlap of maxillary anterior teeth. (A) Vertical overlap (overbite). (B) Horizontal overlap (overjet). (From Friedman, M. H., and J. Weisberg: The temporomandibular joint. In Gould, J. A. III (ed.): Orthopedics and Sports Physical Therapy. St. Louis, C. V. Mosby Co., 1990, p 578.)*

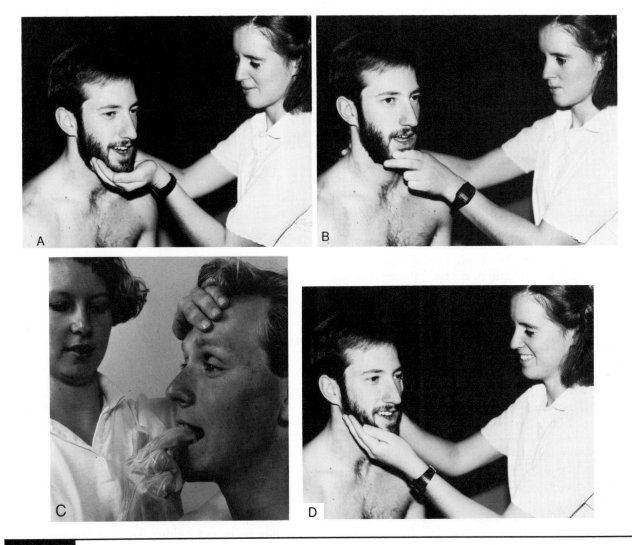

FIGURE 3–20. *Resisted isometric movements for the muscles controlling the temporomandibular joint. (A) Opening of the mouth (depression). (B) Closing of the mouth (elevation or occlusion). (C) Closing of the mouth (method 2). (D) Lateral deviation of the jaw.*

TABLE 3–1. Muscles of the Temporomandibular Joint: Their Action and Nerve Supply

Action	Muscles Acting	Nerve Supply
Opening of mouth (depression of mandible)	1. Lateral (external) pterygoid 2. Mylohyoid* 3. Geniohyoid* 4. Digastric*	Mandibular (CN V) Inferior alveolar (CN V) Hypoglossal (CN XII) Inferior alveolar (CN V) Facial (CN VII)
Closing of mouth (elevation of mandible or occlusion)	1. Masseter 2. Temporalis 3. Medial (internal) pterygoid	Mandibular (CN V) Mandibular (CN V) Mandibular (CN V)
Protrusion of mandible	1. Lateral (external) pterygoid 2. Medial (internal) pterygoid 3. Masseter* 4. Mylohyoid* 5. Geniohyoid* 6. Digastric* 7. Stylohyoid* 8. Temporalis (anterior fibers)*	Mandibular (CN V) Mandibular (CN V) Mandibular (CN V) Inferior alveolar (CN V) Hypoglossal (CN XII) Inferior alveolar (CN V) Facial (CN VII) Facial (CN VII) Mandibular (CN V)
Retraction of mandible	1. Temporalis (posterior fibers) 2. Masseter* 3. Digastric* 4. Stylohyoid* 5. Mylohyoid* 6. Geniohyoid*	Mandibular (CN V) Mandibular (CN V) Inferior alveolar (CN V) Facial (CN VII) Inferior alveolar (CN VII) Inferior alveolar (CN V) Hypoglossal (CN XII)
Lateral deviation of mandible	1. Lateral (external) pterygoid (ipsilateral muscle) 2. Medial (internal) pterygoid (contralateral muscle) 3. Temporalis* 4. Masseter*	Mandibular (CN V) Mandibular (CN V) Mandibular (CN V) Mandibular (CN V)

*Act only when assistance is required. CN = Cranial nerve.

Resisted Isometric Movements

Resisted isometric movements of the temporomandibular joints are relatively difficult to test. The jaw should be in the resting position. The examiner applies firm but gentle resistance to the joints by asking the patient to hold the position; the patient is not to let the examiner move it. The movements tested are shown in Figure 3–20 and Table 3–1:

1. Opening of the mouth (depression). This movement may be tested by applying resistance at the chin or, using a rubber glove, over the teeth with one hand while the other hand rests behind the head or neck or over the forehead to stabilize the head.
2. Closing of the mouth (elevation or occlusion). One hand is placed over the back of the head or neck to stabilize the head while the other hand is placed under the chin of the patient's slightly open mouth to resist the movement.
3. Lateral deviation of the jaw. One hand is placed over the side of the head above the temporomandibular joint to stabilize the head. The other hand is placed along the jaw of the patient's slightly open mouth, and the patient pushes out against it. Both sides are tested individually.

Special Tests

The *Chvostek test* is used to determine whether there is pathology involving the seventh cranial (facial) nerve (Fig. 3–21). The examiner taps the parotid gland overlying the masseter muscle. If the facial muscles twitch, the result is positive.

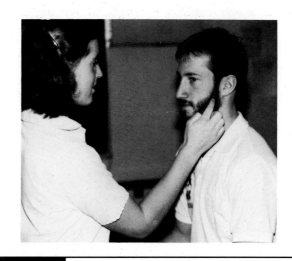

FIGURE 3–21. Chvostek test.

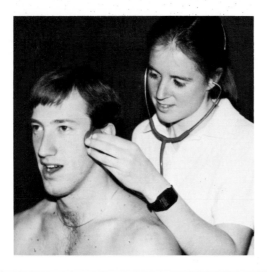

FIGURE 3–22. Auscultation of the temporomandibular joint.

The examiner can listen to (auscultate) the temporomandibular joints during movement (Fig. 3–22). The movements "listened to" include opening and closing of the mouth, lateral deviation of the mandible to the right and left, and mandibular protrusion and occlusion. Normally, only on occlusion would a sound be heard. This is a single, solid sound, not a "slipping" sound. A slipping sound could occur when the teeth are not "hitting" simultaneously. The most common joint noise is reciprocal clicking (see Fig. 3–7), which occurs when the mouth opens and when it closes. It is clinical evidence that the disc is self-reducing. The opening click results when the condyle slips under the posterior aspect of the disc (reduces) or anterior to the disc (subluxes) on opening. The second click, which is quieter, occurs when the condyle slips posterior

to the disc (subluxes) or into its proper position and reduces. A single click may occur when the condyle gets caught behind the disc on opening (see Fig. 3–6) or when the condyle slips behind the disc on closing. On opening, the later the click occurs, the more anterior lies the disc. The later the opening click, the more the disc is displaced anteriorly and the more likely it is to lock. A closing click is usually due to loosening of the structures attaching the disc to the condyle. Clicking is more likely to occur in hypermobile joints.[4, 5]

Grating noise (crepitus) is usually indicative of degenerative joint disease or a hole in the disc. Painful crepitus usually means that the disc has eroded, the condyle bone and temporal bone are rubbing together, and much of the fibrocartilage has been lost. When the examiner is listening, each movement should be done four or five times to ensure a correct diagnosis.

Reflexes and Cutaneous Distribution

The reflex of the temporomandibular joint is called the *jaw reflex* (Fig. 3–23). The examiner's thumb is placed on the chin of the patient with the patient's mouth relaxed and open in the resting position. The examiner then taps the thumbnail with a neurological hammer. The jaw reflex may also be tested by using a tongue depressor (Fig. 3–23). The examiner holds the tongue depressor firmly against the bottom teeth; while the patient relaxes the jaw muscles, the examiner taps the tongue depressor with the reflex hammer. If the reflex occurs, it will close the mouth and is an indication of the test of cranial nerve V.

The examiner must be aware of the dermatomal patterns for the head and neck (Fig. 3–24) as well

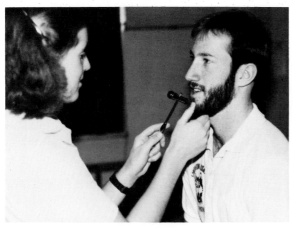

A

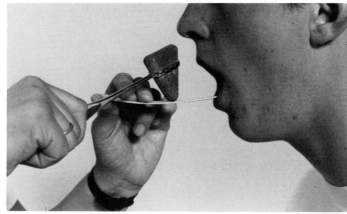

B

FIGURE 3–23. Testing of the jaw reflex. (A) Hitting examiner's thumb. (B) Hitting tongue depressor.

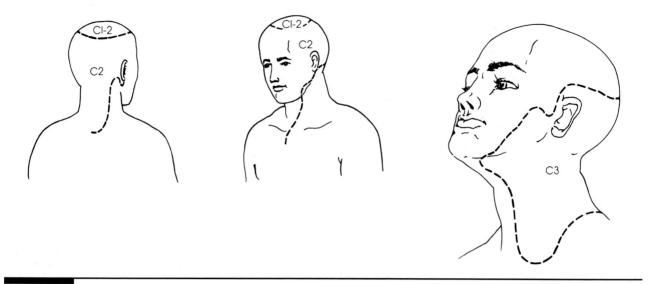

FIGURE 3–24. *Dermatomes of the head.*

as peripheral nerve distribution (Fig. 2–23A). The examiner must remember that pain may be referred to or from the temporomandibular joint from or to the teeth, neck, or head (Fig. 3–25).

Joint Play Movements

The joint play movements of the temporomandibular joints are then determined. Wearing rubber gloves, the examiner places both thumbs on the lower teeth inside the mouth and both index fingers on the mandible outside the mouth. The mandible is then distracted by pushing down with the thumbs and pulling down and forward with the index fingers while the other fingers push against the chin, acting

as a pivot point. When doing this, the examiner should feel the tissue stretch of the joint. Each joint may also be done individually while the other hand and arm stabilize the head. This individual technique is the one more commonly used (Fig. 3–26). Lateral movements may also be accomplished by pushing on the side of first one mandible and then the other.

Palpation

To palpate the temporomandibular joint, the examiner places the finger (padded part anteriorly) in the external auditory canal and asks the patient to actively open and close the mouth. As this is being done, the examiner determines whether both sides

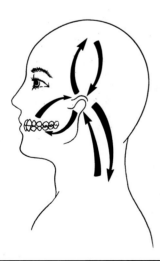

FIGURE 3–25. *Referred pain patterns to and from the temporomandibular joint from and to the teeth, head, or neck.*

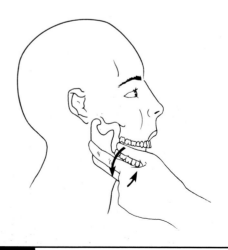

FIGURE 3–26. *Joint play of the temporomandibular joint when the examiner tests temporomandibular joints individually.*

are moving simultaneously and whether the movement is smooth. If the patient feels pain on closing, the posterior capsule is usually involved. The freeway space may be palpated in a similar fashion; the examiner's fingers feel the condyle during closing.

The examiner then places the index fingers over the mandibular condyles and feels for elicited pain or tenderness on opening and closing of the mouth. The examiner may also palpate the pterygoid, the temporalis, and the masseter muscles and any other soft tissues for tenderness or indications of pathology. This procedure is followed by palpation of the following structures:

Mandible. The examiner palpates the mandible along its entire length, feeling for any differences between the left and right sides. As the examiner moves along the superior aspect of the angle of the mandible, the fingers will pass over the parotid gland. Normally, the gland is not palpable, but with pathology (e.g., mumps) the site will feel "boggy" rather than hard and bony, which is normal.

Teeth. The examiner should note the position, absence, or tenderness of the teeth. The examiner wears a rubber glove and palpates inside the mouth. At the same time, the interior cheek region and gums may be palpated for pathology.

Hyoid Bone (Anterior to C2–C3 Vertebrae). While palpating the hyoid bone (Fig. 2–27), the examiner asks the patient to swallow. Normally, the bone should move and cause no pain. The hyoid bone is part of the superior trachea.

Thyroid Cartilage (Anterior to C4–C5 Verte-

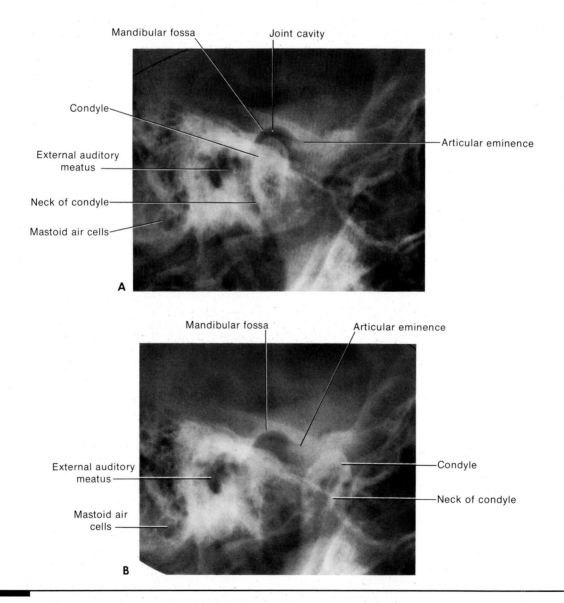

FIGURE 3–27. Radiographs of the right temporomandibular joint. (A) Mouth closed. (B) Mouth open. (From Liebgott, B.: The Anatomical Basis of Dentistry. St. Louis, C. V. Mosby, 1986, p. 295. Courtesy of Dr. Fireman.)

brae). When the neck is in the neutral position, the thyroid cartilage can be easily moved; while in extension, it is tight and the examiner may feel crepitations. The thyroid gland, which is adjacent to the cartilage, may be palpated at the same time. If abnormal or inflamed, it will be tender and enlarged.

Mastoid Processes. The examiner should palpate the skull following the posterior aspect of the ear. The examiner will come to a point on the skull where the finger dips inward (see Fig. 2–27). The point just before the dip is the mastoid process.

Cervical Spine. Beginning on the posterior aspect at the occiput, the examiner should systematically palpate the posterior structures of the neck (spinous processes, facet joints, and muscles of the suboccipital region), working from the head toward the shoulders. On the lateral aspect, the transverse processes of the vertebrae, the lymph nodes (palpable only if swollen), and the muscles should be palpated. Anteriorly, the sternocleidomastoid muscles should be palpated for tenderness. A more detailed description of the palpation of these structures is given in Chapter 2.

Neck side flexion (left and right)
Neck rotation (left and right)
Extend neck by opening mouth
Assess functional opening
Assess freeway space
Open mouth
Close mouth
Measure mandibular length
Measure protrusion of mandible
Measure retrusion of the mandible
Measure lateral deviation of mandible (left and right)
Passive movements (as in active movements, if necessary)
Resisted isometric movements
  Open mouth
  Close mouth
  Lateral deviation of jaw
Special tests
Reflexes and cutaneous distribution
Joint play movements
Palpation
Radiographic examination

After any examination, the patient should always be warned of the possibility of exacerbation of symptoms resulting from the assessment.

---

*Usually the entire assessment is done with the patient sitting.

Radiographic Examination

Anteroposterior View. The examiner should look for condylar shape and normal contours.

Lateral View. The examiner should look for a condylar shape and contours, position of condylar heads in the opened and closed positions (see Fig. 3–27), amount of condylar movement (closed versus open), and relation of temporomandibular joint to other bony structures of the skull and cervical spine (Fig. 3–28).

MRI. This technique is used to differentiate the soft tissue of the joint, mainly the disc, and the bony structures. It has the advantage of using nonionizing radiation (Fig. 3–29).

PRÉCIS OF THE TEMPOROMANDIBULAR JOINT ASSESSMENT*

History
Observation
Examination
  Active movements
    Neck flexion
    Neck extension

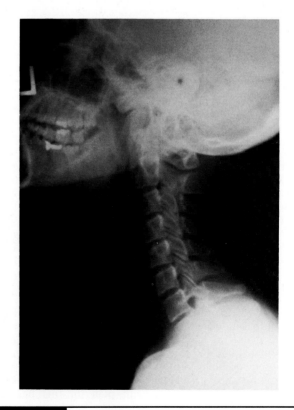

FIGURE 3–28. *Lateral radiograph of the skull, left temporomandibular joint, and cervical spine.*

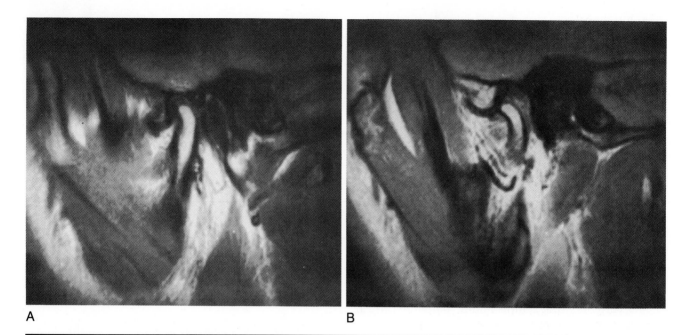

A   B

FIGURE 3–29. *Anterior disc displacement with reduction. (A) The T1-weighted image (SE 250/25) demonstrates anterior displacement of the articular disc in the closed-mouth position. The posterior band lies at approximately 9 o'clock with respect to the condyle. (B) The T1-weighted image (SE 250/25) shows reduction of the disc in the open-mouth position. (Adapted from Bassett, L. W., et al.: MRI Atlas of the Musculoskeletal System. London, Martin Dunitz Ltd., 1989, p. 67.)*

CASE STUDIES

When doing these case studies, the examiner should list the appropriate questions to be asked and why they are being asked, what to look for and why, and what things should be tested and why. Depending on the answers of the patient (and the examiner should consider different responses), several possible causes of the patient's problem may become evident (examples given in parentheses). If so, a differential diagnosis chart should be made up. The examiner can then decide how different diagnoses may affect the treatment plan.

1. A 49-year-old woman comes to you complaining of neck and left temporomandibular joint pain. The pain is worse when she eats, especially if she chews on the left. Describe your assessment plan for this patient (cervical spondylosis versus temporomandibular dysfunction).

2. A 33-year-old woman comes to you complaining of pain and clicking when opening her mouth, especially when the mouth is open wide. She states that there is a small click on closing but minimal pain. Describe your assessment plan for this patient (temporomandibular joint arthritis versus temporomandibular joint disc).

3. An 18-year-old male hockey player comes to you stating that he was hit in the jaw while playing. He is in severe pain and has difficulty speaking. Describe your assessment plan for this patient (cervical sprain versus temporomandibular joint dysfunction).

4. A 35-year-old man comes to you with his jaw locked open. Describe your assessment plan for this patient (temporomandibular disc dysfunction versus temporomandibular arthritis).

5. A 42-year-old woman comes to you complaining of jaw pain and headaches. She slipped on some wet stairs 3 days ago and fell, hitting her chin on the stairs. Describe your assessment plan for this patient (temporomandibular joint dysfunction versus head injury).

6. A 27-year-old nervous woman with long hair comes to you complaining of jaw pain. She has recently had a new dental plate installed. Describe your assessment plan for this patient (cervical sprain versus temporomandibular joint dysfunction).

REFERENCES

CITED REFERENCES

1. Rocabado, M.: Course notes, Course on temporomandibular joints. Edmonton, Canada, 1979.
2. Trott, P. H.: Examination of the temporomandibular joint. In Grieve, G. (ed.): Modern Manual Therapy of the Vertebral Column. Edinburgh, Churchill Livingstone, 1986.
3. Friedman, M. H., and J. Weisberg: The temporomandibular joint. In Gould, J. A. (ed.): Orthopedic and Sports Physical Therapy. St. Louis, C. V. Mosby Co., 1990.
4. Friedman, M. H., and J. Weisberg: Application of orthopedic principles in evaluation of the temporomandibular joint. Phys. Ther. 62:597–603, 1982.
5. Rocabado, M.: Arthrokinematics of the temporomandibular joint. Dent. Clin. North Am. 27:573–594, 1983.

GENERAL REFERENCES

Anthony, C. P., and N. J. Kotthoff: Textbook of Anatomy and Physiology. St. Louis, C. V. Mosby Co., 1971.

Bassett, L. W., R. H. Gold, and L. L. Seeger: MRI Atlas of the Musculoskeletal System. London, Martin Dunitz Ltd., 1989.

Busch, R. M., J. H. Butler, and D. M. Abbott: The relationship of TMJ clicking to palpable facial pain. J. Craniomand. Pract. 1:44–48, 1983.

Clarke, G. T.: Examining temporomandibular disorder patients for cranio-cervical dysfunction. J. Craniomand. Pract. 2:56–63, 1984.

Crouch, J. E.: Functional Human Anatomy. Philadelphia, Lea & Febiger, 1973.

Dawson, P. E.: Evaluation, Diagnosis, and Treatment of Occlusal Problems. St. Louis, C. V. Mosby Co., 1984.

Eversaul, G. A.: Dental Kinesiology. Las Vegas, G. A. Eversaul, 1977.

Fain, W. D., and J. M. McKinney: The TMJ examination form. J. Craniomand. Pract. 3:139, 1985.

Farrar, W. B., and W. L. McCarty: Inferior joint space arthrography and characteristics of condylar paths in internal derangements of the TMJ. J. Prosth. Dent. 41:548–555, 1979.

Farrar, W. B., and W. L. McCarty: The TMJ dilemma. J. Alabama Dent. Assoc. 63:19–26, 1979.

Friedman, M. H., and J. Weisberg: Joint play movements of the temporomandibular joint: Clinical considerations. Arch. Phys. Med. Rehabil. 65:413–417, 1984.

Gelb, H.: Clinical Management of Head, Neck and TMJ Pain and Dysfunction. Philadelphia, W. B. Saunders Co., 1977.

Gelb, H.: An orthopaedic approach to occlusal imbalance and temporomandibular joint dysfunction. Dent. Clin. North Am. 23:181, 1979.

Gelb, H., and J. Tarte: A two-year clinical dental evaluation of 200 cases of chronic headache: The craniocervical-mandibular syndrome. J. Am. Dent. Assoc. 91:1230, 1975.

Helland, M. M.: Anatomy and function of the temporomandibular joint. J. Orthop. Sports Physical Ther. 1:145–152, 1980.

Helland, M. M.: Anatomy and function of the temporomandibular joint. In Grieve, G. (ed.): Modern Manual Therapy of the Vertebral Column. Edinburgh, Churchill Livingstone, 1986.

Hollinshead, W. H., and D. B. Jenkins: Functional Anatomy of the Limbs and Back. Philadelphia, W. B. Saunders Co., 1981.

Hoppenfeld, S.: Physical Examination of the Spine and Extremities. New York, Appleton-Century-Crofts, 1976.

Isberg-Holm, A. M., and P. L. Westesson: Movement of disc and condyle in temporomandibular joints with clicking. Acta. Odont. Scand. 40:151–164, 1982.

Isberg-Holm, A. M., and P. L. Westesson: Movement of disc and condyle in temporomandibular joints with and without clicking. Acta. Odont. Scand. 40:165–177, 1982.

Liebgott, B.: The Anatomical Basis of Dentistry. Philadelphia, W. B. Saunders Co., 1982.

Maitland, G. D.: The Peripheral Joints: Examination and Recording Guide. Adelaide, Australia, Virgo Press, 1973.

Palmer, M. L., and M. Epler: Clinical Assessment Procedures in Physical Therapy. Philadelphia, J. B. Lippincott Co., 1990.

Silver, C. M., S. D. Simon, and A. A. Savastano: Meniscus injuries of the temporomandibular joint. J. Bone Joint Surg. 38A:541, 1956.

Stein, J. L.: The temporomandibular joint. In Little, H. (ed.): Rheumatological Physical Examination. Orlando, Grune & Stratton, 1986.

Talley, R. L., G. J. Murphy, S. D. Smith, M. A. Baylin, and J. L. Hadon: Standards for the history, examination, diagnosis and treatment of temporomandibular disorders—A position paper. J. Craniomand. Pract. 8:60–77, 1990.

Thilander, B.: Innervation of the temporomandibular joint capsule in man. Transactions of the Royal Schools of Dentistry No. 7, 1961.

Travell, J.: Temporomandibular joint pain referred muscles of the head & neck. J. Prosthet. Dent. 10:745, 1960.

Travell, J. G., and D. G. Simons: Myofacial Pain and Dysfunction: The Trigger Point Manual. Baltimore, Williams & Wilkins, 1983.

Trott, P. H.: Examination of the temporomandibular joint. In Grieve, G. (ed.): Modern Manual Therapy of the Vertebral Column. Edinburgh, Churchill Livingstone, 1986.

Watt, D. M.: Temporomandibular joint sounds. J. Dent. 8:119–127, 1980.

Weinberg, L. A.: Temporomandibular joint injuries. In Foreman S. M., and A. C. Croft (eds.): Whiplash Injuries. Baltimore, Williams & Wilkins, 1988.

Williams, P., and R. Warwick (eds.): Gray's Anatomy, 36th British ed. Philadelphia, W. B. Saunders Co., 1980.

CHAPTER 4 Shoulder

The prerequisite to any treatment of a patient with pain in the shoulder region is a precise and comprehensive picture of the signs and symptoms as they present at the examination and how they behaved until that time. This knowledge ensures that the techniques used will be suited to the condition and that the degree of success will be estimated against this understood background. Shoulder pain can be due to intrinsic disease of the shoulder joints or pathology in the periarticular structures, or it may originate from the spine, chest, or visceral structures. The shoulder complex is difficult to assess because of its many structures (most of which are located in a small area), its many movements, and the many lesions that can occur either inside or outside the joints. Influences such as referred pain plus the possibility of more than one lesion at one time, as well as the difficulty in deciding what weight to give to each response, make the examination even more difficult to understand. Assessment of the shoulder region often necessitates an evaluation of the cervical spine to rule out referred symptoms, and the examiner must always be prepared to include the cervical spine in any shoulder assessment.

APPLIED ANATOMY

The *glenohumeral joint* is a multiaxial ball-and-socket synovial joint that depends on muscles rather than bones or ligaments for its support and integrity. The *labrum,* which is a ring of fibrocartilage, surrounds and slightly deepens the glenoid cavity of the scapula. Only part of the humeral head is in contact with the glenoid at any one time. This joint has three axes and three degrees of freedom. The resting position of the glenohumeral joint is 55° of abduction and 30° of horizontal adduction. The close packed position of the joint is full abduction and external rotation. When relaxed, the humerus sits in the upper part of the glenoid cavity; with contraction

of the rotator cuff muscles, it is pulled down into the lower, wider part of the glenoid cavity. If this "dropping down" does not occur, full abduction is impossible. The rotator cuff muscles play an integral role in shoulder movement. Their positioning on the humerus may be visualized by "cupping" the shoulder with the thumb anteriorly as shown in Figure 4–1. The biceps tendon runs between the thumb and index finger just anterior to the index finger. The capsular pattern of the glenohumeral joint is lateral rotation most limited, followed by abduction and medial rotation. Branches of the posterior cord and the suprascapular, axillary, and lateral pectoral nerves innervate the joint.

The *acromioclavicular joint* is a plane synovial joint that augments the range of motion in the humerus. The bones making up this joint are the acromion process of the scapula and the lateral end of the clavicle. The joint has three degrees of freedom. The capsule, which is fibrous, surrounds the joint. An articular disc may be found within the joint. Rarely does it separate the acromion and clavicular articular surfaces. This joint depends on ligaments (primarily the acromioclavicular and coracoclavicular) for its strength. In the resting position of the joint, the arm rests by the side in the normal standing position. In the close packed position of the acromioclavicular joint, the arm is abducted to 90°. The indication of a capsular pattern in the joint is pain at the extreme range of motion. This joint is innervated by branches of the suprascapular and lateral pectoral nerve.

The *sternoclavicular joint,* along with the acromioclavicular joint, enables the humerus to move through a full 180° of abduction. It is a saddle-shaped synovial joint with three degrees of freedom and is made up of the medial end of the clavicle, the manubrium sternum, and the cartilage of the first rib. There is a substantial disc between the two bony joint surfaces, and the capsule is thicker anteriorly than posteriorly. The disc separates the articular surfaces of the clavicle and sternum and

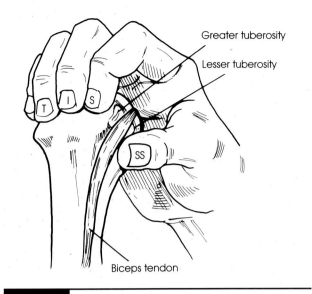

Greater tuberosity

Lesser tuberosity

Biceps tendon

FIGURE 4–1. *Positioning of the rotator cuff with thumb over subscapularis, index finger over supraspinatus, middle finger over infraspinatus, and ring finger over teres minor. (Redrawn from Anderson, J. E.: Grant's Atlas of Anatomy. Baltimore, Williams & Wilkins, 1983, p. 6.48B.)*

adds significant strength to the joint because of attachments, thus preventing medial displacement of the clavicle. Like the acromioclavicular joint, it depends on ligaments for its strength. The movements possible at this joint and the acromioclavicular joint are elevation, depression, protrusion, retraction, and rotation. The close packed position of the sternoclavicular joint is full or maximum rotation of the clavicle, which occurs when the upper arm is in full elevation. The resting position and capsular pattern are the same as with the acromioclavicular joint. The joint is innervated by branches of the anterior supraclavicular nerve and the nerve to the subclavius muscle.

Although the *scapulothoracic "joint"* is not a true joint, it functions as an integral part of the shoulder complex and must be considered in any assessment. Some texts call this structure the *scapulocostal joint.* This joint consists of the body of the scapula and the muscles covering the posterior chest wall. Because it is not a true joint, it does not have a capsular pattern or a close packed position. The resting position of this joint would be the same as for the acromioclavicular joint.

PATIENT HISTORY

In addition to the general history questions that were presented in Chapter 1, there are a number of questions to be asked that apply to the shoulder:

1. What is the patient unable to do functionally? Is the patient able to talk or swallow? Is the patient hoarse? These last signs could indicate an injury to the sternoclavicular joint if there is swelling or a posterior dislocation.

2. What is the extent and behavior of the patient's pain? For example, deep, boring, toothache-like pain in the neck and/or shoulder region may be indicative of *thoracic outlet syndrome* (Fig. 4–2). Strains of the rotator cuff usually cause dull toothache, as in pain that is worse at night, whereas acute calcific tendinitis usually causes a "red-hot," burning type of pain.

3. Are there any movements that cause the patient pain or problems? If so, which ones? The examiner must always keep in mind that cervical spine movements may also cause pain in the shoulder. Persons who have had recurrent dislocations of the shoulder may find that any movement involving lateral rotation will bother them because this movement is involved in anterior dislocations of the shoulder. Excessive abduction and lateral rotation may lead to "dead arm" syndrome in which the patient feels a sudden "paralyzing" pain and weakness in the shoulder. This finding is an indication of anterior shoulder instability. Acromioclavicular pain is especially evident above 90° abduction.

4. What is the patient's age? Many problems of the shoulder can be age related. For example, rotator cuff degeneration usually occurs when the patients are in their 40s and 50s. Calcium deposits may occur between the ages of 20 and 40. Chondrosarcomas may be seen in those over the age of 30 years, whereas *frozen shoulder* is seen in individuals between the ages of 45 and 60 if it is due to causes other than trauma.

5. Are there any activities that cause or increase the pain? For example, bicipital tendinitis is often seen in skiers and may be the result of holding on to a ski tow; in cross-country skiing it may be the result of poling (using the pole for propulsion). Elite swimmers may train for more than 15,000 m daily, which may lead to stress overload of the structures of the shoulder. Does throwing or reaching alter the pain? If so, what positions cause pain or discomfort? These questions may give an indication of the structures that are injured.

6. Do any positions relieve the pain? Patients with nerve root pain may find that elevation of the arm over the head gives relief of symptoms.

7. Is there any indication of muscle spasm, deformity, bruising, wasting, paresthesia, or numbness?

8. If there was an injury, what exactly was the mechanism of injury? Did the patient fall on an outstretched hand, which could indicate a fracture or dislocation of the glenohumeral joint? Did the

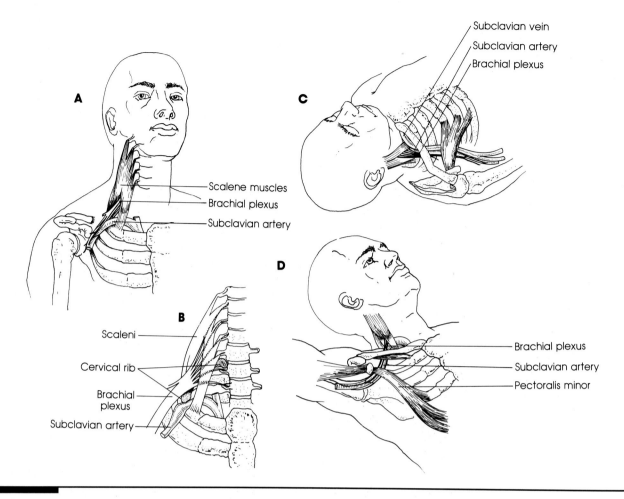

FIGURE 4–2. *Location and causes of thoracic outlet syndrome. (A) Scalenus anterior syndrome. (B) Cervical rib syndrome. (C) Costoclavicular space syndrome. (D) Hyperabduction syndrome.*

patient fall on or receive a blow to the tip of the shoulder? This finding may indicate an acromioclavicular dislocation or subluxation.

9. Does the patient support the upper limb or hesitate to move it? This action could mean that one of the joints of the shoulder complex is unstable or that there is an acute problem in the shoulder.

10. How long has the problem bothered the patient? For example, idiopathic frozen shoulder will go through three stages, each of which lasts 3 to 5 months. The condition becomes progressively worse over a 3- to 5-month period, stays the same for a 3- to 5-month period, and then progressively improves over a 3- to 5-month period.[1]

11. Does the patient complain of the limb feeling weak and heavy after activity? Does the limb tire easily? Are there any *venous* symptoms, such as swelling or stiffness, which may extend all the way to the fingers? Are there any *arterial* symptoms, which may be indicated by coolness or pallor in the upper limb? These complaints may be the result of pressure on an artery, a vein, or both. An example is thoracic outlet syndrome (Fig. 4–2), in which

pressure may be applied to the vascular and/or neurological structures as they enter the upper limb in three locations: at the scalene triangle, at the costoclavicular space, and under pectoralis minor and the coracoid process.[2, 3]

12. Is there any indication of nerve injury? The examiner should evaluate the nerves and the muscles supplied by the nerves to determine this. Any history of weakness, numbness, or paresthesia may indicate nerve injury. For example, the suprascapular nerve may be injured as it passes through the suprascapular notch under the transverse scapular ligament, leading to atrophy and paralysis of the supraspinatus and infraspinatus muscles. The examiner should listen to the history carefully, since this condition could mimic a third-degree (rupture) strain of the supraspinatus tendon. Another potential nerve injury is one to the circumflex (axillary) nerve (Fig. 4–3) after dislocation of the glenohumeral joint. In this case, the deltoid muscle and the teres minor muscle will be atrophied and weak or paralyzed. The radial nerve (Fig. 4–3) is sometimes injured as it winds around the posterior aspect of

the shaft of the humerus. The injury is frequently seen when the humeral shaft is fractured. If the nerve is damaged in this location, the extensors of the elbow, wrist, and fingers will be affected and an altered sensation will occur in the radial nerve sensory distribution.

13. Which hand is dominant? Often the dominant shoulder will be lower than the nondominant shoulder and the range of motion may not be the same for both. Usually, the dominant shoulder will show greater muscularity.

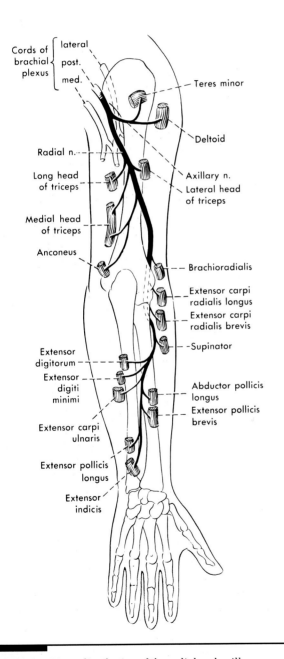

FIGURE 4–3. *Motor distribution of the radial and axillary nerves. (From Hollinshead, W. H., and D. B. Jenkins: Functional Anatomy of the Limbs and Back, 5th ed. Philadelphia, W. B. Saunders Co., 1981, p. 132.)*

OBSERVATION

The patient must be suitably undressed so that the examiner can observe the normal bony and soft-tissue contours of both shoulders and determine whether they are normal and symmetric. When observing the shoulder, the examiner looks at the entire upper limb because the hand may show some vasomotor changes that may be the result of problems in the shoulder. These changes may include shiny skin, loss of hair, swelling, and muscle atrophy.

It is important to watch the patient when the patient removes clothes from the upper body. Is the affected arm undressed last or dressed first? This action by the patient will give some indication of functional restriction, pain, and/or weakness in the upper limb.

Anterior View

When looking at the patient from the anterior view (Fig. 4–4), the examiner should begin by ensuring that the head and neck are in the midline of the body and then observe the shoulders. The examiner should look for the possibility of a *step deformity* (Fig. 4–5) over the shoulder area. Such a deformity may be due to an acromioclavicular dislocation, with the distal end of the clavicle lying superior to the acromion process. If the deformity appears when traction is applied to the arm, it may be due to multidirectional instability, leading to inferior subluxation of the glenohumeral joint. This sign is referred to as a *sulcus sign* because of the appearance of a sulcus below the acromion process. Flattening of the normally round deltoid muscle may indicate an anterior dislocation of the glenohumeral joint or paralysis of the deltoid muscle (Fig. 4–6). The examiner should note any abnormal bumps or alignment in the bones that may indicate past injury such as a fracture of the clavicle.

As mentioned earlier, in most individuals the dominant side will be lower than the nondominant side. This difference may be due to the extra use of the dominant side, resulting in the ligaments, joint capsules, and muscles becoming stretched, allowing the arm to "sag" slightly. Individuals such as tennis players[4] and others who stretch their upper limbs will show even greater differences along with gross hypertrophy of the muscles on the dominant side (Fig. 4–7).

The examiner notes whether the patient is able to assume the normal functional position for the shoulder, which is forward flexion to 45° and abduction to 60°, with the arm in neutral or no rotation. The

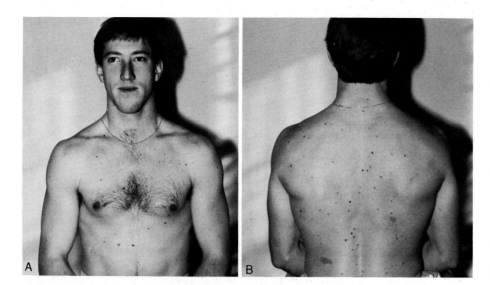

FIGURE 4–4. Anterior (A) and posterior (B) views of the shoulder.

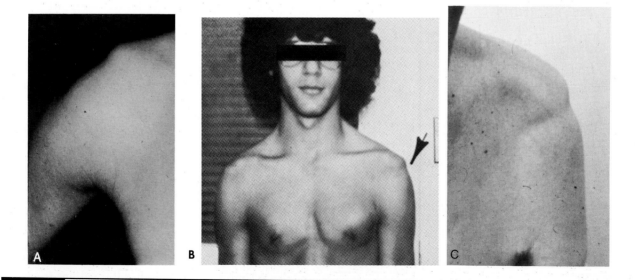

FIGURE 4–5. (A) Step deformity resulting from acromioclavicular dislocation. (B) Sulcus sign for shoulder instability. (From Warren, R. F.: Clin. Sports Med. 2:339, 1983.) (C) Subluxation of glenohumeral joint after stroke (paralysis of deltoid muscle).

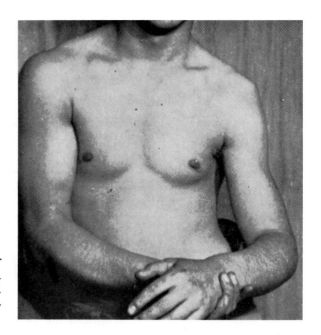

FIGURE 4–6. Subcoracoid dislocation of the shoulder. Note the prominent acromion, the arm held away from the side, and the flat deltoid. (From McLaughlin, H. L.: Trauma. Philadelphia, W. B. Saunders Co., 1959, p. 246.)

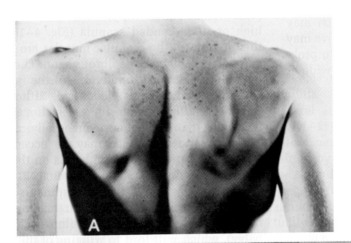

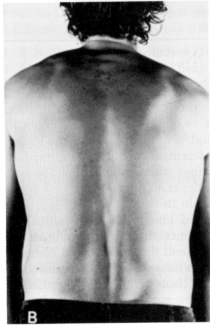

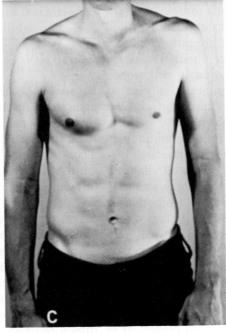

FIGURE 4–7. Depressed right shoulder in a right dominant individual—in this case, a tennis player. (A) Hypertrophy of playing shoulder muscles. (B) With muscles relaxed, the distance between spinous processes and medial border of scapula is widened on the right. (C) Depressed shoulder. (From Priest, J. D., and D. A. Nagel: Am. J. Sports Med. 4:33, 1976.)

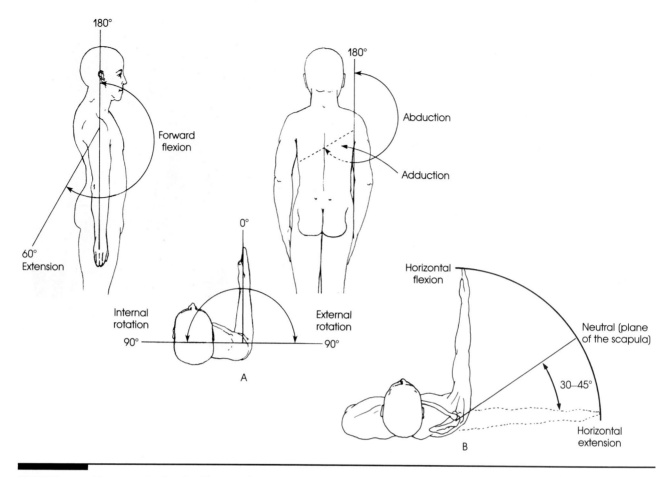

FIGURE 4–11. *Movement in the shoulder complex. (A) Range of motion of the shoulder. (B) Axes of arm elevation. (Adapted from Perry, J.: Clin. Sports Med. 2:255, 1983.)*

45°. After abducting the arm to 90°, the patient moves the straight arm in a backward direction. Circumduction is normally approximately 200° and involves taking the arm in a circle on the vertical plane.

When examining these movements, the examiner may ask the patient to do the movements in combination. For example, *Apley's scratch test* combines medial rotation with adduction and lateral rotation with abduction (Fig. 4–12). By doing the examination this way, many examiners feel they are decreasing the time taken to do the assessment. In addition, by doing the combined movements, the examiner is given some idea of the functional capacity of the patient. For example, for one to comb the hair, for a woman to zip a back zipper, or for a man to reach his wallet in his back pocket, abduction combined with lateral rotation and adduction combined with medial rotation are needed. When using this method, however, the examiner must take care to notice which movements are restricted and which ones are not, because several movements are performed at the same time. Often, the dominant shoul-

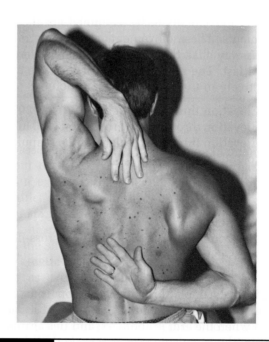

FIGURE 4–12. *Apley scratch test. The left arm is in lateral rotation and abduction, and the right arm is in medial rotation and adduction.*

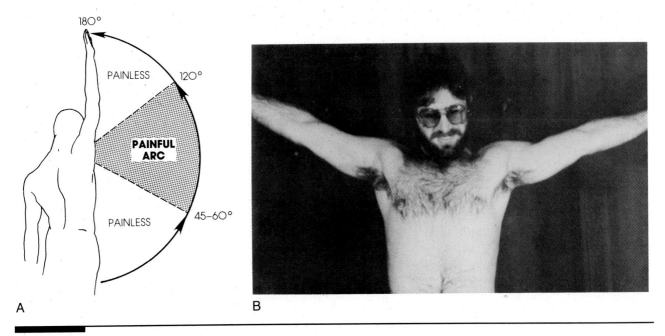

FIGURE 4–13. *Painful arc in the shoulder. (A) In the case of acromioclavicular joint problems only, the range of 120 to 180° would elicit pain. (B) This athlete demonstrates a painful arc—in this case, maximal at approximately 115° of adduction in the coronal plane. This is indicative of impingement. (From Hawkins, R. J., and P. E. Hobeika: Clin. Sports Med. 2:391, 1983.)*

der will show greater restriction than the nondominant shoulder, even in "normal" individuals.

As the patient elevates the upper extremity by abducting the shoulder, the examiner should note whether a painful arc is present (Fig. 4–13).[10] A painful arc may be due to subacromial bursitis, calcium deposits, or a tendinitis of the rotator cuff muscles. The pain is the result of pinching inflamed or tender structures under the acromion process and the coracoacromial ligament. Initially, the structures are not pinched under the acromion process, so the patient is able to abduct 45 to 60° with little difficulty. As the patient abducts further (60 to 120°), the structures become pinched and the patient is often unable to abduct fully because of pain. If full abduction is possible, however, the pain will dimin-

ish after approximately 120° as the pinched soft tissues have passed under the acromion process and are no longer being pinched. Often, the pain is greater going up (against gravity) than coming down, and there is more pain on active abduction than passive abduction. If the movement is very painful, the individual often elevates the arm through forward flexion in an attempt to decrease the pain. If the examiner finds the pain is greater as the patient reaches full elevation, this finding would lead the examiner to consider the possibility of an acromioclavicular joint problem. Table 4–1 presents the signs and symptoms of three types of painful arc in the shoulder, with the superior type being the most common. The examiner may find that the arc of pain may also be present during elevation through for-

TABLE 4–1. Classification of Glenohumeral Painful Arcs*

	Anterior	Posterior	Superior
Night pain	Yes	Yes	Maybe
Age	50 +	50 +	40 +
Sex ratio	F > M	F > M	M > F
Aggravated by	Lateral rotation and abduction	Medial rotation and abduction	Abduction
Tenderness	Lesser tuberosity	Posterior aspect of greater tuberosity	Greater tuberosity
Acromioclavicular joint involvement	No	No	Often
Calcification (if present)	Supraspinatus, infraspinatus, and/or subscapularis	Supraspinatus and/or infraspinatus	Supraspinatus and/or subscapularis
Third-degree strain biceps brachii (long-head)	No	No	Occasional
Prognosis	Good	Very good	Poor (without surgery)

*From Kessel, L., and M. Watson: J. Bone Joint Surg. 59B:166, 1977.[10]

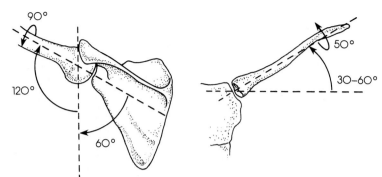

ward flexion, although the pain is usually less severe on this movement. The interconnection of the sub-acromial, subcoracoid, and subscapularis bursae with each other and with the glenohumeral joint capsule will often give a broad area of signs and symptoms.

When examining the movement of elevation through abduction, the examiner must take time to observe the *scapulohumeral rhythm* (Fig. 4–14) anteriorly and posteriorly.[11, 12] That is, during 180° of abduction, there is a 2:1 ratio of movement of the humerus to the scapula, with 120° of movement occurring at the glenohumeral joint and 60° occur-ring at the scapulothoracic joint. During this total movement, there are three phases:

1. In the first phase of 30° of movement, the outer end of the clavicle elevates 12 to 15° while the scapula is said to be "setting." This setting phase means that the scapula may rotate in, rotate out, or not move at all. The angle between the scapular spine and the clavicle will also increase 10°, but there will be no rotation of the clavicle.

2. During the next 60° of elevation (second phase), the clavicle will elevate 30 to 36° and there will be a 2:1 ratio of scapulohumeral movement. There still is no rotation of the clavicle at this stage.

3. During the final 90° of motion (third phase), there continues to be a 2:1 ratio of scapulohumeral movement and the angle between the scapular spine and the clavicle increases an additional 10°. It is in this stage that the clavicle will elevate 30 to 60°. At the same time, the clavicle will rotate posteriorly 50° on a long axis. Also during this final stage, the humerus laterally rotates 90° so that the greater tuberosity of the humerus avoids the acromion proc-ess.

If the clavicle does not rotate and elevate, eleva-tion through abduction at the glenohumeral joint is limited to 120°. If the glenohumeral joint does not move, elevation through abduction is limited to 60°, which occurs totally in the scapulothoracic joint. If there is no lateral rotation of the humerus during abduction, the total movement available is 120°, 60°

of which occurs at the glenohumeral joint and 60° of which occurs at the scapulothoracic articulation. The normal end of range of motion is reached when there is contact of a surgical neck of humerus against the acromion process. *Reverse scapulohumeral rhythm* (Fig. 4–15) means that the scapula moves more than the humerus. This is seen in conditions such as frozen shoulder; the patient appears to "hitch" the entire shoulder complex rather than produce a smooth coordinated abduction movement.

It must be remembered that the biceps tendon does not move in the bicipital groove during move-ment but that the humerus moves over the fixed tendon. From adduction to full elevation of abduc-tion, a given point in the groove moves along the tendon at least 4 cm. If the examiner wanted to keep excursion of the biceps tendon to a minimum, the arm should be elevated with the humerus in medial rotation. Elevation of the arm with the humerus laterally rotated causes maximum excursion of the biceps tendon.

As the patient does the various movements, the examiner watches to see whether the various com-ponents of the shoulder complex move in normal sequence and whether the patient exhibits any ap-prehension when doing the movement. With ante-rior instability of the shoulder, the shoulder girdle often droops, and excessive scapulothoracic move-ment may be seen on abduction. With posterior instability, horizontal adduction (cross-flexion) may cause excessive scapulothoracic movement. Any ap-prehension suggests the possibility of instability. The examiner should also watch for winging of the scapula, which is indicative of injury to the serratus anterior muscle or the long thoracic nerve. If the scapula appears to wing, the examiner asks the patient to forward flex the shoulder to 90°. The examiner then pushes the straight arm toward the patient's body while the patient resists. If there is weakness of the serratus anterior muscle or its nerve, this movement will cause the scapula to wing, which means the medial border of the scapula will move away from the chest wall and protrude posteriorly. Winging of the scapula may also be tested by having

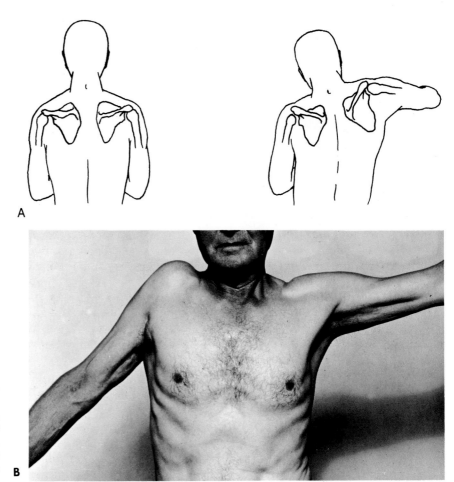

FIGURE 4–15. Reverse scapulohumeral rhythm (notice shoulder hiking). The cause is frozen shoulder (A) and tear of rotator cuff (B). (B is from Beetham, W. P., et al.: Physical Examination of the Joints. Philadelphia, W. B. Saunders Co., 1965, p. 41.)

the patient stand and lean against the wall. The patient is then asked to do a "push-up" away from the wall while the examiner watches for possible winging of the scapula (Fig. 4–9).

Injury to other nerves in the shoulder region must not be overlooked. As previously mentioned, damage to the suprascapular nerve will affect the supraspinatus and infraspinatus muscles, whereas injury to the musculocutaneous nerve will lead to paralysis of the coracobrachialis, biceps, and brachialis muscles. These changes will affect elbow flexion and supination and forward flexion of the shoulder. There will also be a loss of the biceps reflex. Injury to the circumflex (axillary) nerve will lead to paralysis of the deltoid and teres minor muscles, thus affecting abduction and lateral rotation of the shoulder. There will also be a sensory loss over the deltoid insertion area. Damage to the radial nerve will affect all of the extensor muscles of the upper limb. The triceps muscles, which assist extension at the shoulder, may be paralyzed so that the patient will be unable to actively extend the elbow against gravity.

Passive Movements

If the range of motion is not full during the active movements and the examiner is unable to test the end feel, all passive movements of the shoulder should be performed to determine the end feel and passive range of motion. These movements include:

1. Elevation through forward flexion of the arm.
2. Elevation through abduction of the arm.
3. Elevation through abduction of the glenohumeral joint only (Fig. 4–16).
4. Lateral rotation of the arm.
5. Medial rotation of the arm.
6. Extension of the arm.
7. Adduction of the arm.
8. Horizontal adduction/abduction of the arm.
9. Quadrant test.

Particular attention is paid to the passive medial and lateral rotation if the examiner suspects a problem with the glenohumeral joint capsule. The examiner must remember that *subcoracoid bursitis*

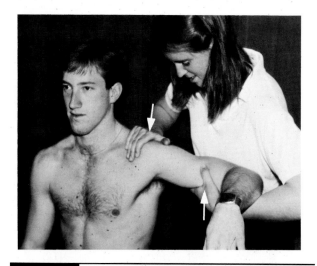

FIGURE 4–16. *Passive abduction of the glenohumeral joint.*

may limit full lateral rotation whereas *subacromial bursitis* may limit full abduction because of compression or pinching of these structures. Even if overpressure has been applied on active movement, it is still necessary for the examiner to perform elevation through abduction of the glenohumeral joint only and the quadrant test. The examiner should find these end feels on passive movements of the shoulder:

1. Elevation through forward flexion: tissue stretch.
2. Elevation through abduction: bone-to-bone or tissue stretch.
3. Lateral rotation: tissue stretch.
4. Medial rotation: tissue stretch.
5. Extension: tissue stretch.
6. Adduction: tissue approximation.

7. Horizontal adduction: tissue stretch or approximation.
8. Horizontal abduction: tissue stretch.
9. Elevation through abduction of glenohumeral joint: bone-to-bone or tissue stretch.

To test the *quadrant position*,[13] the examiner stabilizes the scapula and clavicle by placing the forearm under the patient's scapula of the arm to be tested and extending the hand over the shoulder to hold the trapezius muscle to prevent shoulder shrugging (Fig. 4–17). To test the position, the upper limb is elevated to rest alongside the patient's head with the shoulder externally rotated. The patient's shoulder is then adducted. As adduction occurs on the coronal plane, a point (quadrant position) will be reached where the arm will move forward slightly from the coronal plane. At approximately 60° of adduction (from the arm beside the head), this position of maximum forward movement will occur even if a backward pressure is applied. As the shoulder is further adducted, it will fall back to the previous coronal plane. The quadrant position indicates the position at which the arm has medially rotated during its descent to the patient's side. The rotation of the humerus in the quadrant position demonstrates Codman's "pivotal paradox"[9, 14] and MacConaill's[15] conjunct rotation in diadochal movement. For example, if the arm, with the elbow flexed, is laterally rotated when the arm is at the side and then abducted in the coronal plane to 180°, the shoulder will be in 90° of medial rotation even though no apparent rotation has occurred. The path traced by the humerus during the quadrant test in which the humerus moves forward at approximately 120° of abduction is the unconscious rotation occurring at the glenohumeral joint. When doing the

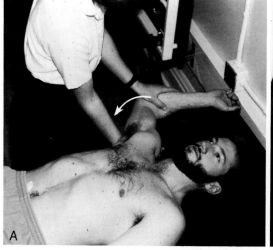
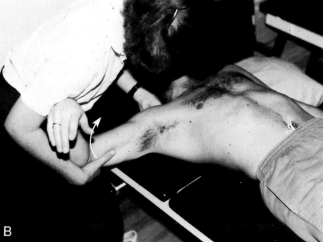

FIGURE 4–17. *Quadrant position. (A) Adduction test. (B) Abduction test (locked quadrant).*

movement, the examiner should not only feel the movement but also determine the quality of the movement and the amount of anterior humeral movement. This test and the following locked quadrant test assess one area or quadrant of the 360° of circumduction. It is the quadrant of the circumduction movement in which the humerus must rotate to allow full pain-free movement. Thus, the tests should normally be pain free. If movement is painful and restricted, the tests indicate early stages of shoulder pathology.[16]

Similarly, the quadrant position may be found by abducting the medially rotated shoulder while maintaining extension. In this case, the quadrant position is reached (approximately 120° abduction) when the shoulder will no longer abduct because it is prevented from laterally rotating due to the catching of the greater tuberosity in the subacromial space. This position is referred to as the *locked quadrant position*. If the arm is allowed to move forward, lateral rotation will occur and full abduction can be achieved. In addition to these movements, passive elevation through abduction of the glenohumeral joint with the clavicle and scapula fixed is also performed by the examiner to determine the amount of abduction in the glenohumeral joint alone. Normally, this movement should be 120°.

The *capsular pattern* of the shoulder is lateral rotation showing the greatest restriction, followed by abduction and medial rotation. Each of these movements has a capsular end feel. Other movements may be limited, but not in the same order and not with as much restriction. Finding of limitation, but not in the order described, is indicative of a *noncapsular pattern*.

Resisted Isometric Movements

Having completed the active and passive movements, which are done while the patient is standing, sitting, or lying supine (in the case of quadrant test), the patient lies supine to do the resisted isometric movements (Fig. 4–18). During the active movements, the examiner should have noted which movements caused discomfort or pain so that this information can be correlated with those of resisted isometric movements. By carefully noting which movements cause pain when doing the tests isometrically, the examiner should be able to determine which muscle or muscles are at fault (Table 4–2). For example, if the patient experiences pain primarily on medial rotation but also on abduction and adduction, a suspected problem would be in the subscapularis muscle, since the other muscles involved in these actions are involved in actions that

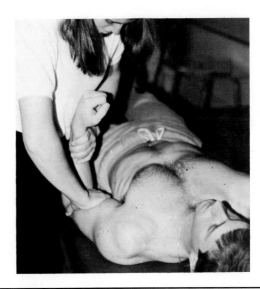

FIGURE 4–18. *Positioning of the patient for resisted isometric movements.*

were found to be pain free. To do the resisted isometric tests, the examiner positions the patient's arm at the side with the elbow flexed to 90°. The movements tested isometrically are:

1. Forward flexion of the shoulder.
2. Extension of the shoulder.
3. Adduction of the shoulder.
4. Abduction of the shoulder.
5. Medial rotation of the shoulder.
6. Lateral rotation of the shoulder.
7. Flexion of the elbow.
8. Extension of the elbow.

Resisted isometric elbow flexion and extension must be performed because some of the muscles act over the elbow as well as the shoulder. The examiner should watch for the possibility of a third-degree strain (rupture) of the long head of biceps tendon when testing isometric elbow flexion (Fig. 4–19).

During the testing, the examiner will find differences in the relative strengths of the various muscle groups around the shoulder. As a general guide, the following proportions can be used:

1. Abduction should be 50 to 60% of adduction.
2. Forward flexion should be 50 to 60% of adduction.
3. Medial rotation should be 45 to 50% of adduction.
4. Lateral rotation should be 65 to 70% of medial rotation.
5. Forward flexion should be 50 to 60% of extension.
6. Horizontal flexion should be 70 to 80% of horizontal extension.

TABLE 4–2. Muscles About the Shoulder: Their Actions and Nerve Supply (Including Nerve Root Derivation)

Action	Muscles Performing Action	Nerve Supply	Nerve Root Derivation
Forward flexion	1. Deltoid (anterior fibers) 2. Pectoralis major (clavicular fibers) 3. Coracobrachialis 4. Biceps (when strong contraction required)	Circumflex (axillary) Lateral pectoral Musculocutaneous Musculocutaneous	C5–C6 (posterior cord) C5–C6 (lateral cord) C5–C7 (lateral cord) C5–C7 (lateral cord)
Extension	1. Deltoid (posterior fibers) 2. Teres major 3. Teres minor 4. Latissimus dorsi 5. Pectoralis major (sternocostal fibers) 6. Triceps (long head)	Circumflex (axillary) Subscapular Circumflex (axillary) Thoracodorsal Lateral pectoral Medial pectoral Radial	C5–C6 (posterior cord) C5–C6 (posterior cord) C5–C6 (posterior cord) C6–C8 (posterior cord) C5–C6 (lateral cord) C8, T1 (medial cord) C5–C8, T1 (posterior cord)
Horizontal adduction	1. Pectoralis major 2. Deltoid (anterior fibers)	Lateral pectoral Circumflex (axillary)	C5–C6 (lateral cord) C5–C6 (posterior cord)
Horizontal abduction	1. Deltoid (posterior fibers) 2. Teres major 3. Teres minor 4. Infraspinatus	Circumflex (axillary) Subscapular Circumflex (axillary) Suprascapular	C5–C6 (posterior cord) C5–C6 (posterior cord) C5–C6 (brachial plexus trunk) C5–C6 (brachial plexus trunk)
Abduction	1. Deltoid 2. Supraspinatus 3. Infraspinatus 4. Subscapularis 5. Teres minor 6. Long head of biceps (if arm externally rotated first, trick movement)	Circumflex (axillary) Suprascapular Suprascapular Subscapular Circumflex (axillary) Musculocutaneous	C5–C6 (posterior cord) C5–C6 (brachial plexus trunk) C5–C6 (brachial plexus trunk) C5–C6 (posterior cord) C5–C6 (posterior cord) C5–C7 (lateral cord)
Adduction	1. Pectoralis major 2. Latissimus dorsi 3. Teres major 4. Subscapularis	Lateral pectoral Thoracodorsal Subscapular Subscapular	C5–C6 (lateral cord) C6–C8 (posterior cord) C5–C6 (posterior cord) C5–C6 (posterior cord)
Medial rotation	1. Pectoralis major 2. Deltoid (anterior fibers) 3. Latissimus dorsi 4. Teres major 5. Subscapularis (when arm is by side)	Lateral pectoral Circumflex (axillary) Thoracodorsal Subscapular Subscapular	C5–C6 (lateral cord) C5–C6 (posterior cord) C6–C8 (posterior cord) C5–C6 (posterior cord) C5–C6 (posterior cord)
Lateral rotation	1. Infraspinatus 2. Deltoid (posterior fibers) 3. Teres minor	Suprascapular Circumflex (axillary) Circumflex (axillary)	C5–C6 (brachial plexus trunk) C5–C6 (posterior cord) C5–C6 (posterior cord)
Elevation of scapula	1. Trapezius (upper fibers) 2. Levator scapulae 3. Rhomboid major 4. Rhomboid minor	Accessory C3–C4 nerve roots C3–C4 nerve roots Dorsal scapular Dorsal scapular Dorsal scapular	Cranial nerve XI C3–C4 C5 (C4), C5 (C4), C5
Depression of scapula	1. Serratus anterior 2. Pectoralis major 3. Pectoralis minor 4. Latissimus dorsi 5. Trapezius (lower fibers)	Long thoracic Lateral pectoral Medial pectoral Thoracodorsal Accessory C3–C4 nerve roots	C5–C6 (C7) C5–C6 (lateral cord) C8, T1 (medial cord) C6–C8 (posterior cord) Cranial nerve XI C3–C4
Protraction (forward movement) of scapula	1. Serratus anterior 2. Pectoralis major 3. Pectoralis minor 4. Latissimus dorsi	Long thoracic Lateral pectoral Medial pectoral Thoracodorsal	C5–C6 (C7) C5–C6 (lateral cord) C8, T1 (medial cord) C6–C8 (posterior cord)
Retraction (backward movement) of scapula	1. Trapezius 2. Rhomboid major 3. Rhomboid minor	Accessory Dorsal scapular Dorsal scapular	Cranial nerve XI (C4), C5 (C4), C5
Lateral (upward) rotation of inferior angle of scapula	1. Trapezius (upper and lower fibers) 2. Serratus anterior	Accessory C3–C4 nerve roots Long thoracic	Cranial nerve XI C3–C4 C5–C6 (C7)
Medial (downward) rotation of inferior angle of scapula	1. Levator scapulae 2. Rhomboid major 3. Rhomboid minor 4. Pectoralis minor	C3–C4 nerve roots Dorsal scapular Dorsal scapular Dorsal scapular Medial pectoral	C3–C4 C5 (C4), C5 (C4), C5 C8, T1 (medial cord)
Flexion of elbow	1. Brachialis 2. Biceps brachii 3. Brachioradialis 4. Pronator teres 5. Flexor carpi ulnaris	Musculocutaneous Musculocutaneous Radial Median Ulnar	C5–C6, (C7) C5–C6 C5–C6, (C7) C6–C7 C7–C8
Extension of elbow	1. Triceps 2. Anconeus	Radial Radial	C6–C8 C7–C8, (T1)

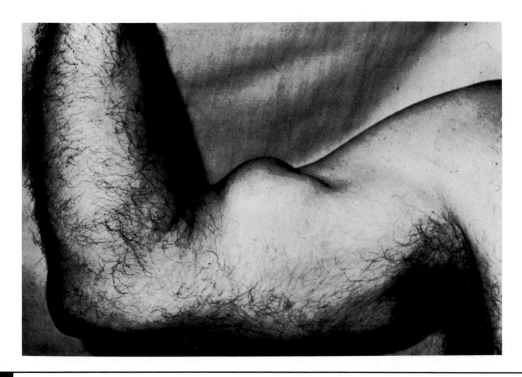

FIGURE 4–19. *Rupture of the long head of the biceps brachii caused by the patient's awkward catch of partner in gymnastics. Bunching of muscle is attended by complete loss of function of the long head. (From O'Donoghue, D. H.: Treatment of Injuries to Athletes, 4th ed. Philadelphia, W. B. Saunders Co., 1984, p. 53.)*

Functional Assessment

The shoulder complex plays an integral role in the activities of daily living, sometimes acting as part of an open kinetic chain and sometimes acting as part of a closed kinetic chain. Assessment of function plays an important part of the shoulder assessment (Fig. 4–20). Limitation of function can greatly affect the patient. For example, placing the hand behind the head (e.g., to comb the hair) requires full lateral rotation, whereas placing the hand in the small of the back (e.g., to get a wallet out of a back pocket or undo a bra) requires full medial rotation. Table 4–3 provides the examiner with a method of determining the patient's functional shoulder strength and endurance.

Special Tests

Some of these tests should always be done, and others need be done only if the examiner wants to confirm findings. Four tests—one each for anterior, posterior, and inferior instability and the upper limb tension test—should always be done, and the examiner should learn to use them proficiently. The other tests need to be done only as confirming tests.

Tests for Anterior Shoulder Instability

Anterior Drawer Test of the Shoulder.[17] The patient lies supine. The examiner places the hand of the affected shoulder in the examiner's axilla, holding the patient's hand with the arm so that the patient remains relaxed. The shoulder to be tested is abducted between 80 and 120°; forward flexed, 0 and 20°; and laterally rotated, 0 and 30°. The examiner then stabilizes the patient's scapula with the opposite hand, pushing the spine of the scapula forward with the index and middle fingers. The examiner's thumb exerts counterpressure on the patient's coracoid process. Using the arm that holds the patient's hand, the examiner places the hand around the patient's relaxed upper arm and draws the humerus forward. The movement may be accompanied by a click and/or patient apprehension. The amount of movement available is compared with that of the normal side. A positive test is indicative of anterior instability (Fig. 4–21).

Protzman Test for Anterior Instability.[18] The patient is sitting. The examiner abducts the patient's arm to 90° and supports the arm against the examiner's hip so that the patient's shoulder muscles are relaxed. The examiner palpates the anterior aspect of the head of the humerus with the fingers of one hand deep in the patient's axilla while the fingers of the other hand are placed over the posterior aspect of the humeral head. The examiner then pushes the humeral head anteriorly and inferiorly (Fig. 4–22). If this movement causes pain and palpation indicates abnormal anteroinferior movement, the test is positive for anterior instability. Normally, anterior translation should be no more than 25% of the

Name _____ Hosp # _____ Date _____ Shoulder: R/L

I. PAIN: (5 = none, 4 = slight, 3 = after unusual activity, 2 = moderate, 1 = marked, 0 = complete disability, NA = not
available) _____

II. MOTION:

    A. Patient Sitting
       1. Active total elevation of arm: _____ degrees*
       2. Passive internal rotation:
       (Circle segment of posterior anatomy reached by thumb)
       (Note if reach restricted by limited elbow flexion)

1 = less than trochanter	5 = L5	9 = L1	13 = T9	17 = T5
2 = Trochanter	6 = L4	10 = T12	14 = T8	18 = T4
3 = Gluteal	7 = L3	11 = T11	15 = T7	19 = T3
4 = Sacrum	8 = L2	12 = T10	16 = T6	20 = T2
				21 = T1

       3. Active external rotation with arm at side: _____ degrees
       4. Active external rotation at 90° abduction: _____ degrees
       (Enter "NA" if cannot achieve 90° of abduction)

    B. Patient Supine
       1. Passive total elevation of arm: _____ degrees*
       2. Passive external rotation with arm at side: _____ degrees

*Total elevation of arm measured by viewing patient from side and using goniometer to determine angle between <u>arm</u> and <u>thorax</u>.

III. STRENGTH: (5 = normal, 4 = good, 3 = fair, 2 = poor, 1 = trace, 0 = paralysis)

    A. Anterior deltoid   _____   C. External rotation   _____
    B. Middle deltoid   _____   D. Internal rotation   _____

IV. STABILITY: (5 = normal, 4 = apprehension, 3 = rare subluxation, 2 = recurrent subluxation, 1 = recurrent dislocation, 0 =
fixed dislocation, NA = not available)

    A. Anterior _____   B. Posterior _____   C. Inferior _____

V. FUNCTION: (4 = normal, 3 = mild compromise, 2 = difficulty, 1 = with aid, 0 = unable, NA = not available)

A. Use back pocket	_____	I. Sleep on affected side	_____
B. Perineal care	_____	J. Pulling	_____
C. Wash opposite axilla	_____	K. Use hand overhead	_____
D. Eat with utensil	_____	L. Throwing	_____
E. Comb hair	_____	M. Lifting	_____
F. Use hand with arm at shoulder level	_____	N. Do usual work (specify _____)	_____
G. Carry 10–15 lb with arm at side	_____	O. Do usual sport (specify _____)	_____
H. Dress	_____		

VI. PATIENT RESPONSE: (3 = much better, 2 = better, 1 = same, 0 = worse, NA = not available/applicable)

FIGURE 4–20. *American Shoulder and Elbow Surgeons' shoulder evaluation form. (Courtesy of the American Shoulder and Elbow Surgeons.)*

TABLE 4–3. Functional Strength Testing of the Shoulder

Starting Position	Action	Functional Test*
Sitting	Forward flex arm to 90°	Lift 4 to 5 lb weight: Functional Lift 1 to 3 lb weight: Functionally Fair Lift arm weight: Functionally Poor Cannot lift arm: Nonfunctional
Sitting	Shoulder extension	Lift 4 to 5 lb weight: Functional Lift 1 to 3 lb weight: Functionally Fair Lift arm weight: Functionally Poor Cannot lift arm: Nonfunctional
Side lying (may be done in sitting with pulley)	Shoulder medial rotation	Lift 4 to 5 lb weight: Functional Lift 1 to 3 lb weight: Functionally Fair Lift arm weight: Functionally Poor Cannot lift arm: Nonfunctional
Side lying (may be done in sitting with pulley)	Shoulder lateral rotation	Lift 4 to 5 lb weight: Functional Lift 1 to 3 lb weight: Functionally Fair Lift arm weight: Functionally Poor Cannot lift arm: Nonfunctional
Sitting	Shoulder abduction	Lift 4 to 5 lb weight: Functional Lift 1 to 3 lb weight: Functionally Fair Lift arm weight: Functionally Poor Cannot lift arm: Nonfunctional
Sitting	Shoulder adduction (using wall pulley)	Lift 4 to 5 lb weight: Functional Lift 1 to 3 lb weight: Functionally Fair Lift arm weight: Functionally Poor Cannot lift arm: Nonfunctional
Sitting	Shoulder elevation (shoulder shrug)	5 to 6 Repetitions: Functional 3 to 4 Repetitions: Functionally Fair 1 to 2 Repetitions: Functionally Poor 0 Repetitions: Nonfunctional
Sitting	Sitting push-up (shoulder depression)	5 to 6 Repetitions: Functional 3 to 4 Repetitions: Functionally Fair 1 to 2 Repetitions: Functionally Poor 0 Repetitions: Nonfunctional

*Younger, more fit patients should easily be able to do more than the values given for these tests. A comparison between the good side and the injured side will give the examiner some idea about the patient's functional strength capacity.

Adapted from Palmer, M. L., and M. Epler: Clinical Assessment Procedures in Physical Therapy. Philadelphia, J. B. Lippincott, 1990, pp. 68–73.

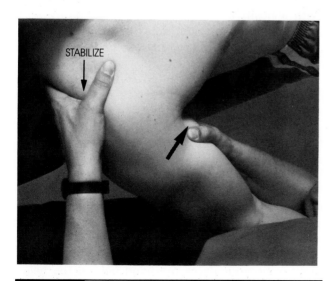

FIGURE 4–21. *Anterior drawer test of the shoulder.*

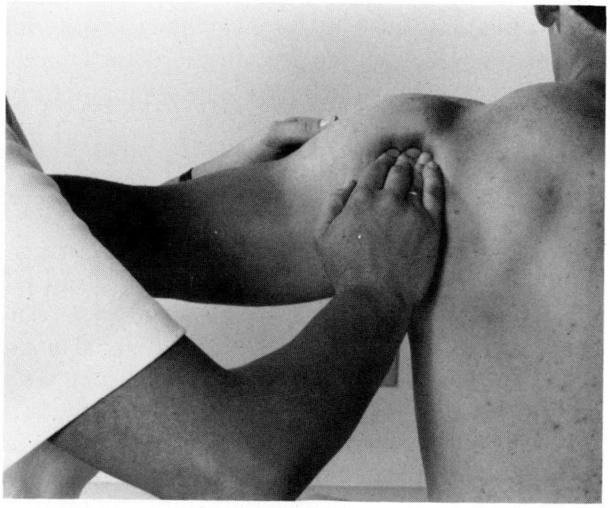

FIGURE 4–22. *Protzman test for anterior instability.*

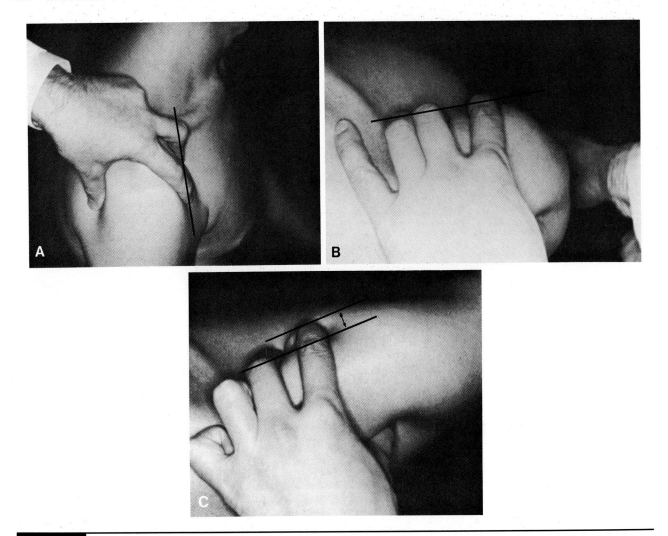

FIGURE 4–23. *Anterior instability test. (Adapted from Leffert, R. D. and G. Gumbey: Clin. Orthop. Relat. Res. 223:22–23, 1987.)*

humeral head.[19] A click may sometimes be palpated as the humeral head slides over the glenoid rim. The test may also be done with the patient in the supine lying position with the elbow supported on a pillow.

Anterior Instability Test.[20] The examiner stands behind the shoulder being examined while the patient sits. The examiner places the examiner's "inside" hand over the shoulder so that the index finger is over the head of the humerus anteriorly and the middle finger is over the coracoid process. The thumb is placed over the posterior humeral head. The examiner's other hand grasps the patient's wrist and carefully abducts and laterally rotates the arm (Fig. 4–23). If, on movement of the arm, the finger palpating the anterior humeral head moves forward, the test is said to be positive for anterior instability. Normally, the two fingers remain in the same plane.

With a positive test, when the arm is returned to the starting position, the index finger will return to the starting position as the humeral head glides backward.

Rockwood Test for Anterior Instability.[21] The examiner stands behind the seated patient. With the arm by the side, the examiner laterally rotates the shoulder. The arm is abducted to 45°, and passive lateral rotation is repeated. The same procedure is repeated at 90° and 120° (Fig. 4–24). For the test to be positive, the patient must show marked apprehension with posterior pain when the arm is tested at 90°. At 45° and 120°, the patient will show some uneasiness and some pain. At 0°, there is rarely apprehension.

Rowe Test for Anterior Instability.[22] The patient lies supine and places the hand behind the head. The examiner places one hand (clenched fist) against

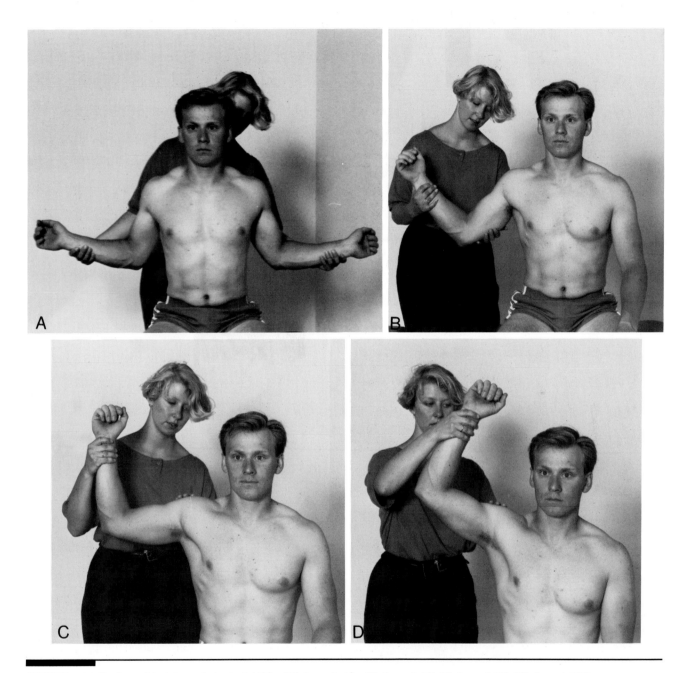

FIGURE 4–24. Rockwood test for anterior instability. (A) Arm at side. (B) Arm at 45°. (C) Arm at 90°. (D) Arm at 120°.

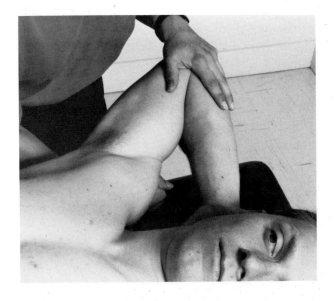

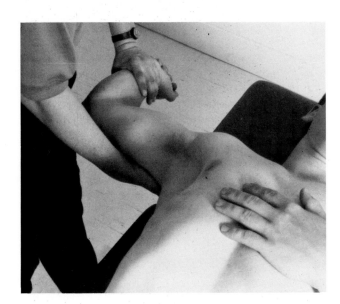

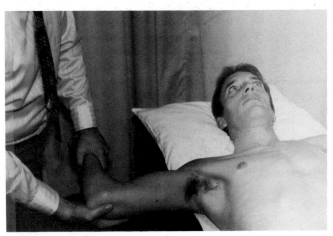

FIGURE 4–25. *Rowe test for anterior instability.*

FIGURE 4–26. *Fulcrum test.*

FIGURE 4–27. *Anterior apprehension (crank) test.*

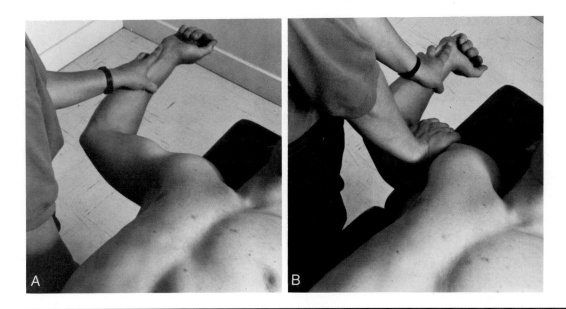

FIGURE 4–28. *Relocation test. (A) Abduction and external rotation. (B) Abduction and external rotation combined with posterior translation of the humerus.*

the posterior humeral head and pushes up while extending the arm slightly (Fig. 4–25). A look of apprehension or pain is indicative of a positive test.

Fulcrum Test.[23] The patient lies supine with the arm abducted to 90°. The examiner places one hand under the glenohumeral joint to act as a fulcrum. The examiner then extends and laterally rotates the arm gently over the fulcrum (Fig. 4–26). A positive test for anterior instability is a look of apprehension by the patient.

Apprehension (Crank) Test for Anterior Shoulder Dislocation. The examiner abducts and laterally rotates the patient's shoulder slowly (Fig. 4–27). A positive test is indicated by a look or feeling of apprehension or alarm on the patient's face, and the patient's resistance to further motion. The patient may also state that the feeling experienced is what it felt like when the shoulder was previously dislocated. It is imperative that this test be done slowly. If the test is done too quickly, the humerus might

dislocate. Hawkins and Bokor[24] noted that the examiner should observe the amount of external rotation possible when the patient becomes apprehensive. If the examiner then applies a posterior stress to the arm (*relocation test*), the patient will lose the apprehension, and further external rotation will be possible before the apprehension returns (Fig. 4–28).

Clunk Test. The patient lies supine. The examiner places one hand on the posterior aspect of the shoulder over the humeral head. The examiner's other hand holds the humerus at the elbow. The examiner fully abducts the arm over the patient's head. The examiner then pushes anteriorly with the hand over the humeral head while the other hand rotates the humerus into lateral rotation (Fig. 4–29). A "clunk" or grinding indicates a positive test and is indicative of a tear of the labrum.[25] The test may also cause apprehension if anterior instability is present. Walsh[26] indicated that if the examiner fol-

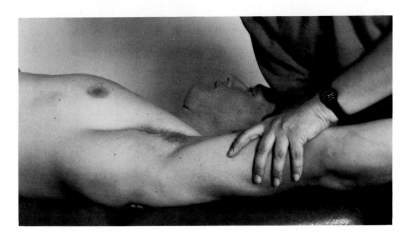

FIGURE 4–29. *Clunk test.*

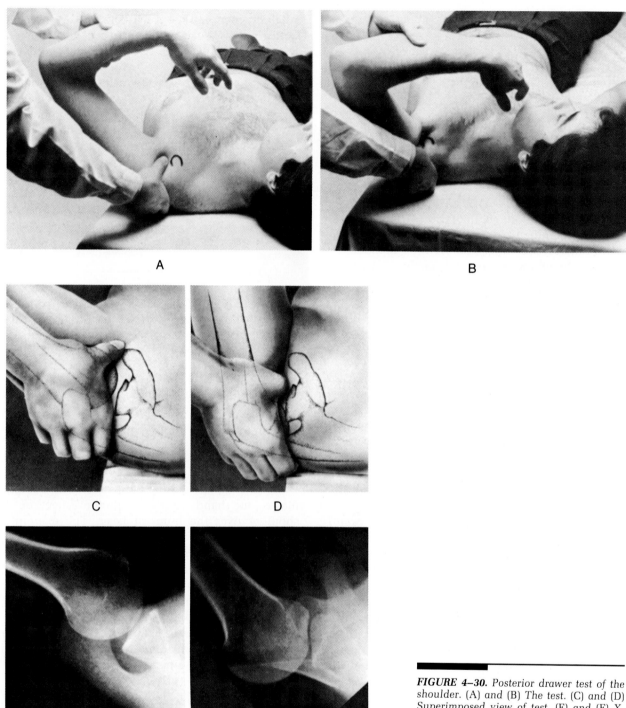

A

B

C

D

E

F

FIGURE 4–30. *Posterior drawer test of the shoulder. (A) and (B) The test. (C) and (D) Superimposed view of test. (E) and (F) X-rays of test. (From Gerber, C., and R. Ganz: J. Bone Joint Surg. 66B:554, 1984.)*

lows the above maneuvers with horizontal adduction that will relocate the humerus, a clunk or click may also be heard, indicating a tear of the labrum as well.

Tests for Posterior Shoulder Instability

Posterior Drawer Test of the Shoulder.[17] The patient lies supine. The examiner stands at the level of the shoulder and grasps the patient's proximal forearm with one hand, flexing the patient's elbow to 120° and the shoulder to 80 to 120° of abduction and 20 to 30° of forward flexion. With the other hand, the examiner stabilizes the scapula by placing the index and middle fingers on the spine of the scapula and the thumb on the coracoid process. The examiner then rotates the forearm medially and forward flexes the shoulder to 60 to 80° while at the same time taking the thumb of the other hand off the coracoid process and pushing the head of the humerus posteriorly. The head of the humerus can be felt by the index finger of the same hand (Fig. 4–30). The test is usually pain free, but the patient may exhibit apprehension. A positive test is indicative of posterior instability.

Norwood Stress Test for Posterior Instability.[27] The patient lies supine with the shoulder abducted 60 to 100° and laterally rotated 90° with the elbow flexed to 90° so the arm is horizontal. The examiner stabilizes the scapula with one hand, palpating the posterior humeral head with the fingers, and stabilizes the upper limb by holding the forearm and elbow at the elbow. The examiner then brings the arm into forward flexion (Fig. 4–31). Cofield and Irving[28] recommend medially rotating the forearm approximately 20° after the forward flexion, then pushing the elbow posteriorly to enhance the effect of the test. A positive test is indicated by the humeral head's slipping posteriorly relative to the glenoid. Care must be taken because the test does not cause apprehension but may cause subluxation or dislocation. The patient confirms that the sensation felt is the same sensation felt during activities. The arm

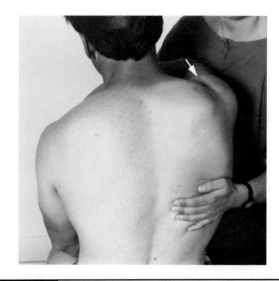

FIGURE 4–32. *Jerk test.*

is returned to the starting position, and the humeral head will be felt to reduce. A clicking may accompany either subluxation or reduction.

Jerk Test.[23] The patient sits with the arm medially rotated and forward flexed to 90°. The examiner grasps the patient's elbow and axially loads the humerus in a proximal direction. While maintaining the axial loading, the examiner moves the arm horizontally (cross-flexion) across the body (Fig. 4–32). A positive test for recurrent posterior instability is the production of a sudden jerk as the humeral head slides off (subluxes) the back of the glenoid (Fig. 4–33). When the arm is returned to the original 90° abduction position, a second jerk may be felt as the head reduces.

Push-Pull Test.[23] The patient lies supine. The examiner holds the patient's arm at the wrist, abducts the arm 90°, and forward flexes it 30°. The examiner places the other hand over the humerus close to the humeral head. The examiner then pulls up on the arm at the wrist while pushing down on the humerus with the other hand (Fig. 4–34). Normally, 50% posterior translation can be accomplished. If more than 50% posterior translation occurs or the patient becomes apprehensive, the examiner should suspect posterior instability.

Posterior Apprehension Test. The examiner forward flexes and medially rotates the patient's shoulder (Fig. 4–35). The examiner then applies a posterior force on the patient's elbow. A positive result is indicated by a look of apprehension or alarm on the patient's face and the patient's resistance to further motion. The test is indicative of a posterior dislocation of the humerus. The test should also be performed with the arm in 90° of abduction. The examiner palpates the head of the humerus with

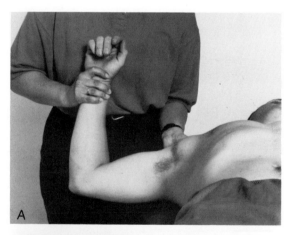

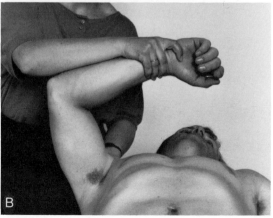

FIGURE 4–31. *Norwood stress test for posterior shoulder instability. (A) Arm abducted 90°. (B) Arm forward flexed.*

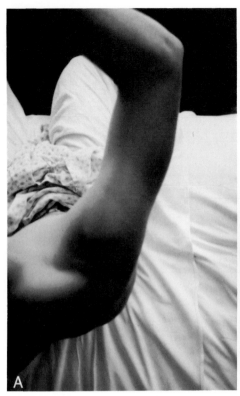

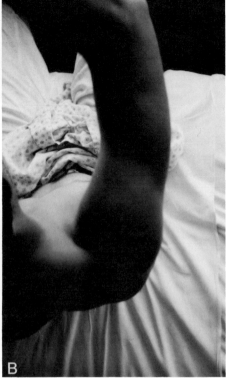

FIGURE 4–33. Positive jerk test. (A) Normal appearance of the shoulder before the patient performs a jerk test. (B) With axial loading and movement of the arm horizontally across the body, the humeral head slides off the back of the glenoid, as demonstrated by the prominence in the anterior aspect of the patient's shoulder. This maneuver resulted in a sudden jerk and some discomfort. (From Matsen, F. A., S. C. Thomas, and C. A. Rockwood: Glenohumeral Instability. In Rockwood, C. A., and F. A. Matsen (eds.): The Shoulder. Philadelphia, W. B. Saunders Co., 1990, p. 551.)

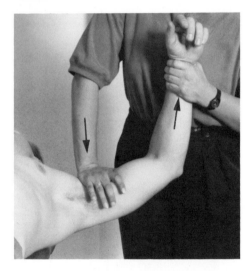

FIGURE 4–34. Push-pull test.

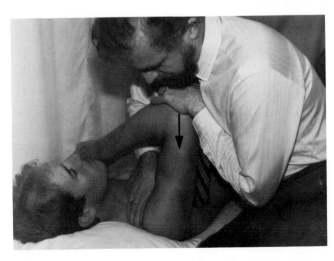

FIGURE 4–35. Posterior apprehension test.

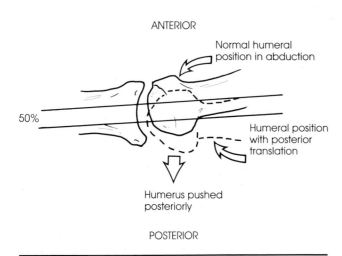

FIGURE 4–36. The posterior stress examination should produce no translation beyond 50% of the diameter of the humeral head in the glenoid.

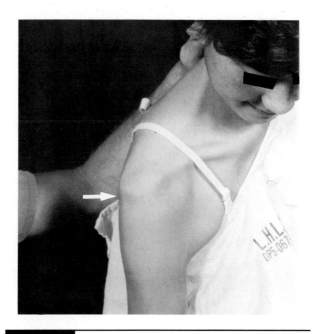

FIGURE 4–38. Positive sulcus sign. (Adapted from Hawkins, R. J., and D. J. Bokor: Clinical evaluation of shoulder problems. In Rockwood, C. A., and R. A. Matsen (eds.): The Shoulder. Philadelphia, W. B. Saunders Co., 1990, p. 169.)

one hand while the other hand pushes the head of the humerus posteriorly (Fig. 4–36). In either case, if the humeral head moves posteriorly more than 50% of its size, posterior instability is evident.[19] The movement may be accompanied by a clunk.

Tests for Inferior and Multidirectional Shoulder Instability

It is believed that if a patient demonstrates inferior instability, multidirectional instability will also be present.

Test for Inferior Shoulder Instability (Sulcus Sign).[17, 23] The patient stands with the arm by the side and shoulder muscles relaxed. The examiner grasps the patient's forearm below the elbow and pushes the arm distally (Fig. 4–37). The presence of a sulcus sign (Figs. 4–5B and 4–38) is indicative of inferior instability.

Feagin Test.[21] The patient stands with the arm abducted to 90° and the elbow extended resting on the top of the examiner's shoulder. The examiner's hands are clasped together over the patient's humerus between the upper and middle thirds. The examiner pushes the humerus down and forward (Fig. 4–39). A look of apprehension on the patient's

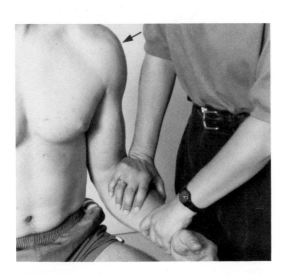

FIGURE 4–37. Test for inferior shoulder instability (sulcus test). Arrow indicates where to look for sulcus, which is not evident in this patient.

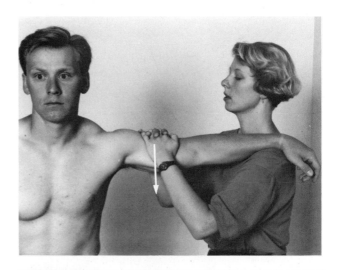

FIGURE 4–39. Feagin test.

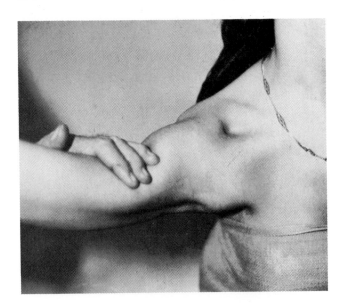

FIGURE 4–40. A 21-year-old woman whose shoulder could be dislocated inferiorly and anteriorly and subluxated posteriorly. She was unable to carry books, reach overhead, or use the arm for activities such as tennis or swimming. There were associated episodes of numbness and weakness of the entire upper extremity that at times lasted for 1 or 2 days. (From Neer, C. S., and C. R. Foster: J. Bone Joint Surg. 62A:900, 1980.)

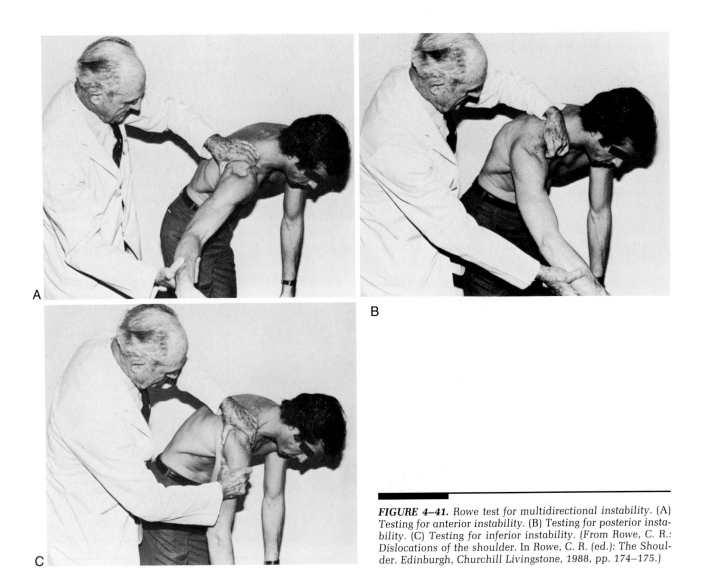

FIGURE 4–41. Rowe test for multidirectional instability. (A) Testing for anterior instability. (B) Testing for posterior instability. (C) Testing for inferior instability. (From Rowe, C. R.: Dislocations of the shoulder. In Rowe, C. R. (ed.): The Shoulder. Edinburgh, Churchill Livingstone, 1988, pp. 174–175.)

face indicates a positive test and indicates anteroinferior instability (Fig. 4–40).

Rowe Test for Multidirectional Instability.[22] The patient stands forward flexed 45° at the waist with the arms relaxed, pointing at the floor. The examiner places one hand over the shoulder so the index and middle fingers sit over the anterior aspect of the humeral head and the thumb sits over the posterior aspect of the humeral head. The examiner then pulls the arm down slightly (Fig. 4–41). To test for anterior instability, the humeral head is pushed anteriorly with the thumb while the arm is extended 20 to 30° from the vertical position. To test for posterior instability, the humeral head is pushed posteriorly with the index and middle fingers while the arm is flexed 20 to 30° from the vertical position. For inferior instability, more traction is applied to the arm, and the sulcus sign is evident.

Test for Other Shoulder Joints

Acromioclavicular Shear Test.[19] With the patient in the sitting position, the examiner cups the hands over the deltoid muscle with one hand on the clavicle and one hand on the spine of the scapula. The examiner then squeezes the heels of the hands together (Fig. 4–42). A positive test is indicated by pain or abnormal movement at the acromioclavicular joint and is indicative of acromioclavicular joint pathology.

Tests for Muscle/Tendon Pathology

Yergason's Test. With the patient's elbow flexed to 90° and stabilized against the thorax with the forearm pronated, the examiner resists supination while the patient also laterally rotates the arm against resistance (Fig. 4–43).[29] A positive result

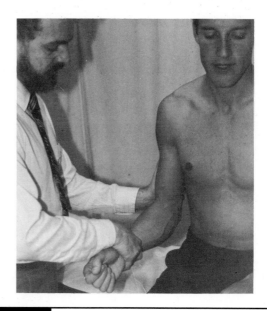

FIGURE 4–43. Yergason's test.

elicits tenderness in the bicipital groove, or the tendon may pop out of the groove and is indicative of bicipital tendinitis. This test is not particularly effective, because the tendon does not move in the bicipital groove during the test and because biceps tendon pain tends to occur with motion or palpation rather than with tension.

Speed's Test (Biceps or Straight Arm Test). The examiner resists shoulder forward flexion by the patient while the patient's forearm is supinated and the elbow is completely extended (Fig. 4–44). A positive test elicits increased tenderness in the bicipital groove and is indicative of bicipital tendinitis. Speed's test is more effective than Yergason's

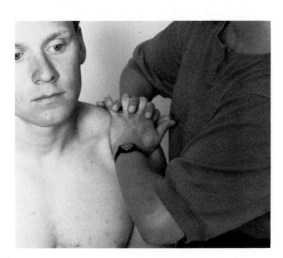

FIGURE 4–42. Acromioclavicular shear test.

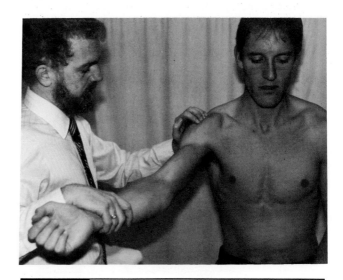

FIGURE 4–44. Biceps test (Speed's test).

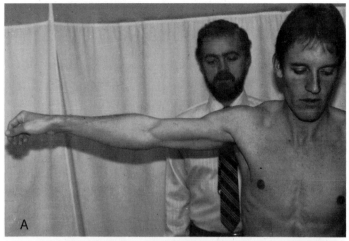

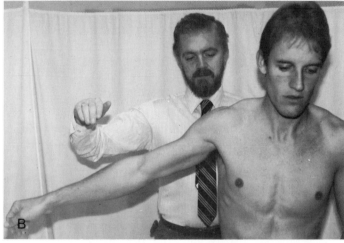

FIGURE 4–45. Drop-arm test. (A) *The patient abducts the arm to 90°.* (B) *The patient tries to lower the arm slowly and is unable to do so; instead, the arm drops to his side. Examiner's hand is illustrating the start position.*

test because the bone moves over the tendon during the test.

Drop Arm Test. The examiner abducts the patient's shoulder to 90° and then asks the patient to slowly lower it to the side in the same arc of movement (Fig. 4–45). A positive test is indicated if the patient is unable to return the arm to the side slowly or has severe pain when attempting to do so. A positive result indicates a tear in the rotator cuff complex.[30]

Ludington's Test.[31] The patient clasps both hands on top of the head, allowing the interlocking fingers to support the weight of the upper limbs (Fig. 4–46). This action allows maximum relaxation of the biceps tendon in its resting position. The patient then alternately contracts and relaxes the biceps muscles. While the patient does the contractions and relaxations, the examiner palpates the biceps tendon, which will be felt on the uninvolved side but not on the affected side if the test result is positive. A positive result indicates a rupture of the long head of biceps tendon.

Supraspinatus Test. The patient's shoulder is abducted to 90° with neutral (no) rotation, and resistance to abduction is provided by the examiner. The shoulder is then medially rotated and angled forward 30° so that the patient's thumbs point toward the floor (Fig. 4–47). Resistance to abduction is again given while the examiner looks for weakness or pain, reflecting a positive test result. A positive test result indicates a tear of the supraspinatus

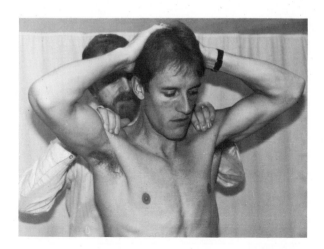

FIGURE 4–46. Ludington's test.

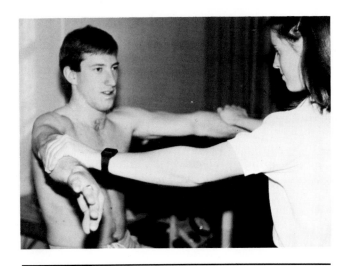

FIGURE 4–47. Supraspinatus test.

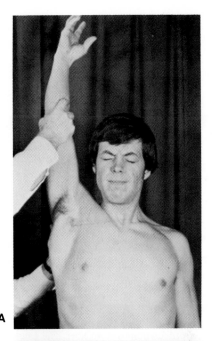

A

B

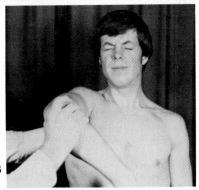

FIGURE 4–48. Impingement sign. (A) A positive impingement sign is present if pain and its resulting facial expression are produced when the arm is forcibly flexed forward by the examiner, jamming the greater tuberosity against the anteroinferior surface of the acromium. (B) An alternative method (Hawkins-Kennedy impingement test) of demonstrating the impingement sign is by forcibly internally rotating the proximal humerus when the arm is forward flexed to 90°. (From Hawkins, R. J., and J. C. Kennedy: Am. J. Sports Med. 8:391, 1980.)

tendon or muscle or neuropathy of the suprascapular nerve.

Impingement Test.[32] The patient's arm is forcibly elevated through forward flexion by the examiner's causing a "jamming" of the greater tuberosity against the anteroinferior acromial surface. The patient's face will show pain, reflecting a positive test result (Fig. 4–48A). The test is indicative of an overuse injury to the supraspinatus muscle and sometimes to the biceps tendon.

Hawkins-Kennedy Impingement Test.[33] The patient stands while the examiner forward flexes the arms to 90° and then forcibly internally rotates the shoulder (Fig. 4–48B). This movement pushes the supraspinatus tendon against the anterior surface of the coracoacromial ligament (Fig. 4–49). Pain indicates a positive test for supraspinatus tendinitis.

Gilchrest Sign.[19, 34] While standing, the patient lifts a 2 to 3 kg weight over the head. The arm is externally rotated fully and lowered to the side in the coronal plane. A positive test is indicated by discomfort or by pain in the bicipital groove. A positive test indicates bicipital tendinitis. In some cases, an audible snap or pain may be felt between 100 and 90° abduction.

Lippman Test. The patient sits or stands while the examiner holds the arm flexed to 90° with one hand. With the other hand, the examiner palpates the biceps tendon 7 to 8 cm below the glenohumeral joint and moves the biceps tendon from side to side in the bicipital groove. A sharp pain is a positive test and indicates bicipital tendinitis.

Heuter's Sign.[34] Normally, if elbow flexion is resisted when the arm is pronated, some supination will occur as the biceps attempts to help the brachialis muscle flex the elbow. This supination movement is called Heuter's sign. If it is absent, the biceps tendon has been disrupted.

Pectoralis Major Contracture Test. The patient lies supine and clasps the hands together behind the head. The arms are then lowered until the elbows touch the examining table (Fig. 4–50). A positive test occurs when the elbows do not reach the table and indicates a tight pectoralis major muscle.

Tests for Neurological Function

Upper Limb Tension (Brachial Plexus Tension) Test.[35] This test is the upper limb equivalent of the straight leg raising test of the lower limb. The patient

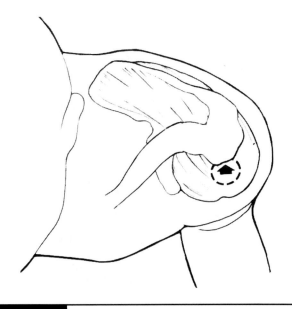

FIGURE 4–49. *The functional arc of elevation of the proximal humerus is forward, as proposed by Neer. The greater tuberosity impinges against the anterior one third of the acromial surface. This critical area comprises the supraspinatus and bicipital tendons and the subacromial bursa. (From Hawkins, R. J., and J. S. Abrams: Orthop. Clin. North Am. 18:374, 1987.)*

is positioned to stress the brachial plexus, primarily the median nerve and C5–C7 nerve roots. The patient lies supine. To perform the test, the examiner takes the patient's arm into abduction and lateral rotation behind the coronal plane at the shoulder. The shoulder girdle is fixed in depression. The elbow is then passively extended with the wrist held in extension and the forearm in supination (Fig. 4–51). Pain in the form of a stretch or ache in the cubital fossa or of tingling in the thumb and first three fingers indicates stretching of the dura mater in the cervical spine and tension on the median nerve. The available range of passive extension of the elbow when compared with the "normal" side can give an indication of the restriction. Lateral flexion of the cervical spine to the opposite side can enhance the effect. If full range of motion is not available in the shoulder, the test can still be performed by taking the shoulder to the point just short of pain in abduction and lateral rotation and performing the other maneuvers of the arm or by passive lateral gliding of the cervical spine.

Tinel's Sign (at the Shoulder). The area of the brachial plexus above the clavicle in the area of the scalene triangle is tapped. A positive sign is indicated by a tingling sensation in one or more of the nerve roots.

Tests for Thoracic Outlet Syndrome

It must be remembered when doing any thoracic outlet test that the examiner must find the pulse before positioning the patient's arm or cervical spine, and that even in a "normal" individual, the pulse may be diminished.

Allen Test.[36] The examiner flexes the patient's elbow to 90° while the shoulder is extended horizontally and rotated laterally (Fig. 4–52). The patient then rotates the head away from the test side. The examiner palpates the radial pulse, which will become absent (disappear) when the head is rotated away from the test side. The pulse disappearance indicates a positive test result for *thoracic outlet syndrome.*

Wright Test or Maneuver. Wright[37] advocated "hyperabducting" the arm so that the hand is brought over the head with the elbow and arm in the coronal plane. He advocated doing the test in the sitting and then the supine positions. Taking a

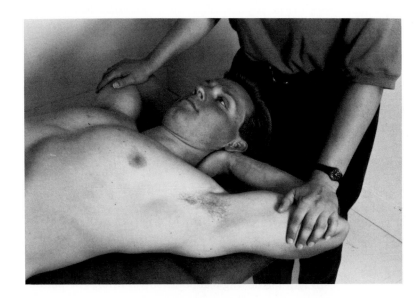

FIGURE 4–50. *Pectoralis major flexibility test. Examiner is testing end feel.*

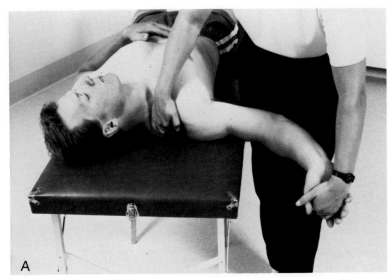

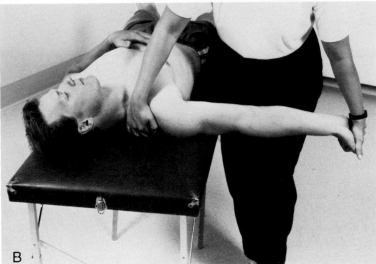

FIGURE 4–51. Upper limb tension test (brachial plexus tension test). (A) Commencing position of brachial plexus tension test. Fixation of the shoulder girdle in depression, glenohumeral abduction, and external rotation. (B) Brachial plexus tension test is completed by extension of the elbow. In less sensitive conditions the wrist would be extended and the cervical spine would be placed into lateral flexion to the contralateral side.

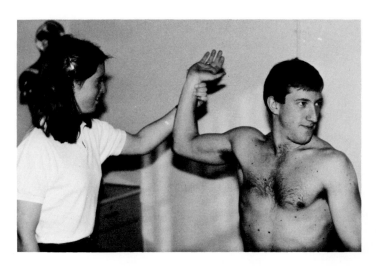

FIGURE 4–52. Allen maneuver.

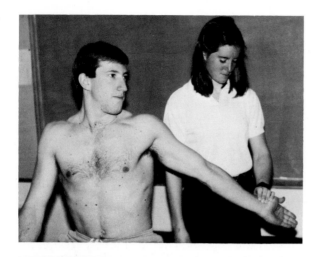

FIGURE 4–53. Adson maneuver.

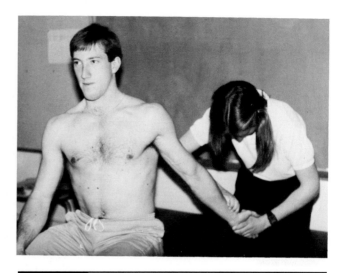

FIGURE 4–55. Costoclavicular syndrome test.

breath, rotating, or extending the head and neck may have an additional effect. The pulse is again palpated for differences.

Adson Maneuver.[38] This test is probably the most common method of testing for thoracic outlet syndrome. The examiner locates the radial pulse. The patient's head is rotated to face the test shoulder (Fig. 4–53). The patient then extends the head while the examiner laterally rotates and extends the patient's shoulder. The patient is instructed to take a deep breath and hold it. A disappearance of the pulse indicates a positive test.

Halstead Maneuver. The examiner finds the radial pulse and applies a downward traction on the test extremity while the patient's neck is hyperextended and the head is rotated to the opposite side (Fig. 4–54). Absence or disappearance of a pulse indicates a positive test for thoracic outlet syndrome.

Costoclavicular Syndrome Test. The examiner palpates the radial pulse and then draws the pa-

tient's shoulder down and back (Fig. 4–55). A positive test is indicated by an absence of the pulse and indicates thoracic outlet syndrome. This test is particularly effective in patients who complain of symptoms while wearing a backpack or heavy coat.

Roos Test.[39] The patient stands and abducts the arms to 90°, externally rotates the shoulders, and flexes the elbows to 90°. The patient then opens and closes the hands slowly for 3 minutes (Fig. 4–56). If the patient is unable to keep the arms in the starting position for 3 minutes or suffers ischemic pain, heaviness of the arm, or numbness and tingling of the hand during the 3 minutes, the test is positive for thoracic outlet syndrome on the affected side.

Provocative Elevation Test.[24] The patient elevates both arms above the horizontal and is asked to rapidly open and close the hands 15 times. If fatigue, cramping, or tingling occurs during the test, the test is positive for vascular insufficiency and thoracic outlet syndrome.

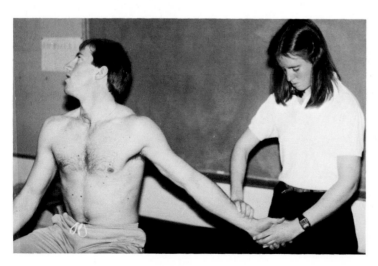

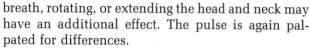

FIGURE 4–54. Halstead maneuver.

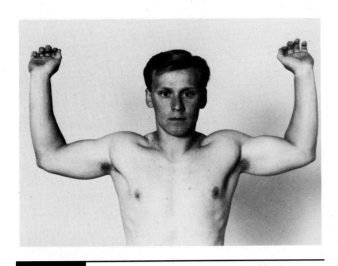

FIGURE 4-56. Roos test.

Reflexes and Cutaneous Distribution

The reflexes in the shoulder region that are often assessed include the pectoralis major clavicular portion (C5–C6), sternocostal portion (C7–C8 and T1), the biceps (C5–C6), and the triceps (C7–C8) (Fig. 4–57). The examiner must also be aware of the dermatomal patterns of the nerve roots (Fig. 4–58) as well as the cutaneous distribution of the peripheral nerves (Fig. 4–59). The examiner should remember that dermatomes will vary from person to person; thus, the accompanying diagrams are estimations only. A test for altered sensation is performed by running the relaxed hands and fingers over the neck, shoulder, and anterior and posterior chest area. Any difference in sensation should be noted. These differences can be mapped out more exactly using a pinwheel, pin, brush, and/or cotton batting.

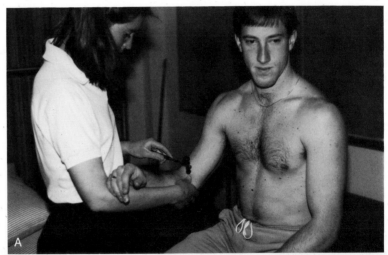

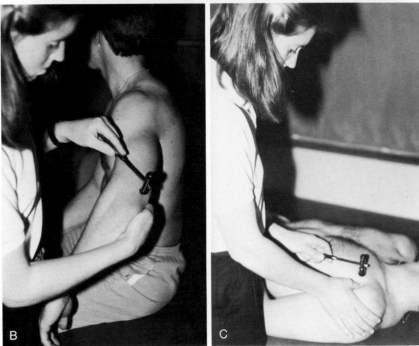

FIGURE 4-57. Positioning to test the reflexes around the shoulder. (A) Biceps. (B) Triceps. (C) Pectoralis major.

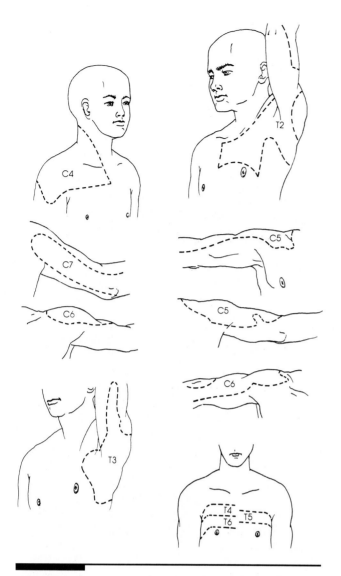

FIGURE 4–58. Dermatomal pattern of the shoulder. Dermatomes on one side only are illustrated.

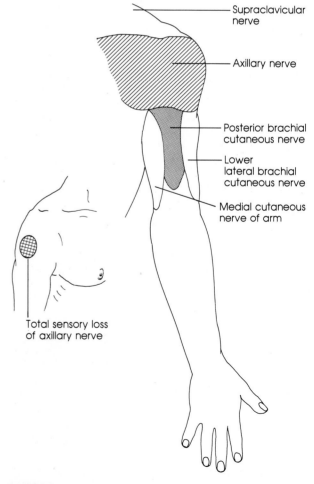

Supraclavicular nerve

Axillary nerve

Posterior brachial cutaneous nerve

Lower lateral brachial cutaneous nerve

Medial cutaneous nerve of arm

Total sensory loss of axillary nerve

FIGURE 4–59. Cutaneous distribution of peripheral nerves around the shoulder.

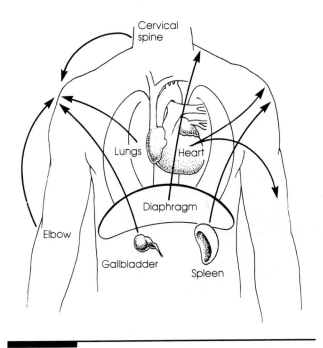

FIGURE 4–60. *Structures referring pain to the shoulder.*

True shoulder pain rarely extends below the elbow. Pain in the acromioclavicular and sternoclavicular joints tends to be localized to the affected joint and usually does not spread or radiate. Pain can be referred to the shoulder from many structures,[40] including the cervical spine, elbow, lungs, heart, diaphragm, gallbladder, and spleen (Fig. 4–60).

Joint Play Movements

Joint play movements[13, 41] are usually performed with the patient lying supine. The examiner compares the amount of available movement on the affected side with the movement on the unaffected side.

The joint play movements performed at the shoulder are shown in Figure 4–61 and include the following:

1. Backward glide of the humerus.
2. Forward glide of the humerus.
3. Lateral distraction of the humerus.
4. Caudal glide of the humerus (long arm traction).
5. Backward glide of the humerus in abduction.
6. Lateral distraction of the humerus in abduction.
7. Anteroposterior and cephalocaudal movements of the clavicle at the acromioclavicular joint.
8. Anteroposterior and cephalocaudal movements of the clavicle at the sternoclavicular joint.
9. General movement of the scapula to determine mobility.

To perform the backward joint play movement of the humerus, the examiner grasps the patient's upper limb, placing one hand around the humerus as high up in the axilla as possible. The other hand is placed around the humerus above and near the elbow (Fig. 4–61A). The examiner then applies a backward force, keeping the patient's arm parallel to the body so that no rotation or torsion occurs at the glenohumeral joint.

Forward joint play movement of the humerus is carried out in a similar fashion, with the examiner's hands as shown in Figure 4–61B. The examiner applies an anterior force, keeping the patient's arm parallel to the body so that no rotation or torsion occurs at the glenohumeral joint.

To apply a lateral distraction joint play movement to the humerus, the examiner's hands are placed as shown in Figure 4–61C. Then, a lateral distraction force is applied to the glenohumeral joint, with the patient's arm kept parallel to the body so that no rotation or torsion occurs at the glenohumeral joint.

Caudal glide joint play movement is performed with the patient in the same supine position. The examiner grasps above the patient's wrist with one hand and palpates below the distal spine of the scapula posteriorly and below the distal clavicle anteriorly over the glenohumeral joint line with the other hand (Fig. 4–61E). The examiner then applies a traction force to the shoulder while palpating to see whether the head of the humerus drops down (moves distally) in the glenoid cavity as it normally should. If the patient complains of pain in the elbow, the test may be done with the hands positioned as in Figure 4–61D.

The examiner then abducts the patient's arm to 90°, grasping above the patient's wrist with one hand while stabilizing the thorax with the other hand. The examiner then applies a "long arm" traction force to determine joint play in this position.

With the patient's arm abducted to 90°, the examiner then grasps the humerus with both hands as close to the thorax as possible and applies a backward force, keeping the patient's arm parallel to the body. This movement is a backward joint play movement of the humerus in abduction (Fig. 4–61F).

To assess the acromioclavicular and sternoclavicular joints, the examiner gently grasps the clavicle as close to the joint to be tested as possible and moves it in and out and up and down while palpating the joint with the other hand. A comparison of the amount of movement available is made between the two sides (Figs. 4–61G and 4–61H).

For a determination of mobility of the scapula, the patient lies on one side to fixate the thorax with the arm relaxed by the side. The uppermost scapula is tested in this position. The examiner faces the patient, placing the lower hand (farthest from the

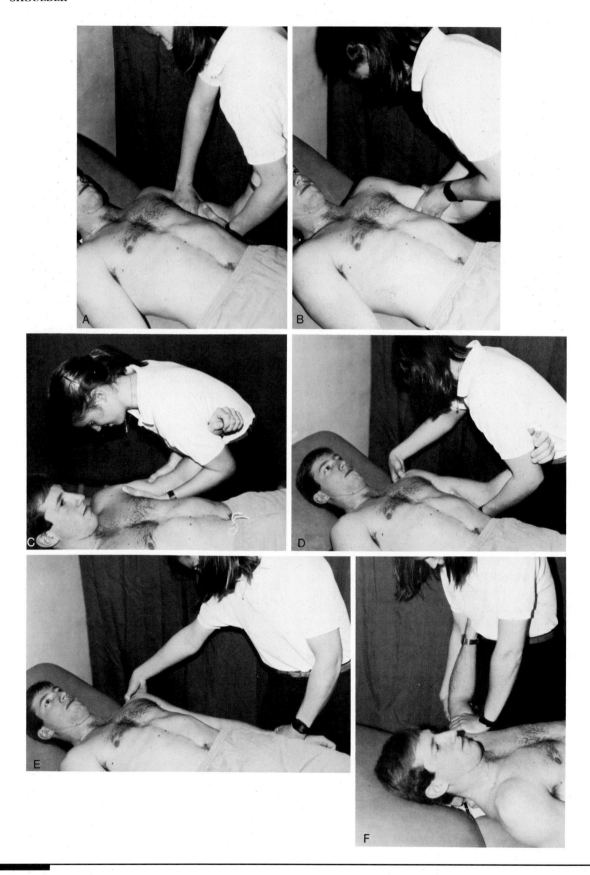

FIGURE 4–61. *Joint play movements of the shoulder complex. (A) Backward glide of the humerus. (B) Forward glide of the humerus. (C) Lateral distraction of the humerus. (D) Long arm traction. (E) Long arm traction applied below elbow. (F) Backward glide of the humerus in abduction.*

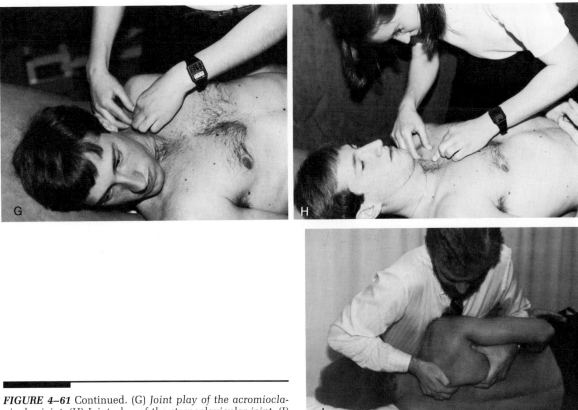

FIGURE 4–61 Continued. (G) *Joint play of the acromiocla-vicular joint.* (H) *Joint play of the sternoclavicular joint.* (I) *General movement of the scapula to determine mobility.*

head) under the patient's arm so that the patient's arm rests on the examiner's forearm. The hand of the examiner's same arm holds the upper (cranial) dorsal surface of the patient's scapula. By holding the scapula in this way, the examiner is able to move it medially, laterally, caudally, cranially, and away from the thorax (Fig. 4–61*I*).

Palpation

When palpating the shoulder complex, the examiner should note any muscle spasm, tenderness, abnormal "bumps," or other signs and symptoms that may indicate the source of pathology. The examiner should perform palpation in a systematic manner, beginning with the anterior structures and working around to the posterior structures. Findings on the injured side should be compared with those on the unaffected, or "uninjured," side. Any differences between the two sides should be noted because they may give an indication of the cause of the patient's problems.

Anterior Structures

The anterior structures of the shoulder may be palpated with the patient in the supine lying or sitting position (Fig. 4–62A).

Clavicle. The clavicle should be palpated along its full length for tenderness or abnormal bumps, such as a callus formation following a fracture, and to ensure that it is in its resting position relative to the uninjured side. That is, it may be rotated ante-riorly or posteriorly more than the unaffected side or one end may be higher than that of the uninjured side, indicating a possible subluxation or dislocation at the sternoclavicular or acromioclavicular joint.

Sternoclavicular Joint. The sternoclavicular joint should be palpated for normal positioning relative to the sternum and first rib. Palpation should also include supporting ligaments and sternocleidomas-toid muscle. Adjacent to the joint, the suprasternal notch may be palpated. From the notch, the exam-iner moves the fingers laterally and posteriorly to palpate the first rib. The examiner should apply slight caudal pressure to the first rib on both sides

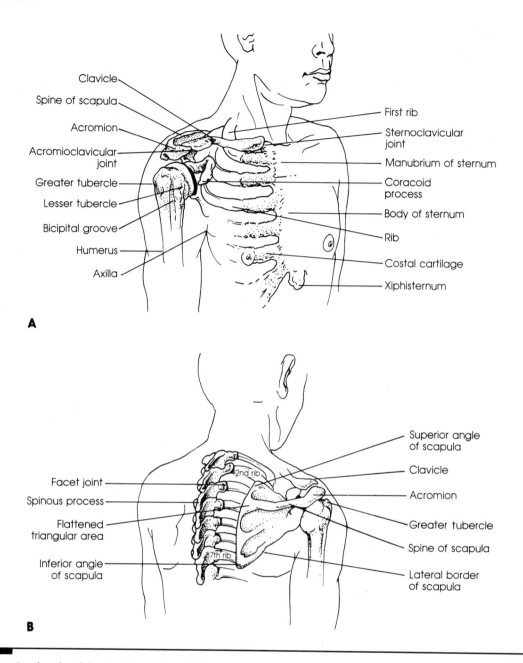

A

B

FIGURE 4–62. Landmarks of the shoulder region. (A) Anterior view. (B) Posterior view.

and note any difference. Spasm of the scalene muscles or pathology in the area may result in elevation of the first rib on the affected side.

Acromioclavicular Joint. Like the sternoclavicular joint, the acromioclavicular joint should be palpated for normal positioning and tenderness. Likewise, supporting ligaments (acromioclavicular and coracoclavicular) and the trapezius, subclavius, and deltoid (anterior, middle, and posterior fibers) muscles should be palpated for tenderness and spasm.

Coracoid Process. The coracoid process may be palpated approximately 2.5 cm below the junction of the lateral one third and medial two thirds of the clavicle. The short head of the biceps and coracobrachialis muscles originate from and the pectoralis minor inserts into this process.

Sternum. In the midline of the chest, the examiner should palpate the three portions of the sternum (manubrium, body, and xiphoid process), noting any abnormality or tenderness.

Ribs and Costal Cartilage. Adjacent to the sternum, the examiner should palpate the sternocostal and costochondral articulations, noting any swelling, tenderness, or other abnormality. These "articulations" are sometimes sprained or subluxed or a costochondritis (Tietze's syndrome) may be evident. The examiner should palpate the ribs as they extend around the chest wall, looking for any potential pathology.

Humerus and Rotator Cuff Muscles. Moving laterally from the chest and caudally from the acromion process, the examiner should palpate the humerus

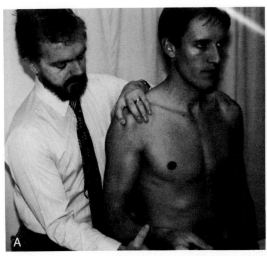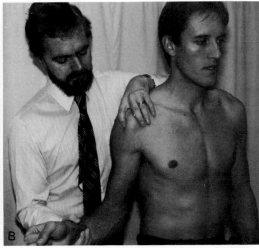

FIGURE 4–63. *Palpation around the shoulder—greater tuberosity (A) and lesser tuberosity (B). Bicipital groove lies between (A) and* (B).

and its surrounding structures for potential pathology. The examiner first palpates the lateral tip of the acromion process and then moves inferiorly to the greater tuberosity of the humerus. The examiner should then laterally rotate the humerus. During palpation, the long head of the biceps in the bicipital groove will slip under the fingers, followed by the lesser tuberosity of the humerus (Fig. 4–63). As with all palpation, the testing should be done gently and carefully to prevent causing the patient undue pain. By alternately rotating the humerus laterally and medially, the smooth progression over the three structures will normally be noted. It will also be noted that the lesser tuberosity is at the level of the coracoid process. If the examiner then palpates along the lesser tuberosity and the lip of the bicipital groove, the fingers will rest on the tendon of subscapularis muscle. If the examiner places the thumb over the lesser tuberosity and "grips" the shoulder between the second, third, and fourth fingers as shown in Figure 4–1, the fingers will be over the insertion of the other three rotator cuff muscles—supraspinatus, infraspinatus, and teres minor. Moving laterally over the bicipital groove to its other lip, the examiner may then palpate the insertion of pectoralis major muscle. The patient is then asked to further medially rotate the humerus so that the forearm rests behind the back, and the examiner palpates just inferior to the anterior aspect of the acromion process for the supraspinatus tendon. Any tenderness of the tendon should be noted. The examiner then passively abducts the patient's shoulder to 80 to 90° and palpates the notch formed by the acromion-spine of the scapula and the clavicle. In the notch, the examiner will be palpating the musculotendinous junction of the supraspinatus muscle.

Axilla. With the shoulder slightly abducted (20 to 30°), the examiner may palpate the structures of the axilla-latissimus dorsi muscle (posterior wall), pectoralis major muscle (anterior wall), serratus anterior muscle (medial wall), lymph nodes (palpable only if swollen), and brachial artery. The patient is then asked to lie prone "on the elbows" with the shoulders slightly laterally rotated and the elbow slightly adducted in relation to the shoulder. The examiner then palpates just inferior to the most lateral aspect of the scapula for the insertion of the infraspinatus muscle. Just distal to this insertion, the examiner may be able to palpate the insertion of teres minor.

Posterior Structures

To complete the palpation, the patient may be either sitting or lying prone with the upper limb by the trunk (Fig. 4–63B).

Spine of Scapula. From the acromion process the examiner moves along the spine of the scapula, noting any tenderness or abnormality.

Scapula. The examiner follows the spine of the scapula to the medial border of the scapula and then the outline of the scapula, which normally extends from the spinous process of T2 to the spinous process of T7. The examiner then moves around the inferior angle of the scapula and along the lateral border of the scapula. After the borders of the scapula have been palpated, the posterior surface (supraspinatus and infraspinatus muscles) may be palpated for tenderness, atrophy, or spasm.

Spinous Processes of Lower Cervical and Thoracic Spine. In the midline, the examiner may palpate the cervical and thoracic spinous processes for any abnormality. This is followed by palpation of the trapezius muscle.

Triceps Tendon. Inferior to the posterior aspect of the acromion process, the examiner may palpate

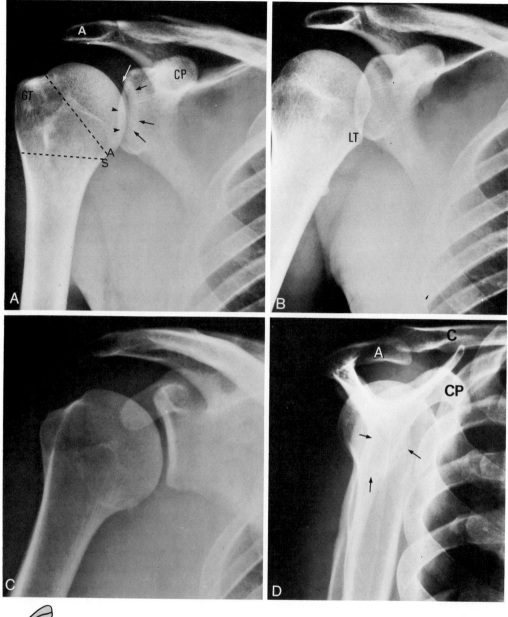

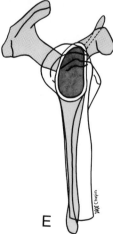

FIGURE 4-64. *Normal radiographic examination. (A) External rotation. The greater tuberosity (GT) is seen in profile. The humeral head normally overlaps the glenoid on this view. The anterior (small arrows) and posterior (arrowheads) glenoid margins are well seen and do not overlap owing to the anterior tilt of the glenoid. The anatomic (A, black) and surgical (S) necks of the humerus are indicated. CP = Coracoid process, A (white) = acromion process. A vacuum phenomenon (white arrow) is present. (B) Internal rotation. The overlap of the greater tuberosity and the humeral head produces a rounded appearance of the proximal humerus. LT = Lesser tuberosity. A small exostosis is noted projecting from the humeral metaphysis. (C) Posterior oblique. The glenohumeral cartilage space is seen in profile with no overlap of the humerus and glenoid. (D) Normal scapular "Y" view. This true lateral view of the scapula (anterior oblique of the shoulder) shows the humeral head centered over the glenoid (arrows). A = Acromion, C = clavicle, CP = coracoid process. (E) Diagram of normal scapular Y.*

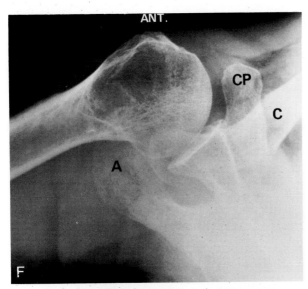

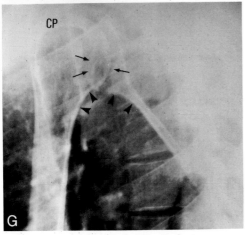

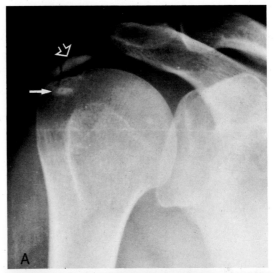

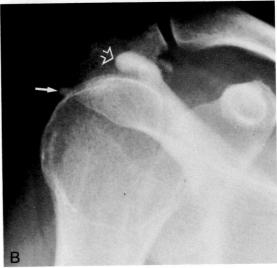

2. The relation of the clavicle to the acromion process.
3. Whether the epiphyseal plate of the humeral head is present and, if so, whether it is normal.
4. Whether there are any calcifications in any of the tendons (Fig. 4–65), especially those of the supraspinatus or infraspinatus muscles.

A stress anteroposterior radiograph may be used to "gap" the injured acromioclavicular joint to see whether there has been a third-degree sprain or to show an inferior laxity at the glenohumeral joint

FIGURE 4–64 Continued (F) *Axillary view. CP = Coracoid process, A = acromion, ANT. = anterior, C = clavicle. (G) Normal transthoracic view. The smooth arch formed by the inferior border of the scapula and the posterior aspect of the humerus is indicated (arrowheads). The coracoid process (CP) is faintly seen. The margins of the glenoid are indicated (arrows). This view is slightly oblique, allowing the glenoid to be seen more en face than usual. (From Weissman, B. N. W., and C. B. Sledge: Orthopedic Radiology. Philadelphia, W. B. Saunders Co., 1986, p. 219.)*

the tendon of the long head of triceps as it originates from the infraglenoid tubercle.

Radiographic Examination

Anteroposterior View. With this view (Fig. 4–64), the examiner should note:

1. The relation of the humerus to the glenoid cavity.

FIGURE 4–65. *Calcific tendinitis—supraspinatus and infraspinatus. (A) External rotation view shows calcification projected over the base of the greater tuberosity (arrow) and above the greater tuberosity (open arrow). (B) Internal rotation view projects the infraspinatus calcification (arrow) in profile and documents its posterior location. The supraspinatus calcification (open arrow) is rotated medially and maintains its superior location. (From Weissman, B. N. W., and C. B. Sledge: Orthopedic Radiology. Philadelphia, W. B. Saunders Co., 1986, p. 227.)*

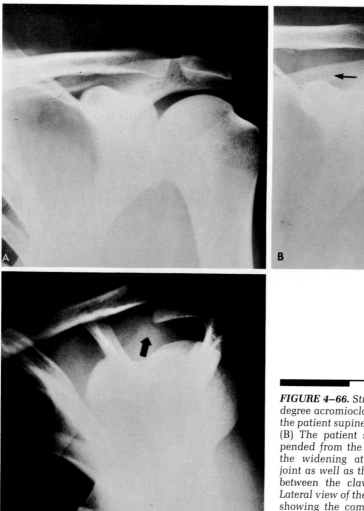

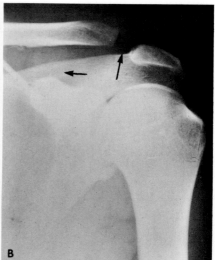

FIGURE 4–66. Stress radiograph for third-degree acromioclavicular sprain. (A) With the patient supine, no dislocation is noted. (B) The patient standing with 4 lb suspended from the wrist. Note particularly the widening at the acromioclavicular joint as well as the difference in distance between the clavicle and coracoid. (C) Lateral view of the acromioclavicular joint showing the complete separation. (From O'Donoghue, D. H.: Treatment of Injuries to Athletes, 4th ed. Philadelphia, W. B. Saunders Co., 1984, p. 142.)

(Fig. 4–66). Medial rotation of the humerus with this view may show a defect on the lateral aspect of the humeral head from recurrent dislocations. This defect is called a Hill-Sach lesion. The examiner should look at the *acromiohumeral interval* (the distance between the acromion process and the humerus) and see whether it is normal.[42] The normal interval is 7 to 14 mm (Fig. 4–67). If this distance decreases, it may be an indication of rotator cuff tears.

Axial Lateral View. For this view to be obtained, the patient must be able to abduct the shoulder. The examiner should note:

1. The relation of the glenoid cavity, humerus, scapula, and clavicle.
2. The acromioclavicular joint. This view is the best for observing this joint.

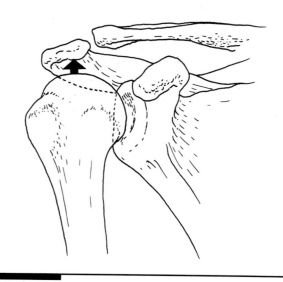

FIGURE 4–67. Acromiohumeral interval.

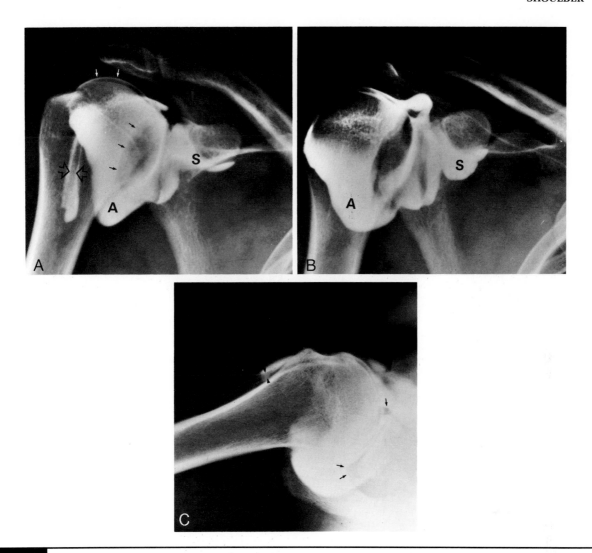

FIGURE 4–68. *Normal single-contrast arthrogram. (A) External rotation. (B) Internal rotation. A = Axillary recess, S = subscapularis recess, open arrows = tendon of long head of biceps within biceps sheath. The humeral articular cartilage is coated with contrast medium (white arrows). There is no contrast agent in the subacromial-subdeltoid bursa. The defect created by the glenoid labrum (arrows) is seen. Filling of the subscapularis recess is often poor on external rotation views because of bursal compression by the subscapularis muscle. In the axillary view (C), the anterior (single arrow), and posterior (double arrow) glenoid labral margins are seen. The biceps tendon (arrowheads) can be seen surrounded by contrast medium in the biceps tendon sheath. No contrast agent overlies the surgical neck of the humerus. (From Weissman, B. N. W., and C. B. Sledge: Orthopedic Radiology. Philadelphia, W. B. Saunders Co., 1986, p. 222.)*

3. Any calcification in the subscapularis, infraspinatus, and teres minor muscles.

Arthrogram. An arthrogram of the shoulder is useful for delineating many of the soft tissues and recesses around the glenohumeral joint (Figs. 4–68 and 4–69).[43–45] For example, the glenohumeral joint will normally hold approximately 16 to 20 ml of solution. With adhesive capsulitis (idiopathic frozen shoulder), the amount the joint will hold may decrease to 5 to 10 ml. The arthrogram will show a decrease in the capacity of the joint and obliteration of the axillary fold. Also, there is an almost complete lack of filling of the subscapular bursa with adhesive capsulitis (Fig. 4–70). Tearing of any structures such as the supraspinatus tendon may result in extravasation of the radiopaque dye.

CT Scans. This technique, especially when combined with radiopaque dye (*computed tomoarthrogram*, or CTA), is effective in diagnosing bone and soft-tissue anomalies and injuries around the shoulder, including tears of the labrum (Fig. 4–71).

MRI. This technique is proving to be useful in delineating soft-tissue injuries to the shoulder. It is possible to differentiate bursitis, tendinitis, and muscle strains, especially with injuries to the rotator cuff. Labial tears and the state of bone marrow can also be diagnosed in the shoulder by using MRI (Figs. 4–72, 4–73, 4–74, and 4–75).

Angiogram. In the case of thoracic outlet syndromes and other arterial impingement-type syndromes, angiograms are sometimes used to demonstrate blockage of the subclavian artery during certain moves (Fig. 4–76).

Text continued on page 139

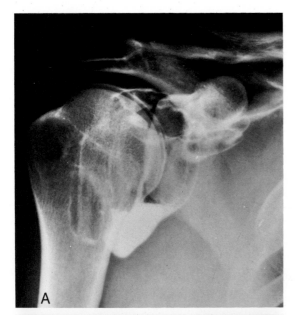

A

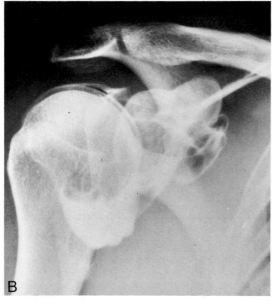

B

FIGURE 4–69. *Normal double-contrast arthrogram. Upright views of the patient with a sandbag suspended from the wrist and the humerus in external rotation (A) and internal rotation (B) show the structures noted on single-contrast examination and allow better appreciation of the articular cartilages. (From Weissman, B. N. W., and C. B. Sledge: Orthopedic Radiology. Philadelphia, W. B. Saunders Co., 1986, p. 223).*

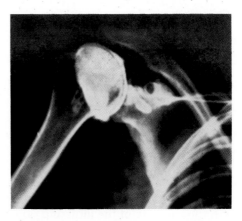

FIGURE 4–70. *Typical arthrographic picture in adhesive capsulitis. Note the absence of dependent axillary fold and poor filling of the biceps. (From Neviaser, J. S.: J. Bone Joint Surg. 44A:1328, 1962.)*

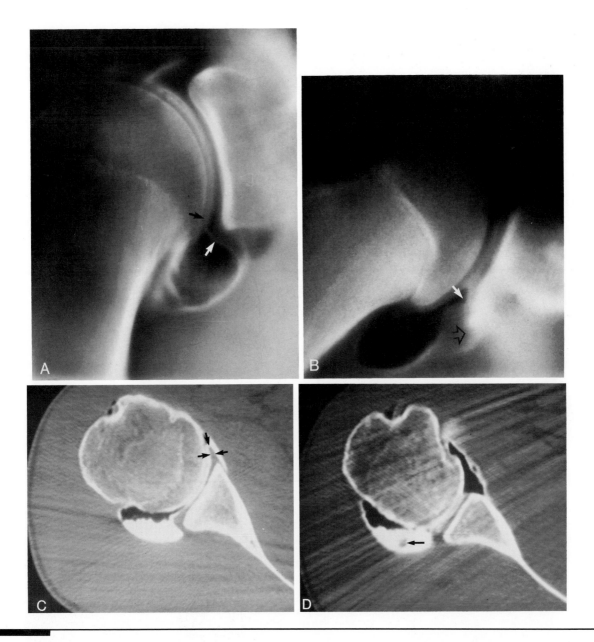

FIGURE 4–71. Tomogram and CT scan of the glenoid labrum. (A) Normal glenoid labrum on posterior oblique double-contrast arthrotomography. Tomographic section through the anterior margin of the glenoid in the posterior oblique position shows smooth articular cartilage on the humeral head and glenoid and a smooth contour to the glenoid labrum (arrows). (B) Abnormal glenoid labrum. Tomographic section shows a triangular defect in the labrum (arrow). The bony margin of the glenoid is also noted to be irregular (open arrow). The patient had suffered a single anterior dislocation. (Courtesy of Dr. Ethan Braunstein, Brigham and Women's Hospital, Boston, Mass.) (C) Normal glenoid labrum on CT after double-contrast arthrography. The sharply pointed anterior (arrows) and the slightly rounder posterior margins of the labrum are well seen. (D) CTA shows absence of the anterior labrum and a loose body (arrow) posteriorly. (C and D courtesy of Arthur Newberg, M.D., Boston, Mass.) (From Weissman, B. N. W., and C. B. Sledge: Orthopedic Radiology. Philadelphia, W. B. Saunders Co., 1986, p. 257.)

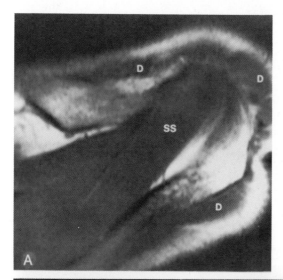

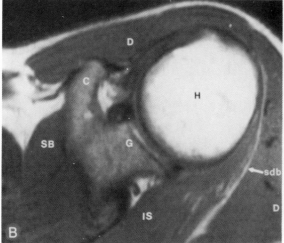

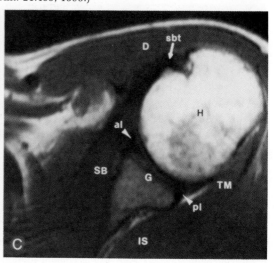

FIGURE 4–72. MRI of T1-weighted axial images from cranial (A) to caudal (C). D = Deltoid muscle, SS = supraspinatus muscle, C = coracoid, H = humerus, SB = subscapularis muscle, G = glenoid of scapula, sdb = subdeltoid-subacromial bursa, IS = infraspinatus muscle, sbt = subscapularis tendon, al = anterior labrum, TM = teres minor muscle, pl = posterior labrum. (From Meyer, S. J. F., and M. K. Dalinka: Orthop. Clin. North Am. 21:499, 1990.)

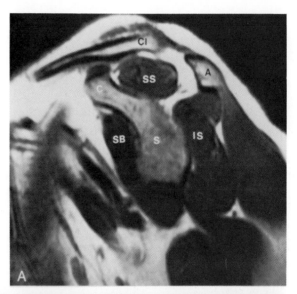

FIGURE 4–73. MRI of T1-weighted sagittal oblique images from medial (A) to lateral (C). Cl = Clavicle, C = coracoid, SS = supraspinatus muscle, A = acromion, SB = subscapularis muscle, S = scapula, IS = infraspinatus muscle, D = deltoid muscle, sst = supraspinatus tendon, ist = infraspinatus tendon, H = humerus, CB = coracobrachialis and biceps (short head) muscle, TM = teres minor muscle. (From Meyer, S. J. F., and M. K. Dalinka: Orthop. Clin. North Am. 21:501, 1990.)

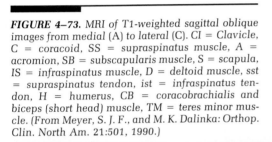

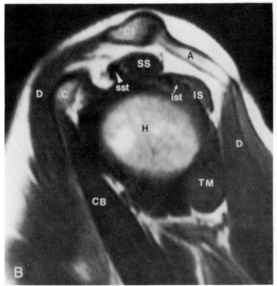

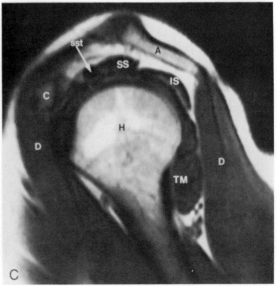

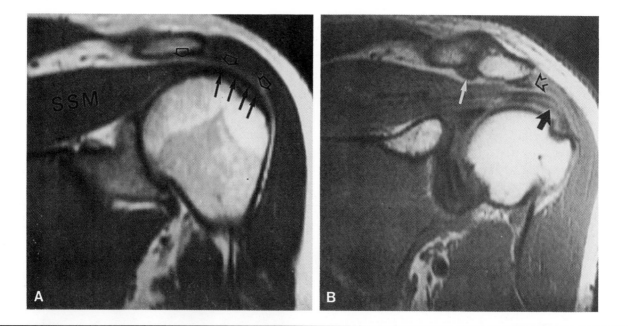

FIGURE 4–74. MRI. (A) Midplane coronal oblique image (repetition time, 800 msec; echo time, 20 msec) of a normal shoulder, illustrating the intermediate signal intensity of the supraspinatus muscle (SSM) and the homogeneous signal void of the supraspinatus tendon (black arrows). The subacromial-subdeltoid peribursal fat plane, which has a high signal intensity, is also clearly defined (open arrows). (B) Anterior coronal oblique image (repetition time, 800 msec; echo time, 20 msec) showing tendinitis. Diffuse high signal intensity is seen in the distal portion of the supraspinatus tendon (black arrow). The tendon is neither thinned nor irregular. The peribursal fat plane is normal. A small acromial spur is present anteriorly (open arrow), and the capsule of the acromioclavicular joint is mildly hypertrophic (white arrow). (From Iannotti, J. P., et al.: J. Bone Joint Surg. 73A:20, 1991.)

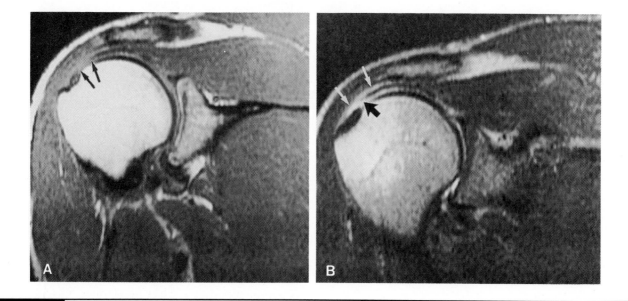

FIGURE 4–75. MRI of midplane coronal oblique images showing a small tear of the cuff. (A) On an image made with a short repetition time and echo time (800 and 20 msec), a small focus of discontinuity is seen in the supraspinatus tendon (arrows). The peribursal fat plane is lost. (B) On an image made with a long repetition time and echo time (2,500 and 70 msec), the intensity of the signal within the small region of discontinuity in the tendon is increased further (black arrow). High signal intensity fluid is seen in the subacromial-subdeltoid bursa (white arrows). (From Iannotti, J. P., et al.: J. Bone Joint Surg. 73A:21, 1991.)

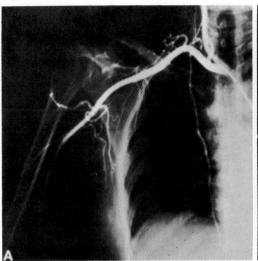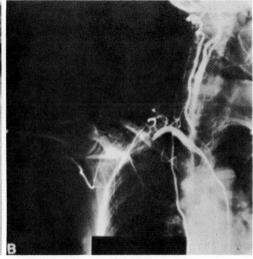

FIGURE 4–76. Angiograms of the subclavian artery with the arm at rest (A) and abducted (B). Note complete obstruction of the subclavian artery (B). (From Brown, C.: Clin. Orthop. Relat. Res. 173:55, 1983.)

PRÉCIS OF THE SHOULDER COMPLEX ASSESSMENT*

History (sitting)
Observation (sitting or standing)
Examination
  Active movements (sitting or standing)
    Elevation through forward flexion of the arm
    Elevation through abduction of the arm
    Elevation through the plane of the scapula
    Medial rotation of the arm
    Lateral rotation of the arm
    Adduction of the arm
    Horizontal adduction/abduction of the arm
    Circumduction of the arm
  Passive movements (sitting)
    Elevation through abduction of the arm
    Elevation through forward flexion of the arm
    Elevation through abduction at the glenohumeral joint only
    Lateral rotation of the arm
    Medial rotation of the arm
    Extension of the arm
    Adduction of the arm
    Horizontal adduction/abduction of the arm
  Special tests (sitting)
  Reflexes and cutaneous distribution (sitting)
  Palpation (sitting)
  Resisted isometric movements (supine lying)
    Forward flexion of the shoulder
    Extension of the shoulder
    Abduction of the shoulder
    Adduction of the shoulder
    Medial rotation of the shoulder
    Lateral rotation of the shoulder
    Flexion of the elbow
    Extension of the elbow
  Special tests (supine lying)
  Joint play movements (supine lying)
    Backward glide of the humerus
    Forward glide of the humerus
    Lateral distraction of the humerus
    Long arm traction
    Backward glide of the humerus in abduction
    Anteroposterior and cephalocaudal movements of the clavicle at the acromioclavicular joint
    Anteroposterior and cephalocaudal movements of the clavicle at the sternoclavicular joint
    General movement of the scapula to determine mobility
Radiographic examination

After any examination, the patient should always be warned of the possibility of exacerbation of symptoms resulting from the assessment.

---

*The précis is shown in an order that will limit the amount of moving that the patient has to do but ensure that all necessary structures are tested.

CASE STUDIES

When doing these case studies, the examiner should list the appropriate questions to be asked and why they are being asked, what to look for and why, and what things should be tested and why. Depending on the answers of the patient (and the examiner should consider several different responses), several possible causes of the patient's problem may become evident (examples given in parentheses). If so, a differential diagnosis chart should be made up. The examiner can then decide how different diagnoses may affect the treatment plan.

1. A 47-year-old man comes to you complaining of pain in the left shoulder. There is no history of overuse activity. The pain that occurs when he elevates his shoulder is referred to his neck and sometimes down his arm to his wrist. Describe your assessment plan for this patient (cervical spondylosis versus subacromial bursitis).

2. An 18-year-old woman recently had a Putti-Platt procedure for a recurring dislocated left shoulder. When you see her she is still in a sling, but the surgeon wants

you to begin treatment. Describe your assessment plan for this patient.

3. A 68-year-old woman comes to you complaining of pain and restricted range of motion in the right shoulder. She tells you that 3 months ago she slipped on a rug on a tile floor and landed on her elbow. Both her elbow and shoulder hurt at that time. Describe your assessment plan for this patient (olecranon bursitis versus adhesive capsulitis).

4. A 23-year-old man comes to you complaining of shoulder pain. He says that 2 days ago he was playing catch with a football; when his friend threw the ball, he reached for it, lost his balance, and fell on the tip of his shoulder but managed to hang onto the ball. Describe your assessment plan for this patient (acromioclavicular sprain versus supraspinatus tendinitis).

5. A 5-year-old boy is brought to you by his parents. They state that he was running around the recreation room chasing a friend when he tripped over a stool and landed on his shoulder. He refuses to move his arm and is crying as the accident occurred only 2 hours ago. Describe your assessment plan for this patient (clavicular fracture versus humeral epiphyseal injury).

6. A 35-year-old female master swimmer comes to you complaining of shoulder pain. She states she has been swimming approximately 2,000 m per day in two training sessions; she recently increased her swimming from 1,500 m per day to get ready for a competition in 3 weeks. Describe your assessment plan for this patient (subacromial bursitis versus biceps tendinitis).

7. A 20-year-old male tennis player comes to you complaining that when he serves the ball, his arm "goes dead." He has had this problem for 3 weeks and has never had the problem before. He has increased his training during the past month. Describe your assessment plan for this patient (thoracic outlet syndrome versus brachial plexus lesion).

8. A 15-year-old female competitive swimmer comes to you complaining of diffuse shoulder pain. She notices the problem most when she does the backstroke. She complains that her shoulder sometimes feels unstable when doing this stroke. Describe your assessment plan for this patient (anterior instability versus supraspinatus tendinitis).

9. A 48-year-old man comes to you complaining of neck and shoulder pain. He states that he has difficulty abducting his right arm. There is no history of trauma, but he remembers being in a car accident 10 years ago. Describe your assessment plan for this patient (cervical spondylosis versus adhesive capsulitis).

REFERENCES

CITED REFERENCES

1. Cyriax, J.: Textbook of Orthopaedic Medicine, vol. I: Diagnosis of Soft Tissue Lesions. London, Bailliere Tindall, 1982.
2. Nichols, H. M.: Anatomic structures of the thoracic outlet syndrome. Clin. Orthop. Relat. Res. 51:17, 1967.
3. Riddell, D. H. Thoracic outlet syndrome: Thoracic and vascular aspects. Clin. Orthop. Relat. Res. 51:53, 1967.
4. Priest, J. D., and D. A. Nagel: Tennis shoulder. Am. J. Sports Med. 4:28, 1976.
5. Hitchcock, H. H., and C. O. Bechtol: Painful shoulder: Observation on the role of the tendon of the long head of the biceps brachii in its causation. J. Bone Joint Surg. 30A:263, 1948.
6. Carson, W. C., W. W. Lovell, and T. E. Whitesides: Congenital elevation of the scapula. J. Bone Joint Surg. 63A:1199, 1981.
7. Cavendish, M. E.: Congenital elevation of the scapula. J. Bone Joint Surg. 54B:395, 1972.
8. Perry, J.: Biomechanics of the shoulder. In Rowe, C. R. (ed.): The Shoulder. Edinburgh, Churchill Livingstone, 1988.
9. Kapandji, I. A.: The Physiology of Joints, vol. 1: Upper Limb. New York, Churchill Livingstone, 1970.
10. Kessel, L., and M. Watson: The painful arc syndrome. J. Bone Joint Surg. 59B:166, 1977.
11. Reid, D. C.: The shoulder girdle: Its function as a unit in abduction. Physiotherapy 55:57, 1969.
12. Saha, S. K.: Mechanics of shoulder movements and a plea for the recognition of "zero position" of glenohumeral joint. Clin. Orthop. Relat. Res. 173:3, 1983.
13. Maitland, G. D.: Peripheral Manipulation. London, Butterworths, 1977.
14. Rowe, C. R.: Unusual shoulder conditions. In Rowe, C. R. (ed.): The Shoulder. Edinburgh, Churchill Livingstone, 1988.
15. MacConaill, M. A., and J. V. Basmajian: Muscles and Movements—A Basis for Human Kinesiology. Baltimore, Williams & Wilkins, 1969.
16. Corrigan, B., and G. D. Maitland: Practical Orthopedic Medicine. London, Butterworths, 1985.
17. Gerber, C., and R. Ganz: Clinical assessment of instability of the shoulder. J. Bone Joint Surg. 66B:551–556, 1984.
18. Protzman, R. R.: Anterior instability of the shoulder. J. Bone Joint Surg. 62A:909–918, 1980.
19. Davies, G. J., J. A. Gould, and R. L. Larson: Functional examination of the shoulder girdle. Phys. Sports Med. 9:82–104, 1981.
20. Leffert, R. D., and G. Gumley: The relationship between dead arm syndrome and thoracic outlet syndrome. Clin. Orthop. Relat. Res. 223:20–31, 1987.
21. Rockwood, C. A.: Subluxations and dislocations about the shoulder. In Rockwood, C. A., and D. P. Green (eds.): Fractures in Adults—1. Philadelphia, J. B. Lippincott Co., 1984.
22. Rowe, C. R.: Dislocations of the shoulder. In Rowe, C. R. (ed.): The Shoulder. Edinburgh, Churchill Livingstone, 1988.
23. Matsen, F. A., S. C. Thomas, and C. A. Rockwood: Glenohumeral instability. In Rockwood, C. A., and F. A. Matsen (eds.): The Shoulder. Philadelphia, W. B. Saunders Co., 1990.
24. Hawkins, R. J., and D. J. Bokor: Clinical evaluation of shoulder problems. In Rockwood, C. A., and F. A. Matsen (eds.): The Shoulder. Philadelphia, W. B. Saunders Co., 1990.
25. Andrews, J. R., and S. Gillogly: Physical examination of the shoulder in throwing athletes. In Zarins, B., J. R. Andrews, and W. G. Carson (eds.): Injuries to the Throwing Arm. Philadelphia, W. B. Saunders Co., 1985.
26. Walsh, D. A.: Shoulder evaluation of the throwing athlete. Sports Med. Update 4:24–27, 1989.
27. Norwood, L. A., and G. C. Terry: Shoulder posterior and subluxation. Am. J. Sports Med. 12:25–30, 1984.
28. Cofield, R. H., and J. F. Irving: Evaluation and classification of shoulder instability. Clin. Orthop. Relat. Res. 223:32–43, 1987.
29. Yergason, R. M.: Supination sign. J. Bone Joint Surg. 13:160, 1931.
30. Moseley, H. F.: Disorders of the shoulder. Clinical Symposia 12:1–30, 1960.
31. Ludington, N. A.: Rupture of the long head of the biceps flexor cubiti muscle. Ann. Surg. 77:358–363, 1923.
32. Neer, C. S., and R. P. Welsh: The shoulder in sports. Orthop. Clin. North Am. 8:583–591, 1977.
33. Hawkins, R. J., and J. C. Kennedy: Impingement syndrome in athletics. Am. J. Sports Med. 8:151–163, 1980.
34. Post, M.: Physical Examination of the Musculoskeletal System. Chicago, Year Book Medical Publishers Inc., 1987.
35. Elvey, R. L.: The investigation of arm pain. In Grieve, G. P. (ed.): Modern Manual Therapy of the Vertebral Column. Edinburgh, Churchill Livingstone, 1986.
36. Allen, E. V.: Thromboangiitis obliterans: Methods of diagnosis of chronic occlusive arterial lesions distal to the wrist with illustrative cases. Am. J. Med. Sci. 178:237–244, 1929.
37. Wright, I. S.: The neurovascular syndrome produced by hyperabduction of the arms. Am. Heart J. 29:1–19, 1945.

38. Adson, A. W., and J. R. Coffey: Cervical rib—A method of anterior approach for relief of symptoms by division of the scalenus anticus. Ann. Surg. 85:839–857, 1927.
39. Roos, D. B.: Congenital anomalies associated with thoracic outlet syndrome. J. Surg. 132:771–778, 1976.
40. Brown, C.: Compressive, invasive referred pain to the shoulder. Clin. Orthop. Rel. Res. 173:55, 1983.
41. Kaltenborn, E. M.: Mobilization of the Extremity Joints. Oslo, Olaf Norlis Bokhandle, 1980.
42. Weiner, D. S., and I. Macnab: Superior migration of the humeral head. J. Bone Joint Surg. 52B:524, 1970.
43. Kernwein, G. A., B. Rosenberg, and W. R. Sneed: Arthrographic studies of the shoulder joint. J. Bone Joint Surg. 39A:1267, 1957.
44. Neviaser, J. S.: Arthrography of the shoulder joint: Study of the findings of adhesive capulitis of the shoulder. J. Bone Joint Surg. 44A:1321, 1962.
45. Reeves, B.: Arthrography of the shoulder. J. Bone Joint Surg. 48B:424, 1966.

GENERAL REFERENCES

Adams, J. C.: Outline of Orthopaedics. London, E & S Livingstone, 1968.
Albert, M. S., and M. J. Wooden: Isokinetic evaluation and treatment of the shoulder. In Physical Therapy of the Shoulder. Edinburgh, Churchill Livingstone, 1991.
American Orthopaedic Association: Manual of Orthopaedic Surgery. Chicago, 1972.
Anderson, J. E.: Grant's Atlas of Anatomy. Baltimore, Williams and Wilkins, 1983.
Bassett, L. W., R. H. Gold, and L. L. Seeger: MRI Atlas of the Musculoskeletal System. London, Martin Dunitz Ltd., 1989.
Bateman, J. E.: The Shoulder and Neck, 2nd ed. Philadelphia, W. B. Saunders Co., 1978.
Bateman, J. E.: Neurologic painful conditions affecting the shoulder. Clin. Orthop. Relat. Res. 173:44, 1983.
Beetham, W. P., H. F. Polley, C. H. Slocum, and W. F. Weaver: Physical Examination of the Joints. Philadelphia, W. B. Saunders Co., 1965.
Bernageau, J.: Roentgenographic assessment of the rotator cuff. Clin. Orthop. Relat. Res. 254:87–91, 1990.
Black, K. P., and J. A. Lombardo: Suprascapular nerve injuries with isolated paralysis of the infraspinatus. Am. J. Sports Med. 18:225–228, 1990.
Boissonnault, W. G., and S. C. Janos: Dysfunction, evaluation and treatment of the shoulder. In Donatelli, R. A., and M. J. Wooden (eds.): Orthopedic Physical Therapy. Edinburgh, Churchill Livingstone, 1989.
Booth, R. E., and J. P. Marvel: Differential diagnosis of shoulder pain. Orthop. Clin. North Am. 6:353–379, 1975.
Cailliet, R.: Shoulder Pain. Philadelphia, F. A. Davis Co., 1966.
Clarkson, H. M., and G. B. Gilewich: Musculoskeletal Assessment—Joint Range of Motion and Manual Muscle Strength. Philadelphia, Williams & Wilkins, 1989.
Constant, C. R., and A. H. G. Murley: A clinical method of functional assessment of the shoulder. Clin. Orthop. Relat. Res. 214:160–164, 1987.
Dempster, W. T.: Mechanisms of shoulder movement. Arch. Phys. Med. Rehabil. 436:49, 1965.
Deutsch, A. L., D. Resnick, and J. H. Mink: Computed tomography of the glenohumeral and sternoclavicular joints. Orthop. Clin. North Am. 16:497–511, 1985.
Fallcel, J. E., T. C. Murphy, and T. R. Malone: Shoulder Injuries: Sports Injury Management. Baltimore, Williams & Wilkins, 1988.
First Aid. St. John's Ambulance. Ottawa, The Runge Press Ltd., 1963.
Forrester, D. M., and J. C. Brown: The Radiology of Joint Disease. Philadelphia, W. B. Saunders Co., 1987.
Foster, C. R.: Multidirectional instability of the shoulder in the athlete. Clin. Sports Med. 2:355, 1983.
France, M. K.: Anatomy and biomechanics of the shoulder. In Donatelli, R. A. (ed.): Physical Therapy of the Shoulder. Edinburgh, Churchill Livingstone, 1991.

Garrick, J. G., and D. R. Webb: Sports Injuries: Diagnosis and Management. Philadelphia, W. B. Saunders Co., 1990.
Gartland, J. J.: Fundamentals of Orthopaedics. Philadelphia, W. B. Saunders Co., 1979.
Greenfield, B. H., R. Donatelli, M. J. Wooden, and J. Wilkes: Isokinetic evaluation of shoulder rotational strength between the plane of the scapula and the frontal plane. Am. J. Sports Med. 18:124–128, 1990.
Halback, J. W., and R. T. Tank: The shoulder. In Gould, J. A. (ed.): Orthopedic and Sports Physical Therapy. St. Louis, C. V. Mosby Co., 1990.
Hawkins, R. J., and J. S. Abrams: Impingement syndrome in the absence of rotator cuff tear (stage 1 and 2). Orthop. Clin. North Am. 18:373–382, 1987.
Hawkins, R. J., and P. E. Hobeika: Impingement syndrome in the athletic shoulder. Clin. Sports Med. 2:391, 1983.
Hollinshead, W. H., and D. B. Jenkins: Functional Anatomy of the Limb and Back. Philadelphia, W. B. Saunders Co., 1981.
Hoppenfeld, S.: Physical Examination of the Spine and Extremities. New York, Appleton-Century-Crofts, 1976.
Iannotti, J. P., M. B. Zlatkin, J. L. Esterhai, H. Y. Kressel, M. K. Dalinka, and K. P. Spindler: Magnetic resonance imaging of the shoulder. J. Bone Joint Surg. 73A:17–29, 1991.
Jobe, F. W.: Painful athletic injuries of the shoulder. Clin. Orthop. Relat. Res. 173:117, 1983.
Judge, R. D., G. D. Zuidema, and F. T. Fitzgerald: Clinical Diagnosis: A Physiological Approach. Boston, Little, Brown & Co., 1982.
Leffert, R. D.: Clinical diagnoses, testing and electromyographic study in brachial plexus traction injuries. Clin. Orthop. Relat. Res. 237:24–31, 1988.
Lippman, R. K.: Frozen shoulder; periarthritis; bicipital tenosynovitis. Arch. Surg. 47:283, 1943.
Maki, N. J.: Cineradiographic studies with shoulder instabilities. Am. J. Sports Med. 16:362–364, 1988.
McMaster, W. C.: Painful shoulder in swimmers: A diagnostic challenge. Phys. Sportsmed. 14(12):108–122, 1986.
Meyer, S. J. F., and M. K. Dalinka: Magnetic resonance imaging of the shoulder. Orthop. Clin. North Am. 21:497–513, 1990.
Moran, C. A., and S. R. Saunders: Evaluation of the shoulder: A sequential approach. In Donatelli, R. A. (ed.): Physical Therapy of the Shoulder. Edinburgh, Churchill Livingstone, 1991.
Naffzinger, H. C., and W. T. Grant: Neuritis of the brachial plexus mechanical in origin: The scalenus syndrome. Clin. Orthop. Relat. Res. 51:7, 1967.
Neer, C. S.: Impingement lesions. Clin. Orthop. Relat. Res. 173:70, 1983.
Neer, C. S., and C. R. Foster: Inferior capsular shift for involuntary inferior and multidirectional instability of the shoulder. J. Bone Joint Surg. 62A:897–908, 1980.
Neviaser, J. S.: Adhesive capsulitis and the stiff and painful shoulder. Orthop. Clin. North Am. 11:327, 1980.
Neviaser, R. J.: Anatomic considerations and examination of the shoulder. Orthop. Clin. North Am. 11:187, 1980.
Neviaser, R. J.: Lesions of the biceps and tendinitis of the shoulder. Orthop. Clin. North Am. 11:343, 1980.
Neviaser, R. J.: Painful conditions affecting the shoulder. Clin. Orthop. Relat. Res. 173:63, 1983.
Neviaser, R. J.: Tears of the rotator cuff. Orthop. Clin. North Am. 11:295, 1980.
Norris, T. R.: History and physical examination of the shoulder. In Nicholas, J. A., and E. B. Hershman (eds.): The Upper Extremity in Sports Medicine. St. Louis, C. V. Mosby Co., 1990.
O'Donoghue, D. H.: Treatment of Injuries to Athletes, 4th ed. Philadelphia, W. B. Saunders Co., 1984.
Overton, L. M.: The causes of pain in the upper extremities: A differential diagnosis study. Clin. Orthop. Relat. Res. 51:27, 1967.
Palmer, M. L., and M. Epler: Clinical Assessment Procedures in Physical Therapy. Philadelphia, J. B. Lippincott Co., 1990.
Patla, C. E.: Upper extremity. In Payton, O. D., et al. (eds.): Manual of Physical Therapy. Edinburgh, Churchill Livingstone, 1989.
Perry, J.: Anatomy and biomechanics of the shoulder in throwing, swimming, gymnastics, and tennis. Clin. Sports Med. 2:247, 1983.

Post, M., R. Silver, and M. Singh: Rotator cuff tear: Diagnosis and treatment. Clin. Orthop. Relat. Res. 173:78, 1983.

Rathburn, J. B., and I. Macnab: The microvascular pattern of the rotator cuff. J. Bone Joint Surg. 52B:540, 1970.

Reid, D. C.: Functional Anatomy and Joint Mobilization. Edmonton, University of Alberta Press, 1970.

Rockwood, C. A., E. A. Szalay, R. J. Curtis, D. C. Young, and S. P. Kay: X-ray evaluation of shoulder problems. In Rockwood, C. A., and F. A. Matsen (eds.): The Shoulder. Philadelphia, W. B. Saunders Co., 1990.

Rowe, C. R.: Examination of the shoulder. In Rowe, C. R. (ed.): The Shoulder. Edinburgh, Churchill Livingstone, 1988.

Rowe, C. R.: Recurrent transient anterior subluxation of the shoulder—The "dead arm" syndrome. Clin. Orthop. Relat. Res. 223:11–19, 1987.

Saha, A. K.: Mechanism of shoulder movements and a plea for the recognition of "zero position" of glenohumeral joint. Clin. Orthop. Relat. Res. 173:3–10, 1983.

Sarrafian, S. K.: Gross and functional anatomy of the shoulder. Clin. Orthop. Relat. Res. 173:44, 1983.

Schenkman, M., and V. R. de Cartaya: Kinesiology of the shoulder complex. J. Orthop. Sports Phys. Ther. 8:438–450, 1987.

Schwartz, E., R. F. Warren, S. J. O'Brien, and J. Fronek: Posterior shoulder instability. Orthop. Clin. North Am. 18:409–419, 1987.

Seeger, L. L.: Magnetic resonance imaging of the shoulder. Clin. Ortho. Rel. Res. 244:48–59, 1989.

Tank, R., and J. Halbach: Physical therapy evaluation of the shoulder complex in athletes. J. Orthop. Sports Phys. Ther. 3:108, 1982.

Wadsworth, C. T.: Manual Examination and Treatment of the Spine and Extremities. Baltimore, Williams & Wilkins, 1988.

Weissman, B. N. W., and C. B. Sledge: Orthopedic Radiology. Philadelphia, W. B. Saunders Co., 1986.

Wiles, P., and R. Sweetnam: Essentials of Orthopaedics. London, J. A. Churchill Ltd., 1965.

Williams, A., R. Evans, and P. D. Shirley: Imaging of Sports Injuries. London, Bailliere Tindall, 1989.

Wood, V. E., R. Twito, and J. M. Verska: Thoracic outlet syndrome. Orthop. Clin. North Am. 19:131–146, 1988.

Yocum, L. A.: Assessing the shoulder: History, physical examination, differential diagnosis, and special tests used. Clin. Sports Med. 2:281, 1983.

Zarins, B.: Anterior subluxation and dislocation of the shoulder. In AAOSS on Upper Extremity Injuries in Athletes. St. Louis, C. V. Mosby Co., 1986.

Elbow Joints

The elbow's primary role in the upper limb complex is to help position the hand in the appropriate location to perform its function. Once the shoulder has positioned the hand in a gross fashion, the elbow allows for adjustments in height and length of the limb to position the hand correctly. In addition, the forearm rotates, in part at the elbow, to place the hand in the most effective position to perform its function.

APPLIED ANATOMY

The elbow consists of a complex set of joints that require careful assessment for proper treatment. The treatment must be geared to the pathology of the condition because the joint responds poorly to trauma, harsh treatment, or incorrect treatment.

Because they are closely related, the joints of the elbow complex make up a compound synovial joint, with injury to any one part affecting the other components as well. The elbow articulations are made up of the ulnohumeral joint and the radiohumeral joint. In addition, the complexity of the elbow articulations is further increased by the superior radioulnar joint, which has continuity with the elbow articulations. These three joints make up the *cubital articulations*. The capsule and joint cavity are continuous for all three joints. The combination of these joints allows two degrees of freedom at the elbow. The *trochlear joint* allows one degree of freedom (flexion-extension), and the radiohumeral and superior radioulnar joints allow the other degree of freedom (rotation).

The *ulnohumeral*, or *trochlear*, *joint* is found between the trochlea of the humerus and the trochlear notch of the ulna and is classified as a *uniaxial hinge joint*. The bones of this joint are shaped so that the axis of movement is not horizontal but instead passes downward and medially, going through an arc of movement. This position leads to

the carrying angle at the elbow[1] (Fig. 5–1). The resting position of this joint is with the elbow flexed to 70° and the forearm supinated 10°. The neutral position (0°) is midway between supination and pronation in the "thumb-up" position (Fig. 5–2). The capsular pattern is flexion more limited than extension, and the close packed position is extension with the forearm in supination. On full extension, the medial part of the olecranon process is not in contact with the trochlea; on full flexion, the lateral part of the olecranon process is not in contact with the trochlea. This change allows the side-to-side joint play movement necessary for supination and pronation. A small amount of rotation occurs at this joint. In early flexion, 5° of medial rotation occurs; in late flexion, 5° of lateral rotation occurs.

The *radiohumeral joint* is a uniaxial hinge joint between the capitulum of the humerus and the head of the radius. The resting position is with the elbow fully extended and the forearm fully supinated. The close packed position of the joint is with the elbow flexed to 90° and the forearm supinated 5°. As with the trochlear joint, the capsular pattern is flexion more limited than extension.

The ulnohumeral and radiohumeral joints are supported medially by the *ulnar collateral ligament*, a fan-shaped structure, and laterally by the *radial collateral ligament*, a cordlike structure. The ulnar collateral ligament has two parts, which along with the flexor carpi ulnaris muscle form the *cubital tunnel* through which passes the *ulnar nerve* (Fig. 5–3). Any injury or blow to the area or injury that increases the carrying angle will put an abnormal stress on the nerve as it passes through the tunnel. This can lead to problems such as *tardy ulnar palsy*, a condition that can occur many years after the original injury.

The *superior radioulnar joint* is a uniaxial pivot joint. The head of the radius is held in proper relation to the ulna and humerus by the *annular ligament*, which makes up four fifths of the joint. The resting position of this joint is supination of 35°

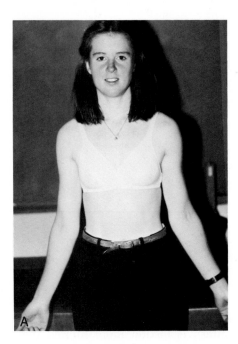

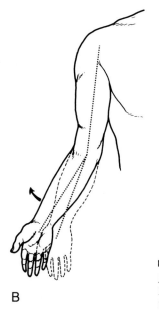

B

FIGURE 5–1. (A) Carrying angle of the elbow. (B) Excessive valgus carrying angle. (From American Orthopaedic Association: Manual of Orthopaedic Surgery. Chicago, 1979, p. 146.)

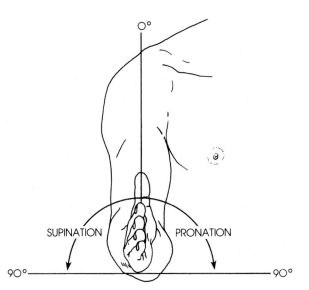

0°

SUPINATION   PRONATION

90°———————————————————90°

FIGURE 5–2. "Thumb-up" or neutral (zero) position between supination and pronation.

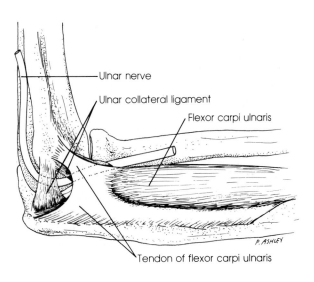

Ulnar nerve
Ulnar collateral ligament
Flexor carpi ulnaris

P. ASHLEY

Tendon of flexor carpi ulnaris

FIGURE 5–3. Cubital tunnel.

and elbow flexion of 70°. The close packed position is supination of 5°. The capsular pattern of this joint is equal limitation of supination and pronation.

The three elbow articulations are innervated by branches from the musculocutaneous, median, ulnar, and radial nerves.

The *middle radioulnar articulation* is not a true joint but is made up of the radius and ulna and the *interosseous membrane* between the two bones. The interosseous membrane is tense only midway between supination and pronation (neutral position). Although this "joint" is not part of the elbow joint complex, it is affected by injury to the elbow joints; conversely, injury to this area can affect the mechanics of the elbow articulations. The interosseous membrane prevents proximal displacement of the radius on the ulna. The displacement is most likely to occur with pushing movements. The *oblique cord* connects the radius and ulna, running from the lateral side of the *ulnar tuberosity* to the radius slightly below the *radial tuberosity*. Its fibers run at right angles to those of the interosseous membrane. The cord assists in preventing displacement of the radius on the ulna, especially movements involving pulling.

PATIENT HISTORY

In addition to the general history questions presented in Chapter 1, the following information should be ascertained:

1. What is the patient's usual activity or pastime?
2. What are the details of the present pain and other symptoms? What are the sites and boundaries of the pain? The pain may be radiating and could ache or be worse at night. Aching pain over the lateral epicondyle that radiates may be indicative of a "tennis elbow" problem.
3. How old is the patient? What is the patient's occupation? Tennis elbow (lateral epicondylitis) problems usually occur in persons 35 years of age or older and in those who use a great deal of wrist flexion and extension in their occupations. If the patient is a child who complains of pain in the elbow and lacks supination on examination, the examiner could suspect a dislocation of the head of the radius. This type of injury is often seen in young children. A parent may give the child a sharp "come-along" tug on the arm, leading to a dislocation of the head of the radius.
4. Does the patient complain of any abnormal nerve distribution pain? The examiner should note whether there is any tingling or numbness and, if so, where it is for reference when checking dermatomes and peripheral nerve distribution later in the examination.

5. Are any movements impaired? Which movements does the patient feel are restricted? If flexion or extension is limited, two joints may be involved—the ulnohumeral and radiohumeral. If supination or pronation is problematic, any one of five joints could be involved—the radiohumeral, superior radioulnar, middle radioulnar, inferior radioulnar, or ulnomeniscocarpal.

6. Does the patient have any history of previous injury or trauma? This question is especially important in regard to the elbow because the ulnar nerve may be affected by tardy ulnar palsy.

OBSERVATION

The patient must be suitably undressed so that both arms are exposed to allow comparison of the two sides.

The examiner first places the patient's arms in the anatomic position to determine whether there is a normal carrying angle[1] (see Fig. 5–1). It is the angle formed by the long axis of the humerus and the long axis of the ulna and is most evident when the elbow is straight and the forearm is fully supinated (Fig. 5–4). In the adult, this would be a slight valgus

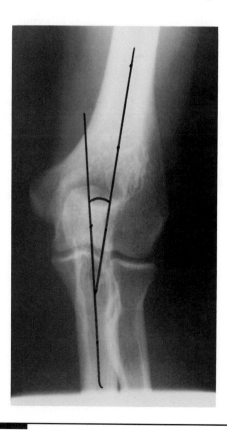

FIGURE 5–4. *Carrying angle. The carrying angle may be determined by noting the angle of intersection between a line connecting midpoints in the distal humerus and a line connecting midpoints in the proximal ulna.*

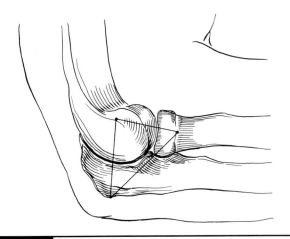

FIGURE 5–5. *The triangular area in which intra-articular swelling is most evident in the elbow.*

deviation between the humerus and the ulna when the forearm is supinated and the elbow is extended. In males, the normal carrying angle is 5 to 10°; in females, it is 10 to 15°. If the carrying angle is more than 15°, it is called *cubitus valgus;* if it is less than 5 to 10°, it is called *cubitus varus.* Because of the shape of the humeral condyles that articulate with the radius and ulna, the carrying angle changes linearly depending on the degree of extension or flexion. Cubitus valgus is greatest in extension. The angle decreases as the elbow flexes, reaching varus in full flexion.[2]

If swelling exists, all three joints of the elbow complex would be affected because they have a common capsule. Joint swelling is often most evident in the triangular space between the radial head, tip of the olecranon, and lateral epicondyle (Fig. 5–5). Swelling resulting from olecranon bursitis (student's elbow) is more discrete, being more sharply demarcated as a "goose egg" over the olecranon process (Fig. 5–6). With swelling, the joint would be held in its resting position with the elbow held

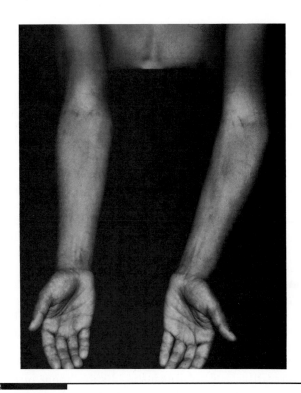

FIGURE 5–7. *Cubitus varus illustrated showing "gun stock" deformity on the left arm. (From Volz, R. C., and B. F. Morrey: The physical examination of the elbow. In Morrey, B. F. (ed.): The Elbow and Its Disorders. Philadelphia, W. B. Saunders Co., 1985, p. 63. Copyright Mayo Clinic Foundation, Rochester, MN.)*

in approximately 70° of flexion. It is in the resting position that the joint has maximum volume.

The examiner should look for normal bony and soft-tissue contours anteriorly and posteriorly. Often, athletes such as pitchers and other throwers will have a much larger arm on their throwing side. If there has been a fracture or epiphyseal injury to the distal humerus and a cubitus varus results, a gun stock deformity may be seen (Fig. 5–7).

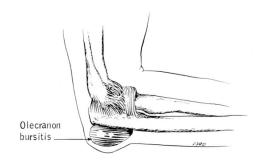

Olecranon bursitis

FIGURE 5–6. *Olecranon bursitis. (From O'Donoghue, D. H.: Treatment of Injuries to Athletes. Philadelphia, W. B. Saunders Co., 1984, p. 243.)*

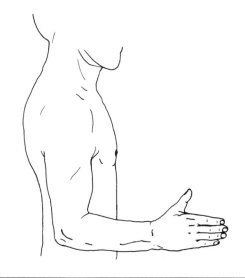

FIGURE 5–8. *Position of function of the elbow.*

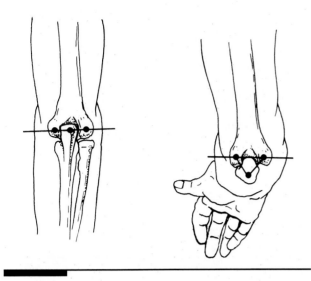

FIGURE 5-9. *Relation of the medial and lateral epicondyles and the olecranon at the elbow in extension and flexion.*

The examiner should note whether the patient can assume the normal position of function of the elbow (Fig. 5-8). A normal functional position is 90° of flexion, with the forearm midway between supination and pronation.[3] In this position, the olecranon process of the ulna and the medial and lateral epicondyles of the humerus will normally form an isosceles triangle (Fig. 5-9). When the arm is fully extended, the three points normally form a straight line.[4] The isosceles triangle is sometimes called the *triangle sign*. If there is a fracture or dislocation or degeneration leading to loss of bone and/or cartilage, the distance between the apex and the base decreases and the isosceles triangle no longer exists. The triangle can be measured on x-rays.[2] The forearm may also be considered to be in a functional position when slightly pronated, as in writing. From this position, forward flexion of the shoulder enables the person to bring food to the mouth; supination of the forearm decreases the amount of shoulder flexion necessary to accomplish this.

EXAMINATION

Active Movements

Examination is performed with the patient in the sitting position. As always, active movements are done first, and it is important to remember that the most painful movements are done last. The active movements include:

1. Flexion of the elbow (140 to 150°).
2. Extension of the elbow (0 to 10°).
3. Supination of the forearm (90°).
4. Pronation of the forearm (80 to 90°).

Active elbow *flexion* is 140 to 150°, and the end feel is usually tissue approximation. In thin individuals, the end feel may be bone to bone as a result of the coronoid process hitting against the coronoid fossa.

Active elbow *extension* is 0°, although up to a 10° hyperextension may be exhibited, especially in women. This hyperextension is considered normal if it is equal on both sides and there is no history of trauma. The end feel of active elbow extension is bone to bone. Loss of elbow extension is a sensitive indicator of intra-articular pathology. It is the first movement lost after injury to the elbow and the first regained with healing. However, terminal flexion loss is more disabling than the same degree of terminal extension loss. Loss of either motion affects the area of reach of the hand, which may in turn affect function.

Active *supination* should be 90°, and the end feel should be tissue stretch (Fig. 5-10).

For active *pronation*, the range of motion is approximately the same (80 to 90°), and the end feel is tissue stretch. It should be noted, however, that for both supination and pronation only 75° (approx-

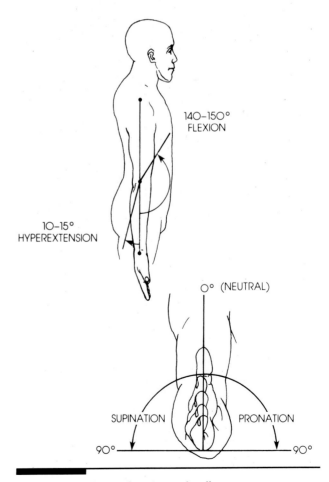

FIGURE 5-10. *Range of motion at the elbow.*

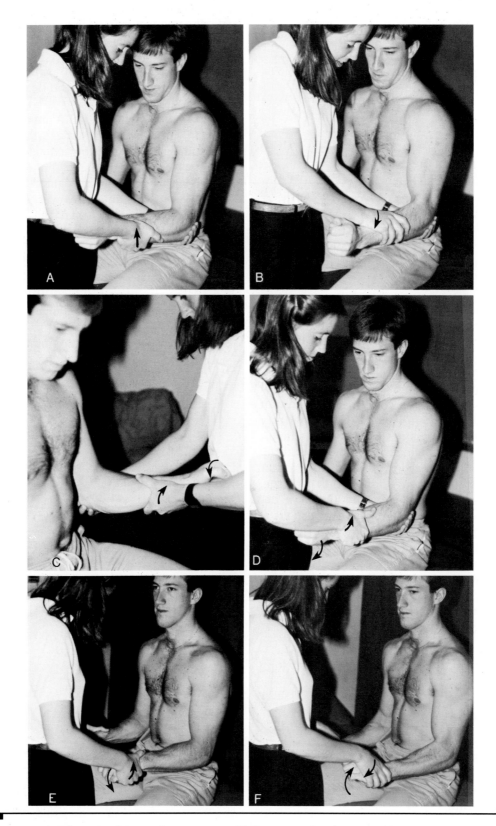

FIGURE 5–11. *Positioning for resisted isometric movements.* (A) Extension. (B) Flexion. (C) Pronation. (D) Supination. (E) Wrist flexion. (F) Wrist extension.

imately) occurs in the forearm articulations. The remaining 15° is the result of wrist action. The examiner should watch the patient closely when testing supination and pronation. The patient may try to compensate for loss of range of motion in these directions by adducting or abducting the shoulder.

Passive Movements

If the range of motion is full on active movements, overpressure may be gently applied to test the end feel in each direction. If the movement is not full, passive movements should be carried out to test the end feel, including:

1. Flexion of the elbow.
2. Extension of the elbow.
3. Supination of the forearm.
4. Pronation of the forearm.

In addition to the end feel tests during passive movements, the examiner should note whether a capsular pattern is present. The capsular pattern for the elbow complex as a whole is more limitation of flexion than extension.

Resisted Isometric Movements

For proper testing of the muscles of the elbow complex, the movement must be resisted and isometric. Muscle flexion power around the elbow is greatest in the range of 90 to 110° with the forearm supinated. At 45° or 135°, flexion power is only 75% of maximum.[3] The patient is seated, and the following movements are tested (Fig. 5–11 and Table 5–1):

1. Elbow flexion.
2. Elbow extension.
3. Supination.
4. Pronation.
5. Wrist flexion.
6. Wrist extension.

It is necessary to carry out wrist extension and flexion because there is a large number of muscles that act over the wrist as well as the elbow.

Functional Assessment

When assessing the elbow, it is important to remember that the elbow is the middle portion of an integral kinetic chain. It allows the hand to be positioned in space; it helps stabilize the upper extremity for power and detailed work activities; and it provides power to the arm for lifting activities.[5] Motion in the elbow allows the hand to be positioned so that daily functions can be easily performed. The full range of elbow movements is not necessary to perform these activities; most activities of daily living are performed between 30° and 130° flexion and between 50° of pronation and 50° of supination (Figs. 5–12 and 5–13). To reach the head, approximately 140° of flexion is needed. The activities of combing or washing the hair, reaching a back zipper, and walking on crutches require a greater range of motion. Activities such as pouring fluid, drinking from a container, cutting with a knife, reading a newspaper, and using a screwdriver require an adequate range of supination and pronation. Figures 5–14 and 5–15 show the range of motion or arc of movement necessary to do certain activities or the range of motion needed to touch parts of the body. It must be remembered that elbow injuries

TABLE 5–1. Muscles about the Elbow: Their Actions and Nerve Supply, Including Root Derivations

Action	Muscles Involved	Nerve Supply	Nerve Root Derivation
Flexion of elbow	1. Brachialis	Musculocutaneous	C5–C6 (C7)
	2. Biceps brachii	Musculocutaneous	C5–C6
	3. Brachioradialis	Radial	C5–C6 (C7)
	4. Pronator teres	Median	C6–C7
	5. Flexor carpi ulnaris	Ulnar	C7–C8
Extension of elbow	1. Triceps	Radial	C6–C8
	2. Anconeus	Radial	C7–C8, (T1)
Supination of forearm	1. Supinator	Posterior interosseous (radial)	C5–C6
	2. Biceps brachii	Musculocutaneous	C5–C6
Pronation of forearm	1. Pronator quadratus	Anterior interosseous (median)	C8, T1
	2. Pronator teres	Median	C6–C7
	3. Flexor carpi radialis	Median	C6–C7
Flexion of wrist	1. Flexor carpi radialis	Median	C6–C7
	2. Flexor carpi ulnaris	Ulnar	C7–C8
Extension of wrist	1. Extensor carpi radialis longus	Radial	C6–C7
	2. Extensor carpi radialis brevis	Posterior interosseous (radial)	C7–C8
	3. Extensor carpi ulnaris	Posterior interosseous (radial)	C7–C8

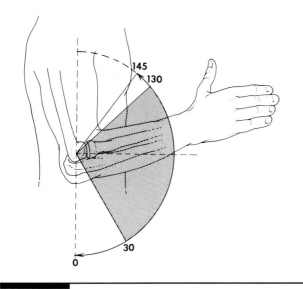

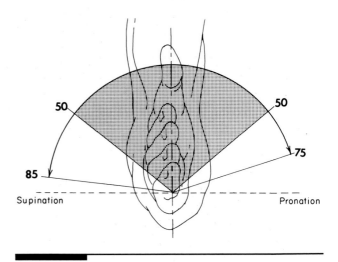

FIGURE 5–12. Normal range of elbow flexion is approximately 0 to 145°. However, functional arc of motion is somewhat less, and most activities can be performed with flexion of 30 to 130°. (From Volz, R. C., and B. F. Morrey: The physical examination of the elbow. In Morrey, B. F. (ed.): The Elbow and Its Disorders. Philadelphia, W. B. Saunders Co., 1985, p. 68. Copyright Mayo Clinic Foundation, Rochester, MN.)

FIGURE 5–13. Pronation and supination motions average 75° and 85°, respectively. Most activities of daily living, however, can be accomplished with 50° of each motion. (From Volz, R. C., and B. F. Morrey: The physical examination of the elbow. In Morrey, B. F. (ed.): The Elbow and Its Disorders. Philadelphia, W. B. Saunders Co., 1985, p. 68. Copyright Mayo Clinic Foundation, Rochester, MN.)

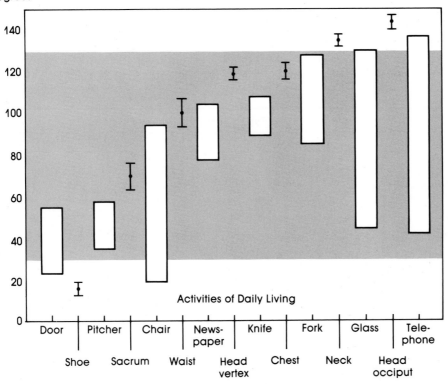

FIGURE 5–14. Fifteen daily activities demonstrating the arc and position of elbow flexion required. Most of these activities are accomplished within a flexion range of 30 to 130°. (Modified from Morrey, B. F.: The Elbow and Its Disorders. Philadelphia, W. B. Saunders Co., 1985, p. 77. Copyright Mayo Clinic Foundation, Rochester, MN.)

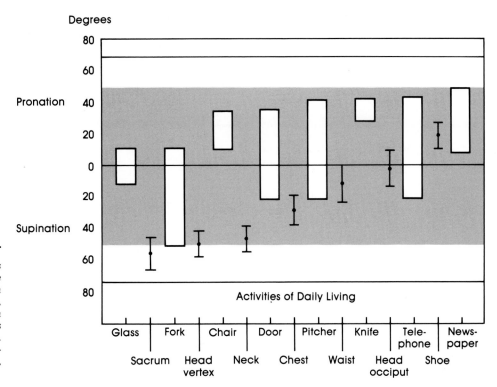

FIGURE 5-15. Fifteen activities of daily living are noted to be accomplished with pronation and supination of 50° and 50°, respectively. (Modified from Morrey, B. F.: The Elbow and Its Disorders. Philadelphia, W. B. Saunders Co., 1985, p. 78. Copyright Mayo Clinic Foundation, Rochester, MN.)

may preclude lifting objects as light as a cup of coffee, owing to lifting mechanics. Because of the length of the lever arm of the forearm, when the elbow is at 90°, loads at the hand are magnified 10-fold at the elbow.[6] Figure 5-16 is an assessment form that can be used to assess the elbow and includes an important functional component. Table 5-2 demonstrates functional tests of strength for the elbow.

Special Tests

Only those special tests that the examiner feels have relevance or will help to confirm the diagnosis should be performed.

Ligamentous Test

Ligamentous Instability Test. The patient's arm is stabilized with one of the examiner's hands at the elbow and the other hand placed above the patient's wrist. With the patient's elbow slightly flexed (20 to 30°) and stabilized with the examiner's hand, an adduction or varus force is applied by the examiner to the distal forearm to test the lateral collateral ligament (Fig. 5-17). Volz and Morrey[6] advocate doing the varus stress test with the humerus in full medial rotation. The examiner applies the force several times with increasing pressure while noting any alteration in pain or range of motion. An abduction or valgus force at the distal forearm is then applied in a similar fashion to test the medial

collateral ligament. Volz and Morrey[6] advocate doing the valgus stress test with the humerus in full lateral rotation. The examiner should note any laxity, decreased mobility, or altered pain that may be present compared with the uninvolved elbow.

Tests for Epicondylitis

Lateral Epicondylitis (Tennis Elbow or Cozen's) Test (Method 1). The patient's elbow is stabilized by the examiner's thumb, which rests on the patient's lateral epicondyle (Fig. 5-18). The patient is then asked to make a fist, pronate the forearm, and radially deviate and extend the wrist while the examiner resists the motion. A positive sign is indicated by a sudden severe pain in the area of the lateral epicondyle of the humerus. The epicondyle may be palpated to indicate the origin of the pain.

Lateral Epicondylitis (Tennis Elbow) Test (Method 2). While palpating the lateral epicondyle, the examiner pronates the patient's forearm, flexes the wrist fully, and extends the elbow (see Fig. 5-18). A positive test is indicated by pain over the lateral epicondyle of the humerus. The examiner may simultaneously palpate the epicondyle.

Lateral Epicondylitis (Tennis Elbow) Test (Method 3). The examiner resists extension of the third digit of the hand distal to the proximal interphalangeal joint, stressing the extensor digitorum muscle and tendon. A positive test is indicated by pain over the lateral epicondyle of the humerus.

Medial Epicondylitis (Golfer's Elbow) Test. While the examiner palpates the patient's medial

Elbow Evaluation

Name: _____ UH#: _____ Elbow: R/L

Procedure: _____ Date: _____ Dominant: R/L

Date of Exam (month/day/year)	/ /	/ /	/ /	/ /	/ /
Pain (maximum points) 5 = none (30); 4 = slight—with continuous activity, no medication (25); 3 = moderate—with occasional activity, some medication (15); 2 = moderately severe—much pain, frequent medication (10); 1 = severe—constant pain, markedly limited activity (5); 0 = complete disability (0)	____ ( )				
Motion degrees (37 points maximum)					
Extension (8 pts max) Flexion (17 pts max)	Extension ____° ( ) Flexion ____° ( )				
Pronation/Supination	Pronation ____° ( )				
(pt) = 0.1 per degree—6 maximum	Supination ____° ( )				
Strength (15 points maximum) 5 = normal; 4 = good; 3 = fair; 2 = poor; 1 = trace; 0 = paralysis; NA = not available					
Flex. Ext. Pro. Sup. Normal 5 (5) (4) (3) (3) Good 4 (4) (3) (2) (2) Fair 3 (3) (2) (1) (1) Poor 2 (2) (1) (0) (0) Trace 1 (1) (0) (0) (0) None 0 (0) (0) (0) (0)	Extension ____ ( ) Flexion ____ ( ) Pronation ____ ( ) Supination ____ ( )				
Instability (6 points maximum)					
Ant./Post. Med./Lat. None 3 3 Mild <5 mm, <5° 2 2 Moderate <10 mm, <10° 1 1 Severe >10 mm, >10° 0 0	Ant./Post. _____ Med./Lat. _____				
Function (12 points maximum) 4 = normal (1); 3 = mild compromise (0.75); 2 = difficulty (0.5); 1 = with aid (0.25); 0 = unable (0); NA = not applicable (Index—multiply × 0.25)					
1. Use back pocket	_____ ( )				
2. Rise from chair	_____ ( )				
3. Perineal care	_____ ( )				
4. Wash opposite axilla	_____ ( )				
5. Eat with utensil	_____ ( )				
6. Comb hair	_____ ( )				
7. Carry 10–15 pounds with arm at side	_____ ( )				
8. Dress	_____ ( )				
9. Pulling	_____ ( )				
10. Throwing	_____ ( )				
11. Do usual work Specify work:	_____ ( )				
12. Do usual sport Specify sport:	_____ ( )				
Patient Response 3 = much better; 2 = better; 1 = same; 0 = worse; NA = not available/not applicable	_____				
Completed By: Name of Examiner					
Index					
Key: 95–100 = excellent; 80–95 = good; 50–80 = fair; <50 = poor	( )	( )	( )	( )	( )

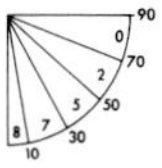

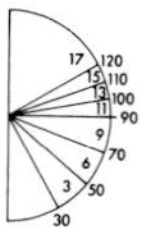

FIGURE 5–16. *Clinically useful elbow evaluation sheet providing objective data retrieval and grading as well as information about function. The use of such a rating index in the clinical setting provides an objective means of comparing different treatment options. (From Morrey, B. F., K. N. An, and E. Y. S. Chao: In Functional Evaluation of the Elbow. In Morrey, B. F. (ed.): The Elbow and Its Disorders. Philadelphia, W. B. Saunders Co., 1985, pp. 88–89. Copyright Mayo Clinic Foundation, Rochester, MN.)*

TABLE 5–2. Functional Testing of the Elbow†

Starting Position	Action	Functional Test*
Sitting	Bring hand to mouth lifting weight (elbow flexion)	Lift 5 to 6 lb: Functional Lift 3 to 4 lb: Functionally Fair Lift 1 to 2 lb: Functionally Poor Lift 0 lb: Nonfunctional
Standing 3 ft from wall, leaning against wall	Push arms straight (elbow extension)	5 to 6 Repetitions: Functional 3 to 4 Repetitions: Functionally Fair 1 to 2 Repetitions: Functionally Poor 0 Repetitions: Nonfunctional
Standing, facing closed door	Open door starting with palm down (supination of arm)	5 to 6 Repetitions: Functional 3 to 4 Repetitions: Functionally Fair 1 to 2 Repetitions: Functionally Poor 0 Repetitions: Nonfunctional
Standing, facing closed door	Open door starting with palm up (pronation of arm)	5 to 6 Repetitions: Functional 3 to 4 Repetitions: Functionally Fair 1 to 2 Repetitions: Functionally Poor 0 Repetitions: Nonfunctional

*Younger patients should be able to lift more (6 to 10 lb) more often (6 to 10 repetitions). With age, weight and repetitions will decrease.
†Adapted from Palmer, M. L., and M. Epler: Clinical Assessment Procedures in Physical Therapy. Philadelphia, J. B. Lippincott, 1990, pp. 109–111.

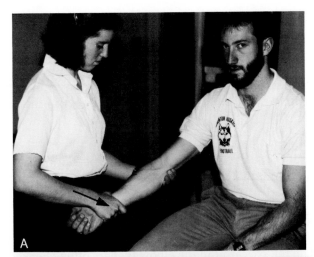
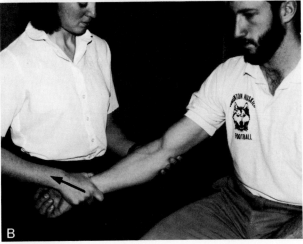

FIGURE 5–17. Testing the collateral ligaments of the elbow. (A) Lateral collateral ligament. (B) Medial collateral ligament.

epicondyle, the patient's forearm is supinated and the elbow and wrist are extended by the examiner. A positive sign is indicated by pain over the medial epicondyle of the humerus.

Tests for Neurological Dysfunction

Tinel's Sign (at the Elbow). The area of the ulnar nerve in the groove (between the olecranon process and medial epicondyle) is tapped. A positive sign is indicated by a tingling sensation in the ulnar distribution of the forearm and hand distal to the

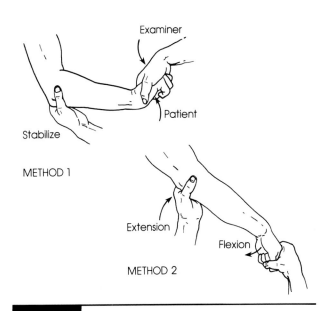

FIGURE 5–18. Tests for tennis elbow.

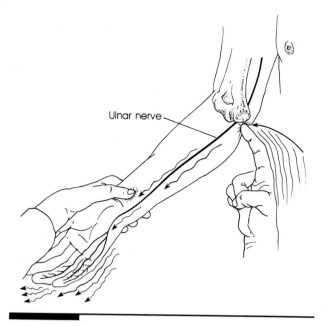

FIGURE 5–19. *Tinel's sign at the elbow for the ulnar nerve.*

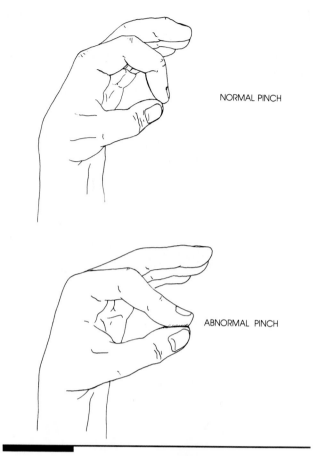

FIGURE 5–20. *Normal versus abnormal pinch seen in anterior interosseous nerve syndrome.*

point of compression of the nerve (Fig. 5–19). The test indicates the rate of regeneration of the sensory fibers of a nerve. The most distal point at which the abnormal sensation is felt represents the limit of nerve regeneration.

Wartenberg's Sign. The patient sits with the hands resting on the table. The examiner passively spreads the fingers apart and asks the patient to bring the fingers together. Inability to squeeze the little finger to the remainder of the hand indicates a positive test for ulnar neuritis.[6]

Elbow Flexion Test. The patient is asked to completely flex the elbow and hold it in the flexed position for 5 minutes. A positive test is indicated by tingling or paresthesia in the ulnar nerve distribution of the forearm and hand. The test helps to determine whether a cubital tunnel syndrome is present.

Test for Pronator Teres Syndrome.[6] The patient sits with the elbow flexed to 90°. The examiner strongly resists pronation as the elbow is extended. A positive test is indicated by tingling or paresthesia in the median nerve distribution in the forearm and hand.

Pinch Grip Test. The patient is asked to pinch the tips of the index finger and thumb together. Normally, there should be a tip-to-tip pinch. If the patient is unable to pinch tip to tip and instead has an abnormal pulp-to-pulp pinch of the index finger and thumb, the test is indicative of a positive sign for pathology to the anterior interosseous nerve, a branch of the median nerve. This finding may indicate an entrapment of the anterior interosseous nerve

as it passes between the two heads of the pronator teres muscle (Fig. 5–20).[17]

Reflexes and Cutaneous Distribution

The reflexes around the elbow that are often checked include the biceps (C5–C6), brachioradialis (C5–C6), and triceps (C7–C8) (Fig. 5–21). The examiner should also check the dermatomes around the elbow and the cutaneous distribution of the various nerves, noting any difference (Figs. 5–22 and 5–23). Pain may be referred to the elbow from the neck (often mimicking tennis elbow), the shoulder, or the wrist (Fig. 5–24).

Anterior Interosseous Nerve

The examiner must know about potential injury to or pinching of the various nerves around the elbow. The anterior interosseous nerve, which is a branch of the median nerve, is sometimes pinched or entrapped as it passes between the two heads of the pronator teres muscle, leading to functional impairment of flexor pollicis longus, the lateral half of

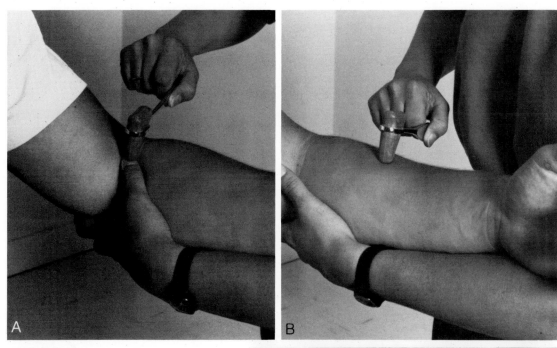

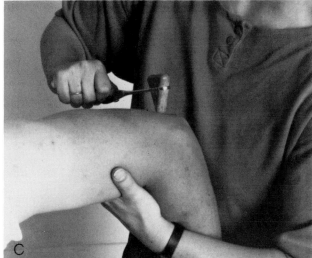

FIGURE 5–21. *Reflexes around the elbow.* (A) *Biceps.* (B) *Brachioradialis.* (C) *Triceps.*

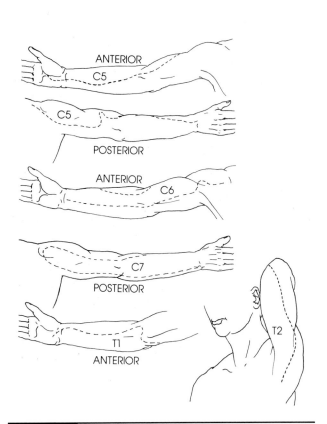

FIGURE 5–22. *Dermatomes around the elbow.*

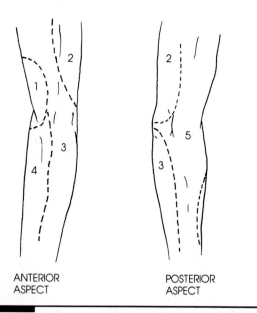

ANTERIOR
ASPECT

POSTERIOR
ASPECT

FIGURE 5–23. *Sensory nerve distribution around the elbow. (1) Lower lateral cutaneous nerve of arm (radial). (2) Medial cutaneous nerve of arm. (3) Medial cutaneous nerve of forearm. (4) Lateral cutaneous nerve of forearm (musculocutaneous nerve). (5) Posterior cutaneous nerve of forearm (radial nerve).*

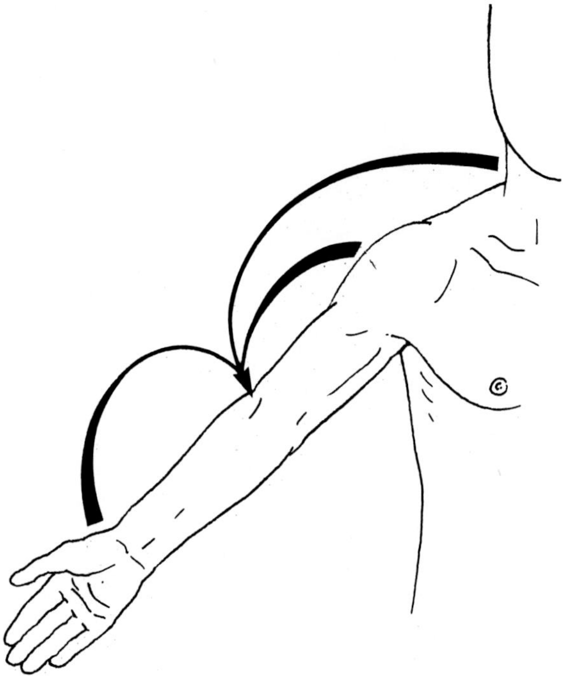

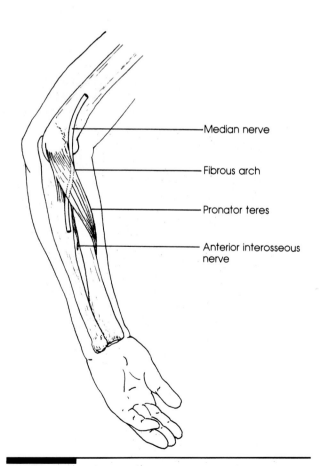

Median nerve

Fibrous arch

Pronator teres

Anterior interosseous nerve

FIGURE 5–25. *Anterior interosseous syndrome.*

FIGURE 5–24. *Referred pain to the elbow.*

flexor digitorum profundus, and pronator quadratus muscles. The condition is called *anterior interosseous nerve syndrome* (Fig. 5–25)[17] and is characterized by a pinch deformity (see Fig. 5–20). The deformity results from the paralysis of the flexors of the index finger and thumb. This leads to extension of the distal interphalangeal joint of the index finger and the interphalangeal joint of the thumb. The resulting pinch is pulp to pulp rather than tip to tip. If the median nerve is damaged or pinched just before the anterior interosseous branch, it may be called *pronator syndrome*; in this case, the flexor carpi radialis, palmaris longus, and flexor digitorum muscles are affected in addition to those affected by the anterior interosseous nerve syndrome. In both cases, the sensory distribution of the median nerve will be affected.

Median Nerve

The median nerve may also be pinched or compressed above the elbow as it passes under the *ligament of Struthers*, an anomalous structure found in approximately 1 per cent of the population (Fig. 5–26).[8] The ligament runs from an abnormal spur on the shaft of the humerus to the medial epicondyle of the humerus. Because the brachial artery sometimes accompanies the nerve through this tunnel, it may also be compressed, resulting in possible vascular as well as neurological symptoms. In this case, the neurological involvement would include the pronator teres muscle as well as those muscles affected by the pronator syndrome. The condition may also be called the *humerus supracondylar process syndrome*.

Ulnar Nerve

In the elbow region, the ulnar nerve is most likely to be injured, compressed, or stretched in the cubital tunnel (see Fig. 5–3).[8] This tunnel, which is relatively long, can cause trapping of the nerve as the nerve passes through it or between the two heads of the flexor carpi ulnaris muscle. When the elbow is flexed, greater stretch is placed on the nerve. Thus, symptoms are more likely to occur when the elbow is flexed. It is usually in the cubital tunnel area that the ulnar nerve is affected, leading to tardy ulnar palsy.

Radial Nerve

The major branch of the radial nerve in the forearm is the *posterior interosseous nerve*, which is given off in front of the lateral epicondyle of the humerus.[8, 9] This branch may be compressed as it passes between the two supinator heads in the *arcade* or *canal of Frohse*, a fibrous arch in the supinator muscle occurring in 30 per cent of the population (Fig. 5–27). Compression leads to functional involvement of the forearm extensor muscles. There is no sensory deficit. This condition, called *radial tunnel syndrome*, may mimic tennis elbow.

Joint Play Movements

When examining the joint play movements (Fig. 5–28), the examiner must compare the injured side with the normal side. The following joint play movements should be performed on the elbow:

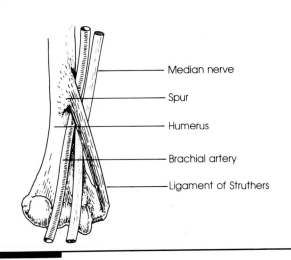

FIGURE 5–26. *Compression of the median nerve by ligament of Struthers.*

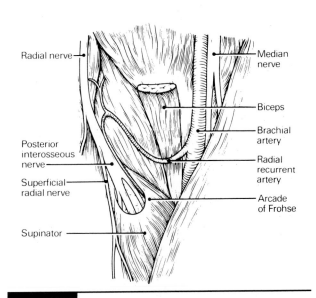

FIGURE 5–27. *Canal or arcade of Frohse. (From Wadsworth, T. G.: The Elbow. New York, Churchill Livingstone, 1982.)*

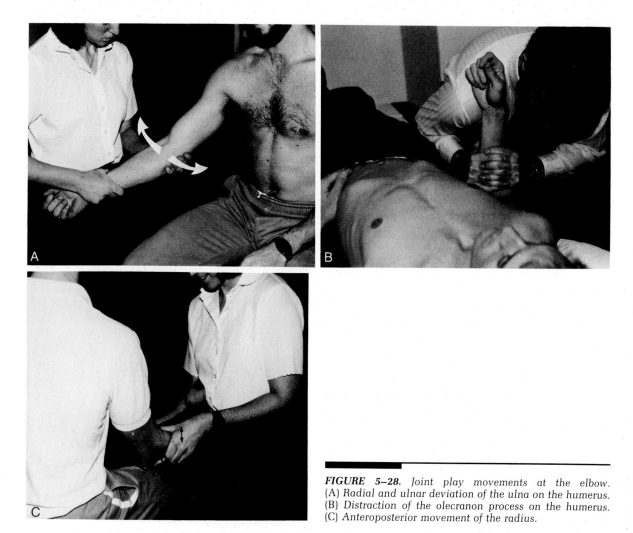

FIGURE 5–28. *Joint play movements at the elbow. (A) Radial and ulnar deviation of the ulna on the humerus. (B) Distraction of the olecranon process on the humerus. (C) Anteroposterior movement of the radius.*

1. Radial deviation of the ulna and radius on the humerus.
2. Ulnar deviation of the ulna and radius on the humerus.
3. Distraction of the olecranon process on the humerus in 90° of flexion.
4. Anteroposterior glide of the radius on the humerus.

The first two movements are performed in a fashion similar to those in the collateral ligament tests. The examiner stabilizes the patient's elbow by holding the patient's humerus firmly and places the other hand above the patient's wrist, abducting and adducting the patient's forearm. The patient's elbow is straight (extended) during the movement, and the end feel should be bone to bone.

To distract the olecranon process, the examiner flexes the patient's elbow to 90°. Wrapping both hands around the patient's forearm close to the elbow, the examiner then applies a distractive force at the elbow, ensuring that no torque is applied.

To test anteroposterior glide of the radius on the humerus, the examiner stabilizes the patient's forearm. The patient's arm is held between the examiner's body and arm. The examiner places the thumb of the other hand over the anterior radial head while the index finger is over the posterior radial head. The examiner then pushes the radial head posteriorly with the thumb and anteriorly with the index finger. This movement must be performed with care because it can be very painful to the patient.

Palpation

With the patient's arm relaxed, the examiner begins palpation on the anterior aspect and moves to the medial aspect, the lateral aspect, and finally the posterior aspect (Fig. 5–29). The patient may sit or lie supine, whichever is more comfortable. The examiner is looking for any tenderness, abnormality, change in temperature or in texture of the tissues, or abnormal "bumps." As with all palpation, the

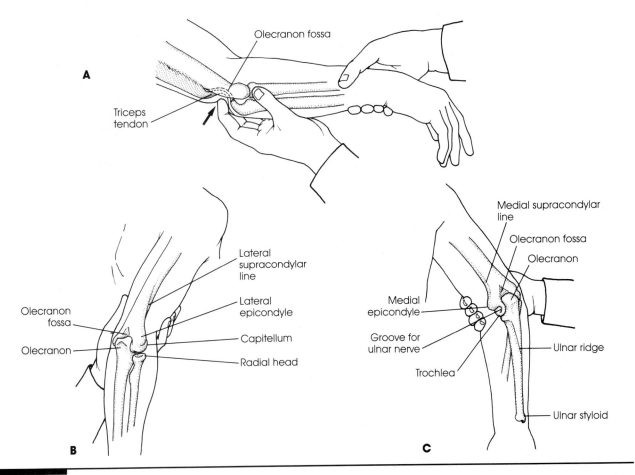

FIGURE 5-29. *Palpation around the elbow.* (A) *Olecranon fossa.* (B) *Posterolateral view of the elbow.* (C) *Posteromedial view of the elbow.*

injured side must be compared with the normal, or uninjured, side.

Anterior Aspect

The following structures are palpated.

Cubital Fossa. The fossa is bound by the pronator teres muscle medially, the brachioradialis muscle laterally, and an imaginary line joining the two epicondyles superiorly. Within the fossa, the biceps tendon and brachial artery may be palpated. After crossing the elbow joint, the brachial artery divides into two branches—the radial artery and the ulnar artery. The examiner must be aware of the brachial artery because it has the potential of being injured as a result of severe trauma (e.g., fracture or dislo-

cation). Trauma to this area may lead to compartment syndromes such as *Volkmann's ischemic contracture.* The median and musculocutaneous nerves are also found in the fossa, but they are not palpable. Pressure on the median nerve may cause symptoms in its cutaneous distribution.

Coronoid Process and Head of Radius. Within the cubital fossa, if the examiner palpates carefully so as not to hurt the patient, the coronoid process of the ulna and the head of the radius may be palpated. Palpation of the radial head will be facilitated by supinating and pronating the forearm. The examiner may palpate the head of the radius from the posterior aspect at the same time by placing the fingers over the head on the posterior aspect and the thumb over it on the anterior aspect. In addition to the muscles previously mentioned, the biceps and brachialis muscles may be palpated for potential abnormality.

Medial Aspect

Moving to the medial aspect of the elbow, the examiner palpates the following structures.

Medial Epicondyle. Originating from the medial epicondyle are the *wrist flexor–forearm pronator* groups of muscles. Both the muscle bellies and their insertions into the bone should be palpated. Tenderness over the epicondyle where the muscles insert is sometimes called *golfer's elbow* or *tennis elbow* of the medial epicondyle.

Medial (Ulnar) Collateral Ligament. This fanshaped ligament may be palpated as it extends from the medial epicondyle to the medial margin of the coronoid process anteriorly and olecranon process posteriorly.

Ulnar Nerve. If the examiner moves posteriorly behind the medial epicondyle, the fingers will rest over the ulnar nerve in the cubital tunnel (proximal part). Usually, the nerve is not directly palpable, but pressure on the nerve will often cause abnormal sensations in its cutaneous distribution. It is this nerve that is struck when one "hits the funny bone."

Lateral Aspect

The following structures are palpated.

Lateral Epicondyle. The wrist extensor muscles originate from the lateral epicondyle, and their muscle bellies, as well as their insertions into the epicondyle, should be palpated. It is at this point of insertion of the common extensor tendon that lateral tennis elbow originates. When palpating, the examiner should remember that the extensor carpi radialis longus muscle inserts above the epicondyle along a short ridge extending from the epicondyle

to the humeral shaft. At the same time, the examiner palpates the brachioradialis and supinator muscles on the lateral aspect of the elbow.

Lateral (Radial) Collateral Ligament. This cord-like ligament may be palpated as it extends from the lateral epicondyle of the humerus to the annular ligament and lateral surface of the ulna.

Annular Ligament. Distal to the lateral epicondyle, the annular ligament and head of the radius may be palpated if not previously done. The palpation is facilitated by supination and pronation of the forearm.

Posterior Aspect

Finally, the following structures should be palpated, as in Figure 5–29.

Olecranon Process and Olecranon Bursa. The olecranon process is best palpated with the elbow flexed to 90°. If the examiner then grasps the skin overlying the process, the olecranon bursa can be palpated. The examiner should note any synovial thickening or the presence of any *rice bodies*, which are small seeds of fragmented fibrous tissue that can act as further irritants to the bursa should it be affected.

Triceps Muscle. The triceps muscle, which inserts into the olecranon process, should be palpated both at its insertion and along its length for any signs of abnormality.

Radiographic Examination

Anteroposterior View. The examiner should note the relations of the epicondyles, trochlea, capitulum, radial head, radial tuberosity, coronoid process, and olecranon process (Fig. 5–30). Any loose bodies,

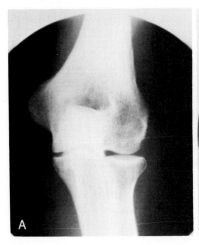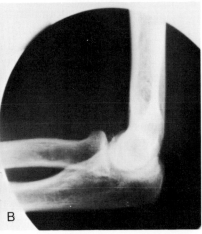

FIGURE 5–30. *Posteroanterior* (A) *and lateral* (B) *radiographs of the elbow.*

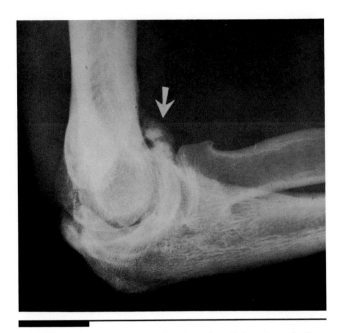

FIGURE 5–31. Excessive ossification after dislocation of elbow treated by early active use. (From O'Donoghue, D. H.: Treatment of Injuries to Athletes, 4th ed. Philadelphia, W. B. Saunders Co., 1984, p. 232.)

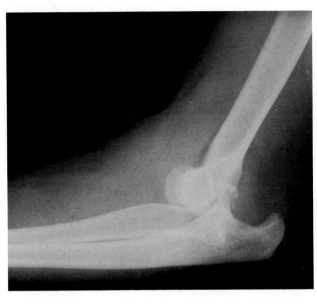

FIGURE 5–32. Lateral film of a dislocated elbow, showing the lower end of the humerus resting on the ulna in front of the coronoid. Note fragmentation of the coronoid. (From O'Donoghue, D. H.: Treatment of Injuries to Athletes, 4th ed. Philadelphia, W. B. Saunders Co., 1984, p. 227.)

calcification, myositis ossificans, joint space narrowing, or osteophytes should be identified. If the examiner is looking at a young child, the epiphysial plate should be noted to see if it is normal for each bone.

Lateral View. The examiner should note the relations of the epicondyles, trochlea, capitulum, radial head, radial tuberosity, coronoid process, and olecranon process. As with the anteroposterior view, any loose bodies, calcifications of the joint (Fig. 5–31), myositis ossificans, dislocations (Fig. 5–32), joint space narrowing, or osteophytes should be noted. The presence of the "fat pad" sign (Fig. 5–33) occurs with elbow joint effusion and may indicate, for example, a fracture, acute rheumatoid arthritis, infection, or osteoid osteoma. Plain radiographs may also be used to visualize the cubital tunnel (Fig. 5–34) and measure the carrying angle (see Fig. 5–4).

Arthrograms. Figure 5–35 illustrates the views seen in normal elbow arthrograms.

MRI. MRI is used to differentiate bone and soft tissue. Because of its high soft-tissue contrast, MRI, a noninvasive technique, is able to discriminate among bone marrow, cartilage, tendons, nerves, and vessels without the use of a contrast medium (Fig. 5–36).

Xerography. Figure 5–37 illustrates the detailed borders of the various structures around the elbow.

Text continued on page 166

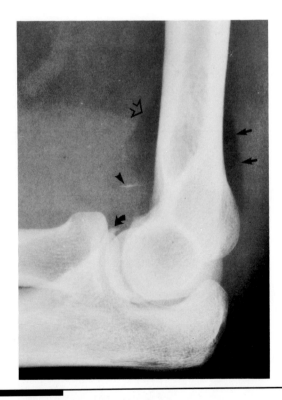

FIGURE 5–33. Coronoid process fracture with hemarthrosis. The posterior fat pad (arrows) is clearly seen on this lateral view with the arm flexed to 90°, indicating joint effusion. The anterior fat pad (open arrow) is clearly visible. There is a fracture of the coronoid process (curved arrow) and a loose body (arrowhead). (From Weissman, B. N. W., and C. B. Sledge: Orthopedic Radiology. Philadelphia, W. B. Saunders Co., 1986, p. 179.)

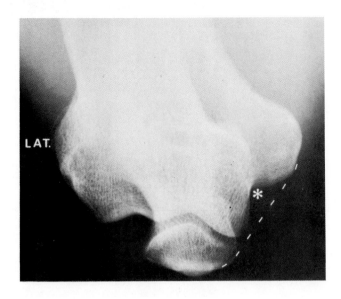

FIGURE 5–34. Cubital tunnel. The ulnar nerve (asterisk) lies in a tunnel bridged by the arcuate ligament (dashed line), which extends from the medial epicondyle to the olecranon process. (After Wadsworth, T. G.: The Elbow. Edinburgh, Churchill Livingstone, 1982.)

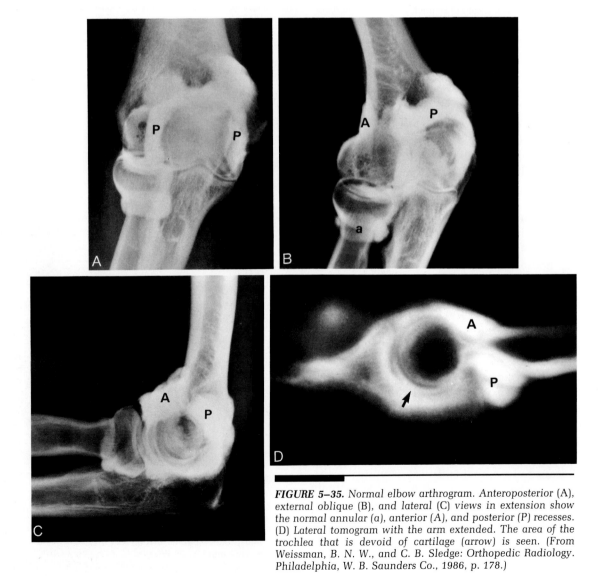

FIGURE 5–35. Normal elbow arthrogram. Anteroposterior (A), external oblique (B), and lateral (C) views in extension show the normal annular (a), anterior (A), and posterior (P) recesses. (D) Lateral tomogram with the arm extended. The area of the trochlea that is devoid of cartilage (arrow) is seen. (From Weissman, B. N. W., and C. B. Sledge: Orthopedic Radiology. Philadelphia, W. B. Saunders Co., 1986, p. 178.)

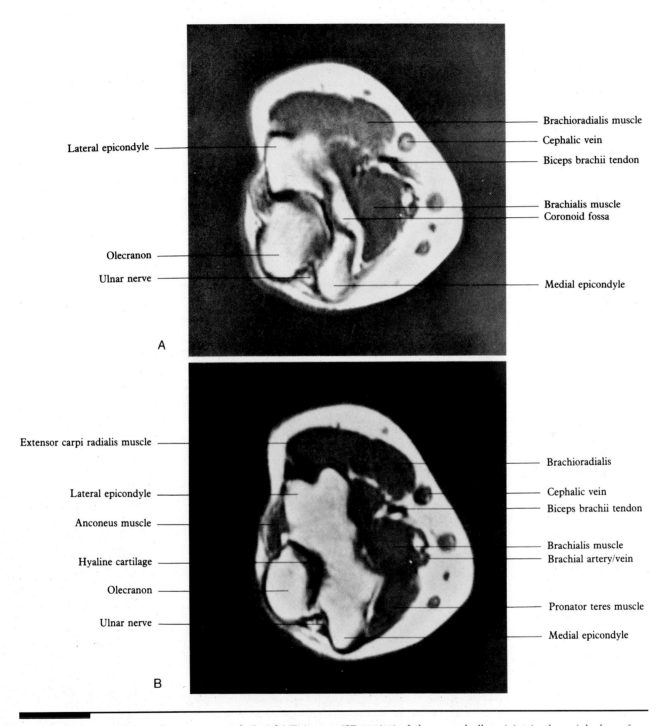

Lateral epicondyle

Olecranon

Ulnar nerve

Brachioradialis muscle

Cephalic vein

Biceps brachii tendon

Brachialis muscle

Coronoid fossa

Medial epicondyle

A

Extensor carpi radialis muscle

Lateral epicondyle

Anconeus muscle

Hyaline cartilage

Olecranon

Ulnar nerve

Brachioradialis

Cephalic vein

Biceps brachii tendon

Brachialis muscle

Brachial artery/vein

Pronator teres muscle

Medial epicondyle

B

FIGURE 5–36. (A–D) Normal anatomy, axial. Serial MR images (SE 500/28) of the normal elbow joint in the axial plane, from superior to inferior.

Illustration continued on following page

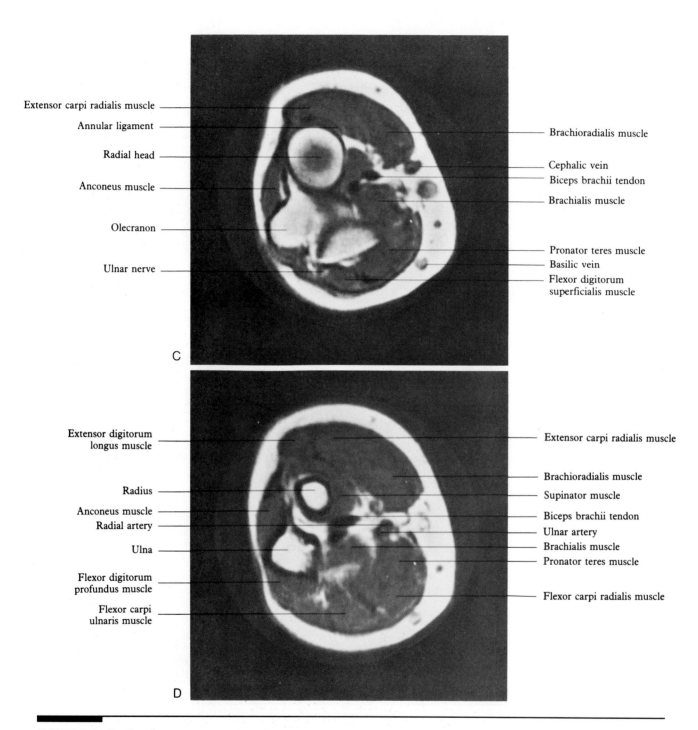

Extensor carpi radialis muscle

Annular ligament

Radial head

Anconeus muscle

Olecranon

Ulnar nerve

Brachioradialis muscle

Cephalic vein

Biceps brachii tendon

Brachialis muscle

Pronator teres muscle

Basilic vein

Flexor digitorum superficialis muscle

C

Extensor digitorum longus muscle

Radius

Anconeus muscle

Radial artery

Ulna

Flexor digitorum profundus muscle

Flexor carpi ulnaris muscle

Extensor carpi radialis muscle

Brachioradialis muscle

Supinator muscle

Biceps brachii tendon

Ulnar artery

Brachialis muscle

Pronator teres muscle

Flexor carpi radialis muscle

D

FIGURE 5–36 Continued

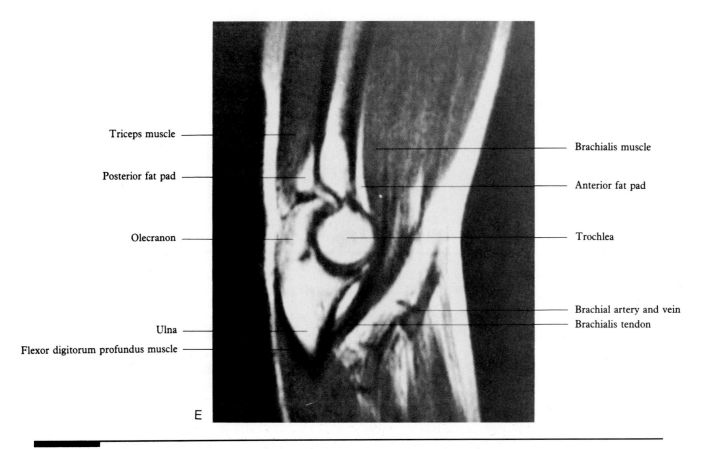

Triceps muscle

Posterior fat pad

Olecranon

Ulna

Flexor digitorum profundus muscle

Brachialis muscle

Anterior fat pad

Trochlea

Brachial artery and vein
Brachialis tendon

E

FIGURE 5–36 Continued (E) Normal anatomy, sagittal. Serial MR images (SE 500/28) of the normal elbow joint in the sagittal plane, from medial to lateral. (From Bassett, L. W., R. H. Gold, and L. L. Seeger: MRI Atlas of the Musculoskeletal System. London, Martin Dunitz Ltd., 1989, p. 133.)

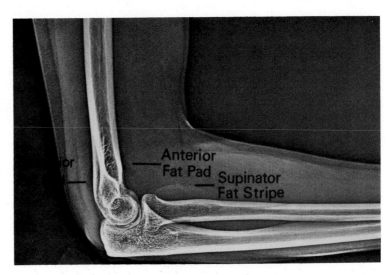

FIGURE 5–37. Xerogram of the elbow demonstrating the fat pads and supinator fat stripe resulting from subtle radial head fracture. (From Berquist, T. H.: Diagnostic radiographic techniques of the elbow. In Morrey, B. F. (ed.): The Elbow and Its Disorders. Philadelphia, W. B. Saunders Co., 1985, p. 100. Copyright Mayo Clinic Foundation, Rochester, MN.)

PRÉCIS OF THE ELBOW ASSESSMENT*

History (sitting)
Observation (sitting)
Examination (sitting)
  Active movements
    Elbow flexion
    Elbow extension
    Supination
    Pronation
  Passive movements (as in active movements, if necessary) (sitting)
  Resisted isometric movements (sitting)
    Elbow flexion
    Elbow extension
    Supination
    Pronation
    Wrist flexion
    Wrist extension
  Special tests (sitting)
  Reflexes and cutaneous distribution (sitting)
  Joint play movements (sitting)
    Radial deviation of ulna and radius on humerus
    Ulnar deviation of ulna and radius on humerus
    Distraction of olecranon process on humerus in 90° of flexion
    Anteroposterior glide of radius on humerus
  Palpation (sitting)
  Radiographic examination

After any examination, the patient should always be warned of the possibility of exacerbation of symptoms as a result of the assessment.

*The entire assessment may be done with the patient in sitting position.

CASE STUDIES

When doing these case studies, the examiner should list the appropriate questions to be asked and why they are being asked, what to look for and why, and what things should be tested and why. Depending on the answers of the patient (and the examiner should consider several different responses), several possible causes of the patient's problems may become evident (examples given in parentheses). If so, a differential diagnosis chart should be made up. The examiner can then decide how different diagnoses may affect the treatment plan.

1. A 52-year-old man is referred to you with a history of right elbow pain. He complains of tenderness over the lateral epicondyle. He informs you that he has not been doing any repetitive forearm activity and does not play tennis. He has some restriction of neck movement. Describe your assessment plan for this patient (cervical spondylosis versus lateral epicondylitis).

2. A 26-year-old male football player is referred to you after surgery for a ruptured (third-degree strain) left biceps tendon at its insertion. His cast has been removed, and you have been asked to restore the patient to normal function. Describe your assessment plan for this patient.

3. A 4-year-old girl is brought to you by her parents. They state that about 2 hours ago they were out shopping and the mother was holding the little girl's arm. The little girl tripped, and the mother "yanked" her up as she fell. The little girl started to cry and would not move her elbow. Describe your assessment plan for this patient (radial head dislocation versus ligamentous sprain).

4. A 46-year-old man comes to you complaining of diffuse left elbow pain. When he carries a briefcase for three or four blocks, his elbow becomes stiff and sore. When he picks up things with his left hand, the pain increases dramatically. Describe your assessment plan for this patient (lateral epicondylitis versus osteoarthritis).

5. A 24-year-old woman comes to you complaining of pain in her right elbow on the medial side. The pain sometimes extends into the forearm and is often accompanied by tingling into the little finger and half of the ring finger. The pain and paresthesia are particularly bothersome when she plays recreational volleyball, which she enjoys very much. Describe your assessment plan for this patient (ulnar neuritis versus medial epicondylitis).

6. A 31-year-old man comes to you complaining of posterior elbow pain. He says he banged his elbow on the table 10 days ago, and he has had posterior swelling for 8 or 9 days. Describe your assessment plan for this patient (olecranon bursitis versus joint synovitis).

7. A 14-year-old female gymnast comes to you complaining of elbow pain. She explains she was doing a vault and bent her elbow backward when she heard a snap. The injury occurred 1 hour ago, and there is some swelling; she does not want to move the elbow. Describe your assessment plan for this patient (biceps tendon rupture versus epiphyseal fracture).

REFERENCES

CITED REFERENCES

1. Beals, R. K.: The normal carrying angle of the elbow. Clin. Orthop. Relat. Res. 119:194, 1976.
2. Charton, A.: The Elbow: The Rheumatological Physical Examination. Orlando, Fla, Grune & Stratton, Inc., 1986.
3. Kapandji, A. I.: The Physiology of the Joints, vol. I: Upper Limb. New York: Churchill Livingstone, 1970.
4. American Orthopaedic Association: Manual of Orthopaedic Surgery. Chicago, 1972.
5. Morrey, B. F., K. N. An, and E. Y. S. Chao: Functional evaluation of the elbow. In Morrey, B. F. (ed.): The Elbow and Its Disorders. Philadelphia, W. B. Saunders Co., 1985.
6. Volz, R. C., and B. F. Morrey: The physical examination of the elbow. In Morrey, B. F. (ed.): The Elbow and Its Disorders. Philadelphia, W. B. Saunders Co., 1985.
7. Wiens, E., and S. Lane: The anterior interosseous nerve syndrome. Can. J. Surg. 21:354, 1978.
8. Spinner, M., and P. S. Spencer: Nerve compression lesions of the upper extremity: A clinical and experimental review. Clin. Orthop. Relat. Res. 104:46, 1974.
9. Wadsworth, T. G.: The Elbow. New York, Churchill Livingstone, 1982.

GENERAL REFERENCES

An, K. N., and B. F. Morrey: Biomechanics of the elbow. In Morrey, B. F. (ed.): The Elbow and Its Disorders. Philadelphia, W. B. Saunders Co., 1985.
Anderson, T. E.: Anatomy and physical examination of the elbow. In Nicholas, J. A., and E. B. Hershman (eds.): The Upper Extremity in Sports Medicine. St. Louis, C. V. Mosby Co., 1990.

Bassett, L. W., R. H. Gold, and L. L. Seeger: MRI Atlas of the Musculoskeletal System. London, Martin Dunitz Ltd., 1989.

Beals, R. K.: The normal carrying angle of the elbow—a radiographic study of 422 patients. Clin. Orthop. Relat. Res. 119:194–196, 1976.

Belhobek, G. H.: Roentgenographic evaluation of the elbow. In Nicholas, J. A., and E. B. Hershman (eds.): The Upper Extremity in Sports Medicine. St. Louis, C. V. Mosby Co., 1990.

Berquist, T. H.: Diagnostic radiographic techniques of the elbow. In Morrey, B. F. (ed.): The Elbow and Its Disorders. Philadelphia, W. B. Saunders Co., 1985.

Bledsoe, R. C., and J. L. Izenstark: Displacement of fat pads in disease and injury of the elbow. Radiology 73:717–724, 1959.

Booker, J. M., and G. A. Thibodeau: Athletic Injury Assessment. St. Louis, Time Mirror/Mosby, 1989.

Bowling, R. W., and P. A. Rockar: The elbow complex. In Gould, J. A. (ed.): Orthopedic and Sports Physical Therapy. St. Louis, C. V. Mosby Co., 1990.

Bunnell, D. H., D. A. Fisher, L. W. Bassett, R. H. Gold, and H. Ellman: Elbow joint: Normal anatomy on MR images. Radiology 165:527–531, 1987.

Cabrera, J. M., and F. C. McCue: Nonosseous athletic injuries of the elbow, forearm, and hand. Clin. Sports Med. 5:681–700, 1986.

Chusid, J. G., and J. J. McDonald: Correlative Neuroanatomy and Functional Neurology. Los Altos, Lange Medical Publications, 1961.

Clarkson, H. M., and G. B. Gilewich: Musculoskeletal Assessment—Joint Range of Motion and Manual Muscle Strength. Baltimore, Williams & Wilkins, 1989.

Conwell, H. E.: Injuries to the elbow. Clin. Symp., 22:35, 1970.

Cyriax, J.: Textbook of Orthopaedic Medicine, vol. I: Diagnosis of Soft Tissue Lesions. London, Bailliere Tindall, 1982.

Forrester, D. M., and J. C. Brown: The Radiology of Joint Disease. Philadelphia, W. B. Saunders Co., 1987.

Garrick, J. G., and D. R. Webb: Sports Injuries: Diagnosis and Management. Philadelphia, W. B. Saunders Co., 1990.

Hollinshead, W. H., and D. B. Jenkins: Functional Anatomy of the Limbs and Back. Philadelphia, W. B. Saunders Co., 1981.

Hoppenfeld, S.: Physical Examination of the Spine and Extremities. New York, Appleton-Century-Crofts, 1976.

Ishizuki, M.: Functional anatomy of the elbow joint and three-dimensional quantitative motion analysis of the elbow joint. J. Jpn. Orthop. Assoc. 53:989, 1979.

Judge, R. D., G. D. Zuidema, and F. T. Fitzgerald: Clinical Diagnosis: A Physiological Approach. Boston, Little, Brown and Co., 1982.

Kaltenborn, F. M.: Mobilization of the Extremity Joints. Oslo, Olaf Norlis Bolchandel, 1980.

Leach, R. E., and J. K. Miller: Lateral and medial epicondylitis of the elbow. Clin. Sports Med. 6:259–272, 1987.

London, J. T.: Kinematics of the elbow. J. Bone Joint Surg. 63A:529, 1981.

Maitland, G. D.: The Peripheral Joints: Examination and Recording Guide. Adelaide, Australia, Virgo Press, 1973.

Morrey, B. F.: Physical examination of the elbow. In Post, M. (ed.): Physical Examination of the Musculoskeletal System. Chicago, Year Book Medical Publishers Inc., 1987.

O'Donoghue, D. H.: Treatment of Injuries to Athletes. Philadelphia, W. B. Saunders Co., 1976, 1984.

Palmer, M. L., and M. Epler: Clinical Assessment Procedures in Physical Therapy. Philadelphia, J. B. Lippincott Co., 1990.

Reid, D. C., and S. Kushner: The elbow region. In Donatelli, R., and M. J. Wooden (eds.): Orthopedic Physical Therapy. Edinburgh, Churchill Livingstone, 1989.

Roles, N. C., and R. H. Maudsley: Radial tunnel syndrome: Resistant tennis elbow as a nerve entrapment. J. Bone Joint Surg. 54B:499, 1972.

Spinner, M.: The arcade of Frohse and its relationship to posterior interosseous nerve paralysis. J. Bone Joint Surg. 50B:809–812, 1968.

Tullos, H. S., and W. J. Bryan: Examination of the throwing elbow. In Zarins, B., J. R. Andrews, and W. G. Carson (eds.): Injuries to the Throwing Arm. Philadelphia, W. B. Saunders Co., 1985.

Wadsworth, C. T.: Manual Examination and Treatment of the Spine and Extremities. Baltimore, Williams & Wilkins, 1988.

Weissman, B. N. W., and C. B. Sledge: Orthopedic Radiology. Philadelphia, W. B. Saunders Co., 1986.

Williams, P. L., and R. Warwick (eds.): Gray's Anatomy. Philadelphia, W. B. Saunders Co., 1980.

CHAPTER 6

Forearm, Wrist, and Hand

The hand and wrist are the most active and intricate parts of the upper extremity. Because of this, they are vulnerable to injury and do not respond well to serious trauma. Their mobility is enhanced by a wide range of movement at the shoulder and complementary movement at the elbow. In addition, the 10 bones, 17 articulations, and 19 intrinsic and 20 extrinsic muscles of the wrist and hand provide a tremendous variability of movement. In addition to being an expressive organ of communication, the hand acts as both a motor and a sensory organ, providing information such as temperature, thickness, texture, depth, and shape as well as the motion of an object. It is this sensual acuity that enables the examiner to accurately examine and palpate during an assessment.

The assessment of the hand should be done with two objectives in mind. First, the injury or lesion should be assessed as accurately as possible to ensure proper treatment. Second, the examiner should evaluate the remaining function to determine whether the patient will have any incapacity in everyday life.

Although the joints of the forearm, wrist, and hand are discussed separately, it must be remembered that these joints do not act in isolation but rather as functional groups. Thus, the position of one joint will influence the position and action of another joint. For example, if the wrist is flexed, the interphalangeal joints will not fully flex, primarily because of passive insufficiency of the finger extensions. In addition, the entire upper limb should be considered a kinetic chain so the hand can be properly positioned. The actions of the shoulder, elbow, and wrist joints enable the hand to be placed on almost any area of the body.

APPLIED ANATOMY

The *distal radioulnar joint* is a uniaxial pivot joint that has one degree of freedom. Although the radius moves over the ulna, the ulna does not remain stationary. It moves back and laterally during pronation and forward and medially during supination. The resting position of the joint is 10° of supination, and the close packed position is 5° of supination. The capsular pattern of the distal radioulnar joint is equal limitation of supination and pronation.

The *radiocarpal (wrist) joint* is a biaxial ellipsoid joint. The radius articulates with the scaphoid and lunate. The lunate and triquetrum also articulate with the cartilaginous disc (triangular-shaped) and not the ulna. The disc extends from the ulnar side of the distal radius and attaches to the ulna at the base of the ulnar styloid process. The disc adds stability to the wrist. It creates a close relation between the ulna and carpal bones and binds together the distal ends of the radius and ulna. With the disc in place, the radius bears 60 per cent of the load and the ulna bears 40 per cent. If the disc is removed, the radius transmits 95 per cent of the axial load and the ulna transmits 5 per cent.[1] Thus, the cartilaginous disc acts as a cushion for the wrist joint. The disc can be damaged by forced extension and pronation. The distal end of the radius is concave and the proximal row of carpals is convex, but the curvatures are not equal. The joint has two degrees of freedom, and the resting position is neutral with slight ulnar deviation. The close packed position is extension, and the capsular pattern is equal limitation in all directions.

The *intercarpal joints* are considered to be the joints between the individual bones of the proximal row of carpal bones (scaphoid, lunate, and triquetrum) and the joints between the individual bones of the distal row of carpal bones (trapezium, trapezoid, capitate, and hamate). They are bound together by small intercarpal ligaments (dorsal, palmar, and interosseous) that allow only a slight amount of gliding movement between the bones. The close packed position is extension, and the resting position is neutral or slight flexion. The *pisotriquetral joint* is considered separately because the pisiform sits on the triquetrum and does not take a direct part in the other intercarpal movements.

The *midcarpal joints* form a compound articulation between the proximal and distal rows of carpal bones with the exception of the pisiform bone. On the medial side, the scaphoid, lunate, and triquetrum articulate with the capitate and hamate, forming a compound *sellar joint*. On the lateral aspect, the scaphoid articulates with the trapezoid and trapezium, forming another compound sellar joint. As with the intercarpal joints, these articulations are bound together by dorsal and palmar ligaments; however, there are no interosseous ligaments between the proximal and distal rows of bones. Therefore, greater movement exists at the midcarpal joints than at the intercarpal joints. The close packed position of these joints is extension with ulnar deviation, and the resting position is neutral or slight flexion with ulnar deviation.

At the thumb, the *carpometacarpal (CMC) joint* is a saddle-shaped (sellar) joint that has three degrees of freedom, whereas the second to fifth carpometacarpal joints are plane joints.[2] The capsular pattern of the carpometacarpal joint of the thumb is abduction most limited followed by extension. The resting position is midway between abduction and adduction and midway between flexion and extension. The close packed position of the carpometacarpal joint of the thumb is full opposition. For the second to fifth carpometacarpal joints, the capsular pattern of restriction is equal limitation in all directions. The bones of these joints are held together by dorsal and palmar ligaments. In addition, the thumb articulation has a strong lateral ligament extending from the lateral side of the trapezium to the radial side of the base of the first metacarpal, and the medial four articulations have an interosseous ligament similar to that found in the carpal articulations.

The carpometacarpal articulations of the fingers allow only gliding movement. The carpometacarpal articulation of the thumb is unique in that it allows flexion, extension, abduction, adduction, rotation, and circumduction. It is able to do this because this articulation, as previously mentioned, is saddle shaped. Because of the many movements possible at this joint, the thumb is able to adopt any position relative to the palmar aspect of the hand.[2]

The plane *intermetacarpal joints* have only a small amount of gliding movement between them and do not include the thumb articulation. They are bound together by palmar, dorsal, and interosseous ligaments.

The *metacarpophalangeal (MCP) joints* are condyloid joints. The second and third metacarpophalangeal joints tend to be immobile and are the primary stabilizing factor of the hand, whereas the fourth and fifth joints are more mobile. The collateral ligaments of these joints are tight on flexion and relaxed on extension. These articulations are also bound by palmar ligaments and deep transverse metacarpal ligaments. Each joint has two degrees of freedom. The first metacarpophalangeal joint has three degrees of freedom, thus facilitating the movement of the carpometacarpal joint of the thumb.[2] The close packed position of the first metacarpophalangeal joint is maximum opposition, and the close packed position for the second to fifth metacarpophalangeal joints is maximum flexion.[3] The resting position of the metacarpophalangeal joints is slight flexion, whereas the capsular pattern is more limitation of flexion than extension.

The *interphalangeal (IP) joints* are uniaxial hinge joints with each joint having one degree of freedom. The close packed position of the *proximal interphalangeal (PIP) joints* and *distal interphalangeal (DIP) joints* is full extension; the resting position is slight flexion. The capsular pattern of these joints is flexion more limited than extension. The bones of these joints are bound together by a fibrous capsule and by the palmar and collateral ligaments. During flexion, there is some rotation in these joints so that the pulp of the fingers faces more fully the pulp of the thumb (Fig. 6–1).

PATIENT HISTORY

In addition to the general history questions presented in Chapter 1, the following information should be determined:

1. What is the patient's usual activity or pastime?

2. What is the patient's occupation?

3. What are the sites and boundaries of pain and any abnormal sensations that are present?

4. Are the symptoms improving, getting worse, or staying the same?

5. When did the injury or onset occur, and how long has the patient been incapacitated? These two questions are not necessarily the same; for instance, a burn may occur at a certain time, but incapacity may not occur until hypertrophic scarring appears.

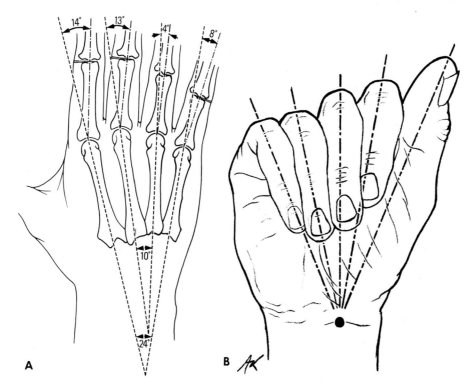

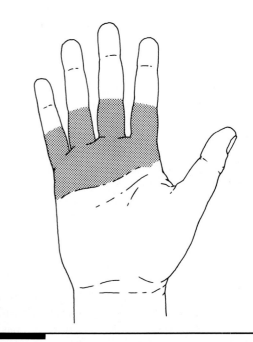

FIGURE 6–1. Alignment of the fingers. (A) Normal physiological alignment. (B) Oblique flexion of the last four digits. Only the index ray flexes toward the median axis. Thus, when the last four digits are flexed separately at the metacarpophalangeal and proximal interphalangeal joints, their axes converge toward the scaphoid tubercle. (From Tubiana, R.: The Hand. Philadelphia, W. B. Saunders Co., 1981, pp. 197 and 22.)

6. What things is the patient functionally unable to do? Which hand is the patient's dominant hand?

7. Has the person ever injured the forearm, wrist, or hand before?

8. Which part of the forearm, wrist, or hand is injured? If the flexor tendons (which are round, have synovial sheaths, and have a longer excursion than the extensor tendons) are injured, they respond much more slowly to treatment than do extensor tendons (which are flat or ovoid). Within the hand, there is a surgical "no man's land" (Fig. 6–2), which is a region between the distal palmar crease and the midportion of the middle phalanx of the fingers. Damage to the flexor tendons in this area requiring surgical repair usually leads to the formation of adhesive bands that restrict gliding. In addition, the tendons may become ischemic in this area, being replaced by scar tissue. Because of this, the prognosis after surgery in this area is poor.

9. What is the mechanism of injury? For example, a fall on the outstretched hand may lead to a lunate dislocation, or extension of the fingers may cause dislocation of the fingers. A rotational force applied to the wrist or near it may lead to a *Galleazzi fracture*, which is a fracture of the radius and dislocation of the distal end of the ulna.

10. What tasks is the patient able or unable to do perform? For example, is there any problem with buttoning, dressing, tying shoelaces, or any other everyday activity?

OBSERVATION

While observing the patient and viewing the hands from both the anterior and posterior aspects, the examiner should note the patient's willingness and ability to use the hand. Normally, when the hand is

FIGURE 6–2. Surgical "no-man's land" (palmar view).

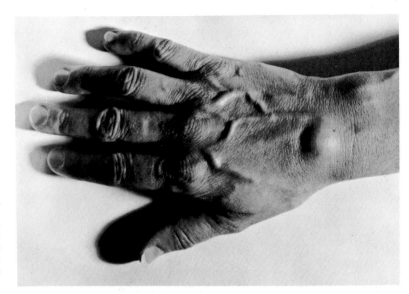

FIGURE 6–3. Ganglion or small cystic swelling on the dorsum of the right hand just distal to the wrist joint. (From Polley, H. F., and G. G. Hunder: Rheumatologic Interviewing and Physical Examination of the Joints. Philadelphia, W. B. Saunders Co., 1978, p. 96.)

in the resting position and the wrist is in the neutral position, the fingers are progressively more flexed as one moves from the radial side of the hand to the ulnar side. Loss of this normal attitude may be due to a lacerated tendon or a contracture such as *Dupuytren's contracture.*

The bone and soft-tissue contours of the forearm, wrist, and hand should be normal, and any deviation should be noted. The cosmetic appearance of the hand is very important to some patients. Thus, the examiner should also note the patient's reaction to the hand and be prepared to provide a cosmetic evaluation, noting the patient's, and potentially society's, reaction to the hand's cosmetic appearance. This evaluation should always be included with the more important functional assessment. The posture of the hand at rest will often demonstrate common deformities. Are the normal skin creases present? Skin creases occur because of movement at the various joints. The examiner should note any muscle wasting on the thenar eminence (median nerve), first dorsal interosseous muscle (C7 nerve root), or hypothenar eminence (ulnar nerve) that may be indicative of nerve or nerve root injury.

Any localized swellings (such as a ganglion) that are usually seen on the dorsum of the hand should be recorded (Fig. 6–3). In the wrist and hand, effusion and synovial thickening are most evident on the dorsal and radial aspects. Swelling of the metacarpophalangeal and interphalangeal joints is most obvious on the dorsal aspect.

The dominant hand tends to be larger than the nondominant hand, and the examiner should remember that if the patient has an area on the fingers that lacks sensation, this area will be avoided when lifting or identifying objects, and the patient will instead use another finger with normal sensitivity.

Any vasomotor, sudomotor, pilomotor, and trophic changes should be recorded. These changes may be indicative of a peripheral nerve injury, peripheral vascular disease, diabetes mellitus, Raynaud's disease, or reflex neurovascular syndromes such as shoulder-hand syndrome or Sudeck's atrophy. The changes seen could include loss of hair on the hand, brittle fingernails, increase or decrease in sweating of the palm, shiny skin, radiographic evidence of osteoporosis, or any difference in temperature between the two limbs. Table 6–1 illustrates

TABLE 6–1. Sympathetic Changes After Nerve Injury*

Sympathetic Function	Early Changes		Late Changes
Vasomotor	Skin color	Rosy	Mottled or cyanotic
	Skin temperature	Warm	Cool
Sudomotor	Sweat	Dry skin	Dry or overly moist
Pilomotor	Gooseflesh response	Absent	Absent
Trophic	Skin texture	Soft, smooth	Smooth, nonelastic
	Soft-tissue atrophy	Slight	More pronounced, especially in finger pulps
	Nail changes	Blemishes	Curved in longitudinal and horizontal planes, "talonlike"
	Hair growth	May fall out or become longer and finer	May fall out or become longer and finer
	Rate of healing	Slowed	Slowed

*From Hunter, J., et al. (eds.): Rehabilitation of the Hand: Surgery and Therapy. St. Louis, C. V. Mosby Co., 1990, p. 595.

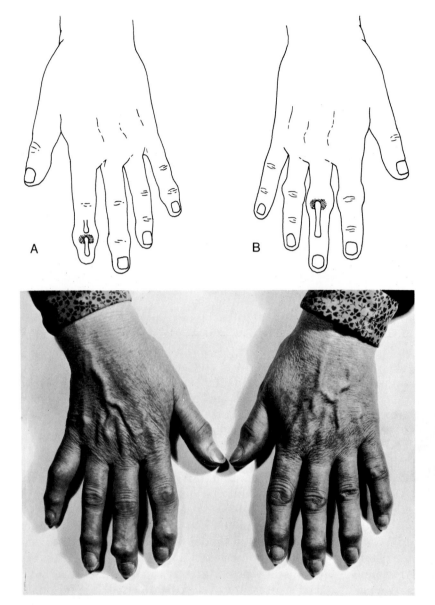

FIGURE 6–4. (A) Heberden's nodes. (B) Bouchard's nodes. (C) Degenerative joint disease (osteoarthritis) of both hands. Osteoarthritic enlargement of the distal interphalangeal joints (Heberden's nodes) and the proximal interphalangeal joints (Bouchard's nodes) is present. The metacarpophalangeal joints are not affected. (C is from Polley, H. F., and G. G. Hunder: Rheumatologic Interviewing and Physical Examination of the Joints. Philadelphia, W. B. Saunders Co., 1978, p. 120.)

vasomotor, sudomotor, pilomotor, and trophic changes that occur in the hand when sympathetic nerve function has been affected.

The examiner should note any hypertrophy of one or more fingers. Hypertrophy of the bone may be seen in Paget's disease, neurofibromatosis, or arteriovenous fistula.

The presence of Heberden's or Bouchard's nodes (Fig. 6–4) should be recorded. Heberden's nodes appear on the dorsal surface of the distal interphalangeal joints and are associated with osteoarthritis. Bouchard's nodes are on the dorsal surface of the proximal interphalangeal joints. They are often associated with gastrectasis and rheumatoid arthritis.

Any ulcerations may indicate neurological or circulatory problems. Any alteration in color of the limb with changes in position may indicate a circulatory problem.

The examiner should note any rotational or angulated deformities of the fingers, which may be indicative of previous fracture. The nail beds are normally parallel to one another. The fingers, when extended, generally are slightly rotated toward the thumb. Ulnar drift may be seen in rheumatoid arthritis owing to the shape of the metacarpophalangeal joints and the pull of the long flexor tendons.

Scars, if present, may indicate recent surgery or past injury. A scar may result in decreased mobility in a joint if the formation of scar tissue is sufficient.

The examiner should take time to observe the fingernails. "Spoon-shaped" nails are often the result of fungal infection, and "clubbed" nails may result from hypertrophy of the underlying soft tissue or respiratory or cardiac problems (Figs. 6–5 and 6–6). Table 6–2 shows other pathological processes that may affect the fingernails.

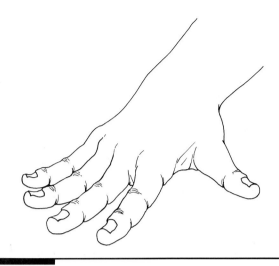

FIGURE 6–5. "Spoon" nails.

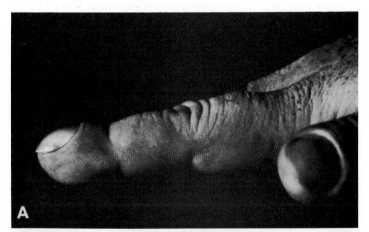

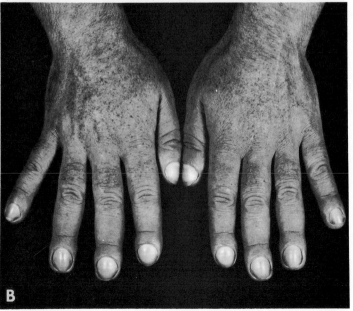

FIGURE 6–6. Clubbing of distal interphalangeal joints and rounding of the nails in a patient with hypertrophic osteoarthropathy. (A) Close-up side view of index finger. (B) Dorsal aspect of both hands. (From Polley, H. F., and G. G. Hunder: Rheumatologic Interviewing and Physical Examination of the Joints. Philadelphia, W. B. Saunders Co., 1978, p. 122.)

TABLE 6–2. Glossary of Nail Pathology*

Condition	Description	Occurrence
Beau's lines	Transverse lines or ridges marking repeated disturbances of nail growth	Systemic diseases, toxic or nutritional deficiency states of many types, trauma (from manicuring)
Defluvium unguium (onychomadesis)	Complete loss of nails	Certain systemic diseases such as scarlet fever, syphilis, leprosy, alopecia areata, and exfoliative dermatitis
Diffusion of lunula unguis	"Spreading" of lunula	Dystrophies of the extremities
Eggshell nails	Nail plate thin, semitransparent bluish-white, with a tendency to curve upward at the distal edge	Syphilis
Fragilitas unguium	Friable or brittle nails	Dietary deficiency, local trauma
Hapalonychia	Nails very soft, split easily	Following contact with strong alkalis; endocrine disturbances, malnutrition, syphilis, chronic arthritis
Hippocratic nails	"Watch-glass nails" associated with "drumstick fingers"	Chronic respiratory and circulatory diseases, especially pulmonary tuberculosis; hepatic cirrhosis
Koilonychia	"Spoon nails"; nails are concave on the outer surface	Dysendocrinisms (acromegaly), trauma, dermatoses, syphilis, nutritional deficiencies, hypothyroidism
Leukonychia	White spots or striations or rarely the whole nail may turn white (congenital type)	Local trauma, hepatic cirrhosis, nutritional deficiencies, and many systemic diseases
Mees' lines	Transverse white bands	Hodgkin's granuloma, arsenic and thallium toxicity, high fevers, local nutritional derangement
Moniliasis of nails	Infections (usually paronychial) caused by yeast forms (*Candida albicans*)	Frequently in food-handlers, dentists, dishwashers, gardeners
Onychatrophia	Atrophy or failure of development of nails	Trauma, infection, dysendocrinism, gonadal aplasia, and many systemic disorders
Onychauxis	Nail plate is greatly thickened	Mild persistent trauma, systemic diseases such as peripheral stasis, peripheral neuritis, syphilis, leprosy, hemiplegia, or at times may be congenital
Onychia	Inflammation of the nail matrix causing deformity of the nail plate	Trauma, infection, many systemic diseases
Onychodystrophy	Any deformity of the nail plate, nail bed, or nail matrix	Many diseases, trauma, or chemical agents (poisoning, allergy)
Onychogryposis	"Claw nails"—extreme degree of hypertrophy, sometimes with horny projections arising from the nail surface	May be congenital or related to many chronic systemic diseases (see onychauxis above)
Onycholysis	Loosening of the nail plate beginning at the distal or free edge	Trauma, injury by chemical agents, many systemic diseases
Onychomadesis	Shedding of all the nails (defluvium unguium)	Dermatoses such as exfoliative dermatitis, alopecia areata, psoriasis, eczema, nail infection, severe systemic diseases, arsenic poisoning
Onychophagia	Nail biting	Neurosis
Onychorrhexis	Longitudinal ridging and splitting of the nails	Dermatoses, nail infections, many systemic diseases, senility, injury by chemical agents, hyperthyroidism
Onychoschizia	Lamination and scaling away of nails in thin layers	Dermatoses, syphilis, injury by chemical agents
Onychotillomania	Alteration of the nail structures caused by persistent neurotic picking of the nails	Neurosis
Pachyonychia	Extreme thickening of all the nails. The nails are more solid and more regular than in onychogryposis	Usually congenital and associated with hyperkeratosis of the palms and soles
Pterygium unguis	Thinning of the nail fold and spreading of the cuticle over the nail plate	Associated with vasospastic conditions such as Raynaud's phenomenon and occasionally with hypothyroidism

*From Berry, T. J.: The Hand As a Mirror of Systemic Disease. Philadelphia, F. A. Davis Co., 1963.

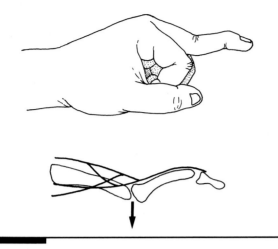

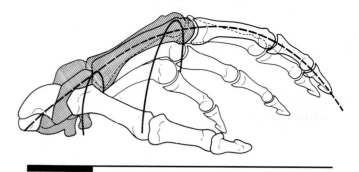

FIGURE 6–9. *Longitudinal and transverse arches of the hand (lateral view). Shaded areas show the fixed part of the skeleton. (From Tubiana, R.: The Hand. Philadelphia, W. B. Saunders Co., 1981, p. 25.)*

FIGURE 6–7. *"Swan neck" deformity.*

Common Hand and Finger Deformities

Deformities of the hand and fingers that may be seen include the following:

Swan Neck Deformity. This deformity usually involves only the fingers. There is flexion of the metacarpophalangeal and distal interphalangeal joints. In addition to this, there is extension of the proximal interphalangeal joint. The condition is a result of contracture of the intrinsic muscles and is often seen in rheumatoid arthritis or after trauma (Fig. 6–7).

Boutonnière Deformity. Extension of the metacarpophalangeal and distal interphalangeal joints and flexion of the proximal interphalangeal joint are seen. The deformity is the result of a rupture of the central tendinous slip of the extensor hood and is most common after trauma or in rheumatoid arthritis (Fig. 6–8).

Claw Fingers. This deformity results from the loss of intrinsic muscle action and the overaction of the extrinsic extensor muscles on the proximal phalanx of the fingers. The metacarpophalangeal joints are hyperextended, and the proximal and distal interphalangeal joints are flexed. When intrinsic function is lost, the hand is called an "intrinsic-minus" hand. The normal cupping of the hand is lost, the arches of the hand disappear, and there is intrinsic muscle wasting. Normally, the hand has two arches—a longitudinal arch and a transverse arch (Fig. 6–9). The deformity is most often due to a combined median and ulnar nerve palsy (Fig. 6–10).

"Trigger Finger." Also known as *digital tenovaginitis stenosans,* this deformity is the result of a thickening of the flexor tendon sheath, which causes sticking of the tendon when the patient attempts to flex the finger. A low-grade inflammation of the proximal fold of the flexor tendon leads to swelling and constriction (stenosis) in the digital flexor tendon. When the patient attempts to flex the finger, the tendon sticks, and the finger "lets go," often with a snap. As the condition worsens, the finger will flex but eventually will not let go, and it will have to be passively extended. The condition is more likely to occur in middle-aged women,

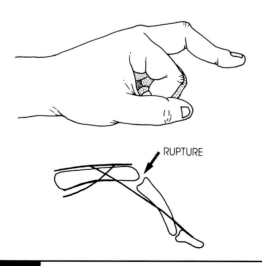

RUPTURE

FIGURE 6–8. *Boutonnière deformity.*

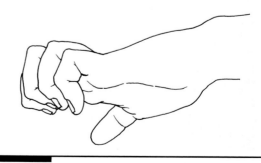

FIGURE 6–10. *"Claw" fingers (intrinsic minus hand).*

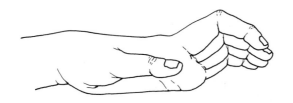

FIGURE 6–11. *"Ape hand" deformity.*

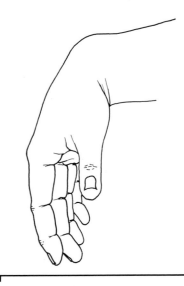

FIGURE 6–13. *Drop-wrist deformity.*

whereas "trigger thumb" is more common in young children. The condition usually occurs in the third or fourth finger. It is most often associated with rheumatoid arthritis and tends to be worse in the morning.

"Ape Hand" Deformity. There is wasting of the thenar eminence of the hand as a result of a median nerve palsy, and the thumb falls back in line with the fingers as a result of the pull of the extensor muscles. The patient is also unable to oppose or flex the thumb (Fig. 6–11).

Bishop's or Benediction Hand Deformity. There is wasting of the hypothenar muscles of the hand, the interossei muscles, and the two medial lumbrical muscles because of ulnar nerve palsy (Fig. 6–12).

Drop-Wrist Deformity. The extensor muscles of the wrist are paralyzed as a result of a radial nerve palsy, and the wrist and fingers cannot be extended (Fig. 6–13).

"Z" Deformity of the Thumb. The thumb is flexed at the metacarpophalangeal joint and extended at the interphalangeal joint (Fig. 6–14). The deformity

may be due to heredity, or it may be associated with rheumatoid arthritis.

Dupuytren's Contracture. This condition is the result of contracture of the palmar fascia. There is a fixed flexion deformity of the metacarpophalangeal and proximal interphalangeal joints (Fig. 6–15). Dupuytren's contracture is usually seen in the ring or little finger, and the skin is often adherent to the fascia. It affects men more often than women and is usually seen in the 50- to 70-year-old age group.

Mallet Finger. A mallet finger deformity is the result of a rupture or avulsion of the extensor tendon where it inserts into the distal phalanx of the finger. The rupture or avulsion results in the distal phalanx resting in a flexed position (Fig. 6–16).

Other Physical Findings

The hand is the terminal part of the upper limb. Many pathological conditions manifest themselves in this structure and may lead the examiner to

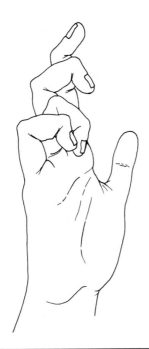

FIGURE 6–12. *"Bishop's hand" or "benediction hand" deformity.*

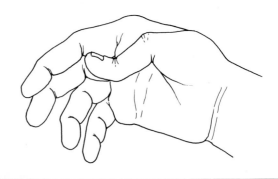

FIGURE 6–14. *"Z" deformity of the thumb.*

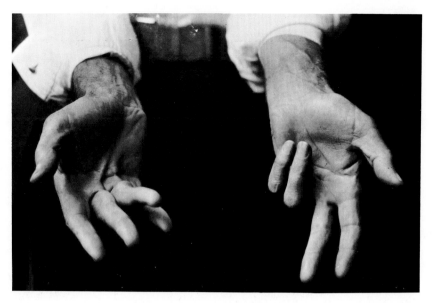

FIGURE 6–15. Dupuytren's contracture in both hands showing flexion contractures of the fourth and fifth digits of the left hand and less severe contractures in the third, fourth, and fifth digits of the right hand. Note the puckering of palmar skin and presence of bands extending from the concavity of the palm to the proximal interphalangeal joints of the third and fourth digits of the right hand. (From Polley, H. F., and G. G. Hunder: Rheumatologic Interviewing and Physical Examination of the Joints. Philadelphia, W. B. Saunders Co., 1978, p. 98.)

suspect pathological conditions elsewhere in the body. Some of these conditions may include:

1. Generalized or continued body exposure to radiation produces brittle nails, longitudinal nail ridges, skin keratosis (thickening), and ulceration.

2. The Plummer-Vinson syndrome produces spoon-shaped nails (Fig. 6–5). This condition is a dysphasia with atrophy in the mouth, pharynx, and upper esophagus.

3. Psoriasis may cause scaling, deformity, and fragmentation and detachment of the nails.

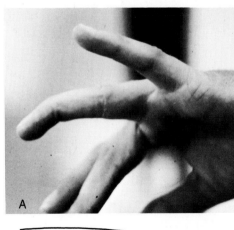
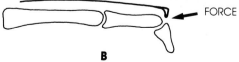

FIGURE 6–16. Mallet finger. (A) Patient actively attempting to extend finger. (B) Mechanism of injury. Tendon is ruptured or avulsed from bone.

4. Hyperthyroidism produces nail atrophy and ridging with warm, moist hands.

5. Vasospastic conditions produce a thin nail fold and *pterygium* (abnormal extension) of the cuticle.

6. Avitaminosis and chronic alcoholism produce transverse, or "Beau's," lines in the nails (Fig. 6–17).

7. Many arterial diseases produce a lack of linear growth with thick, dark nails.

8. Lues (syphilis) produces a hypertrophic overgrowth of the nail plate. The nails break and crumple easily.

9. Chronic respiratory disorders produce clubbing of the nails (Fig. 6–6).

10. Subacute bacterial endocarditis may produce "Osler's nodes," which are small, tender nodes in the finger pads.

11. Congenital heart disease may produce cyanosis and nail clubbing.

12. Neurocirculatory aesthesia (loss of strength and energy) produces cold, damp hands.

13. Parkinson's disease produces a typical hand tremor known as "pill roller hand" (Fig. 6–18).

14. Causalgic states produce a painful, swollen, hot hand.

15. "Opera glove" anesthesia is seen in hysteria, leprosy, and diabetes. It is a condition in which there is numbness from the elbow to the fingers (Fig. 6–19).

16. *Raynaud's disease* produces a cold, mottled, painful hand. It is an idiopathic vascular disorder characterized by intermittent attacks of pallor and cyanosis of the extremities brought on by cold or emotion.

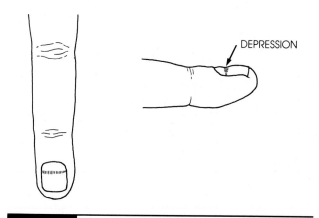

FIGURE 6–17. Beau's lines.

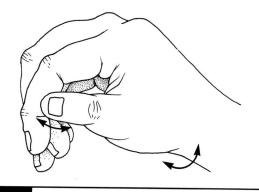

FIGURE 6–18. "Pill rolling" hand seen in Parkinson's disease.

FIGURE 6–19. "Opera glove" anesthesia showing area of abnormal sensation.

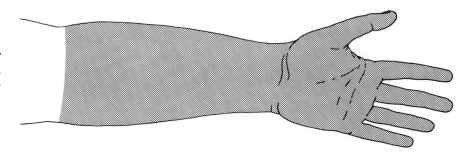

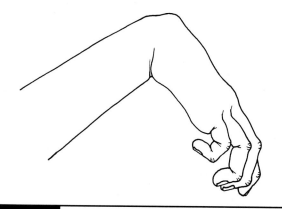

FIGURE 6–20. Deformity seen with Volkmann's ischemic contracture. Note clawed fingers.

17. Rheumatoid arthritis produces a warm, wet hand as well as joint swelling, dislocations, or subluxations and ulnar deviation of the wrist.

18. The deformed hand of Volkmann's ischemic contracture is one that is very typical for a compartment syndrome after a fracture or dislocation of the elbow (Fig. 6–20).

Table 6–3 gives further examples of physical findings of the hand.

EXAMINATION

It is important for the examiner to remember that adduction of the hand (ulnar deviation) is greater than abduction (radial deviation) because of shortness of the ulnar styloid process. Supination of the forearm is stronger than pronation, whereas abduction has a greater range of motion in supination than

---

TABLE 6–3. Outline of Physical Findings of the Hand*

I. Variations in size and shape of hand
  A. Large, blunt fingers (spade hand)
    1. Acromegaly
    2. Hurler's disease (gargoylism)
  B. Gross irregularity of shape and size
    1. Paget's disease of bone
    2. Maffucci's syndrome
    3. Neurofibromatosis
  C. Spider fingers, slender palm (arachnodactyly)
    1. Hypopituitarism
    2. Eunuchism
    3. Ehlers-Danlos syndrome, pseudoxanthoma elasticum
    4. Tuberculosis
    5. Asthenic habitus
    6. Osteogenesis imperfecta
  D. Sausage-shaped phalanges
    1. Rickets (beading of joints)
    2. Granulomatous dactylitis (tuberculosis, syphilis)
  E. Spindliform joints (fingers)
    1. Early rheumatoid arthritis
    2. Systemic lupus erythematosus
    3. Psoriasis
    4. Rubella
    5. Boeck's sarcoidosis
    6. Osteoarthritis
  F. Cone-shaped fingers
    1. Pituitary obesity
    2. Fröhlich's dystrophy
  G. Unilateral enlargement of hand
    1. Arteriovenous aneurysm
    2. Maffucci's syndrome
  H. Square, dry hands
    1. Cretinism
    2. Myxedema
  I. Single, widened, flattened distal phalanx
    1. Sarcoidosis
  J. Shortened fourth and fifth metacarpals (bradymetacarpalism)
    1. Pseudohypoparathyroidism
    2. Pseudopseudohypoparathyroidism
  K. Shortened, incurved fifth finger (symptom of Du Bois)
    1. Mongolism
    2. "Behavioral problem"
    3. Gargoylism (broad, short, thick-skinned hand)
  L. Malposition and abduction, fifth finger
    1. Turner's syndrome (gonadal dysgenesis, webbed neck, etc.)
  M. Syndactylism
    1. Congenital malformations of the heart, great vessels
    2. Multiple congenital deformities
    3. Laurence-Moon-Biedl syndrome
    4. In normal individuals as an inherited trait
  N. Clubbed fingers
    1. Subacute bacterial endocarditis
    2. Pulmonary causes
      a. Tuberculosis
      b. Pulmonary arteriovenous fistula
      c. Pulmonic abscess
      d. Pulmonic cysts

      e. Bullous emphysema
      f. Pulmonary hypertrophic osteoarthropathy
      g. Bronchogenic carcinoma
    3. Alveolocapillary block
      a. Interstitial pulmonary fibrosis
      b. Sarcoidosis
      c. Beryllium poisoning
      d. Sclerodermatous lung
      e. Asbestosis
      f. Miliary tuberculosis
      g. Alveolar cell carcinoma
    4. Cardiovascular causes
      a. Patent ductus arteriosus
      b. Tetralogy of Fallot
      c. Taussig-Bing complex
      d. Pulmonic stenosis
      e. Ventricular septal defect
    5. Diarrheal states
      a. Ulcerative colitis
      b. Tuberculous enteritis
      c. Sprue
      d. Amebic dysentery
      e. Bacillary dysentery
      f. Parasitic infestation (gastrointestinal tract)
    6. Hepatic cirrhosis
    7. Myxedema
    8. Polycythemia
    9. Chronic urinary tract infections (upper and lower)
      a. Chronic nephritis
    10. Hyperparathyroidism (telescopy of distal phalanx)
    11. Pachydermoperiostosis (syndrome of Touraine, Solente, and Golé)
  O. Joint disturbances
    1. Arthritides
      a. Osteoarthritis
      b. Rheumatoid arthritis
      c. Systemic lupus erythematosus
      d. Gout
      e. Psoriasis
      f. Sarcoidosis
      g. Endocrinopathy (acromegaly)
      h. Rheumatic fever
      i. Reiter's syndrome
      j. Dermatomyositis
    2. Anaphylactic reaction—serum sickness
    3. Scleroderma
II. Edema of the hand
  A. Cardiac disease (congestive heart failure)
  B. Hepatic disease
  C. Renal disease
    1. Nephritis
    2. Nephrosis
  D. Hemiplegic hand
  E. Syringomyelia
  F. Superior vena caval syndrome
    1. Superior thoracic outlet tumor
    2. Mediastinal tumor or inflammation
    3. Pulmonary apex tumor
    4. Aneurysm

*Modified from Berry, T. J.: The Hand as a Mirror of Systemic Disease. Philadelphia, F. A. Davis Co., 1963.

Table continued on following page

TABLE 6–3. Outline of Physical Findings of the Hand* *Continued*

Generalized anasarca, hypoproteinemia
- H. Postoperative lymphedema (radical breast amputation)
- I. Ischemic paralysis (cold, blue, swollen, numb)
- J. Lymphatic obstruction
  1. Lymphomatous masses in axilla
- K. Axillary mass
  1. Metastatic tumor, abscess, leukemia, Hodgkin's disease
- L. Aneurysm of ascending or transverse aorta, or of axillary artery
- M. Pressure on innominate or subclavian vessels
- N. Raynaud's disease
- O. Myositis
- P. Cervical rib
- Q. Trichiniasis
- R. Scalenus anticus syndrome
- III. Neuromuscular effects
  - A. Atrophy
    1. Painless
       a. Amyotrophic lateral sclerosis
       b. Charcot-Marie-Tooth peroneal atrophy
       c. Syringomyelia (loss of heat, cold, and pain sensation)
       d. Neural leprosy
    2. Painful
       a. Peripheral nerve disease
          1. Radial nerve (wrist drop)
             a. Lead poisoning, alcoholism, polyneuritis, trauma
             b. Diphtheria, polyarteritis, neurosyphilis, anterior poliomyelitis
          2. Ulnar nerve (benediction palsy)
             a. Polyneuritis, trauma
          3. Median nerve (claw hand)
             a. Carpal tunnel syndrome
                1. Rheumatoid arthritis
                2. Tenosynovitis at wrist
                3. Amyloidosis
                4. Gout
                5. Plasmacytoma
                6. Anaphylactic reaction
                7. Menopause syndrome
                8. Myxedema
  - B. Extrinsic pressure on the nerve (cervical, axillary, supraclavicular, or brachial)
    1. Pancoast tumor (pulmonary apex)
    2. Aneurysms of subclavian arteries, axillary vessels, or thoracic aorta
    3. Costoclavicular syndrome
    4. Superior thoracic outlet syndrome
    5. Cervical rib
    6. Degenerative arthritis of cervical spine
    7. Herniation of cervical intervertebral disc
  - C. Shoulder-hand syndrome
    1. Myocardial infarction
    2. Pancoast tumor
    3. Brain tumor
    4. Intrathoracic neoplasms

- 5. Discogenetic disease
- 6. Cervical spondylosis
- 7. Febrile panniculitis
- 8. Senility
- 9. Vascular occlusion
- 10. Hemiplegia
- 11. Osteoarthritis
- 12. Herpes zoster
- D. Ischemic contractures (sensory loss in fingers)
  1. Tight plaster cast applications
- E. Polyarteritis nodosa
- F. Polyneuritis
  1. Carcinoma of lung
  2. Hodgkin's disease
  3. Pregnancy
  4. Gastric carcinoma
  5. Reticuloses
  6. Diabetes mellitus
  7. Chemical neuritis
     a. Antimony, benzene, bismuth, carbon tetrachloride, heavy metals, alcohol, arsenic, lead, gold, emetine
  8. Ischemic neuropathy
  9. Vitamin B deficiency
  10. Atheromata
  11. Arteriosclerosis
  12. Embolic
- G. Carpodigital (carpopedal spasm) tetany
  1. Hypoparathyroidism
  2. Hyperventilation
  3. Uremia
  4. Nephritis
  5. Nephrosis
  6. Rickets
  7. Sprue
  8. Malabsorption syndrome
  9. Pregnancy
  10. Lactation
  11. Osteomalacia
  12. Protracted vomiting
  13. Pyloric obstruction
  14. Alkali poisoning
  15. Chemical toxicity
     a. Morphine, lead, alcohol
- H. Tremor
  1. Parkinsonism
  2. Familial disorder
  3. Hypoglycemia
  4. Hyperthyroidism
  5. Wilson's disease (hepatolenticular degeneration)
  6. Anxiety
  7. Ataxia
  8. Athetosis
  9. Alcoholism, narcotic addiction
  10. Multiple sclerosis
  11. Chorea (Sydenham's, Huntington's)

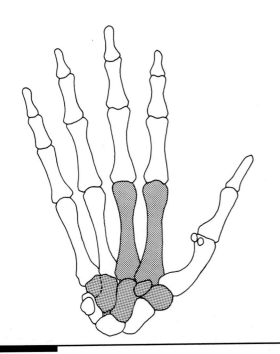

FIGURE 6–21. Palmar view of hand showing stable segment (stippled areas).

The wrist and hand have a fixed and mobile segment. The fixed segment consists of the distal row of carpal bones (trapezium, trapezoid, capitate, and hamate) and the second and third metacarpals. This is the stabilizing segment of the wrist and hand (Fig. 6–21), and movement between these bones is less than that between the bones of the mobile segments. This arrangement allows stability without rigidity and enables the hand to move more discretely and with suppleness. The mobile segment is made up of the five phalanges and the first, fourth, and fifth metacarpal bones.

The functional position of the wrist is extension to 20 to 35° with ulnar deviation of 10 to 15°.[3] This position, sometimes called the *position of rest*, minimizes the restraining action of the long extensor tendons and allows complete flexion of the fingers (Fig. 6–22). In this position, the pulps of the index finger and thumb come into contact to facilitate thumb-finger action. The *position of wrist immobilization* (Fig. 6–23) is extension more than the position of rest, with the metacarpophalangeal joints flexed more and the interphalangeal joint extended. In this way, the joints are immobilized so that the potential for contracture is kept to a minimum.

During extension, most of the movement occurs in the radiocarpal joint (approximately 50°) and less occurs in the midcarpal joint (approximately 35°) (Fig. 6–24). The motion of extension is accompanied by slight radial deviation and pronation of the forearm. During flexion, most of the movement occurs

pronation. Adduction and abduction range of motion is minimal when the wrist is fully extended or flexed. Flexion and extension at the fingers are maximal when the wrist is in neutral (not abducted or adducted); flexion and extension of the wrist are minimal when the wrist is in pronation.

FIGURE 6–22. Position of function of the hand. (A) Normal view. (B) The hand is in the position of function. Notice in particular that a very small amount of motion in the thumb and fingers is useful motion in that it can be used in pinch and grasp. Notice the close relation of the tendons to bone. The flexor tendons are held close to bone by a pulleylike thickening of the flexor sheath as represented schematically. With the hand in this position, intrinsic and extrinsic musculature is in balance, and all muscles are acting within their physiological resting length.
EDC, Extensor digitorum communis
EPL, Extensor pollicis longus
FDP, Flexor digitorum profundus
FDS, Flexor digitorum sublimis
FPL, Flexor pollicis longus
EPB, Extensor pollicis brevis
APL, Abductor pollicis longus
i, Interossei
tm, Transverse metacarpal ligament
l, Lumbrical
ad, Adductor pollicis brevis
ab, Abductor pollicis brevis
(B is from O'Donoghue, D. H.: Treatment of Injuries to Athletes. Philadelphia, W. B. Saunders Co., 1984, p. 287.)

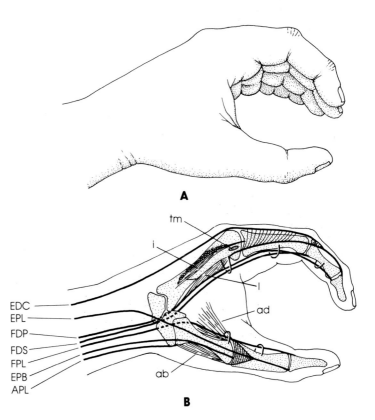

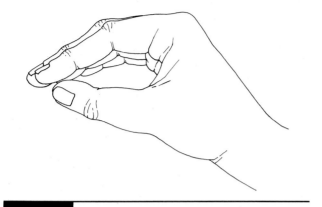

FIGURE 6–23. *Position of immobilization.*

in the midcarpal joint (approximately 50°) and less occurs in the radiocarpal joint (approximately 35°). This movement is accompanied by slight ulnar deviation and supination of the forearm. Radial deviation occurs primarily between the proximal and distal rows of carpal bones (0 to 20°), with the proximal row moving toward the ulna and the distal row moving radially. Ulnar deviation occurs primarily at the radiocarpal joint (0 to 37°).[3]

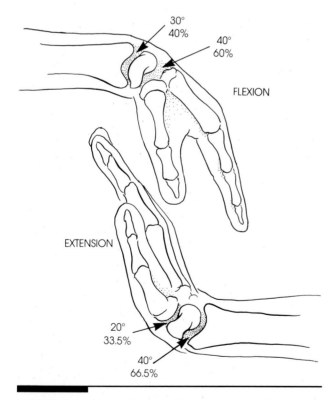

FIGURE 6–24. *During flexion of the wrist, the motion is more midcarpal and less radiocarpal. During extension of the wrist, the motion is more radiocarpal and less midcarpal. (Adapted from Sarrafin, S. K., J. L. Molamed, and G. M. Goshgarian: Clin. Orthop. Relat. Res. 126:156, 1977.)*

Active Movements

Physiological (Anatomic) Movement

Examination is accomplished with the patient in the sitting position. As always, the most painful movements are done last. In determination of the movements of the hand, the middle finger is considered to be midline (Fig. 6–25). Wrist flexion will decrease as the fingers are flexed, and movements of flexion and extension are limited, usually by the antagonistic muscles and ligaments. The patient should actively perform the following movements:

1. Pronation of the forearm (85 to 90°).
2. Supination of the forearm (85 to 90°).
3. Wrist abduction (radial deviation) (15°).
4. Wrist adduction (ulnar deviation) (30 to 45°).
5. Wrist flexion (80 to 90°).
6. Wrist extension (70 to 90°).
7. Finger flexion (MCP, 85 to 90°; PIP, 100 to 115°; DIP, 80 to 90°).
8. Finger extension (MCP, 30 to 45°; PIP, 0°; DIP, 20°).
9. Finger abduction (20 to 30°).
10. Finger adduction (0°).
11. Thumb flexion (CMC, 45 to 50°; MCP, 50 to 55°; IP, 85 to 90°).
12. Thumb extension (MCP, 0°; IP, 0 to 5°).
13. Thumb abduction (60 to 70°).
14. Thumb adduction (30°).
15. Opposition of little finger and thumb (tip to tip).

Active *pronation* and *supination* are approximately 85 to 90°, although there is variability between individuals and it is more important to compare the movement with that of normal side. Approximately 75° of supination and pronation occurs in the forearm articulations. The remaining approximately 15° is the result of wrist action. The normal end feel of both movements is tissue stretch, although in skinny individuals, the end feel of pronation may be bone to bone.

Radial and *ulnar deviations* of the wrist are 15° and 30 to 45°, respectively. The normal end feel of these movements is bone to bone. Wrist flexion is 80 to 90°; wrist extension is 70 to 90°. The end feel of each movement is tissue stretch.

Flexion of the fingers occurs at the metacarpophalangeal joints (85 to 90°), the proximal interphalangeal joints (100 to 115°), and the distal interphalangeal joints (80 to 90°). Extension occurs at the metacarpophalangeal joints (30 to 45°), the proximal interphalangeal joints (0°), and the distal interphalangeal joints (20°). The end feel of finger flexion and extension is tissue stretch. Finger abduction occurs at the metacarpophalangeal joints (20 to 30°).

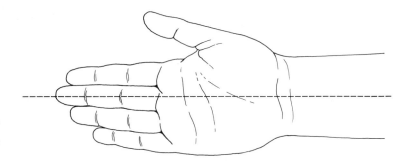

FIGURE 6–25. *Axis or reference position of the hand.*

The end feel is tissue stretch. Finger adduction occurs at the same joint (0°).

The digits are medially deviated slightly in relation to the metacarpal bones (see Fig. 6–1). When the fingers are flexed, they should point toward the scaphoid tubercle. In addition, the metacarpals are at an angle to each other. These positions increase the dexterity of the hand and oblique flexion of the medial four digits but contribute to deformities seen in conditions such as rheumatoid arthritis.

Thumb flexion occurs at the carpometacarpal joint (45 to 50°), the metacarpophalangeal joint (50 to 55°), and the interphalangeal joint (80 to 90°). It is associated with medial rotation of the thumb as a result of the shape of the carpometacarpal joint. Extension of the thumb occurs at the interphalangeal joint (0 to 5°). It is associated with lateral rotation. Flexion-extension takes place in a plane parallel to the palm of the hand. Thumb abduction is 60 to 70°; thumb adduction is 30°. These movements occur in a plane at right angles to the flexion-extension plane.[3]

The examiner must be aware that active movements may be affected because of neurological as well as contractile problems. For example, the median nerve is sometimes compressed as it passes through the carpal tunnel (Fig. 6–26), affecting its motor and sensory distribution in the hand and

fingers. The condition is referred to as *carpal tunnel syndrome*. The nerve may be compressed after trauma (e.g., Colles fracture, lunate dislocation) or by tenosynovitis of the flexor tendons, a ganglion, or collagen disease. As many as 20 per cent of pregnant women may experience some median nerve symptoms caused by fluid retention. If the patient does not have full active range of motion and it is difficult to measure range of motion because of swelling, pain, or contracture, the examiner can use a ruler or tape measure to record the distance from the fingertip to one of the palmar creases (Fig. 6–27).[4] This measurement will provide baseline data

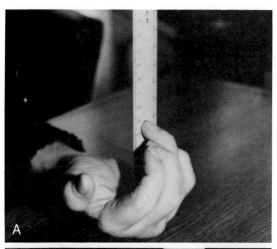

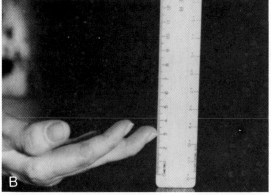

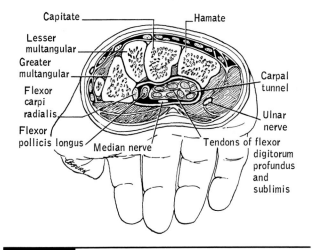

FIGURE 6–26. *Cross section of the wrist showing the carpal tunnel. (O'Donoghue, D. H.: Treatment of Injuries to Athletes, 4th ed. Philadelphia, W. B. Saunders Co., 1984, p. 285.)*

FIGURE 6–27. *(A) Gross flexion is measured as the distance between fingertips and proximal palmar crease. (B) Gross extension is measured as the distance between fingertips and dorsal plane. (From Wadsworth, C. T.: J. O. S. P. T. 5:115, 1983.)*

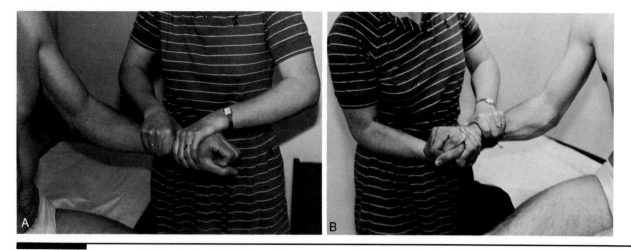

FIGURE 6–28. *Resisted isometric movements of the wrist. (A) Flexion. (B) Extension.*

for any effect of treatment. It is important to note on the chart which crease was used in the measurement. The majority of functional activities of the hand require the fingers and thumb to open at least 5 cm, and the fingers should be able to flex within 1 to 2 cm of the distal palmar crease.[5]

Passive Movements

If, when watching the patient perform the active movements, the examiner feels the range of motion is full, overpressure could be gently applied to test the end feel of the joint in each direction. If the movement is not full, passive movements must be performed by the examiner to test the end feel. At the same time, the examiner must watch for the presence of a capsular pattern. The passive movements are the same as the active movements, and the examiner must remember to test each individual joint.

The capsular pattern of the distal radioulnar joint is full range of motion with pain at the extremes of supination and pronation. At the wrist, the capsular

pattern is equal limitation of flexion and extension. At the metacarpophalangeal and interphalangeal joints, the capsular pattern is flexion more limited than extension. At the trapeziometacarpal joint of the thumb, the capsular pattern is abduction more limited than extension.

Resisted Isometric Movements

As with the active movements, the resisted isometric movements are done in the sitting position. The movements must be isometric and performed in the neutral position (Figs. 6–28 and 6–29):

1. Pronation of the forearm (see Fig. 5–11).
2. Supination of the forearm (see Fig. 5–11).
3. Wrist abduction (radial deviation).
4. Wrist adduction (ulnar deviation).
5. Wrist flexion.
6. Wrist extension.
7. Finger flexion.
8. Finger extension.
9. Finger abduction.

FIGURE 6–29. *Muscles and their actions at the wrist.*
(1) *Flexor carpi ulnaris*
(2) *Flexor digitorum profundus*
(3) *Flexor digitorum superficialis*
(4) *Palmaris longus*
(5) *Flexor carpi radialis*
(6) *Abductor pollicis longus*
(7) *Extensor pollicis brevis*
(8) *Extensor carpi radialis longus*
(9) *Extensor carpi radialis brevis*
(10) *Extensor pollicis longus*
(11) *Extensor digitorum*
(12) *Extensor digiti minimi*
(13) *Extensor carpi ulnaris*
(14) *Flexor pollicis longus*
(15) *Extensor indices*

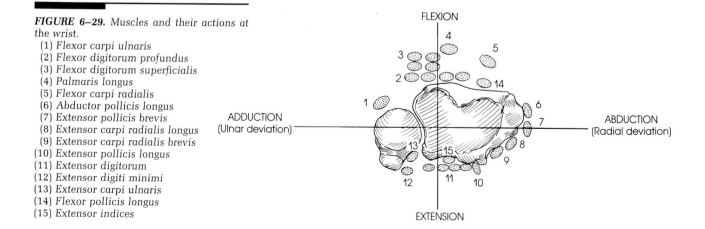

10. Finger adduction.
11. Thumb flexion.
12. Thumb extension.
13. Thumb abduction.
14. Thumb adduction.
15. Opposition of the little finger and thumb.

Table 6–4 shows the muscles and their actions for differentiation during resisted isometric testing. If test instruments are used, the strength ratio of wrist extensors to wrist flexors is approximately 50%, whereas the strength ratio of ulnar deviators to radial deviators is approximately 80%.[6]

TABLE 6–4. Muscles of the Forearm, Wrist, and Hand: Their Actions and Innervation, Including Nerve Root Derivations

Action	Muscles Involved	Innervation	Nerve Root Deviation
Supination of forearm	1. Supinator	Posterior interosseous (radial)	C5–C6
	2. Biceps brachii	Musculocutaneous	C5–C6
Pronation of forearm	1. Pronator quadratus	Anterior interosseous (median)	C8, T1
	2. Pronator teres	Median	C6–C7
	3. Flexor carpi radialis	Median	C6–C7
Extension of wrist	1. Extensor carpi radialis longus	Radial	C6–C7
	2. Extensor carpi radialis brevis	Posterior interosseous (radial)	C7–C8
	3. Extensor carpi ulnaris	Posterior interosseous (radial)	C7–C8
Flexion of wrist	1. Flexor carpi radialis	Median	C6–C7
	2. Flexor carpi ulnaris	Ulnar	C7–C8
Ulnar deviation of wrist	1. Flexor carpi ulnaris	Ulnar	C7–C8
	2. Extensor carpi ulnaris	Posterior interosseous (radial)	C7–C8
Radial deviation of wrist	1. Flexor carpi radialis	Median	C6–C7
	2. Extensor carpi radialis longus	Radial	C6–C7
	3. Abductor pollicis longus	Posterior interosseous (radial)	C7–C8
	4. Extensor pollicis brevis	Posterior interosseous (radial)	C7–C8
Extension of fingers	1. Extensor digitorum communis	Posterior interosseous (radial)	C7–C8
	2. Extensor indices (second finger)	Posterior interosseous (radial)	C7–C8
	3. Extensor digiti minimi (little finger)	Posterior interosseous (radial)	C7–C8
Flexion of fingers	1. Flexor digitorum profundus	Anterior interosseous (median)	C8, T1
		Anterior interosseous (median): lateral two digits	C8, T1
		Ulnar: medial two digits	C8, T1
	2. Flexor digitorum superficialis	Median	C7–C8, T1
	3. Lumbricals	First and second: median; third and fourth: ulnar (deep terminal branch)	C8, T1 / C8, T1
	4. Interossei	Ulnar (deep terminal branch)	C8, T1
	5. Flexor digiti minimi (little finger)	Ulnar (deep terminal branch)	C8, T1
Abduction of fingers (with fingers extended)	1. Dorsal interossei	Ulnar (deep terminal branch)	C8, T1
	2. Abductor digiti minimi (little finger)	Ulnar (deep terminal branch)	C8, T1
Adduction of fingers (with fingers extended)	Palmar interossei	Ulnar (deep terminal branch)	C8, T1
Extension of thumb	1. Extensor pollicis longus	Posterior interosseous (radial)	C7–C8
	2. Extensor pollicis brevis	Posterior interosseous (radial)	C7–C8
	3. Abductor pollicis longus	Posterior interosseous (radial)	C7–C8
Flexion of thumb	1. Flexor pollicis brevis	Superficial head: median (lateral terminal branch)	C8, T1
		Deep head: ulnar	C8, T1
	2. Flexor pollicis longus	Anterior interosseous (median)	C8, T1
	3. Opponens pollicis	Median (lateral terminal branch)	C8, T1
Abduction of thumb	1. Abductor pollicis longus	Posterior interosseous (radial)	C7–C8
	2. Abductor pollicis brevis	Median (lateral terminal branch)	C8, T1
Adduction of thumb	Adductor pollicis	Ulnar (deep terminal branch)	C8, T1
Opposition of thumb and little finger	1. Opponens pollicis	Median (lateral terminal branch)	C8, T1
	2. Flexor pollicis brevis	Superficial head: median (lateral terminal branch)	C8, T1
	3. Abductor pollicis brevis	Median (lateral terminal branch)	C8, T1
	4. Opponens digiti minimi	Ulnar (deep terminal branch)	C8, T1

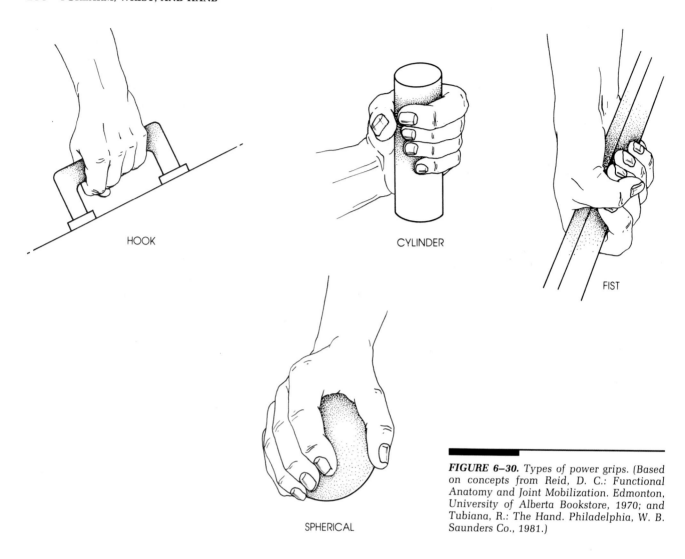

FIGURE 6–30. Types of power grips. (Based on concepts from Reid, D. C.: Functional Anatomy and Joint Mobilization. Edmonton, University of Alberta Bookstore, 1970; and Tubiana, R.: The Hand. Philadelphia, W. B. Saunders Co., 1981.)

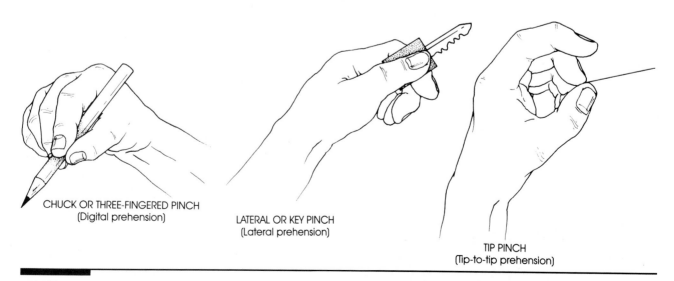

FIGURE 6–31. Types of precision grips or pinches. (Based on concepts from Reid, D. C.: Functional Anatomy and Joint Mobilization. Edmonton, University of Alberta Bookstore, 1970; and Tubiana, R.: The Hand. Philadelphia, W. B. Saunders Co., 1981.)

Functional Assessment (Grip)

Having completed testing of the anatomic or physiological active movements, the examiner then assesses the patient's functional active movements. In terms of functional impairment, the loss of thumb function affects 40 to 50% of hand function. The loss of index finger function accounts for 20% of hand function; the long finger, 20%; the ring finger, 10%; and the little finger, 5%. Loss of the hand accounts for 90% loss of upper limb function.[7]

Although the wrist, hand, and finger joints have the ability to move through the above ranges, most functional daily tasks do not require the full range of motion. For example, functional flexion at the metacarpophalangeal and proximal interphalangeal joints is approximately 60°. Functional flexion at the distal interphalangeal joint is approximately 40°. For the thumb, functional flexion at the metacarpophalangeal and interphalangeal joints is approximately 20°.[5]

Grip, regardless of type, consists of the following four stages[3, 8]:

1. Opening of the hand, which requires the simultaneous action of the intrinsic muscles of the hand and the long extensor muscles.
2. Closing of the fingers to grasp the object and adapt to the object's shape.
3. Exerted force, which will vary depending on the weight, surface characteristics, fragility, and use of the object.
4. Release, in which the hand opens to let go of the object.

The thumb, although not always used in gripping, adds another important dimension when it is used. It both gives stability and helps control the direction in which the object will move. Both of these factors are necessary for precision movements. The thumb also increases the power of a grip by acting as a buttress, resisting the pressure of an object held between it and the fingers.

The nerve supply distribution and the functions of the digits also present interesting patterns. Flexion and sensation of the ulnar digits are controlled by the ulnar nerve and are more related to *power grip*. Flexion and sensation of the radial digits are controlled by the median nerve and are more related to *precision grip*. The muscles of the thumb, often used in both types of grip, are supplied by both nerves. In all cases of gripping, opening of the hand or release depends on the radial nerve.

Power Grip. A power grip requires firm control and gives greater flexor asymmetry to the hand (Fig. 6–30).[3, 8, 9] It is used when strength or force is the primary consideration. With this grip, the digits

maintain the object against the palm. The combined effect of joint position brings the hand into line with the forearm. For a power grip to be formed, the fingers are flexed, and the wrist is in ulnar deviation and extended. Examples of power grips are the *hook grasp*, in which all or the second and third fingers are used as a hook and may involve the interphalangeal joints only or the interphalangeal and metacarpophalangeal joints (the thumb is not involved), and the *cylinder grasp*, or palmar prehension, in which the thumb is used and the entire hand wraps around an object. With the *fist grasp*, or digital palmar prehension, the hand moves around a narrow object. Another type of power grip is the *spherical grasp*, or palmar prehension, in which there is more opposition and the hand moves around the sphere.

Precision or Prehension Grip. The precision grip is an activity limited mainly to the metacarpophalangeal joints (Fig. 6–31).[3, 8, 9] This grip is used when accuracy and precision are required. The palm may or may not be involved, but there is pulp-to-pulp contact between the thumb and fingers and the thumb opposes the fingers. There are three types of pinch grip. The first is called a three-point chuck, three-fingered, or digital prehension in which palmar pinch, or *subterminal opposition*, is achieved. With this grip, there is pulp-to-pulp pinch, and opposition is necessary. An example is holding a pencil. This grip is sometimes called a *precision grip with power*. The second pinch grip is the lateral, key, pulp-to-side pinch, lateral prehension, or *subterminolateral opposition*. The thumb and lateral side of the index finger come into contact and may be called a side, lateral, or key pinch. No opposition is needed. An example of this movement is holding keys or a card. The third pinch grip is the tip pinch or tip-to-tip prehension, or *terminal opposition*. With this positioning, the tip of the thumb is brought into opposition with the tip of another finger. This pinch is used for activities requiring fine coordination rather than power.

Testing Grip Strength

When using the grip dynamometer, the five adjustable hand spacings should be used in consecutive order with the patient grasping the dynamometer with maximum force (Fig. 6–32). Both hands are tested alternately, and each force is recorded.[10, 11] Care must be taken to ensure that the patient does not fatigue. When doing the test, a bell curve will normally be seen (Fig. 6–33) with the greatest strength readings at the middle spacings (second and third spacings) and the weakest readings at the beginning and end. There should be a 5 to 10% difference between the dominant and nondominant hands.[12] With injury, the bell curve should still be

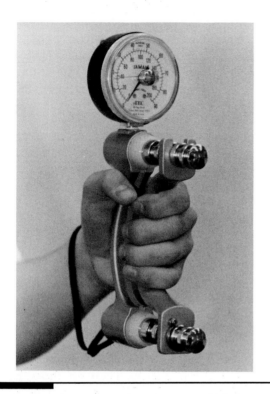

FIGURE 6–32. *Jamar dynamometer. Arm should be held at the patient's side with elbow flexed at approximately 90° when grip is measured.*

present, but the force exerted will be less. An individual who does not exert maximal force for each test will not show the typical bell curve, nor will the values obtained be consistent. Discrepancies of more than 20% in a test-retest situation indicate the patient is not exerting maximal force.[11, 13] Normally, the mean value of three trials is recorded, and both hands are compared.[5] Table 6–5 gives normal values by age group and gender.

Testing Pinch Strength

The strength of the pinch may be tested using a pinch meter (Fig. 6–34). Tables 6–6, 6–7, and 6–8 give average values of pulp pinch, lateral pinch, and chuck pinch. Normally, the mean value of three trials is recorded, and both hands are compared. The three-point chuck or tripod pinch falls between the other two in terms of strength.

Other Functional Testing Methods

In addition to testing grip and pinch strength, the examiner may want to perform a full functional test on the patient. Figure 6–35 gives an example of a

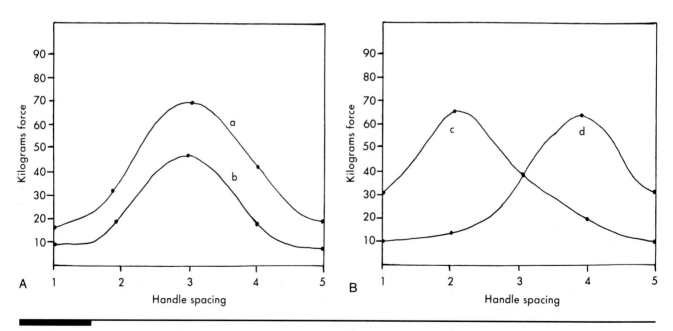

FIGURE 6–33. *(A) The grip strengths of a patient's uninjured hand (a) and injured hand (b) are plotted. Despite the patient's decrease in grip strength because of injury, curve b maintains a bell-shaped pattern and parallels that of the normal hand. These curves are reproducible in repeated examinations, with minimal change in values. A great fluctuation in the size of the curve or absence of a bell-shaped pattern casts doubt on the patient's compliance with the examination and may indicate malingering. (B) If the patient has an exceptionally large hand, the curve will shift to the right (d); with a very small hand, the curve will shift to the left (c). Notice, however, that the bell-shaped pattern is maintained despite the curve's shift in direction. (From Aulicino, P. L. and T. E. DuPuy: Clinical examination of the hand. In Hunter, J., et al. [eds.]: Rehabilitation of the Hand: Surgery and Therapy. St. Louis, C. V. Mosby Co., 1990, p. 45.)*

TABLE 6–5. Normal Values by Age Group and Gender for Combined Right and Left Hand Grip Strength (kg)*

Age (yr)	15 to 19		20 to 29		30 to 39		40 to 49		50 to 59		60 to 69	
	Male	*Female*	*Male*	*Female*	*Male*	*Female*	*Male*	*Female*	*Male*	*Female*	*Male*	*Female*
Excellent	≥113	≥71	≥124	≥71	≥123	≥73	≥119	≥73	≥110	≥65	≥102	≥60
Above average	103–112	64–70	113–123	65–70	113–122	66–72	110–118	65–72	102–109	59–64	93–101	54–59
Average	95–102	59–63	106–112	61–64	105–112	61–65	102–109	59–64	96–101	55–58	86–92	51–53
Below average	84–94	54–58	97–105	55–60	97–104	56–60	94–101	55–58	87–95	51–54	79–85	48–50
Poor	≤83	≤53	≤96	≤54	≤96	≤55	≤93	≤54	≤86	≤50	≤78	≤47

*Modified from Canadian Standardized Test of Fitness: Operations Manual. Ottawa, Fitness and Amateur Sport Canada, 1986, p. 36.

functional assessment form for the hand. Table 6–9 provides a functional strength–testing method.

Functional coordinated movements may be tested by asking the patient to perform simple activities, such as fastening a button, tying a shoelace, or tracing a diagram. Different prehension patterns are used regularly during daily activities. The estimated use of the different grips during activities of daily living are noted below[14]:

Pulp-to-pulp pinch:	20%
Three lateral pinch:	20%
Five-finger pinch:	15%
Fist grip:	15%
Cylinder grip:	14%
Three-fingered pinch:	10%
Spherical grip:	4%
Hook grip:	2%

These tests may also be graded on a four-point scale. This scale is particularly suitable if the patient has difficulty with one of the subtests, and the subtests can be scale-graded:

Unable to perform task:	0
Completes task partially:	1
Completes task but is slow and clumsy:	2
Performs task normally[14]:	3

Special Tests

Only those special tests that the examiner feels have relevance should be performed.

Tests for Ligaments, Tendons, Capsules, and Instability

Finkelstein Test. The Finkelstein test[15] is used to determine the presence of de Quervain's or Hoffman's disease, a tenosynovitis in the thumb. The patient makes a fist with the thumb inside the fingers (Fig. 6–36). The examiner stabilizes the forearm and ulnarly deviates the wrist. A positive test is indicated by pain over the abductor pollicis longus and extensor pollicis brevis tendons at the wrist and is indicative of a tenosynovitis in these two tendons. Because the test may cause some discomfort in normal individuals, the examiner should compare the pain caused on the affected side with that of the normal side.

Bunnel-Littler Test. The metacarpophalangeal joint is held slightly extended while the examiner moves the proximal interphalangeal joint into flexion, if possible (Fig. 6–37).[16] If the test is positive, which is indicated by the proximal interphalangeal joint not being able to be flexed, there is a tight intrinsic muscle or contracture of the joint capsule. If the metacarpophalangeal joints are slightly flexed,

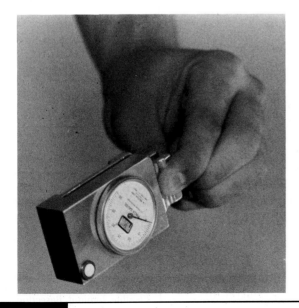

FIGURE 6–34. *Pulp pinch prehension (commercial pinch grip).*

TABLE 6–6. Average Strength of Pulp Pinch With Separate Digits (100 Subjects)*

	Pulp Pinch (kg)			
	Male Hand		*Female Hand*	
Digit	*Major*	*Minor*	*Major*	*Minor*
II	5.3	4.8	3.6	3.3
III	5.6	5.7	3.8	3.4
IV	3.8	3.6	2.5	2.4
V	2.3	2.2	1.7	1.6

*From Hunter J., et al. (eds.): Rehabilitation of the Hand: Surgery and Therapy. St. Louis, C. V. Mosby Co., 1990, p. 115.

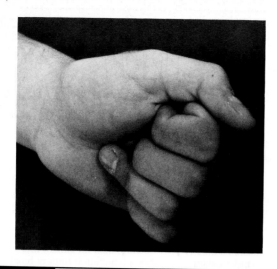

FIGURE 6–40. *Sweater finger sign. Rupture of the flexor profundus tendon in the ring finger of a football player.*

positive test is indicated by instability or subluxation of the scaphoid.[19]

Grind Test. The examiner holds the patient's hand with one hand and grasps the patient's thumb below the metacarpophalangeal joint with the other hand. The examiner then applies axial compression and rotation to the metacarpophalangeal joint. If pain is elicited, the test is positive and indicative of degenerative joint disease in the metacarpophalangeal or metacarpotrapezial joint.[13]

Tests for Neurological Dysfunction

Tinel's Sign (at the Wrist).[15] The examiner taps over the carpal tunnel at the wrist (Fig. 6–42). A

positive test causes tingling or paresthesia into the thumb, index finger (forefinger), and middle and lateral half of the ring finger (median nerve distribution). Tinel's sign at the wrist is indicative of a carpal tunnel syndrome. The tingling or paresthesia must be felt distal to the point of pressure for a positive test. The test gives an indication of the rate of regeneration of the sensory fibers of the median nerve. The most distal point at which the abnormal sensation is felt represents the limit of nerve regeneration.

Phalen's (Wrist Flexion) Test. The examiner flexes the patient's wrists maximally and holds this position for 1 minute by pushing the patient's wrists together (Fig. 6–43). A positive test is indicated by tingling in the thumb, index finger, and middle and lateral half of the ring finger and is indicative of carpal tunnel syndrome caused by pressure on the median nerve.[20]

Reverse Phalen's Test. The examiner extends the patient's wrist while asking the patient to grip the examiner's hand. The examiner then applies direct pressure over the carpal tunnel for 1 minute. A positive test is indicated by the same symptoms as are seen in Phalen's test and is indicative of pathology to the median nerve.[17]

Froment's Sign. The patient attempts to grasp a piece of paper between the thumb and index finger (Fig. 6–44).[21] When the examiner attempts to pull away the paper, the terminal phalanx of the thumb will flex because of paralysis of the adductor pollicis muscle, indicating a positive test. If, at the same time, the metacarpophalangeal joint of the thumb hyperextends, the hyperextension is noted as a positive **Jeanne's sign.**[13] Both tests are indicative of ulnar nerve paralysis.

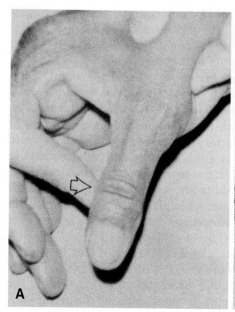
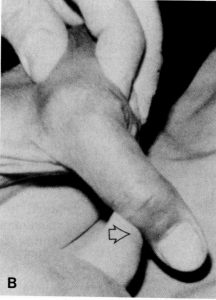

FIGURE 6–41. *(A) and (B) Testing stability of the ulnar collateral ligament in the thumb of a normal individual. In extension, the thumb was stable, but in flexion, it appeared to be unstable. This was caused by the laxity of the dorsal capsule at the metacarpophalangeal joint. (From Nicholas, J. A., and E. B. Hershman: Upper Extremity in Sports Medicine. St. Louis, C. V. Mosby Co., 1990, p. 580.)*

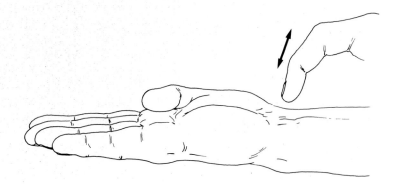

FIGURE 6–42. Tinel's sign at the wrist.

Egawa's Sign. The patient flexes the middle digit and then alternately deviates the finger radially and ulnarly. If the patient is unable to do this, the interossei are affected. A positive sign is indicative of ulnar nerve paralysis.

Wrinkle (Shrivel) Test. The patient's fingers are placed in warm water for approximately 5 to 20 minutes. The examiner then removes the patient's fingers from the water and observes whether the skin over the pulp is wrinkled (Fig. 6–45). Normal fingers will show wrinkling, whereas denervated ones will not. The test is valid only within the first few months after injury.[22]

Ninhydrin Sweat Test. The patient's hand is cleaned thoroughly and wiped with alcohol. The patient then waits 5 to 30 minutes with the fingertips not in contact with any surface. This waiting time allows time for the sweating process to ensue. After the waiting period, the fingertips are pressed with moderate pressure against good-quality bond paper (i.e., 20 lb) that has not been touched. The fingertips are held in place for 15 seconds and traced with a pencil. The paper is then sprayed with triketohydrindene (Ninhydrin) spray reagent and allowed to dry (24 hours). The sweat areas will stain purple. If the change in color (from white to purple) does not occur, it is considered a positive test for a nerve

lesion.[23,24] The reagent must be fixed if a permanent record is required.

Weber's (Moberg's) Two-Point Discrimination Test. The examiner uses a paper clip, two-point discriminator, or calipers (Fig. 6–46) to simultaneously apply pressure on two adjacent points in a longitudinal direction or perpendicular to the long axis of the finger moving proximally to distally in an attempt to find the minimal distance at which the patient can distinguish the two stimuli.[8] This distance is called the *threshold for discrimination.* Coverage values are shown in Figure 6–47. The patient must concentrate on feeling the points and must not be able to see the area being tested. Only the fingertips need to be tested. The patient's hand should be immobile on a hard surface. For accurate results, the examiner must ensure that the two points touch the skin simultaneously. There should be no blanching of the skin when the points are applied. The distance between the points is decreased or increased depending on the response of the patient. The starting distance between the points is one that the patient can easily distinguish (e.g., 15 mm). If the patient is hesitant to respond or becomes inaccurate, the patient is required to respond accurately seven or eight of 10 times before the distance is narrowed and the test repeated.[5,24-26] Normal discrimination distance recognition is less than 6 mm. This test is best for hand sensation involving statically holding an object between the fingers and

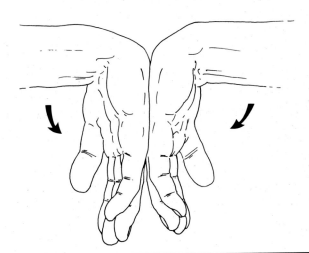

FIGURE 6–43. Phalen's test.

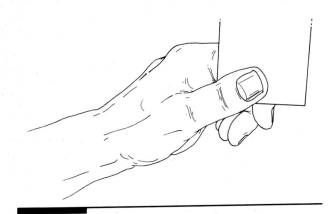

FIGURE 6–44. Froment's sign.

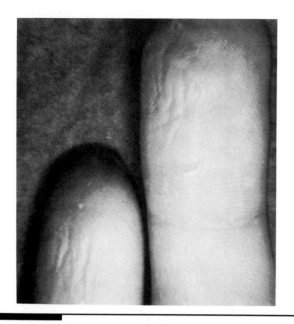

FIGURE 6–45. *The wrinkle test may be reliable for digital nerve sympathetic function if the fingers (in this case, the radial digital nerves of the fourth and fifth digits) are completely denervated. (From Waylett-Rendall, J.: Orthop. Clin. North Am. 19:48, 1988.)*

thumb and requiring pinch strength. Table 6–10 demonstrates some two-point discrimination normal values and distances required for certain tasks.

Dellon's Moving Two-Point Discrimination Test. This test is used to predict functional recovery and measures the quickly adapting fibers/receptor system.[8] The test is similar to Weber's two-point discrimination test except that the two points are moved during the test. The examiner moves two blunt points from proximal to distal along the long axis of the limb or digit starting with a distance of

8 mm between the points. The distance between the points is increased or decreased depending on the response of the patient. The distance between the two points is decreased until the two points can no longer be distinguished. During the test, the patient's eyes are closed and the hand is cradled in the examiner's hand. The two smooth points, whether using a paper clip, two-point discriminator, or calipers, are gently placed longitudinally. There should be no blanching of the skin when the points are applied. The patient is asked whether one or two points are felt. If the patient is hesitant to respond or becomes inaccurate, the patient is required to respond accurately seven or eight of 10 times before the distance is narrowed and the test repeated.[5, 24, 25, 27] The test is used to assess the integrity of rapidly adapting mechanoreceptors. Normal discrimination distance recognition is 2 to 5 mm.[26] The values obtained for this test are slightly lower than those obtained for Weber's static two-point discrimination test.[25] Although the entire hand may be tested, it is more common to test only the anterior digital pulp. This test is best for hand sensation related to activity and movement.

Tests for Manual Dexterity and Coordination

Many standardized tests have been developed to assess manual dexterity and coordination. Each of these tests has its supporters and detractors. Some of the more common tests follow.

Jebson-Taylor Hand Function Test. This easily administered test involves seven functional areas:

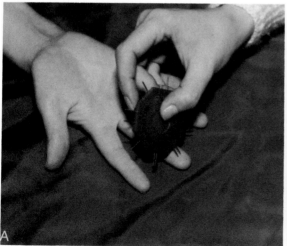
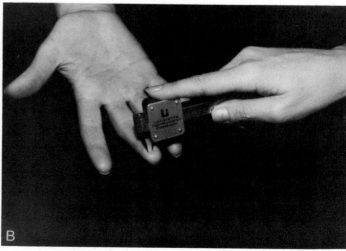

FIGURE 6–46. *Devices used to test two-point discrimination. (A) The Disk-Criminator is a set of two plastic discs, each containing a series of metal rods at varying intervals from 1 to 25 mm apart. This device evaluates both moving and static two-point discrimination and is available from Disk-Criminator, Baltimore, Maryland. (B) Two-point aesthesiometer.*

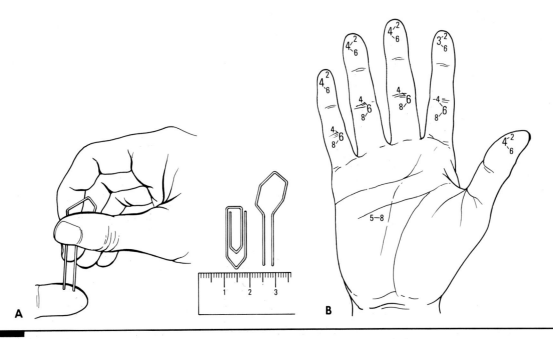

FIGURE 6–47. Two-point discrimination. (A) Technique of performing the two-point discrimination test of Weber (after Moberg). (B) Values of discriminations in the Weber test in millimeters in the different zones of the palm. The largest figure indicates the average values; the two other figures indicate the minimum and maximum values (after Moberg). (Reprinted from Tubiana, R.: The Hand. Philadelphia, W. B. Saunders Co., 1981, pp. 645–646.)

(1) writing, (2) card turning, (3) picking up small objects, (4) simulated feeding, (5) stacking, (6) picking up large, light objects, and (7) picking up large, heavy objects. The subtests are timed for each limb. This test primarily measures gross coordination, assessing prehension and manipulative skills with functional tests. It does not test bilateral integration.[5, 28–30] Anyone wishing to do the test should consult the original article[31] for details of administration.

Minnesota Rate of Manipulation Tests. This test involves five activities: (1) placing, (2) turning, (3) displacing, (4) one-hand turning and placing, and (5) two-hand turning and placing. The activities are timed for both limbs and compared with normal values. The test primarily measures gross coordination and dexterity.[5, 28, 29]

TABLE 6–10. Two-Point Discrimination Normal Values and Discrimination Distances Required for Certain Tasks*

Normal	Less than 6 mm
Fair	6 to 10 mm
Poor	11 to 15 mm
Protective	1 point perceived
Anesthetic	0 points perceived
Winding a watch	6 mm
Sewing	6 to 8 mm
Handling precision tools	12 mm
Gross tool handling	>15 mm

*Adapted from Callahan, A. D.: Sensibility testing. In Hunter, J., et al. (eds.): Rehabilitation of the Hand: Surgery and Therapy. St. Louis, C. V. Mosby Co., 1990, p. 605.

Purdue Pegboard Test. This test measures fine coordination making use of small pins, washers, and collars. The assessment categories of the test are (1) right hand, (2) left hand, (3) both hands, (4) right, left, and both, and (5) assembly. The subtests are timed and compared with normal values based on gender and type of job.[5, 28, 29]

Crawford Small Parts Dexterity Test. This test measures fine coordination including the use of tools such as tweezers and screwdrivers to assemble things, to adjust equipment, and to do engraving.[5, 28]

Simulated Activities of Daily Living Examination. This test consists of 19 subtests, including standing, walking, putting on a shirt, buttoning, zipping, putting on gloves, dialing a telephone, tying a bow, manipulating safety pins, manipulating coins, threading a needle, unwrapping a Band-Aid, squeezing toothpaste, and using a knife and fork. Each subtask is timed.[14]

Moberg Pickup Test. An assortment of nine or 10 objects (e.g., bolts, nuts, screws, buttons, coins, pens, paper clips, and keys) is used. The patient is timed for the following tests:

1. Putting objects in a box with the affected hand.
2. Putting objects in a box with the unaffected hand.
3. Putting objects in a box with the affected hand and eyes closed.

The examiner notes which digits are used for prehension. Digits with altered sensation are less likely

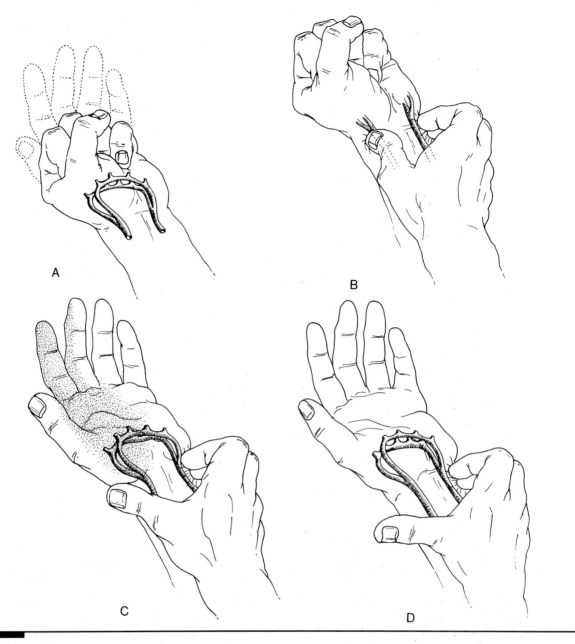

FIGURE 6–48. Allen test.

to be used. The test is used for median or combined median and ulnar nerve lesions.[24]

Box and Block Test. This is a test for gross manual dexterity in which 150 blocks, each measuring 2.5 cm², are used. The patient has 1 minute in which to individually transfer the blocks from one side of a divided box to the other. The number of blocks transferred is given as the score. Patients are given a 15-second practice trial before the test.[30]

Nine-Hole Peg Test. This test is used to test finger dexterity. The patient places nine 3.2-cm pegs in a 12.7-cm² board and removes them. The score is the time taken to do this task. Each hand is tested.[30]

Tests for Circulation and Swelling

Allen Test. The patient is asked to open and close the hand several times as quickly as possible and then squeeze the hand tightly (Fig. 6–48).[20] The examiner's thumb and index finger are placed over the radial and ulnar arteries. The patient then opens the hand while pressure is maintained over the arteries. One artery is tested by releasing the pressure over that artery to see if the hand flushes. The other artery is then tested in a similar fashion. Both hands should be tested for comparison. This test determines the patency of the radial and ulnar

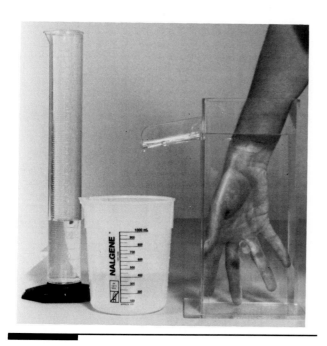

FIGURE 6–49. Volumeter used to measure hand volume.

arteries and determines which artery provides the major blood supply to the hand.

Hand Volume Test. If the examiner is concerned about changes in hand size, a volumeter (Fig. 6–49) may be used. This device can be used to assess changes in hand size resulting from localized swelling, generalized edema, or atrophy.[28] Comparisons with the normal limb will give the examiner an idea of changes occurring in the affected hand. Care must be taken when doing this test to ensure accurate readings. There is often a 10-ml difference between right and left hands and between dominant and nondominant hands. If swelling is the problem, differences of 30 to 50 ml can be noted.[5, 32]

Reflexes and Cutaneous Distribution

The examiner must be aware of the sensory distribution of the ulnar, median, and radial nerves in the hand (Fig. 6–50). Several sensation tests may be carried out in the hand. Table 6–11 illustrates the tests used and the sensation and nerve fibers tested. Pinprick is used to test for pain. Constant light touch, which is a component of fine discrimination, may be tested in the hand using a Semmes-Weinstein pressure esthesiometer (Von Frey test). This kit has 20 probes, each with different thicknesses of nylon monofilament (Fig. 6–51). The patient is blinded to the test, and each filament is applied perpendicularly to the finger with the smallest filament being used first. The filament is pushed against the finger until the filament bends. The next filament is then used and so on until the patient feels one before or just as it bends.[5, 24] The test is repeated three times to ensure a positive result.[26] Normal values vary between 2.36 and 2.83 mg (Table 6–12).

Stereognosis or tactile gnosis, which is the ability to identify common objects by touch, should also be tested. Objects are placed in the patient's hand while the patient is blinded to the test. The time until the object is recognized is noted. Normal subjects can usually name the object within 3 seconds of contact.[25]

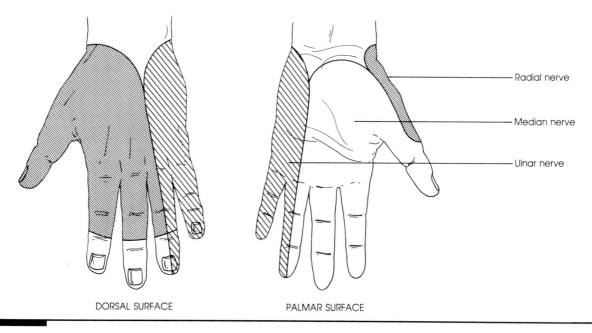

DORSAL SURFACE   PALMAR SURFACE

— Radial nerve

— Median nerve

— Ulnar nerve

FIGURE 6–50. Peripheral nerve distribution in the hand.

TABLE 6–11. Tests for Cutaneous Sensibility*

Test	Sensation	Fiber/Receptor Type
Pin	Pain	Free nerve endings
Warm/cold	Temperature	Free nerve endings
Cotton wool	Moving touch	Quick adapting
Finger stroking	Moving touch	Quick adapting
Dellon test	Moving touch	Quick adapting
Tuning fork	Vibration	Quick adapting
Von Frey	Constant touch	Slow adapting
Weber test	Constant touch	Slow adapting
Pick-up test	Constant touch	Slow adapting
Precision sensory grip	Constant touch	Slow adapting
Gross grip	Constant touch	Slow adapting

*Modified from Dellon, A. L.: The paper clip: Light hardware to evaluate sensibility in the hand. Contemp. Orthop. 1:40, 1979.

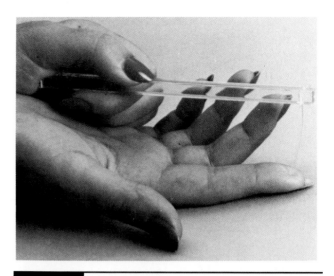

FIGURE 6–51. *The Semmes-Weinstein monofilament is applied perpendicular to the skin for 1 to 1.5 seconds, held in place for 1 to 1.5 seconds, and lifted for 1 to 1.5 seconds. (From Waylett-Rendall, J.: Orthop. Clin. North Am. 19:51, 1988.)*

Vibratory sense is tested using a 30-cps (high frequency) or 256-cps (low frequency) tuning fork. The "blinded" patient indicates when vibration is felt as the examiner touches the skin with the vibrating tuning fork and whether the vibration feels the same. The score is the number of correct responses divided by the total number of presentations.[33]

To test moving touch, the examiner's finger strokes the patient's finger. The patient notes whether the stroking was felt and what it felt like.

It must be remembered that pain may be referred to the wrist and the hand from the cervical or upper thoracic spine, shoulder, and elbow. Seldom is wrist or hand pain referred up the limb (Fig. 6–52).

Neurologically, the examiner must be aware of potential injury to the various nerves around the wrist and hand.

The *median nerve* gives off a sensory branch above the wrist before it passes through the carpal tunnel. This sensory branch supplies the skin of the palm (Fig. 6–53). It is important to remember that carpal tunnel syndrome will not affect the median sensory distribution in the palm but will result in altered sensation in the fingers.

The *ulnar nerve* is sometimes compressed as it passes through the pisohamate, or *Guyon's canal* (Fig. 6–54). The nerve may be compressed from trauma, use of crutches, or chronic pressure, for example, as seen in people who cycle long distances while leaning on the handlebars or extensively use pneumatic jackhammers. The ulnar nerve gives off two sensory branches above the wrist. These branches supply the palmar and dorsal aspects of the hand, as illustrated in Figure 6–50, and do not pass through Guyon's canal. Thus, if the ulnar nerve is compressed in the canal, only the fingers will show an altered sensation.

The examiner can attempt a differential diagnosis of paresthesia in the hand if altered sensation is present. A comparison with a normal dermatome chart should be made, and the examiner should remember that there is a fair amount of variability within the dermatomes (Fig. 6–55). In addition, there are areas of the hand where sensation is more important (Fig. 6–56). Abnormal sensation may mean the following:

1. Numbness in the thumb only may be due to pressure on the digital nerve on the outer aspect of the thumb.

TABLE 6–12. Light Touch Testing Using Semmes-Weinstein Pressure Esthesiometer*

Esthesiometer Probe No.	Calculated pressure (g/mm²)	Interpretation
2.44–2.83	3.25–4.86	Normal light touch
3.22–4.56	11.1–47.3	Diminished light touch, point localization† intact
4.74–6.10	68.0–243.0	Minimal light touch, area localization‡ intact
6.10–6.65	243.0–439.0	Sensation but no localization sensibility

*From Omer, G. E.: Report of the Committee for Evaluation of the Clinical Result in Peripheral Nerve Injury. J. Hand Surg. 8:755, 1983.
†Point localization: the dowel is in contact with the skin point stimulated.
‡Area localization: the dowel is in contact with any point inside the zone of the area being tested (in the hand or foot).

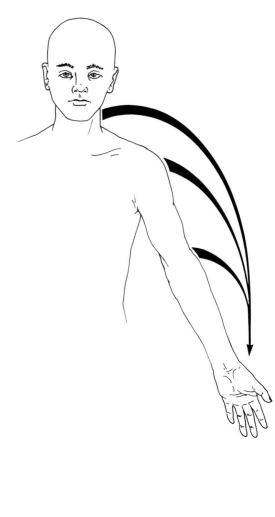

FIGURE 6–52. *Symptoms can be referred to the wrist and hand from the elbow, shoulder, and cervical spine.*

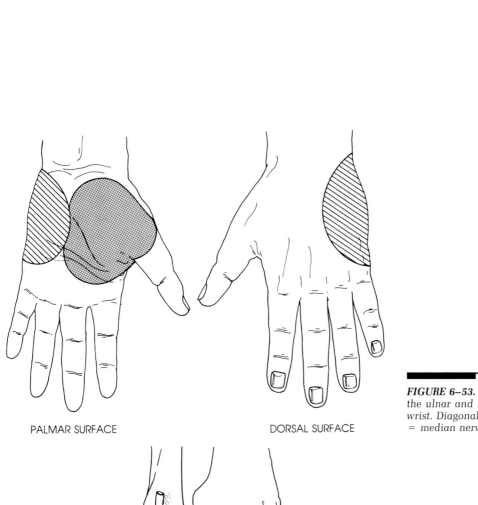

PALMAR SURFACE   DORSAL SURFACE

FIGURE 6–53. *Sensory distribution of branches of the ulnar and median nerves given off above the wrist. Diagonal lines = ulnar nerve; shaded area = median nerve.*

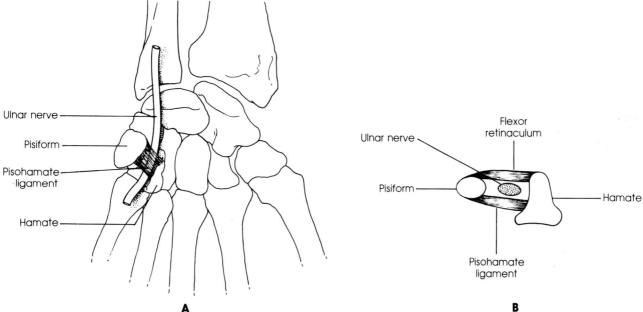

Ulnar nerve

Pisiform

Pisohamate ligament

Hamate

A

Flexor retinaculum

Ulnar nerve

Pisiform

Hamate

Pisohamate ligament

B

FIGURE 6–54. *Guyon's canal. (A) Palmar view. (B) Section view showing position of nerve relative to pisohamate ligament and flexor retinaculum.*

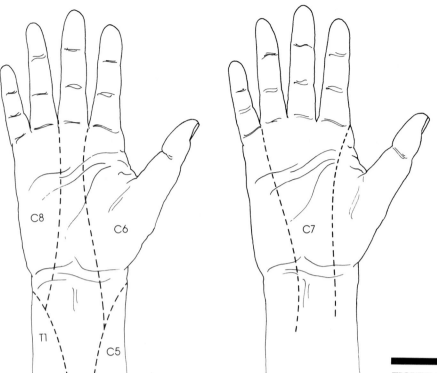

FIGURE 6–55. Dermatomes of the hand. Note overlap at dermatomes. Both views are palmar.

2. Pins and needles in the thumb may be due to a contusion of the thenar branch of the median nerve.

3. Paresthesia in the thumb and index finger may be due to a C5 disc lesion or C6 nerve root palsy.

4. Paresthesia in the thumb, index finger, and middle finger may be due to a C5 disc lesion, C6 nerve root palsy, or thoracic outlet syndrome.

5. Paresthesia of the thumb, index finger, and middle and half of the ring finger on the palmar aspect may be due to an injury to the median nerve, possibly through the carpal tunnel; on the dorsal aspect, it could be due to injury to the radial nerve.

6. Numbness of the thumb and middle finger may be due to a tumor of the humerus.

7. Paresthesia on all five digits in one or both hands may be due to a thoracic outlet syndrome. If it is in both hands, it may be due to a central cervical disc protrusion. The level of protrusion would be indicated by the distribution of the paresthesia.

8. Paresthesia of the index and middle fingers may be due to a trigger finger or "stick" palsy, if it is on the palmar aspect, or C6 disc lesion or C7 nerve root palsy. On the dorsal aspect of the hand, it may be due to a carpal exostosis or subluxation. Stick palsy is the result of an inordinant amount of pressure from a cane on the ulnar nerve as it passes through the palm.

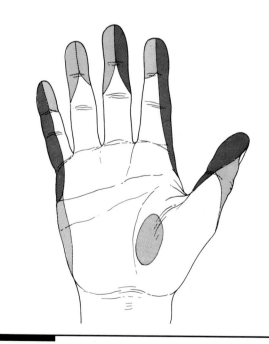

FIGURE 6–56. Importance of hand sensation. Dark areas indicate where sensation is most important; gray, where sensation is a little less important; and white, where sensation is least important. (From Tubiana, R.: The Hand. Philadelphia, W. B. Saunders Co., 1981, p. 74.)

9. Paresthesia of the index, middle, and ring fingers may be due to a C6 disc lesion, C7 nerve root injury, or carpal tunnel syndrome.

10. Paresthesia of all four fingers may be due to a C6 disc lesion or injury to the C7 nerve root.

11. Paresthesia of the middle finger only may be due to a C6 disc lesion or C7 nerve root lesion.

12. Paresthesia of the middle and ring fingers may be due to a C6 disc lesion, C7 nerve root lesion, or stick palsy.

13. Paresthesia of the middle, ring, and little fingers may be due to a C7 disc lesion or C8 nerve root palsy. The same would be true if there were paralysis of the ring and little fingers. This paresthesia may also be the result of a thoracic outlet syndrome.

14. Paresthesia on the ulnar side of the ring finger and the entire little finger may be due to pressure of the ulnar nerve at the elbow or in the palm.

Joint Play Movements

When assessing joint play movements, the examiner should remember that if the patient complains of inability or pain on wrist flexion, the lesion is probably in the midcarpal joints. If the patient complains of inability or pain on wrist extension, the lesion is probably in the radiocarpal joints because it is in these joints that most of the movement occurs during these actions. If the patient complains of pain or inability on supination and pronation, the lesion is probably in the ulnameniscocarpal joint or inferior radioulnar joint.

The following joint play movements are carried out on the *wrist* (Fig. 6–57):

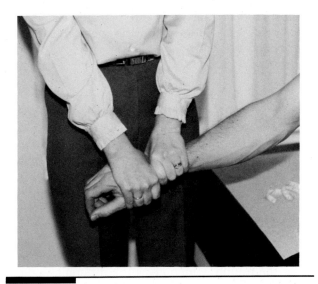

FIGURE 6–57. *Position for joint play movements of the wrist.*

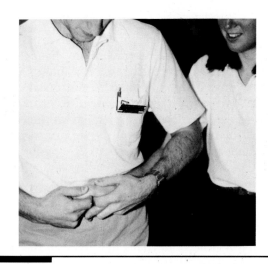

FIGURE 6–58. *Position for joint play movements of the fingers.*

1. Long-axis extension (traction or distraction).
2. Anteroposterior glide.
3. Side glide.
4. Side tilt.

The joint play movement of the *intermetacarpal joints* is anteroposterior glide.

The following joint play movements are carried out on *fingers* (Fig. 6–58):

1. Long-axis extension (traction or distraction).
2. Anteroposterior glide.
3. Rotation.
4. Side glide.

The amount of movement obtained by the joint play should be compared with that of the normal side and considered significant only if there is a difference between the two sides.

Wrist

For the wrist, long-axis extension is performed by the examiner stabilizing the radius and ulna with one hand (the patient's arm may be flexed to 90° and stabilization applied at the elbow if there is no pathology at the elbow) and placing the other hand just distal to the wrist. The examiner then applies a longitudinal traction movement with the distal hand.

Anteroposterior glide is applied at the wrist in two positions. The examiner first places the stabilizing hand around the distal end of the radius and ulna just proximal to the radiocarpal joint and then places the other hand around the proximal row of carpal bones. If the hands are positioned properly, they should touch each other (see Fig. 6–57). The examiner applies an anteroposterior gliding movement of the proximal row of carpal bones on the radius and ulna. Then, the stabilizing hand is moved so that it is around the proximal row of carpal bones. The examiner places the mobilizing hand around the distal row of carpal bones. An anteroposterior gliding movement is applied to the distal row of carpal bones on the proximal row.

Side glide is performed in a similar fashion, except that a side-to-side movement is performed instead of an anteroposterior movement. To perform side tilting of the carpals on the radius and ulna, the examiner stabilizes the radius and ulna by placing the stabilizing hand around the distal radius and ulna just proximal to the radiocarpal joint and the mobilizing hand around the patient's hand and then radially or ulnarly deviates the hand on the radius and ulna. These joint play movements are general ones involving all carpal bones. To check the joint play movements of the individual carpal bones, *Kaltenborn's technique* should be used.[34]

Intermetacarpal Joints

To accomplish anteroposterior glide at the intermetacarpal joints, the examiner stabilizes one metacarpal bone and moves the adjacent metacarpal anteriorly and posteriorly in relation to the fixed bone. The process is repeated for each joint.

Fingers

The joint play movements for the fingers are the same for the metacarpophalangeal, proximal interphalangeal, and distal interphalangeal joints; the hand position of the examiner just moves further distally.

To perform long-axis extension, the examiner stabilizes the proximal segment or bone using one hand while placing the second hand around the distal segment or bone of the particular joint to be tested. With the mobilizing hand, the examiner applies a longitudinal traction to the joint.

Anteroposterior glide is accomplished by stabilizing the proximal bone with one hand. The mobilizing hand is placed around the distal segment of the joint, and the examiner applies an anterior and/or posterior movement to the distal segment, being sure to maintain the joint surfaces parallel to one another. A minimal amount of traction may be applied to bring about slight separation of the joint surfaces.

Rotation of the joints of the fingers is accomplished by stabilizing the proximal segment with one hand. With the other hand, the examiner applies slight traction to the joint to distract the joint surfaces and then rotates the distal segment on the proximal segment.

To perform side glide joint play to the joints of the fingers, the proximal segment is stabilized with

one hand, while the examiner applies slight traction to the joint with the mobilizing hand to distract the joint surfaces and then moves the distal segment sideways, keeping the joint surfaces parallel to one another.

Carpal Bones

Kaltenborn[34] suggests 10 tests to determine the mobility of each of the carpal bones. The movement between each of the bones is determined in a sequential manner, and both sides are to be tested for comparison.

1. Fixate the capitate and move the trapezoid.
2. Fixate the capitate and move the scaphoid.
3. Fixate the capitate and move the lunate.
4. Fixate the capitate and move the hamate.
5. Fixate the scaphoid and move the trapezoid and trapezium.
6. Fixate the radius and move the scaphoid.
7. Fixate the radius and move the lunate.
8. Fixate the ulna and move the triquetrum.
9. Fixate the triquetrum and move the hamate.
10. Fixate the triquetrum and move the pisiform.

Palpation

To palpate the forearm, wrist, and hand, the examiner starts proximally and works distally, first on the dorsal surface and then on the anterior surface (Fig. 6–59). The muscles of the forearm are first palpated for any signs of tenderness or pathology.

Dorsal Surface

On the dorsal aspect, the examiner begins on the thumb side of the hand and palpates the "snuff box," the carpal bones, and the metacarpal bones and phalanges.

Anatomic "Snuff Box." The snuff box is located between the tendons of extensor pollicis longus and extensor pollicis brevis and can be best seen by having the patient actively extend the thumb. The scaphoid bone may be palpated inside the snuff box. Tenderness of the scaphoid bone is often treated as a fracture until proven otherwise because of the possibility of avascular necrosis of the bone. Palpating proximally, one finds the radial styloid on the lateral aspect (in the anatomic position) of the wrist. Moving medially over the radius, the examiner will come to the radial (Lister's) tubercle. The extensor pollicis longus tendon moves around the tubercle to enter the thumb, which gives it a different angle of pull from extensor pollicis brevis. The ulnar styloid is palpated on the medial aspect (in the anatomic

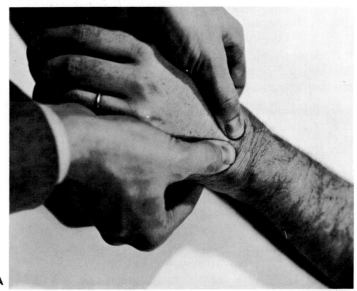

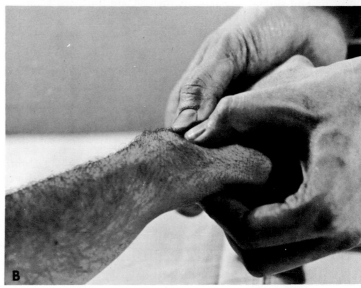

FIGURE 6–59. *Palpation of the left wrist by using both hands. (A) Top view. (B) Side view. The wrist is being palpated firmly (note blanched nails of the examiner's thumbs) by both thumbs and second (index) fingers. The other fingers serve to support and position the patient's hand, as partially shown in B. (From Polley, H. F., and G. G. Hunder: Rheumatologic Interviewing and Physical Examination of the Joints. Philadelphia, W. B. Saunders Co., 1978, p. 101.)*

position) of the wrist. The examiner will note that the radial styloid extends further distally than the ulnar styloid. Palpating over the dorsum of the wrist, crossing the radius and ulna, one should attempt to palpate the six extensor tendon tunnels (noting any crepitus or restriction to movement) moving lateral to medial:

1. Tunnel 1—abductor pollicis longus and extensor pollicis brevis.
2. Tunnel 2—extensor carpi radialis longus and brevis.
3. Tunnel 3—extensor pollicis longus.
4. Tunnel 4—extensor digitorum and extensor indexes.
5. Tunnel 5—extensor digiti minimi.
6. Tunnel 6—extensor carpi ulnaris.

Carpal Bones. In the anatomic snuff box, the examiner can begin palpating the proximal row of

carpal bones, starting with the scaphoid bone. When palpating the carpal bones, the examiner usually palpates them on the anterior and dorsal surfaces at the same time. The proximal row of carpal bones from lateral to medial (in the anatomic position) are the:

1. Scaphoid.
2. Lunate.
3. Triquetrum (just below the ulnar styloid).
4. Pisiform.

On the anterior aspect, the examiner should take care to ensure proper positioning of the lunate bone. If it dislocates or subluxes, it tends to move in an anterior direction into the carpal tunnel, which may lead to carpal tunnel syndrome symptoms. The pisiform is often easier to palpate if the patient's wrist is flexed. The examiner may then palpate the pisiform where the flexor carpi ulnaris tendon inserts into it.

Returning to the anatomic snuff box and moving distally, the examiner palpates the trapezium bone. As this is done, the radial pulse is often palpated in the anatomic snuff box. The carpal bones in distal row from lateral to medial (in the anatomic position) are palpated individually:

1. Trapezium.
2. Trapezoid.
3. Capitate (distal to lunate).
4. Hamate (distal to triquetrum; the hook of the hamate on anterior surface is the easiest part to palpate).

Metacarpal Bones and Phalanges. The examiner returns to the trapezium bone and moves further distally to palpate the trapezium, first metacarpal joint, and the metacarpal bone. Moving medially, the examiner palpates each metacarpal bone on the anterior and dorsal surfaces in turn. A similar procedure is carried out for the metacarpophalangeal and interphalangeal joints and the phalanges. These structures are also palpated on their medial and lateral aspects for tenderness, swelling, altered temperature, or other signs of pathology (Fig. 6–60).

To test distal blood flow, the examiner compresses the nail bed and notes the time taken for color to

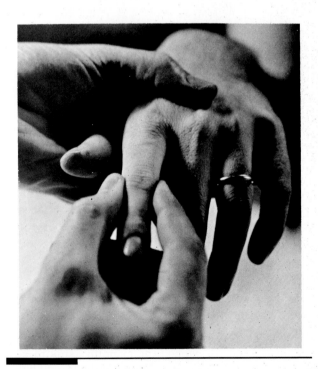

FIGURE 6–60. Palpation of the proximal interphalangeal joint of the left second finger. The examiner's left hand is supporting the patient's hand while the examiner's right thumb and forefinger are used to simultaneously and alternately palpate the medial and lateral aspects of the joint. The other proximal interphalangeal joints are examined in a similar manner. (From Polley, H. F., and G. G. Hunder: Rheumatologic Interviewing and Physical Examination of the Joints. Philadelphia, W. B. Saunders Co., 1978, p. 132.)

return to the nail. Comparison with the normal side will give some indication of restricted flow.

Anterior Surface

The examiner then moves to the anterior surface to complete the palpation.

Pulses. Proximally, the radial and ulnar pulses are first palpated. The radial pulse on the anterolateral aspect of the wrist on top of the radius is easiest to palpate and is the one most frequently used when "taking a patient's pulse." It runs between the tendons of flexor carpi radialis and abductor pollicis longus. The ulnar pulse may be palpated lateral to the tendon of flexor carpi ulnaris. It is more difficult to palpate because it runs deeper and lies under the pisiform and the palmar fascia.

Tendons. Moving across the anterior aspect, the examiner may be able to palpate the long flexor tendons in a lateral-to-medial direction:

1. Flexor carpi radialis.
2. Flexor pollicis longus.
3. Flexor digitorum superficialis.
4. Flexor digitorum profundus.
5. Palmaris longus.
6. Flexor carpi ulnaris (inserts into pisiform).

The palmaris longus (if present) lies over the tendons of the flexor digitorum superficialis, which lie over the tendons of the flexor digitorum profundus.

Palmar Fascia and Intrinsic Muscles. The examiner should then move distally to palpate the palmar fascia and intrinsic muscles of the thenar and hypothenar eminences for indications of pathology.

Skin Flexion Creases. From an anatomic point of view, the examiner should note the various skin flexion creases of the wrist, hand, and fingers (Fig. 6–61). The flexion creases indicate lines of adherence between the skin and fascia with no intervening adipose tissue. The following creases should be noted:

1. The proximal skin crease of the wrist indicates the upper limit of the synovial sheaths of the flexor tendons.
2. The middle skin crease of the wrist indicates the wrist (radiocarpal) joint.
3. The distal skin crease of the wrist indicates the upper margin of the flexor retinaculum.
4. The radial longitudinal skin crease of the palm encircles the thenar eminence. (Palm readers refer to this line as the "life line.")
5. The proximal transverse line of the palm runs across the shafts of the metacarpal bones, indicating the superficial palmar arterial arch (Fig. 6–50). (Palm readers refer to this line as the "head line.")

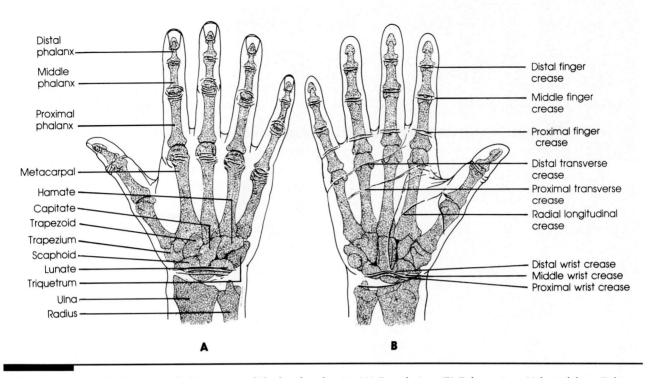

FIGURE 6–61. *Bony landmarks and skin creases of the hand and wrist. (A) Dorsal view. (B) Palmar view. (Adapted from Tubiana, R.: The Hand. Philadelphia, W. B. Saunders Co., 1981, p. 619.)*

6. The distal transverse line of the palm lies over the heads of the second to fourth metacarpals. (Palm readers refer to this line as the "love line.")

7. The proximal skin crease of the fingers is 2 cm distal to the metacarpophalangeal joints.

8. The middle skin crease of the fingers is made up of two lines and lies over the proximal interphalangeal joints.

9. The distal skin crease of the fingers lies over the distal interphalangeal joints.

10. On the flexor and extensor aspects, the skin creases over the proximal and distal interphalangeal joints lie proximal to the joint. On the extensor aspect, the metacarpophalangeal creases lie proximal to the joint; on the flexor aspect, they lie distal to the joint.

Arches. In addition, the examiner should ensure the viability of the arches of the hand (see Fig. 6–9). The carpal transverse arch is the result of the shape of the carpal bones, which in part forms the carpal tunnel. The flexor retinaculum forms the roof for the tunnel. The metacarpal transverse arch is formed by the metacarpal bones, and its shape can have great variability because of the mobility of these bones. This arch is most evident when the palm is cupped. The longitudinal arch is made of the carpal bones, metacarpal bones, and phalanges. The keystone of this arch is the metacarpophalangeal joints, which provide stability and support for the arch.

Weakness or atrophy of the intrinsic muscles of the hand will lead to a loss of these arches. The deformity is most obvious with paralysis of the median and ulnar nerves, resulting in an "ape hand" deformity.

Radiographic Examination

Anteroposterior View. The examiner should note the shape and position of the bones (Fig. 6–62), watching for any (1) evidence of fractures or displacement, (2) decrease in the joint spaces (Fig. 6–63), and (3) change in bone density, which may be due to avascular necrosis. If it is due to avascular necrosis, there will be rarefaction and increased density of the bone and possibly sclerosis of the bone. Avascular necrosis is often seen in the scaphoid bone (Figs. 6–64 and 6–65A) after a fracture or in the lunate in Kienböck's disease (Fig. 6–65B).[30] In some cases, the triangular fibrocartilage or disc may be visualized (Fig. 6–66).

The anteroposterior view of the wrist and hand is used to determine the skeletal age of an individual.[12] The left hand and wrist are used for study because they are thought to be less influenced by environmental factors. The method used in this technique is based on the fact that after an *ossification center*

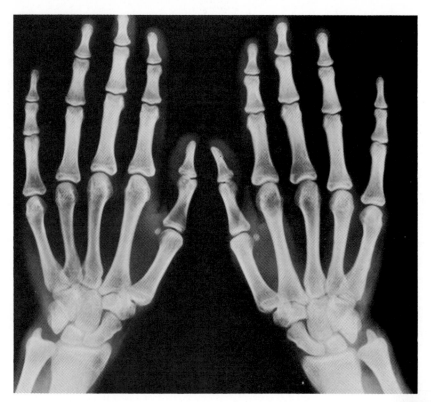

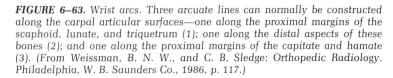

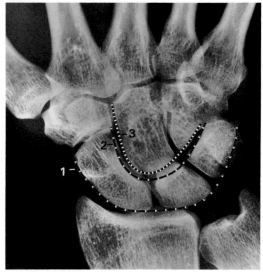

FIGURE 6–62. Radiograph showing the skeletons of both hands. The thumb metacarpal is the shortest, and the index metacarpal is by far the longest. The first and second phalanges of the middle and ring finger are longer than those of the index finger. Note the interlocking design of the carpometacarpal articulations and the saddle shape in opposing planes of the articular surfaces of the trapezium and the base of the first metacarpal. (From Tubiana, R.: The Hand. Philadelphia, W. B. Saunders Co., 1981, p. 21.)

FIGURE 6–63. Wrist arcs. Three arcuate lines can normally be constructed along the carpal articular surfaces—one along the proximal margins of the scaphoid, lunate, and triquetrum (1); one along the distal aspects of these bones (2); and one along the proximal margins of the capitate and hamate (3). (From Weissman, B. N. W., and C. B. Sledge: Orthopedic Radiology. Philadelphia, W. B. Saunders Co., 1986, p. 117.)

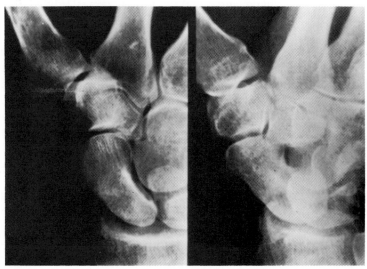

A   B

FIGURE 6–64. Radiograph of the normal scaphoid. (A) Posteroanterior view. (B) Lateral view. (From Tubiana, R.: The Hand. Philadelphia, W. B. Saunders Co., 1981, p. 659.)

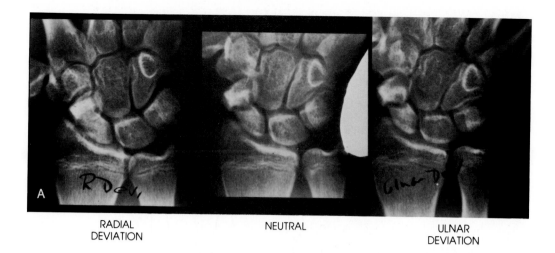

RADIAL
DEVIATION

NEUTRAL

ULNAR
DEVIATION

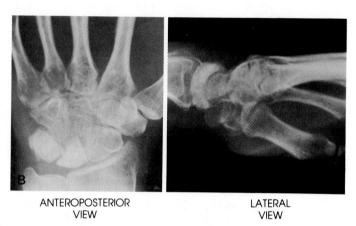

FIGURE 6–65. Avascular necrosis of the carpal bones. (A) Scaphoid fracture shown in three positions. (From Cooney, W. P., et al.: Clin. Orthop. Relat. Res. 149:92, 1980.) (B) Lunate fracture and sclerosis in Kienbock's disease. (From Beckenbaugh, R. D., et al.: Clin. Orthop. Relat. Res. 149:99, 1980.)

ANTEROPOSTERIOR
VIEW

LATERAL
VIEW

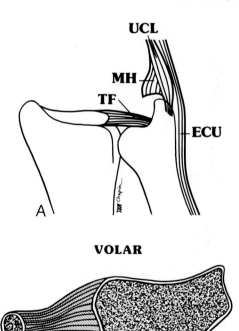

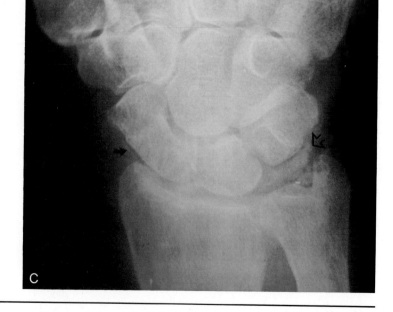

FIGURE 6–66. Triangular fibrocartilage complex. (A) This complex includes the triangular fibrocartilage (articular disc, TF), the meniscus homologue (MH), the ulnar collateral ligament (UCL), and the dorsal and volar radioulnar ligaments (not shown). The extensor carpi ulnaris tendon (ECU) is shown. (B) The triangular fibrocartilage (dotted area) attaches to the ulnar border of the radius and the distal ulna. The triangular shape is evident on this transverse section through the radius and ulnar styloid. The volar aspect of the wrist is labeled. (C) Chondrocalcinosis. There is heavy calcification of the articular cartilage (curved arrow) and the area of the triangular fibrocartilage complex (open arrow). (From Weissman, B. N. W., and C. B. Sledge: Orthopedic Radiology. Philadelphia, W. B. Saunders Co., 1986, p. 115.)

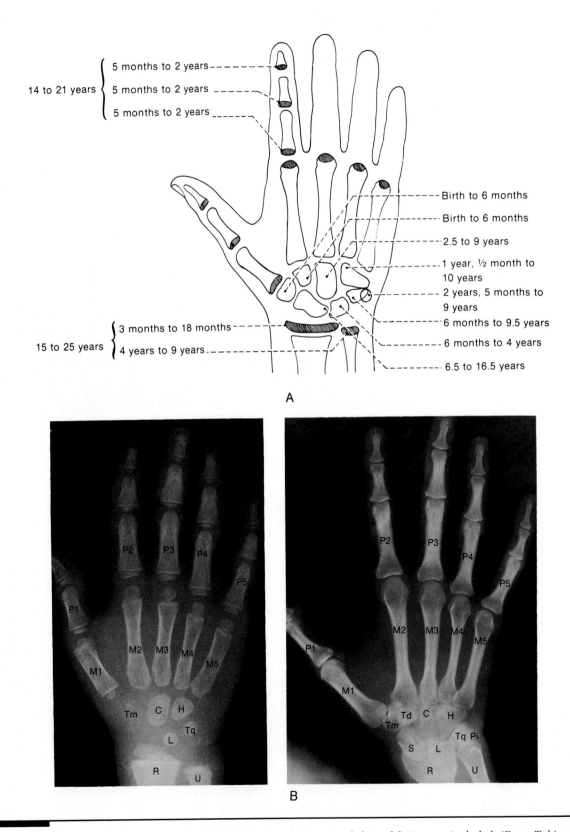

FIGURE 6–67. *Ossification centers of the hand. (A) Date of appearance and date of fusion are included. (From Tubiana, R.: The Hand. Philadelphia, W. B. Saunders Co., 1981, p. 11.) (B) Radiographs of the hand and wrist. Left: Child, 4- to 5-year-old boy or 3- to 4-year-old girl. Right: Adult. C = capitate, H = hamate, L = lunate, M = metacarpal, P = phalanx, Pi = pisiform, R = radius, S = scaphoid, Td = trapezoid, Tm = trapezium, Tq = triquetrum, U = ulna. (From Liebgott, B.: The Anatomical Basis of Dentistry. St. Louis, C. V. Mosby, 1986.)*

appears (Fig. 6–67), it changes its shape and size in a systematic manner as the ossification gradually spreads throughout the cartilaginous parts of the skeleton. The wrist and hand are studied because several bones are available for overall comparison. The patient's hand is compared with standard plates[17] until one plate is found that best approximates that of the patient. There is one standard for males and another for females. In two thirds of the population, skeletal age is no more than 1 year above or below chronologic age. Acceleration or retardation of 3 years or more is considered abnormal. At birth, none of the carpal bones is visible (see Fig. 1–8). This method may be used up to age 20, when the bones of the hand and wrist have fused.

Lateral View. The examiner should note the shape and position of bones for any evidence of fractures and/or displacement (Fig. 6–68A).

Axial View. The axial view is especially useful if the examiner suspects a problem with the carpal bones (Fig. 6–69).

Arthrogram. If the history and clinical assessment suggest a ligament or fibrocartilage problem of the wrist, arthrography helps to confirm the diagnosis (Fig. 6–70).

Computed Tomography (CT) Scan. This technique can be used to visualize bone and soft tissue; by making computer-assisted "slices," tissues can be better visualized (Fig. 6–71).

Magnetic Resonance Imaging (MRI). This non-

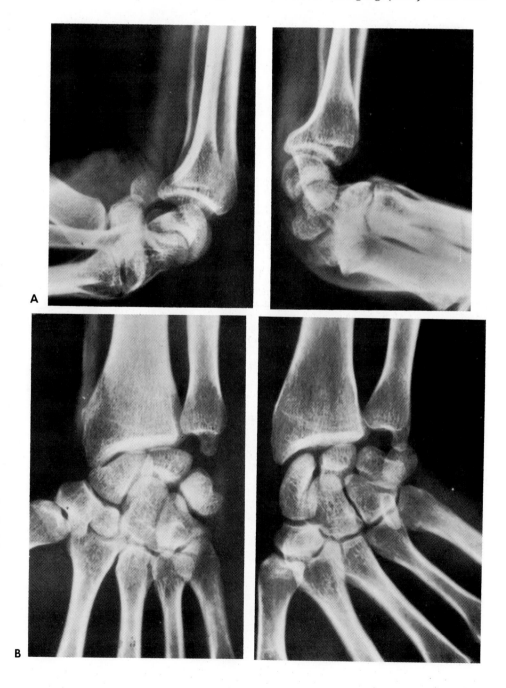

FIGURE 6–68. (A) Radiographs of wrist flexion and extension (lateral views). (B) Posteroanterior views of wrist in radial and ulnar deviation. Note the change in the form of the lunate, indicating a slipping toward the front in the radial slant and toward the rear in the ulnar. (From Tubiana, R.: The Hand. Philadelphia, W. B. Saunders Co., 1981, p. 655.)

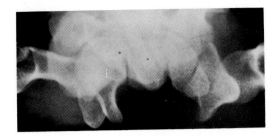

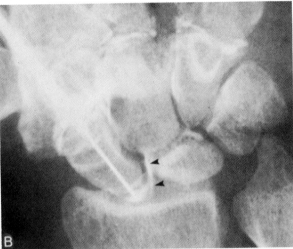

FIGURE 6–69. Radiograph of the carpal tunnel (axial view). (From Tubiana, R.: The Hand. Philadelphia, W. B. Saunders Co., 1981, p. 662.)

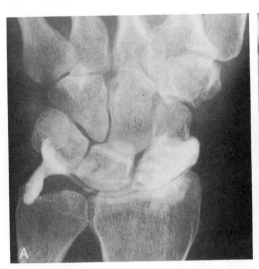

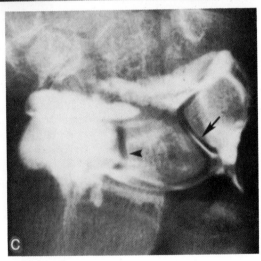

FIGURE 6–70. (A) Posteroanterior view of the wrist following a normal radiocarpal joint arthrogram. Contrast remains confined to the radiocarpal space. (B) After a radiocarpal joint space injection, contrast tracks (arrowheads) through a disrupted scapholunate ligament to fill the midcarpal and carpometacarpal joint spaces. (C) After a radiocarpal joint space arthrogram, the scapholunate ligament is intact because contrast has not yet filled the scapholunate space (arrowhead); however, contrast tracks through the lunotriquetral joint space (arrow) as a result of lunotriquetral ligament disruption. (From Lightman, D. M.: The Wrist and Its Disorders. Philadelphia, W. B. Saunders Co., 1988, p. 89.)

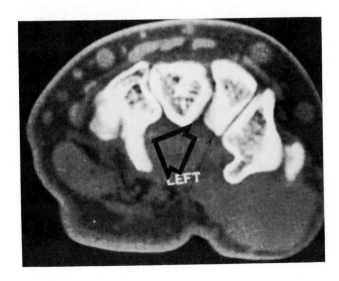

FIGURE 6–71. A fracture of the left hamate hook (arrow) as shown by a CT scan. In this instance, a fracture was suspected on a carpal tunnel view but was not demonstrated as well as it was by CT scan. (From Zemel, N. P., and H. H. Stark: Clin. Sport Med. 5:720, 1986.)

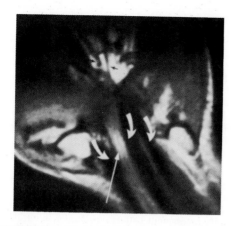

FIGURE 6–72. MRI. SETR = 1,500 msec, TE = 60 msec. Coronal section through palmar aspect of carpal tunnel clearly depicts median nerve (long arrow) coursing between the flexor tendons (curved arrows). Median nerve branches (small arrows) can also be delineated. (From Weiss, K. L., et al.: Height field MRI surface coil imaging of the wrist and hand. Radiology 160:150, 1986.)

invasive technique is useful for visualizing the soft tissues of the wrist and hand and provides the best means of delineating the soft tissues and bone. For example, it can show swelling of the median nerve in carpal tunnel syndrome and thickening of tendon sheaths (Fig. 6–72).

PRÉCIS OF THE FOREARM, WRIST, AND HAND ASSESSMENT

History (sitting)
Observation (sitting)
Examination (sitting)
    Active movements
        Pronation of the forearm
        Supination of the forearm
        Wrist flexion
        Wrist extension
        Radial deviation of wrist
        Ulnar deviation of wrist
        Finger flexion (at MCP, PIP, and DIP joints)
        Finger extension (at MCP, PIP, and DIP joints)
        Finger abduction
        Finger adduction
        Thumb flexion
        Thumb extension
        Thumb abduction
        Thumb adduction
        Opposition of the thumb and little finger
        Functional grip tests
        Pinch tests
        Coordination tests
    Passive movements (as in active movements, except functional grip, pinch tests, and coordination tests, if necessary)
    Resisted isometric movements (as in active movements, in the neutral position)

Special tests (sitting)
Reflexes and cutaneous distribution (sitting)
Joint play movements (sitting)
    Long-axis extension at the wrist and fingers (MCP, PIP, and DIP joints)
    Anteroposterior glide at the wrist and fingers (MCP, PIP, and DIP joints)
    Side glide at the wrist and fingers (MCP, PIP, and DIP joints)
    Side tilt at the wrist
    Anteroposterior glide at the intermetacarpal joints
    Rotation at the MCP, PIP, and DIP joints
    Carpal bone mobility
Palpation (sitting)
Radiographic examination

After any examination, the patient should always be warned of the possibility of exacerbation of symptoms as a result of the assessment.

CASE STUDIES

When doing these case studies, the examiner should list the appropriate questions to be asked and why they are being asked, what to look for and why, and what things should be tested and why. Depending on the answers of the patient (and the examiner should consider different responses), several possible causes of the patient's problem may become evident (examples given in parentheses). If so, a differential diagnosis chart should be made up. The examiner can then decide how different diagnoses may affect the treatment plan.

1. A 31-year-old pregnant woman complains of pain in the right hand of 3 months' duration. The pain awakens her at night and is relieved only by vigorous rubbing of her hand and motion of the fingers and wrist. There is some tingling in the index and middle fingers. Describe your assessment for this patient (carpal tunnel syndrome versus lunate subluxation).

2. An 18-year-old man comes to you after suffering a right scaphoid fracture. He has been in a cast for 12 weeks, and clinical union has been achieved. Describe your assessment for this patient.

3. A 16-year-old girl comes to you complaining of thumb pain. She was skiing during the weekend and fell, landing on her ski pole. She hurt her thumb when she fell. Describe your assessment for this patient (ulnar collateral ligament sprain versus Bennett's fracture).

4. A 48-year-old man comes to you complaining of a painful hand. He happened to hit it against a metal door jam as he was going outside. During the next few days, the hand became swollen and painful, and he has become very protective of it. Describe your assessment of this patient (Sudek's atrophy versus hand aneurysm).

5. A 52-year-old woman who has rheumatoid arthritis comes to you because her hands hurt and she has difficulty doing things functionally. Describe your assessment of this patient.

6. A 14-year-old boy comes to you complaining of wrist pain with swelling on the dorsum of the hand. He says he tripped and fell on the outstretched hand. He states the wrist hurt, the pain decreased, and then the swelling came on over 2 or 3 days. Describe your assessment of this patient (scaphoid fracture versus ganglion).

7. A 28-year-old man was in an industrial accident and lacerated his flexor tendons in the palm of his hand. Describe your assessment of this patient.

8. A 37-year-old woman comes to you complaining of pain and grating on the radial side of the wrist. Describe your assessment of this patient (cartilagenous disc versus scaphoid fracture).

9. A 26-year-old man comes to you complaining of pain and clicking in his wrist. He is a carpenter, and it especially bothers him when he uses a screwdriver. Describe your assessment of this patient (cartilagenous disc versus degenerative arthritis).

10. A 72-year-old woman comes to you with a left Colles fracture. Describe your assessment of this patient.

REFERENCES

CITED REFERENCES

1. Palmer, A. K., and F. W. Werner: The triangular fibrocartilage complex of the wrist: Anatomy and function. J. Hand Surg. 6:152, 1981.
2. Sarrafin, S. K., J. L. Molamed, and G. M. Goshgarian: Study of wrist motion in flexion and extension. Clin. Orthop. Relat. Res. 126:153–159, 1977.
3. Kapandji, I. A.: The Physiology of Joints, vol. I: Upper Limb. New York, Churchill Livingstone, 1970.
4. Wadsworth, C. T.: Wrist and hand examination and interpretation. J. Orthop. Sports Phys. Ther. 5:108, 1983.
5. Blair, S. J., E. McCormick, J. Bear-Lehman, E. E. Fess, and E. Rader: Evaluation of impairment of the upper extremity. Clin. Orthop. Relat. Res. 221:42–58, 1987.
6. Vanswearingen, J. M.: Measuring wrist muscle strength. J. Ortho. Sports Phys. Ther. 4:217–228, 1983.
7. Hume, M. C., H. Gellman, H. McKellop, and R. H. Brumfield: Functional range of motion of the joints of the hand. J. Hand Surg. 15A:240–243, 1990.
8. Tubiana, R.: The Hand. Philadelphia, W. B. Saunders Co., 1981.
9. Reid, D. C.: Functional Anatomy and Joint Mobilization. Edmonton, University of Alberta Press, 1970.
10. Bechtal, C. D.: Grip test: The use of a dynamometer with adjustable handle spacings. J. Bone Joint Surg. 36A:820–832, 1954.
11. Mathiowetz, V., K. Weber, G. Volland, and N. Kashman: Reliability and validity of grip and pinch strength evaluations. J. Hand Surg. 9A:222–226, 1984.
12. Hansman, C. F., and M. M. Mresh: Appearance and fusion of ossification centers in the human skeleton. Am. J. Roentgenol. 88:476, 1962.
13. Aulcino, P. L., and T. E. DuPuy: Clinical examination of the hand. In Hunter, J., et al. (eds.); Rehabilitation of the Hand: Surgery and Therapy. St. Louis, C. V. Mosby Co., 1990.
14. McPhee, S. D.: Functional hand evaluations: A review. Am. J. Occup. Ther. 41:158–163, 1987.
15. Finkelstein, H.: Stenosing tendovaginitis at the radial styloid process. J. Bone Joint Surg. 12:509, 1930.
16. Hoppenfeld, S.: Physical Examination of the Spine and Extremities. New York, Appleton-Century-Crofts, 1976.
17. Post, M.: Physical Examination of the Musculoskeletal System. Chicago, Year Book Medical Pub., 1987.
18. Booher, J. M., and G. A. Thibodeau: Athletic Injury Assessment. St. Louis, C. V. Mosby Co., 1989.
19. Taleisnik, J.: Carpal instability. J. Bone Joint Surg. 70A:1262–1268, 1988.
20. American Society for Surgery of the Hand: The Hand—Examination and Diagnosis. Aurora, Col., 1978.
21. Moldaver, J.: Tinel's sign—Its characteristics and significance. J. Bone Joint Surg. 60A:412, 1978.
22. O'Riain, S.: Shrivel test: A new and simple test of nerve function in the hand. Br. Med. J. 3:615, 1973.
23. Stromberg, W. B., R. M. McFarlane, J. L. Bell, S. L. Koch, and M. L. Mason: Injury of the median and ulnar nerves—150 cases with an evaluation of Moberg's ninhydrin test. J. Bone Joint Surg. 43A:717–730, 1961.
24. Callahan, A. D.: Sensibility testing. In Hunter, J., et al. (eds.): Rehabilitation of the Hand: Surgery and Therapy. St. Louis, C. V. Mosby Co., 1990.
25. Jones, L. A.: The assessment of hand function: A critical review of techniques. J. Hand Surg. 14A:221–228, 1989.
26. Omer, G. E.: Report of the Committee for Evaluation of the Clinical Result in Peripheral Nerve Injury. J. Hand Surg. 8:754–759, 1983.
27. Dellon, A. L., C. H. Kallman: Evaluation of functional sensation in the hand. J. Hand Surg. 8:865–870, 1983.
28. Fess, E. E.: Documentation: Essential elements of an upper extremity assessment battery. In Hunter, J., et al.: Rehabilitation of the Hand: Surgery and Therapy. St. Louis, C. V. Mosby Co., 1990.
29. Baxter-Petralia, P. L., S. M. Blackmore, and P. M. McEntee: Physical capacity evaluation. In Hunter, J., et al.: Rehabilitation of the Hand: Surgery and Therapy. St. Louis, C. V. Mosby Co., 1990.
30. Beckenbaugh, R. D., T. C. Shives, J. H. Dobyns, and R. L. Linschied: Kienbock's disease: The natural history of Kienbock's disease and consideration of lunate fractures. Clin. Orthop. Relat. Res. 149:98, 1980.
31. Jebson, R. H., N. Taylor, R. B. Trieschmann, M. J. Trotter, and L. A. Howard: An objective and standardized test of hand function. Arch. Phys. Med. Rehabil. 50:311–319, 1969.
32. Bell-Krotoski, J. A., D. E. Breger, and R. B. Beach: Application of biomechanics for evaluation of the hand. In Hunter, J., et al. (eds.): Rehabilitation of the Hand: Surgery and Therapy. St. Louis, C. V. Mosby Co., 1990.
33. Trombly, C. A., and A. D. Scott: Evaluation of motor control. In Trombly, C. A. (ed.): Occupational Therapy for Physical Dysfunction. Baltimore, Williams & Wilkins, 1989.
34. Kaltenborn, F. M.: Mobilization of the Extremity Joints. Oslo, Olaf Norlis Bokhandel, 1980.

GENERAL REFERENCES

American Orthopaedic Association: Manual of Orthopaedic Surgery. Chicago, 1972.
Backhouse, K. M.: Functional anatomy of the hand. Physiotherapy 54:114, 1968.
Beach, R. B.: Measurement of extremity volume by water displacement. Phys. Ther. 57:286–287, 1977.
Beetham, W. P., H. F. Polley, C. H. Slocumb, and W. F. Weaver: Physical Examination of the Joints. Philadelphia, W. B. Saunders Co., 1965.
Bell-Krotoski, J., and E. Tomancik: The repeatability of testing with Semmes-Weinstein monofilaments. J. Hand Surg. 12A:155–161, 1987.
Brand, P. W.: Clinical Mechanisms of the Hand. St. Louis, C. V. Mosby Co., 1985.
Brown, D. E., and D. M. Lightman: Physical examination of the wrist. In Lichtman, D. (ed.): The Wrist and Its Disorders. Philadelphia, W. B. Saunders Co., 1988.
Cailliet, R.: Hand Pain and Impairment. Philadelphia, F. A. Davis Co., 1971.
Canadian Standardized Test of Fitness: Operations Manual. Ottawa, Fitness and Amateur Sport Canada, 1986.
Clarkson, H. M., and G. B. Gilewich: Musculoskeletal Assessment—Joint Range of Motion and Manual Muscle Strength. Baltimore, Williams & Wilkins, 1989.
Clawson, D. K., W. A. Souter, C. J. Carthum, and M. L. Hymen: Functional assessment of the rheumatoid hand. Clin. Orthop. Relat. Res. 77:203–210, 1971.
Coleman, H. M.: Injuries of the articular disc at the wrist. Bone Joint Surg. 42B:522, 1960.
Cooney, W. P., J. H. Dobyns, and R. L. Linschied: Fractures of the scaphoid: A rational approach to management. Clin. Orthop. Relat. Res. 149:90, 1980.

Cooney, W. P., M. J. Lucca, E. Y. S. Chao, and R. L. Linscheid: Kinesiology of the thumb trapeziometacarpal joint. J. Bone Joint Surg. 63A:1371, 1981.

Cyriax, J.: Textbook of Orthopaedic Medicine, vol. I: Diagnosis of Soft Tissue Lesions. London, Bailliere Tindall, 1982.

Dellon, A. L.: Clinical use of vibratory stimuli to evaluate peripheral nerve injury and compression neuropathy. Plast. Reconst. Surg. 65:466–475, 1980.

Dellon, A. L.: The moving two point discrimination test: Clinical evaluation of the quickly adapting fiber/receptor system. J. Hand. Surg. 3:474–481, 1978.

Dellon, A. L.: The paper clip: Light hardware to evaluate sensibility in the hand. Contemp. Ortho. 1:39–42, 1979.

Destouet, J. M., L. A. Gilula, and W. R. Reinus: Roentgenographic diagnosis of wrist pain and instability. In Lichtman, D. (ed.): The Wrist and Its Disorders. Philadelphia, W. B. Saunders Co., 1988.

Forrester, D. M., and J. C. Brown: The Radiology of Joint Disease. Philadelphia, W. B. Saunders Co., 1987.

Garrick, J. G., and D. R. Webb: Sports Injuries: Diagnoses and Treatment. Philadelphia, W. B. Saunders Co., 1990.

Gelberman, R. H., R. M. Szabo, R. V. Williamson, and M. P. Dimick: Sensibility testing in peripheral nerve compression syndromes. J. Bone Joint Surg. 65A:632–637, 1983.

Gilula, L. A., and P. M. Weeks: Post-traumatic ligamentous instabilities of the wrist. Diagn. Radiol. 129:641, 1978.

Greulich, W. W., and S. U. Pyle: Radiographic Atlas of Skeletal Development of the Wrist and Hand. Stanford, Calif., Stanford University Press, 1959.

Henderson, W. R.: Clinical assessment of peripheral nerve injuries—Tinel's test. Lancet 2:801–805, 1948.

Hollinshead, W. H., and D. B. Jenkins: Functional Anatomy of the Limbs and Back. Philadelphia, W. B. Saunders Co., 1981.

Jacobs, P.: Atlas of Hand Radiographs. Baltimore, University Park Press, 1973.

Jacobson, C., and L. Sperling: Classification of the hand grip—A preliminary study. J. Occup. Med. 18:395–398, 1976.

Johnson, R. P.: The acutely injured wrist and its residuals. Clin. Orthop. Relat. Res. 140:33, 1980.

Judge, R. D., G. D. Zuidema, and F. T. Fitzgerald: Clinical Diagnosis: A Physiological Approach. Boston, Little, Brown and Co., 1982.

Kauer, J. M. G.: Functional anatomy of the wrist. Clin. Orthop. Relat. Res. 149:9, 1980.

Kendall, E. P., and B. K. McCreary: Muscles: Testing and Function. Baltimore, Williams & Wilkins, 1983.

Kricum, M. E.: Wrist arthrography. Clin. Orthop. Relat. Res. 187:65–71, 1984.

Levin, S., G. Pearsall, and R. J. Ruderman: Von Frey's method of measuring pressure sensibility in the hand: An emergency analysis of the Weinstein-Semmes pressure aesthesiometer. J. Hand Surg. 3:211–216, 1978.

Liebgott, B.: The Anatomical Basis of Dentistry. Philadelphia, W. B. Saunders Co., 1982.

Linn, M. R., F. A. Mann, and L. A. Gilula: Imaging the symptomatic wrist. Orthop. Clin. North Am. 21:515–543, 1990.

Long, C., P. W. Conrad, E. A. Hall, and S. L. Furler: Intrinsic-extrinsic muscle control of the hand in power grip and precision handling—An electromyographic study. J. Bone Joint Surg. 52A:853–867, 1970.

Maitland, G. D.: The Peripheral Joints: Examination and Recording Guide. Adelaide, Australia, Virgo Press, 1973.

Mayer, V.: Evaluation and rehabilitation of athletic injuries of the hand and wrist: Hand and wrist injuries and treatment. Sports Injury Management 2:1–28, 1989.

Mayer, V., and J. H. Gieck: Rehabilitation of hand injuries in athletics. Clin. Sports Med. 5:783–794, 1986.

McMurtry, R. Y.: The wrist. In Little, H. (ed.): The Rheumatological Physical Examination. Orlando, Fla., Grune & Stratton Inc., 1986.

McMurtry, R. Y., Y. Youm, A. E. Flatt, and T. E. Gillespie: Kinematics of the wrist. II: Clinical applications. J. Bone Joint Surg. 60A:955, 1978.

McRae, R.: Clinical Orthopaedic Examination. New York, Churchill-Livingstone, 1976.

Mennell, J. M.: Joint Pain. Boston, Little, Brown and Co., 1964.

Mennell, J. M.: Manipulation of the joints of the wrist. Physiotherapy 57:247, 1971.

Middleton, W. D., J. B. Kneeland, G. M. Kellman, J. D. Cates, J. R. Sanger, A. Jesmanowicz, W. Froncisz, and J. S. Hyde: MRI imaging of the carpal tunnel: Normal anatomy and preliminary findings in the carpal tunnel syndrome. Am. J. Radiol. 148:307–316, 1987.

Mikic, Z. D.: Detailed anatomy of the articular disc of the distal radioulnar joint. Clin. Orthop. Relat. Res. 245:123–132, 1989.

Moberg, E.: Criticism and study of methods for examining sensibility in the hand. Neurology 12:8–19, 1962.

Moran, C. A., and A. D. Callahan: Sensibility measurement and management. In Moran, C. (ed.): Hand Rehabilitation. Clinics in Physical Therapy. Edinburgh, Churchill Livingstone, 1986.

Napier, J. R.: The prehensile movements of the human hand. J. Bone Joint Surg. 38B:902–913, 1956.

Nicholas, J. A., and E. B. Hershman (eds.): The Upper Extremity in Sports. St. Louis, C. V. Mosby Co., 1990.

Nicholas, J. S.: The swollen hand. Physiotherapy 63:285, 1977.

O'Donoghue, D. H.: Treatment of Injuries to Athletes, 4th ed. Philadelphia, W. B. Saunders Co., 1984.

Omer, G. E.: Sensation and sensibility in the upper extremity. Clin. Orthop. Relat. Res. 104:30–36, 1974.

Palmer, A. K., and F. W. Werner: Biomechanics of the distal radioulnar joint. Clin. Orthop. Relat. Res. 187:26–35, 1984.

Palmer, M. L., and M. Epler: Clinical Assessment Procedures in Physical Therapy. Philadelphia, J. B. Lippincott Co., 1990.

Philps, P. E., and E. Walker: Comparison of the finger wrinkling test results to established sensory tests in peripheral nerve injury. Am. J. Occup. Ther. 31:565–572, 1977.

Porter, R. W.: New test for finger-tip sensation. Br. Med. J. 2:927–928, 1966.

Renfrew, S.: Fingertip sensation—A routine neurological test. Lancet 1:396–397, 1969.

Samman, P. D.: The Nails in Disease. London, Wm. Heinemann Medical Books Ltd., 1965.

Smith, H. B.: Smith hand function evaluation. Am. J. Occup. Ther. 27:244–251, 1973.

Sperling, L., and C. Jacobson-Sollerman: The grip pattern of the healthy hand during eating. Scand. J. Rehab. Med. 9:115–121, 1977.

Swanson, A. B., G. de Groof Swanson, and C. Goren-Hagert: Evaluation of impairment of hand function. In Hunter, J., et al. (eds.): Rehabilitation of the Hand: Surgery and Therapy. St. Louis, C. V. Mosby Co., 1990.

Todd, T. W.: Atlas of Skeletal Maturation. St. Louis, C. V. Mosby Co., 1937.

Tucker, W. E.: Manipulative techniques employed in the treatment of injury and osteoarthritis of the fingers and hands. Physiotherapy 57:257, 1971.

Volz, R. G., and J. Benjamin: Biomechanics of the wrist. Clin. Orthop. Relat. Res. 149:112, 1980.

Wadsworth, C. T.: The wrist and hand. In Gould, J. A. (ed.): Orthopedic and Sports Physical Therapy. St. Louis, C. V. Mosby Co., 1990.

Wadsworth, C. T.: Manual Examination and Treatment of the Spine and Extremities. Baltimore, Williams & Wilkins, 1988.

Wadsworth, C. T.: Wrist and hand examination and interpretation. J. Ortho. Sports Phys. Ther. 5:108–120, 1983.

Waylett-Rendall, J.: Sensibility evaluation and rehabilitation. Orthop. Clin. North Am. 19:43–56, 1988.

Weiss, K. L., J. Beltran, and L. M. Lubbers: High-field MR surface-coil imaging of the hand and wrist—Pathologic correlations and clinical relevance. Radiology 160:147–152, 1986.

Weissman, B. N. W., and C. B. Sledge: Orthopedic Radiology. Philadelphia, W. B. Saunders Co., 1986.

Williams, P., and R. Warwick: Gray's Anatomy, 36th British ed. Philadelphia, W. B. Saunders Co., 1980.

Wynn Parry, C. B.: Rehabilitation of the Hand. London, Butterworths, 1981.

Youm, Y., R. Y. McMurtry, A. E. Flatt, and T. E. Gillespie: Kinematics of the wrist: I. An experimental study of radioulnar deviation and flexion-extension. J. Bone Joint Surg. 60A:423, 1978.

Zemel, N. P., and H. H. Stark: Fractures and dislocations of the carpal bones. Clin. Sports Med. 5:709–724, 1986.

Thoracic (Dorsal) Spine

Assessment of the thoracic spine involves examination of the part of the spine that is most rigid because of the associated rib cage. The rib cage in turn provides protection for the heart and lungs. Normally, the thoracic spine, being one of the primary curves, exhibits a mild *kyphosis* (posterior curvature); the *cervical* and *lumbar spines*, being secondary curves, exhibit a mild *lordosis* (anterior curvature). When the examiner assesses the thoracic spine, it is essential that the cervical and lumbar spines be evaluated at the same time (Fig. 7–1).

APPLIED ANATOMY

The *costovertebral joints* are synovial plane joints located between the ribs and the vertebral body. There are 24 of these joints, and they are divided into two parts. Ribs 1, 10, 11, and 12 articulate with a single vertebra. The other articulations have an intra-articular ligament that divides the joint into two parts so that each rib (ribs 2 through 9) articulates with two adjacent vertebrae and the intervening intervertebral disc.

The *costotransverse joints* are synovial joints found between the ribs and the transverse processes of the vertebra of the same level for ribs 1 through 10. Because ribs 11 and 12 do not articulate with the transverse processes, this joint does not exist for these two levels.

The *costochondral joints* lie between the ribs and the costal cartilage. The *sternocostal joints* are found between the costal cartilage and the sternum. Joints 2 through 6 are synovial, whereas the first costal cartilage is united with the sternum by a synchondrosis. Where a rib articulates with an adjacent rib or costal cartilage, a synovial interchondral joint (ribs 5 through 9) exists.

The superior facet of the T1 vertebra is similar to a facet of the cervical spine. Because of this, T1 is classified as a *transitional vertebra*. The T1 superior facet faces up and back; the inferior facet faces down and forward. The T2–T11 superior facets face up, back, and slightly laterally; the inferior facets face down, forward, and slightly medially (Fig. 7–2). This shape enables slight rotation in the thoracic spine. Thoracic vertebrae T11 and T12 are classified as transitional, and the facets of these vertebrae become positioned in a way similar to that of the lumbar facets. The superior facets of these two vertebrae face up, back, and more medially; the inferior facets face forward and slightly laterally. The close packed position of the facet joints in the thoracic spine is extension.

Within the thoracic spine, there are 12 vertebrae, which diminish in size from T1 to T3 and then increase progressively in size to T12. These vertebrae are distinctive in having facets on the body and transverse processes for articulation with the ribs. The spinous processes of these vertebrae face obliquely downward. T7 has the greatest spinous process angulation, whereas the upper three thoracic vertebrae have spinous processes that project directly posteriorly. In other words, the spinous processes of these vertebrae are on the same plane as the transverse processes of the same vertebrae (Fig. 7–3).

T4–T6 vertebrae have spinous processes that project downward slightly. In this case, the tips of the spinous processes are on a plane halfway between their own transverse processes and the transverse processes of the vertebrae below. For T7, T8, and T9 vertebrae, the spinous processes project downward, with the tip of the spinous processes being on a plane of the transverse processes of the verte-

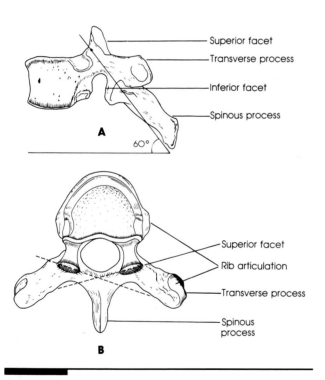

FIGURE 7–2. *Thoracic vertebra. (A) Side view. (B) Superior view.*

Superior facet
Transverse process
Inferior facet
Spinous process

A

60°

Superior facet
Rib articulation
Transverse process
Spinous process

B

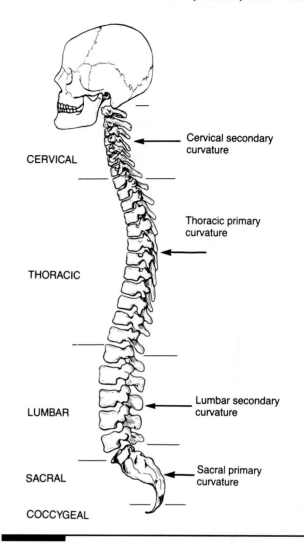

CERVICAL — Cervical secondary curvature

THORACIC — Thoracic primary curvature

LUMBAR — Lumbar secondary curvature

SACRAL — Sacral primary curvature

COCCYGEAL

FIGURE 7–1. *The articulated spine. (Modified from Liebgott, B.: The Anatomical Basis of Dentistry. St. Louis, C. V. Mosby, 1986, p. 454.)*

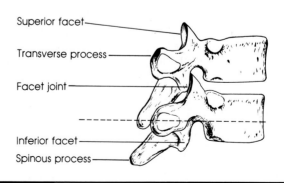

Superior facet
Transverse process
Facet joint
Inferior facet
Spinous process

FIGURE 7–3. *Spinous process of one thoracic vertebra at level of body of vertebra below (T7–T9).*

brae below. For the T10 spinous process, the arrangement is similar to that of the T9 spinous process (i.e., the spinous process is level with the transverse process of the vertebra below). For T11, the arrangement is similar to that of T6 (i.e., the spinous process is halfway between the two transverse processes of the vertebra). T12 is similar to T3 (i.e., the level of the transverse process is level with the spinous process of the same vertebra). The location of the spinous processes becomes important if the examiner wishes to perform posteroanterior central vertebral pressures. For example, if the examiner pushes on the spinous process of T8, the body of T9 will also move. In fact, the vertebral body of T8 will probably arc, whereas T9 will move in an anterior direction. T7 is sometimes classified as a transitional vertebra because it is the point at which the lower limb axial rotation alternates with the upper limb axial rotation (Fig. 7–4).

The ribs, which help to stiffen the thoracic spine, articulate with the demifacets on vertebrae T2–T9. For T1 and T10 vertebrae, there is a whole facet for ribs 1 and 10, respectively. The first rib articulates with T1 only; the second rib articulates with T1 and T2; the third rib articulates with T2 and T3, and so on. Ribs 1 through 7 articulate with the sternum directly and are classified as *true ribs*. Ribs 8 through 10 join with the costocartilage of the rib above and are classified as *false ribs*. Ribs 11 and 12 are classified as *floating ribs* because they do not attach to the sternum or costal cartilages at their distal ends.

Ribs 11 and 12 articulate only with the bodies of T11 and T12 vertebrae, not with the transverse processes of the vertebrae or with the costocartilage of the rib above. The ribs are held by ligaments to the body of the vertebra and to the transverse processes of the same vertebrae. Some of these ligaments also bind the ribs to the vertebra above.

At the top of the rib cage, the ribs are relatively horizontal. As the rib cage descends, they run more and more obliquely downward. By the 12th rib, the ribs are more vertical than horizontal. With inspiration, the ribs are pulled up and forward; this increases the anteroposterior diameter of the ribs. The first six ribs increase the anteroposterior dimension of the chest, mainly by rotating around their long axes. Rotation downward of the rib neck is associated with depression, whereas rotation upward of the same portion is associated with elevation. These movements are known as a "pump handle" action and are accompanied by elevation of the manubrium sternum upward and forward (Fig. 7–5).[1–3]

Ribs 7 through 10 mainly increase lateral, or transverse, dimension. To accomplish this, the ribs move upward, backward, and medially to increase the infrasternal angle or downward, forward, and laterally to decrease the angle. These movements are known as a "bucket handle" action. This action is also performed by ribs 2 through 6 but to a much lesser degree (Fig. 7–5).

The lower ribs (ribs 8 through 12) move laterally in what is known as a "caliper" action that increases lateral diameter[2] (Fig. 7–5).

The ribs are quite elastic in children, but they become increasingly brittle with age. In the anterior half of the chest, the ribs are subcutaneous; in the posterior half, they are covered by muscles.

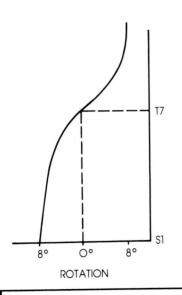

FIGURE 7–4. *Axial rotation of the spine going from left to right on heel strike.*

PATIENT HISTORY

A thorough and complete history should include past and present problems. By listening carefully, the examiner is often able to identify the patient's problem and can then go on to use the observation and examination to confirm or refute the impressions established from the history. All information concerning the present pain and its site, nature, and behavior is important. If any part of the history implicates the cervical or lumbar spine, the examiner must include these areas in the assessment as well.

In addition to the general questions asked in Chapter 1, the following information should be determined:

1. What are the details of the present pain and other symptoms? What are the sites and boundaries of the pain? Have the patient point to the location(s).

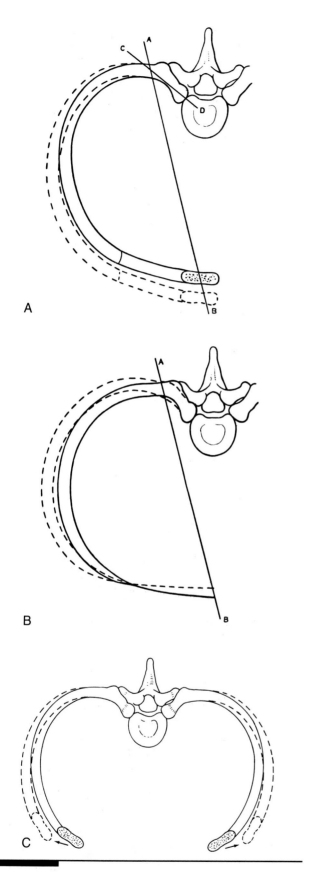

Is there any radiation of pain? The examiner should remember that many of the abdominal structures such as the stomach, liver, and pancreas may refer pain to the thoracic region. Does the pain occur on inspiration, expiration, or both? Pain referred around the chest wall tends to be costovertebral in origin. Thoracic nerve root pain is often severe and is referred in a sloping band along an intercostal space. Pain that the patient describes as passing through the thorax may be spondylitic pain. Is the pain deep, superficial, shooting, burning, or aching?

2. Is there any paresthesia?

3. Which activities aggravate the problem? Active use of the arms will sometimes irritate a thoracic lesion. Pulling and pushing activities can be especially bothersome to a patient with thoracic problems.

4. Which activities ease the problem?

5. Is the condition improving, becoming worse, or staying the same?

6. What are the patient's age and occupation? For example, conditions such as Scheuermann's disease occur in young teenagers between the ages of 13 and 16.

7. Does the patient have any problems with digestion? Pain may be referred to the thoracic spine or ribs from pathological conditions in the thorax or abdomen.

8. Does the patient have any difficulty in breathing? If a breathing problem exists, it may be due to a structural deformity (e.g., scoliosis) or thorax pathology.

9. Are the patient's symptoms referred to the legs, arms, or head and neck? If so, it is imperative that the examiner assess these areas as well. For example, because shoulder movements may be restricted with thoracic spine problems, the examiner must always be aware that problems in one part of the body may affect other parts of the body.

10. Are the symptoms improving or worsening?

11. Is the pain affected by coughing? Sneezing? Straining?

12. Does any particular posture bother the patient?

OBSERVATION

The patient must be suitably undressed so that the body is exposed as much as possible. In the case of a female, the bra is often removed to provide a better view of the spine and rib cage. The patient is usually observed first standing and then sitting.

As with any observation, the examiner should note any alteration in the overall spinal posture (see Chapter 15) because it may lead to problems in the

FIGURE 7–5. Action of the ribs. (A) Pump handle action. (B) Bucket handle action. (C) Caliper action. (A and B from Williams, P., and R. Warwick [eds.]: Gray's Anatomy, 37th ed. Edinburgh, Churchill Livingstone, 1989, p. 498.)

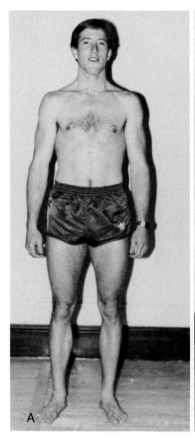 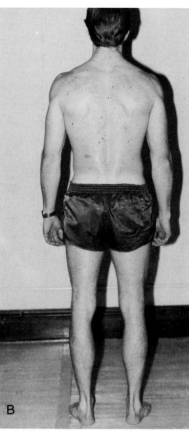

FIGURE 7-6. Normal posture. (A) Front view. (B) Posterior view.

thoracic spine. It is important to observe the total body posture from the head to the toes and look for any deviation from normal (Fig. 7–6). Posteriorly, the spine of the scapula should be level with the T3 spinous process, whereas the inferior angle of the scapula is level with the T7 spinous process. The medial border of the scapula is parallel to the spine and approximately 5 cm lateral to the spinous processes.

Kyphosis. Kyphosis is a condition that is most prevalent in the thoracic spine (Fig. 7–7). The examiner must ensure that a kyphosis is actually present, remembering that a slight kyphosis, or posterior curvature, is normal and is found in every individual. In addition, some individuals have "flat" scapulae, which will give the appearance of an excessive kyphosis. The examiner must ensure that it is actually the spine that has the excessive curvature. Types of kyphotic deformities are shown in Figure 7–8:[4]

1. *Round back*, or decreased pelvic inclination (20°) with a thoracolumbar or thoracic kyphosis (Fig. 7–9).
2. *Hump back*, often a localized, sharp, posterior angulation called *gibbus*.
3. *Flat back*, or decreased pelvic inclination (20°) with a mobile spine.

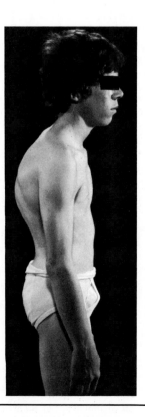

FIGURE 7-7. Congenital thoracic kyphosis. (From Moe, J. H., et al.: Scoliosis and Other Spinal Deformities. Philadelphia, W. B. Saunders Co., 1978, p. 152.)

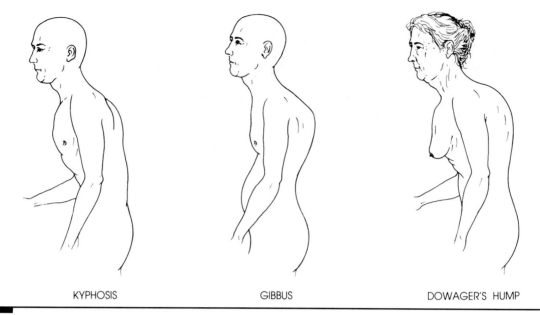

| KYPHOSIS | GIBBUS | DOWAGER'S HUMP |

FIGURE 7–8. Kyphotic deformities.

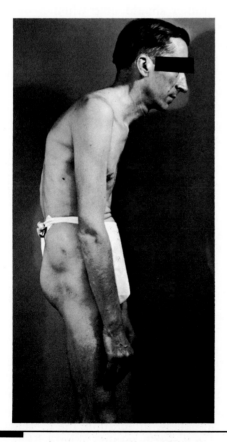

FIGURE 7–9. *Lateral view of patient with ankylosing (rheumatoid) spondylitis showing forward protrusion of head, flattening of anterior chest wall, thoracic kyphosis, protrusion of abdomen, and flattening of lumbar lordosis. This patient also has slight flexion of the hips on the pelvis. (From Polley, H. F., and G. G. Hunder: Rheumatologic Interviewing and Physical Examination of the Joints. Philadelphia, W. B. Saunders, 1978, p. 161.)*

4. *Dowager's hump*, which results from postmenopausal osteoporosis.

Scoliosis. This is a deformity in which there are one or more lateral curvatures of the lumbar or thoracic spine. (In the cervical spine, the condition is called *torticollis*.) The curvature may occur in the thoracic spine alone, in the thoracolumbar area, or in the lumbar spine alone (Fig. 7–10). Scoliosis may be nonstructural or structural. Poor posture, hysteria, nerve root irritation, inflammation in the spine area, leg length discrepancy, or hip contracture can cause nonstructural scoliosis. Structural changes may be genetic, idiopathic, or due to some congenital problem such as a wedge vertebra, hemivertebra, or failure of vertebral segmentation. In other words, there is a structural change in the bone, and normal flexibility of the spine is lost.[5]

A number of curve patterns may be present in the scoliosis (Fig. 7–11).[5] The curve patterns are designated according to the level of the apex of the curve (Table 7–1). A *right thoracic curve* has a convexity toward the right, and the apex of the curve is in the thoracic spine. With a *cervical scoliosis*, or torticollis, the apex is between C1 and C6. For a *cervicothoracic curve*, the apex is at C7 or T1. For a *thoracic curve*, the apex is between T2 and T11. The *thoracolumbar curve* has its apex at T12 or L1. The *lumbar curve* has an apex between L2 and L4, and a *lumbosacral scoliosis* has an apex at L5 or S1. The involvement of the thoracic spine results in a very poor cosmetic appearance or defect as a result of deformation of the ribs along with the spine.

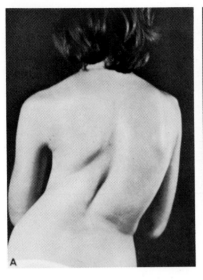 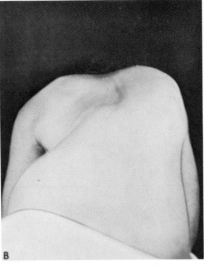

FIGURE 7–10. Idiopathic scoliosis. (A) Postural deformity caused by idiopathic thoracolumbar scoliosis. (B) Asymmetry of posterior thorax accentuated with patient flexed. Note "hump" on the right and "hollow" on the left. (From Gartland, J. J.: Fundamentals of Orthopedics. Philadelphia, W. B. Saunders Co., 1979, p. 341.)

With a structural scoliosis, the vertebral bodies rotate to the convexity of the curve and become distorted.[6] If the thoracic spine is involved, this rotation causes the ribs on the convex side of the curve to push posteriorly, causing a rib "hump" and narrowing the thoracic cage on the convex side. As the vertebral body rotates to the convex side of the curve, the spinous process deviates toward the concave side. The ribs on the concave side move anteriorly, causing a "hollow" and a widening of the thoracic cage on the concave side (Fig. 7–12). Lateral deviation may be more evident if the examiner uses a plumb bob (plummet) from the C7 spinous process or external occipital protuberance (Fig. 7–13).

The examiner should note whether the ribs are symmetric and whether the rib contours are normal and equal on the two sides. In idiopathic scoliosis, the rib contours are not normal, and there is asymmetry of the ribs. Muscle spasm resulting from injury may also be evident. The bony and soft-tissue contours should be observed for equality on both sides or any noticeable difference.

The examiner should note whether the patient sits up properly with the normal spinal curves present and whether the tip of the ear, tip of the acromion process, and high point of the iliac crest are in a straight line as they should be or whether the patient sits in a slumped position (i.e., sag sitting, as in Fig. 7–14B).

The skin should be observed for any abnormality or scars (Fig. 7–15). If there are scars, what were the causes?

Breathing. Does the patient breathe diaphragmatically or apically? Children tend to breath abdominally, whereas women tend to do upper thoracic breathing. Men tend to be upper and lower thoracic breathers. In the aged, breathing tends to be in the lower thoracic and abdominal regions. The examiner should note the quality of the respiratory movements as well as the rate, rhythm, and effort required to inhale and exhale. In addition, the presence of any coughing or noisy breathing should be noted. Because the chest wall movement that occurs during breathing displaces the pleural surfaces, thoracic muscles, nerves, and ribs, pain is accentuated by breathing and coughing if any one of these structures is injured.

RIGHT THORACIC CURVE

RIGHT THORACIC–LUMBAR CURVE

LEFT LUMBAR CURVE

RIGHT THORACIC AND LEFT LUMBAR CURVE (DOUBLE MAJOR CURVE)

FIGURE 7–11. Examples of scoliosis curve patterns.

TABLE 7–1. Curve Patterns and Prognosis in Idiopathic Scoliosis*

	Curve Pattern				
	Primary Lumbar	*Thoracolumbar*	*Combined Thoracic and Lumbar*	*Primary Thoracic*	*Cervicothoracic*
Incidence (%)	23.6	16	37	22.1	1.3
Average age curve noted (yr)	13.25	14	12.3	11.1	15
Average age curve stabilized (yr)	14.5	16	15.5	16.1	16
Extent of curve	T11–L3 (five vertebrae)	T6 or T7–L1 or L1, 2 (six to eight vertebrae)	Thoracic, T6–T10 (five segments) Lumbar, T11–L4 (five segments)	T6–T11 (six segments)	C7 or T1–T4 or T5 (four to six vertebrae)
Apex of curve	L1 or L2	T11 or L2	Thoracic, T7 or T8 Lumbar, L2	T8 or T9 (rotation extreme, convexity usually to right)	T3
Average angular value at maturity (degrees) Standing	36.8	42.7	Thoracic, 51.9; lumbar, 41.4	81.4	34.6
Supine	29.1	35	Thoracic, 41.4; lumbar, 37.7	73.8	32.2
Prognosis	Most benign and least deforming of all idiopathic curves	Not severely deforming Intermediate between thoracic and lumbar curves	Good Body usually well aligned, curves even if severe tend to compensate each other High percentage of very severe scoliosis if onset before age of 10 yr	Worst Progresses more rapidly, becomes more severe, and produces greater clinical deformity than any other pattern Five years of active growth during which could increase	Deformity unsightly Poorly disguised because of high shoulder, elevated scapula, and deformed thoracic cage

*Adapted from Ponseti, I. V., and B. Friedman: J. Bone Joint Surg. *32-A*:381, 1950.

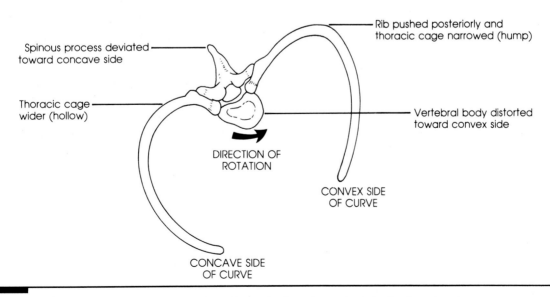

FIGURE 7–12. Pathological changes in the ribs and vertebra with idiopathic scoliosis in the thoracic spine.

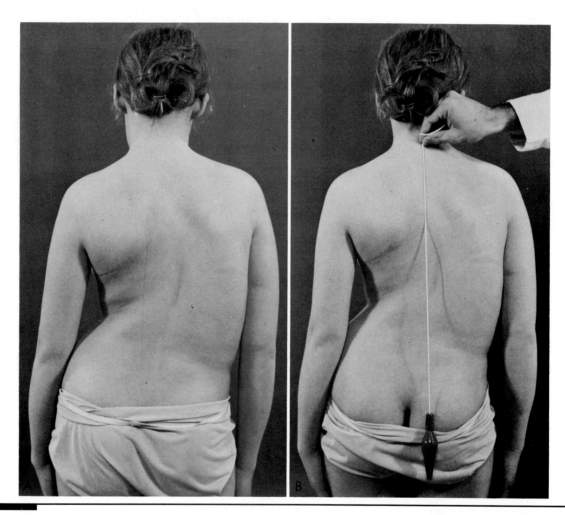

FIGURE 7–13. *Right thoracic idiopathic scoliosis (posterior view). (A) The left shoulder is lower, and the right scapula is more prominent. Note the decreased distance between the right arm and the thorax, with the shift of the thorax to the right. The left iliac crest appears higher, but this is due to the shift of the thorax with fullness on the right and elimination of the waistline. The "high" hip is thus only apparent, not real. (B) Plumbline dropped from the prominent vertebra of C7 (vertebra prominens) measures the decompensation of the thorax over the pelvis. The distance from the vertical plumbline to the gluteal cleft is measured in centimeters and is recorded noting the direction of deviation. When there is a cervical or cervicothoracic curve, the plumb should fall from the occipital protuberance (inion). (From Moe, J. H., et al.: Scoliosis and Other Spinal Deformities. Philadelphia, W. B. Saunders Co., 1978, p. 14.)*

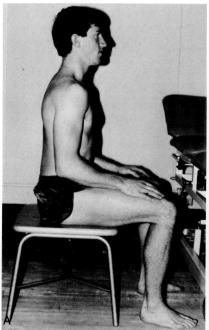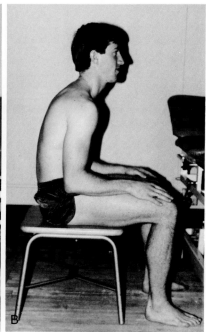

FIGURE 7–14. Sitting posture. (A) Normal position. (B) Sag sitting.

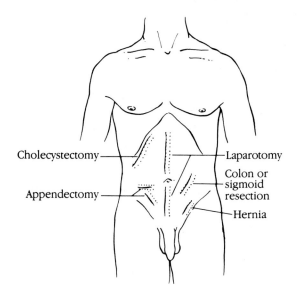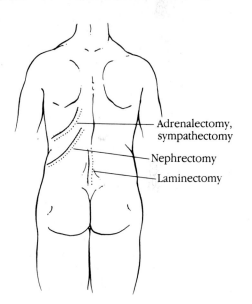

Cholecystectomy

Appendectomy

Laparotomy

Colon or sigmoid resection

Hernia

Adrenalectomy, sympathectomy

Nephrectomy

Laminectomy

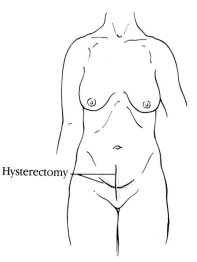

Hysterectomy

FIGURE 7–15. Common surgical scars of the abdomen and thorax. (From Judge, R. D., et al.: Clinical Diagnosis: A Physiologic Approach. Boston, Little, Brown and Co., 1982, p. 295.)

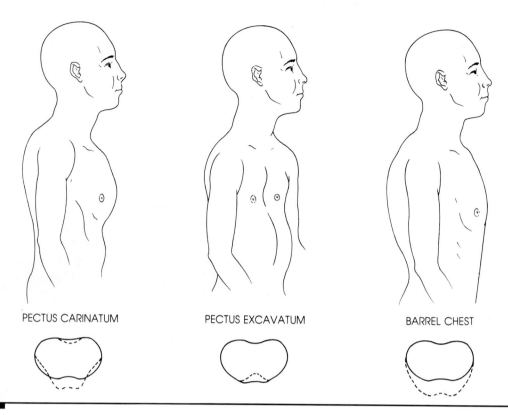

PECTUS CARINATUM   PECTUS EXCAVATUM   BARREL CHEST

FIGURE 7–16. Chest deformities. Lower vertical views show change in chest wall contours with deformity.

Chest Deformities. Are there any chest deformities (Fig. 7–16)?

1. *Pigeon chest* (pectus carinatum). The sternum projects forward and downward like the heel of a boot, increasing the anteroposterior dimension of the chest. This deformity impairs the effectiveness of breathing by restricting ventilation volume.

2. *Funnel chest* (pectus excavatum). This deformity is the result of the sternum's being pushed posteriorly by an overgrowth of the ribs.[7] The anteroposterior dimension of the chest is decreased, and the heart may be displaced. On inspiration, this deformity causes a depression of the sternum that affects respiration and may result in kyphosis.

3. *Barrel chest.* The sternum projects forward and upward so that the anteroposterior diameter is increased. It is seen in conditions such as emphysema.

EXAMINATION

When carrying out an examination of the thorax and thoracic spine, the examiner must remember that although the assessment is primarily of the thoracic spine, if the history, observation, or examination indicates symptoms into or from the neck, upper limb, or lumbar spine and lower limb, these struc-

tures must be examined as well. Thus, the examination of the thoracic spine may be an extensive one. Unless there is a history of specific trauma or injury to the thoracic spine, the examiner must be prepared to assess more than that area alone. If a problem is suspected above the thoracic spine, the scanning examination of the cervical spine and upper limb (as described in Chapter 2) should be performed. If a problem is suspected below the thoracic spine, the scanning examination of the lumbar spine and lower limb (as described in Chapter 8) should be done. Only examination of the thoracic spine is described here.

Active Movements

The active movements of the thoracic spine are usually done with the patient standing. It must be remembered that movement will be limited by the rib cage and the long spinous processes of the thoracic spine. When assessing the thoracic spine, the examiner should be sure to note whether the movement occurs in the spine or in the hips. It must be remembered that an individual can touch the toes with a completely rigid spine if there is sufficient range of motion in the hip joints. Likewise, tight hamstrings may alter the results. The movements may be done with the patient sitting, in which case the effect of hip movement will be eliminated or decreased. As with any examination, the most painful movements are done last.

These active movements should be carried out in the thoracic spine, as shown in Figure 7–17:

1. Forward flexion (20 to 45°).
2. Extension (25 to 45°).
3. Side flexion (left and right) (20 to 40°).

4. Rotation (left and right) (35 to 50°).
5. Costovertebral expansion (3 to 7.5 cm).
6. Rib motion.

Forward Flexion

For forward flexion (forward bending), the normal range of motion in the thoracic spine is 20 to 45° (Fig. 7–18). Because the range of motion at each

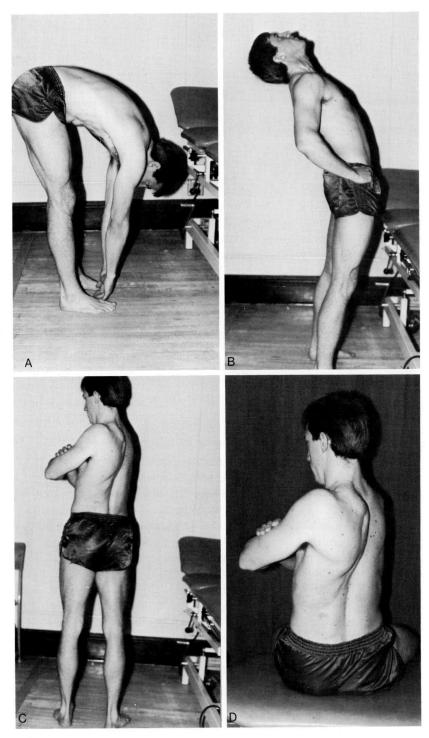

FIGURE 7–17. *Active movement. (A) Forward flexion. (B) Extension. (C) Rotation (standing). (D) Rotation (sitting).*

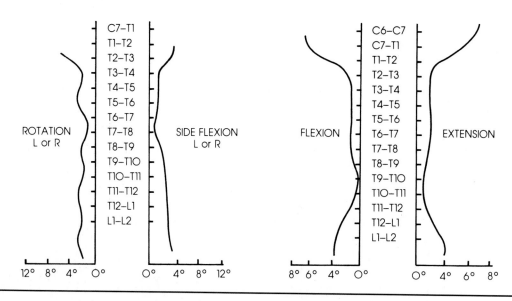

FIGURE 7–18. *Average range of motion in the thoracic spine. (Adapted from Grieve, G. P.: Common Vertebral Joint Problems. Edinburgh, Churchill Livingstone, 1981, pp. 41–42.)*

vertebra is difficult to measure, the examiner can use a tape measure to derive an indication of overall movement (Fig. 7–19). These methods are indirect ones. If one wishes to measure the range of motion at each vertebral segment, a series of radiographs would be necessary. The examiner first measures the length of the spine from the C7 spinous process to the T12 spinous process with the patient in the normal standing posture. The patient is then asked to bend forward, and the spine is again measured. A 2.7-cm difference in tape measure length is considered normal.

If the examiner wishes, the spine may be measured from the C7 to the S1 spinous process with the patient in the normal standing position. The patient is then asked to bend forward, and the spine is again measured. A 10-cm difference in tape measure length is considered normal. In this case, the examiner is measuring movement in the lumbar as well as in the thoracic spine; thus, most movement, approximately 7.5 cm, occurs between T12 and S1.

A third method of measuring spinal flexion is to ask the patient to bend forward and try to touch the toes while keeping the knees straight. The examiner then measures from the fingertips to the floor and records the distance. The examiner must keep in mind that with this method, the movement could occur totally in the hip.

The examiner can decide which method to use. It is of primary importance, however, to note on the patient's chart how the measuring was done and which reference points were used.

While the patient is flexed forward, the examiner can observe the spine from the "skyline" view (Fig. 7–20). With nonstructural scoliosis, the scoliotic curve will disappear on forward flexion; with structural scoliosis, it will remain. With the skyline view, the examiner is looking for a hump on one side (convex side of curve) and a hollow (concave side of curve) on the other. This "hump and hollow" sequence is due to vertebral rotation, which pushes the ribs and muscles out on one side and causes the paravertebral valley on the opposite side. The vertebral rotation is most evident in the flexed position.

When the patient flexes forward, the thoracic spine should curve forward in a smooth, even manner (Fig. 7–21). The examiner should look for any apparent tightness or sharp angulation such as a gibbus when the movement is performed. If the patient has an excessive kyphosis to begin with, very little forward flexion movement will occur in the thoracic spine.

Extension

Extension (backward bending) in the thoracic spine is normally 25 to 45°. As this movement occurs over 12 vertebrae, the movement between the individual vertebrae is difficult to detect visually. As with flexion, the examiner can use a tape measure and obtain the distance between the same two points (the C7 and T12 spinous processes). Again, a 2.5-cm difference in tape measure length between standing and extension is considered normal. McKenzie[8] advocates having the patient place the hands in the small of the back to add stability while performing the backward movement.

As the patient extends, the thoracic curve should curve backward or at least straighten in a smooth, even manner. The examiner should look for any

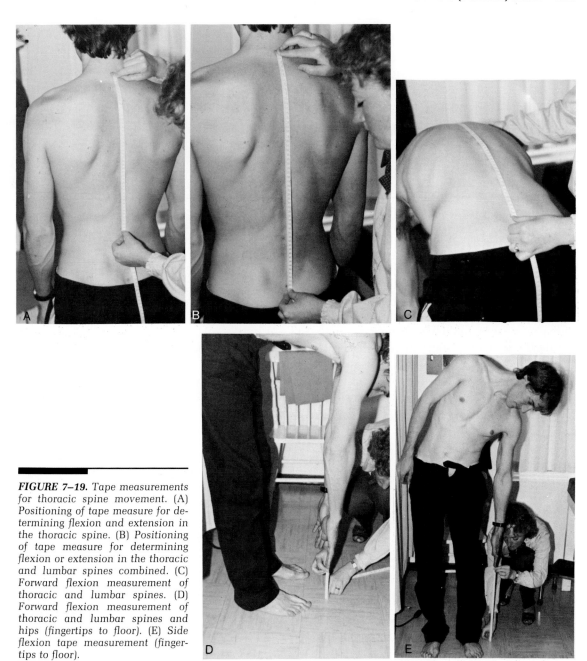

FIGURE 7–19. Tape measurements for thoracic spine movement. (A) Positioning of tape measure for determining flexion and extension in the thoracic spine. (B) Positioning of tape measure for determining flexion or extension in the thoracic and lumbar spines combined. (C) Forward flexion measurement of thoracic and lumbar spines. (D) Forward flexion measurement of thoracic and lumbar spines and hips (fingertips to floor). (E) Side flexion tape measurement (fingertips to floor).

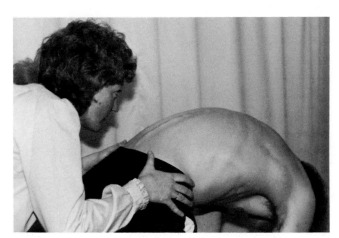

FIGURE 7–20. Examiner performing "skyline" view of spine for assessment of scoliosis.

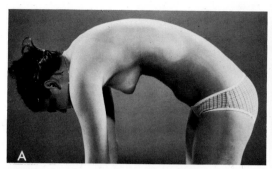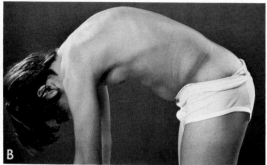

FIGURE 7–21. *Side view in forward bending position for assessment of kyphosis. (A) Normal thoracic roundness is demonstrated with a gentle curve to the whole spine. (B) An area of increased bending is seen in the thoracic spine, indicating structural changes—Scheuermann's disease, in this example. (From Moe, J. H., et al.: Scoliosis and Other Spinal Deformities. Philadelphia, W. B. Saunders Co., 1978, p. 18.)*

apparent tightness or angulation when the movement is performed. If the patient shows excessive kyphosis (Fig. 7–22), the kyphotic curvature will remain on extension whether the movement is tested while the patient is standing or lying prone.

Side Flexion

Side (lateral) flexion is approximately 20 to 40° to the right and left. The patient is asked to run the hand down the side of the leg as far as possible

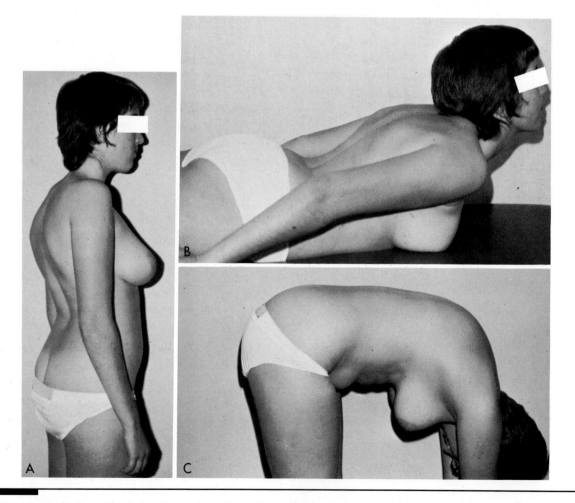

FIGURE 7–22. *Kyphosis and lordosis. (A) On physical examination, definite increases in thoracic kyphosis and lumbar lordosis are visualized. (B) Thoracic kyphosis does not fully correct on thoracic extension. (C) Lumbar lordosis, on the other hand, usually corrects on forward bending; in this case, some lordosis remains. (From Moe, J. H., et al.: Scoliosis and Other Spinal Deformities. Philadelphia, W. B. Saunders Co., 1978, p. 339.)*

without bending forward or backward. The examiner can then "eyeball" the angle of side flexion or use a tape measure to determine the length from the fingertips to the floor and compare it with that of the other side (see Fig. 7–19E). Normally, the distances should be equal. In either case, one must remember that movement in the lumbar spine as well as in the thoracic spine is being measured. As the patient bends sideways, the spine should curve sideways in a smooth, even manner. The examiner should look for any tightness or abnormal angulation, which may indicate hypomobility or hypermobility at a specific segment when the movement is performed.

Rotation

Rotation in the thoracic spine is approximately 35 to 50°. The patient is asked to cross the arms in front or place the hands on opposite shoulders and then rotate to the right and left while the examiner eyeballs the amount of rotation, comparing both ways. Again, the examiner must remember that movement in the lumbar spine as well as in the thoracic spine is occurring.

Costovertebral Expansion

Costovertebral joint movement is usually determined by measuring chest expansion (Fig. 7–23). The examiner places the tape measure around the chest at the level of the fourth intercostal space. The patient is asked to exhale as much as possible, and the examiner takes a measurement. The patient is then asked to inhale as much as possible and hold it while the second measurement is taken. The normal difference between inspiration and expiration is 3 to 7.5 cm.

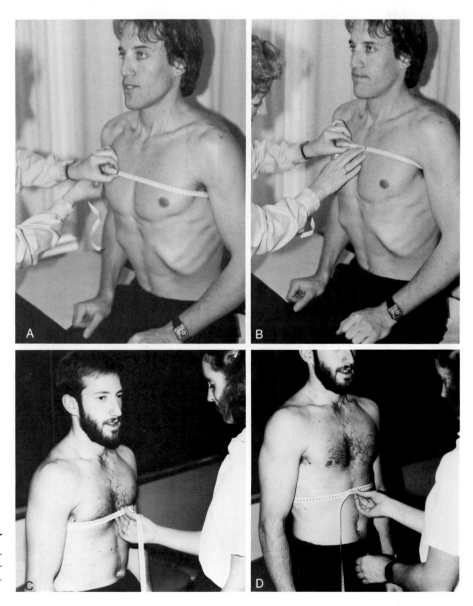

FIGURE 7–23. Measuring chest expansion. (A) Fourth lateral intercostal space. (B) Axilla. (C) Nipple line. (D) Tenth rib.

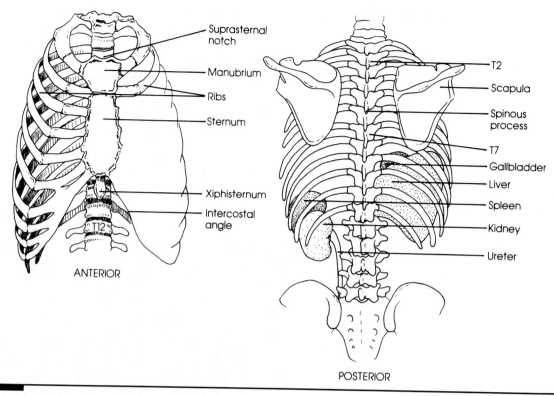

FIGURE 7–33. Landmarks of the thoracic spine.

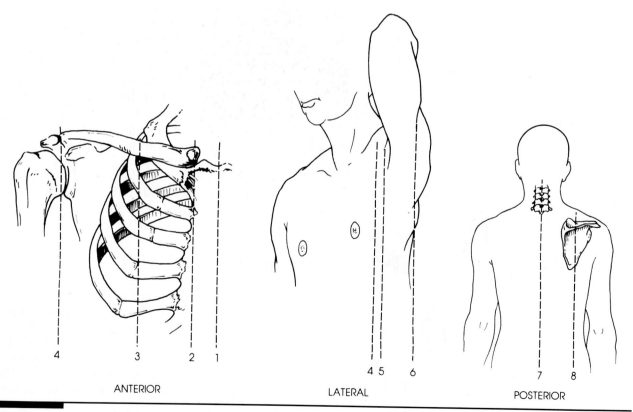

FIGURE 7–34. Lines of reference in the thoracic area.
1. Midsternal line.
2. Parasternal line.
3. Midclavicular line.
4. Anterior axillary line.
5. Midaxillary line.
6. Posterior axillary line.
7. Midspinal (vertebral) line.
8. Midscapular line.

Anterior Aspect

The following structures should be anteriorly palpated:

Sternum. In the midline of the chest, the manubrium sternum, body of the sternum, and xiphoid process should be palpated for any abnormality or tenderness.

Ribs and Costal Cartilage. Adjacent to the sternum, the examiner should palpate the sternocostal and costochondral articulations, noting any swelling, tenderness, or abnormality. These "articulations" are sometimes sprained or subluxed, or a costochondritis (*Tietze syndrome*) may be evident. The ribs should be palpated as they extend around the chest wall, with any potential pathology or crepitations (e.g., subcutaneous emphysema) noted.

Clavicle. The clavicle should be palpated along its length for abnormal bumps (callus) or tenderness.

Abdomen. The abdomen should be palpated for tenderness or other signs indicating pathology. The palpation is done in a systematic fashion, using the fingers of one hand to feel the tissues while the other hand is used to apply pressure. Palpation is carried out to a depth of 1 to 3 cm to reveal areas of tenderness and abnormal masses. Palpation is usu-

ally carried out using the quadrant or the nine-region system (Fig. 7–35).

Posterior Aspect

The examiner then moves to the posterior aspect of the chest wall to complete the palpation.

Scapula. The medial, lateral, and superior borders of the scapula should be palpated for any swelling or tenderness. The scapula normally extends from the spinous process of T2 to that of T7. After the borders of the scapula have been palpated, the examiner palpates the posterior surface of the scapula. Structures palpated will be the supraspinatus and infraspinatus muscles and the spine of the scapula.

Spinous Processes of the Thoracic Spine. In the midline, the examiner may posteriorly palpate the thoracic spinous processes for abnormality. The examiner then moves laterally about 2 to 3 cm to palpate the thoracic facet joints. Because of the overlying muscles, it is usually very difficult to palpate these joints, although the examiner may be able to palpate for muscle spasm and tenderness in the area. Muscle spasm may also be elicited if some internal structures are injured. For example, pathol-

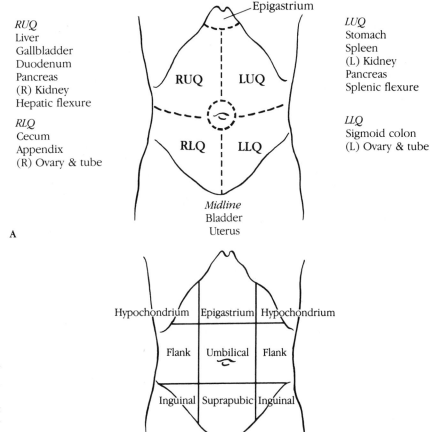

FIGURE 7–35. Superficial topography of the abdomen. (A) Four-quadrant system. (B) Nine-region system. (From Judge, R. D., et al.: Clinical Diagnosis: A Physiological Approach. Boston, Little, Brown and Co., 1982, p. 284.)

ogy affecting the following structures can cause muscle spasm in the surrounding area:

1. *Gallbladder.* Spasm on the right side in the area of the eighth and ninth costal cartilages.
2. *Spleen.* Spasm at the level of ribs 9 through 11 on the left side.
3. *Kidneys.* Spasm at the level of ribs 11 and 12 on both sides at the level of the L3 vertebra.

Evidence of positive findings with no comparable history of musculoskeletal origin could lead the examiner to believe the problem was not of a musculoskeletal origin.

Radiographic Examination

Anteroposterior View. With this view (Fig. 7–36), the examiner should note the following:

1. Any wedging of the vertebrae.
2. Whether the disc spaces appear normal.
3. Whether the ring epiphysis, if present, is normal.
4. Whether there is a "bamboo" spine, indicative of ankylosing spondylitis (Fig. 7–37).
5. Any scoliosis (Fig. 7–38).

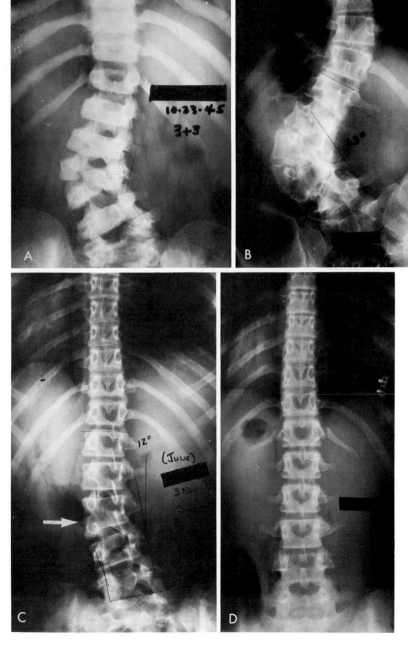

FIGURE 7–36. *Structural scoliosis caused by congenital defect. (A) Left midlumbar and right lumbosacral hemivertebrae in a 3-year-old child (example of hemimetameric shift). (B) A first cousin also demonstrates a midlumbar hemivertebra as well as asymmetric development of the upper sacrum. (C) This girl has a semisegmented hemivertebra (see arrow) in the midlumbar spine with a mild 12° curve. (D) Her identical twin sister showed no congenital anomalies of the spine. (From Moe, J. H., et al.: Scoliosis and Other Spinal Deformities. Philadelphia, W. B. Saunders Co., 1978, p. 134.)*

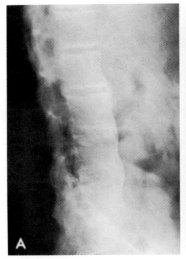 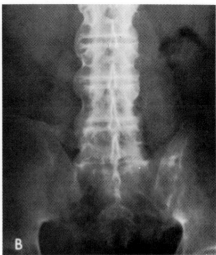

FIGURE 7–37. Ankylosing spondylitis of spine. Note the bamboo effect on the anteroposterior view and bony encasement of vertebral bodies on the lateral view. (From Gartland, J. J.: Fundamentals of Orthopedics. Philadelphia, W. B. Saunders Co., 1979.)

6. Malposition of heart and lungs.
7. Normal symmetry of the ribs.

Lateral View. The examiner should note:

1. A normal mild kyphosis.
2. Any wedging of the vertebrae, which may be an indication of structural kyphosis resulting from conditions such as Scheuermann's disease or wedge fracture (Fig. 7–39).
3. Whether the disc spaces appear normal.
4. Whether the ring epiphysis, if present, is normal.

5. Whether there are any *Schmorl's nodes* (herniation of the intervertebral disc into the vertebral body).
6. Angle of the ribs.
7. Any osteophytes.

Measurement of Spinal Curvature for Scoliosis. With the *Cobb method* (Fig. 7–40), an anteroposterior view is used.[5] A line is drawn parallel to the superior cortical plate of the proximal end vertebra and to the inferior cortical plate of the distal end vertebra. A perpendicular line is erected to each of these lines, and the angle of intersection of the

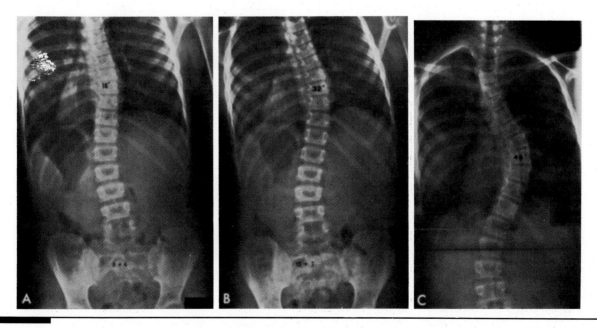

FIGURE 7–38. The natural history of idiopathic scoliosis. (A) Note the mild degree of vertebral rotation and curvature and the imbalance of the upper torso. (B) Note the rather dramatic increase in curvature and the increased rotation of the apical vertebrae 1 year later. (C) Further progression of the curvature has occurred, and the opportunity for brace treatment has been missed. (From Bunnell, W. P.: Orthop. Clin. North Am. 10:817, 1979.)

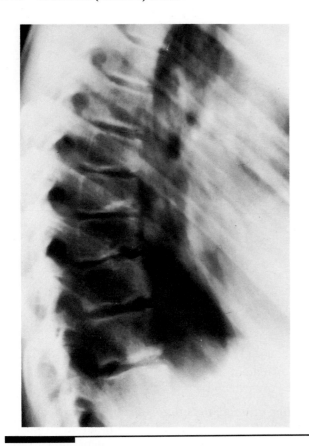

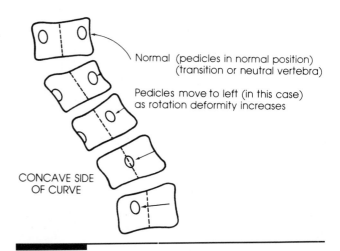

FIGURE 7–41. *Rotation of vertebra seen in scoliosis. On x-ray, the pedicles will appear to be "off center" as the curve progresses.*

perpendicular lines is the angle of spinal curvature resulting from scoliosis. Measurement of the amount of curve has led to a classification of all forms of scoliosis by the Scoliosis Research Society: group 1, 0 to 20° curve; group 2, 21 to 30° curve; group 3, 31 to 50° curve; group 4, 51 to 75° curve; group 5, 76 to 100° curve; group 6, 101 to 125° curve; and group 7, 126° or greater curve.[6]

The rotation of the vertebrae may also be estimated from an anteroposterior view (Fig. 7–41). This estimation is best done by the *pedicle method,* in which

FIGURE 7–39. *Classic radiographic appearance of the spine in a patient with Scheuermann's disease. Note the wedged vertebra, Schmorl's nodules, and marked irregularity of the vertebral endplates. (From Moe, J. H.: Scoliosis and Other Spinal Deformities. Philadelphia, W. B. Saunders Co., 1978, p. 32.)*

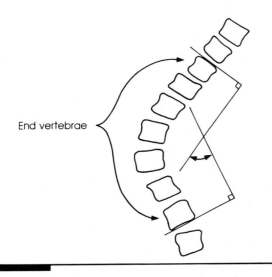

FIGURE 7–40. *Cobb method of measuring scoliotic curve.*

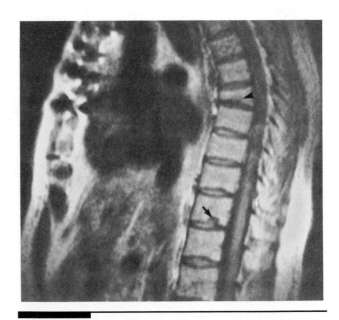

FIGURE 7–42. *Osteoporotic compression fracture of thoracic spine. Midline sagittal T1-weighted image (SE, 500/30) shows compression fracture of upper thoracic vertebral body (arrowhead), indicated by anterior wedging. Marrow signal intensity is maintained (arrowhead). Schmorl's node is incidentally noted at a lower level (arrow). (From Bassett, L. W., et al.: MRI Atlas of the Musculoskeletal System. London, Martin Dunitz Ltd., 1989, p. 49.)*

the examiner determines the relation of the pedicles to the lateral margin of the vertebral bodies. The vertebra is in neutral when the pedicles are equal distances from the lateral margin of the peripheral bodies. If rotation is evident, the pedicles will appear to move laterally toward the concavity of the curve.

MRI. This expensive, noninvasive technique is useful for delineating soft tissue as well as bony tissue (Fig. 7–42).

PRÉCIS OF THE THORACIC SPINE ASSESSMENT*

History
Observation (standing)
Examination
    Active movements (standing or sitting)
        Forward flexion
        Extension
        Side flexion (left and right)
        Rotation (left and right)
    Passive movements (sitting)
        Forward flexion
        Extension
        Side flexion (left and right)
        Rotation (left and right)
    Resisted isometric movements (sitting)
        Forward flexion
        Extension
        Side flexion (left and right)
        Rotation (left and right)
    Special tests (sitting)
    Reflexes and cutaneous distribution (sitting)
    Special tests (prone lying)
    Joint play movements (prone lying)
        Posteroanterior central vertebral pressure
        Posteroanterior unilateral vertebral pressure
        Transverse vertebral pressure
        Rib springing
    Palpation (prone lying)
    Palpation (supine lying)
    Radiographic examination

After any assessment, the patient should always be warned of the possibility of exacerbation of symptoms as a result of examination.

---

*The précis is shown in an order that will limit the amount of moving that the patient has to do but ensure that all necessary structures are tested.

CASE STUDIES

When doing these case studies, the examiner should list the appropriate questions to be asked and why they are being asked, what to look for and why, and what things should be tested and why. Depending on the answers of the patient (and the examiner should consider different responses), several possible causes of the patient's problems may be evident (examples given in parentheses). If so, a differential diagnosis chart should be made up. The examiner can then decide how different diagnoses may affect the treatment plan.

1. A 14-year-old boy presents complaining of a severe aching pain in the middorsal spine of several weeks' duration. He is neurologically normal. X-rays reveal a narrowing and anterior wedging at T5 with a Schmorl's nodule into T4. Describe your assessment plan for this patient (kyphosis versus Scheuermann's disease).

2. A 23-year-old woman has a structural scoliosis with a single "C" curve having its apex at T7. Describe your assessment plan before beginning treatment. How would you measure the curve and amount of rotation?

3. A 38-year-old woman comes to your clinic complaining of chest pain with tenderness at the costochondral junction of two ribs on the left side. Describe your assessment plan for this patient (Tietse syndrome versus rib hypomobility).

4. A 26-year-old male ice hockey player comes to you complaining of back pain that is referred around the chest. He explains that he was "boarded" (hit between another player and the boards). He did not notice the pain and stiffness until the next day. He has had the problem for 2 weeks. Describe your assessment plan for this patient (rib hypomobility versus ligament sprain).

5. A 33-year-old patient comes to you complaining of stiffness in the lower spine that is extending into the thoracic spine. Describe your assessment plan for this patient (ankylosing spondylitis versus thoracic spondylosis).

6. A 21-year-old female synchronized swimmer comes to you complaining of pain in her side. She says she was kicked when she helped boost another athlete out of the water 5 days ago. Describe your assessment plan for this patient (rib fracture versus rib hypomobility).

REFERENCES

CITED REFERENCES

1. Williams, P., and R. Warwick (eds.): Gray's Anatomy, 36th British ed. Philadelphia, W. B. Saunders Co., 1980.
2. MacConaill, M. A., and J. V. Basmajian: Muscles and Movements—A Basis for Human Kinesiology. Baltimore, Williams & Wilkins, 1969.
3. Mitchell, F. L., P. S., Moran, and N. A. Pruzzo: An Evaluation and Treatment Manual of Osteopathic Muscle Energy Procedures. Valley Park, Mo., Mitchell, Moran and Pruzzo, Assoc., 1979.
4. Wiles, P., and R. Sweetnam: Essentials of Orthopaedics. London, J. A. Churchill, 1965.
5. Keim, H. A.: Scoliosis. Clin. Symposia 25:1, 1973.
6. Keim, H. A.: The Adolescent Spine. New York, Springer-Verlag, 1982.
7. Sutherland, I. D.: Funnel chest. J. Bone Joint Surg. 40B:244, 1958.
8. McKenzie, R. A.: The Lumbar Spine: Mechanical Diagnosis and Therapy. Waikanae, New Zealand, Spinal Publications Ltd., 1981.
9. Stoddard, A.: Manual of Osteopathic Technique. London, Hutchinson Medical Publications, 1959.
10. Maitland, G. D.: The slump test: Examination and treatment. Aust. J. Physiother. 31:215, 1985.
11. Cyriax, J.: Textbook of Orthopaedic Medicine, 1: Diagnosis of Soft Tissue Lesions. London, Bailliere Tindall, 1982.
12. Maitland, G. D.: Vertebral Manipulation. London, Butterworths, 1973.

GENERAL REFERENCES

Adams, J. C.: Outline of Orthopaedics. London, E & S Livingstone, 1968.

American Orthopaedic Association: Manual of Orthopaedic Surgery. Chicago, 1972.

Bassett, L. W., R. H. Gold, and L. L. Seeger: MRI Atlas of the Musculoskeletal System. London, Martin Dunitz Ltd., 1989.

Beetham, W. P., H. F. Polley, C. H. Slocumb, and W. F. Weaver: Physical Examination of the Joints. Philadelphia, W. B. Saunders Co., 1965.

Blair, J. M.: Examination of the thoracic spine. In Grieve, G. P. (ed.): Modern Manual Therapy of the Vertebral Column. Edinburgh, Churchill Livingstone, 1986.

Bourdillon, J. R.: Spinal Manipulation, 4th ed. New York, Appleton-Century-Crofts, 1987.

Bradford, D. S.: Juvenile kyphosis. Clin. Orthop. Relat. Res. 128:45, 1977.

Brashear, H. R., and R. B. Raney: Shand's Handbook of Orthopaedic Surgery. St. Louis, C. V. Mosby Co., 1978.

Bunnell, W. P.: Treatment of idiopathic scoliosis. Orthop. Clin. North Am. 10:813, 1979.

Cailliet, R.: Scoliosis: Diagnosis and Management. Philadelphia, F. A. Davis Co., 1975.

Drummond, D. S., E. Rogala, and J. Gurr: Spinal deformity: Natural history and the role of school screening. Orthop. Clin. North Am. 10:751, 1979.

Gartland, J. J.: Fundamentals of Orthopaedics. London, E & S Livingstone, 1968.

Goldstein, L. A., and T. R. Waugh: Classification and terminology of scoliosis. Clin. Orthop. Relat. Res. 93:10, 1973.

Gould, J. A.: The spine. In Gould, J. A. (ed.): Orthopedic and Sports Physical Therapy. St. Louis, C. V. Mosby Co., 1990.

Gregersen, G. G., and D. B. Lucas: An in vivo study of the axial rotation of the human thoracolumbar spine. J. Bone Joint Surg., 49A:247, 1967.

Grieve, G. P.: Common Vertebral Joint Problems. New York, Churchill Livingstone, 1981.

Grieve, G. P.: Mobilization of the Spine. New York, Churchill Livingstone, 1979.

Grieve, G. P.: Thoracic joint problems and simulated visceral disease. In Grieve, G. P. (ed.): Modern Manual Therapy of the Vertebral Column. Edinburgh, Churchill Livingstone, 1986.

Hollingshead, W. H., and D. R. Jenkins: Functional Anatomy of the Limbs and Back. Philadelphia, W. B. Saunders Co., 1981.

Hoppenfeld, S.: Physical Examination of the Spine and Extremities. New York, Appleton-Century-Crofts, 1976.

Houpt, J. B.: The shoulder girdle. In Little, H. (ed.): The Rheumatological Physical Examination. Orlando, Fla., Grune & Stratton, 1986.

James, J. J. P.: The etiology of scoliosis. J. Bone Joint Surg. 52B:410, 1970.

Judge, R. D., G. D. Zuidema, and F. T. Fitzgerald: Clinical Diagnosis: A Physiologic Approach. Boston, Little, Brown and Co., 1982.

Kapandji, I. A.: The Physiology of the Joints, vol. III: The Trunk and Vertebral Column. New York, Churchill Livingstone, 1974.

Levene, D. L.: Chest Pain: An Integrated Diagnostic Approach. Philadelphia, Lea & Febiger, 1977.

Liebgott, B.: The Anatomical Basis of Dentistry. Philadelphia, W. B. Saunders Co., 1982.

Maigne, R.: Orthopaedic Medicine: A New Approach to Vertebral Manipulation. Springfield, Ill., Charles C Thomas, 1972.

Margarey, M. E.: Examination of the cervical and thoracic spine. In Grant, R. (ed.): Physical Therapy of the Cervical and Thoracic Spine. Clinics in Physical Therapy. Edinburgh, Churchill Livingstone, 1988.

Moe, J. H., R. B. Winter, D. S. Bradford, and J. F. Lonstein: Scoliosis and Other Spinal Deformities. Philadelphia, W. B. Saunders Co., 1978.

Moll, J. H., and V. Wright: Measurement of spinal movement. In Jayson, M. (ed.): Lumbar Spine and Back Pain. New York, Grune & Stratton, Inc., 1976.

Moll, J. M. H., and V. Wright: An objective clinical study of chest expansion. Ann. Rheum. Dis. 31:1, 1972.

Nash, C. L., and J. H. Moe: A study of vertebral rotation. J. Bone Joint Surg. 52A:223, 1969.

O'Donoghue, D. H.: Treatment of Injuries to Athletes, 4th ed. Philadelphia, W. B. Saunders Co., 1984.

Papaioannu, T., I. Stokes, and J. Kenwright: Scoliosis associated with limb length inequality. J. Bone Joint Surg. 64A:59, 1982.

Rothman, R. H., and F. A. Simeone: The Spine. Philadelphia, W. B. Saunders Co., 1982.

Simmons, E. H.: Kyphotic deformity of the spine in ankylosing spondylitis. Clin. Orthop. Relat. Res. 128:65, 1977.

Sturrock, R. D., J. A. Wojtulewski, and F. D. Hart: Spondylometry in a normal population and in ankylosing spondylitis. Rheumatol. Rehabil. 12:135, 1973.

Tsou, P. M.: Embryology of congenital kyphosis. Clin. Orthop. Relat. Res. 128:18, 1977.

Tsou, P. M., A. Yau, and A. R. Hodgson: Embryogenesis and prenatal development of congenital vertebral anomalies and their classification. Clin. Orthop. Relat. Res. 152:211, 1980.

White, A. A.: Kinematics of the normal spine as related to scoliosis. J. Biomech. 4:405, 1971.

Whiteside, T. E.: Traumatic kyphosis of the thoracolumbar spine. Clin. Orthop. Relat. Res. 128:78, 1977.

Wyke, B.: Morphological and functional features of the innervation of the costovertebral joints. Folia Morphol. 23:296, 1975.

CHAPTER 8 Lumbar Spine

Back pain is one of the great afflictions of mankind today. Almost anyone born today in Europe or North America has a great chance of suffering a disabling back injury regardless of occupation.

The lumbar spine furnishes support for the upper body and transmits weight of the upper body to the pelvis and lower limbs. Because of the strategic location of the lumbar spine, the examiner must remember that this structure should be included in any examination of the spine as a whole in terms of posture or in any examination of the hip and/or sacroiliac joints. Unless there is a definitive history of trauma, it is difficult to determine whether an injury originates in the lumbar spine, sacroiliac joints, or hip joints; thus, all three should be examined in a sequential fashion.

APPLIED ANATOMY

There are five pairs of, or a total of 10, facet joints in the lumbar spine. These diarthrodial joints consist of superior and inferior facets and a capsule. The facets are located on the vertebral arches. Injury, degeneration, or trauma may lead to *spondylosis* (degeneration of the intervertebral disc), *spondylolysis* (a defect in the pars interarticularis of the arch), or *spondylolisthesis* (a forward displacement of one vertebra over another). The superior facets, or articular processes, face medially and backward and in general are concave; the inferior facets face laterally and forward and are convex. There are, however, abnormalities, or *tropisms*, that can occur in the shape of the facets, especially at the L5–S1 level (Fig. 8–1).

These posterior, apophyseal, or facet joints direct the movement that occurs in the lumbar spine. Because of the shape of the facets, rotation in the lumbar spine is minimal and is accomplished only by a shearing force. Side flexion, extension, and flexion can occur in the lumbar spine, but the direction of movement is controlled by the facet joints. The close packed position of the facet joints in the lumbar spine is extension. Normally, the facet joints are not the weight-bearing type; with increased extension, however, they begin to have a weight-bearing function. The resting position is midway between flexion and extension. The capsular pattern is side flexion and rotation equally limited, followed by extension. The examiner may find, however, that if only one facet joint in the lumbar spine has a capsular restriction, the amount of observable restriction will be minimal. The first sacral segment is usually included when one talks about the lumbar spine, and it is at this joint that the fixed segment of the sacrum joins with the mobile segments of the lumbar spine. In some cases, the S1 segment may be mobile. This occurrence is called *lumbarization* of S1, resulting in a sixth "lumbar" vertebra. At other times, the fifth lumbar segment may be fused to the sacrum or ilium, resulting in a *sacralization* of that vertebra. Sacralization results in four mobile lumbar vertebrae.

The intervertebral discs make up approximately 20 to 25 per cent of the total length of the vertebral column. With age, this percentage will decrease as a result of disc degeneration and loss of hydrophilic action in the disc. The *annulus fibrosus*, the outer laminated portion of the disc, is made up of three zones:

1. The outer zone is made up of fibrocartilage classified as *Sharpey's fibers* that attaches to the outer or peripheral aspect of the vertebral body. The number of cartilage cells in the fibrous strands increases with depth.

2. The intermediate zone is made up of another layer of fibrocartilage.

3. The inner zone is primarily made up of fibrocartilage and has the largest number of cartilage cells.[1]

The annulus fibrosus is made up of 20 concentric collarlike rings of collagenous fibers that criss-cross

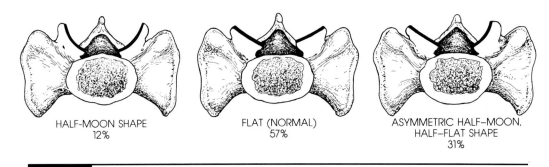

HALF-MOON SHAPE
12%

FLAT (NORMAL)
57%

ASYMMETRIC HALF-MOON,
HALF-FLAT SHAPE
31%

FIGURE 8–1. Facet anomalies (tropisms) at L5–S1.

each other to increase their strength and accommodate torsion movements.[2] The nucleus pulposus is well developed in the cervical and lumbar spine. Initially, at birth, it is made up of a hydrophilic mucoid tissue that is gradually replaced by fibrocartilage. With increasing age, the nucleus pulposus increasingly resembles the annulus fibrosus. The water-binding capacity of the disc decreases with age, and degenerative changes begin to occur in the spine after the second decade of life. (As mentioned, the degeneration of the intervertebral disc is called spondylosis.) Initially, the disc contains approximately 85 to 90 per cent water, but the amount decreases to 65 per cent with age.[3] In addition, it contains a high proportion of mucopolysaccharides, which cause the disc to act as an incompressible fluid. However, these mucopolysaccharides decrease with age and are replaced with collagen. The nucleus pulposus lies slightly posterior to the center of rotation of the disc in the lumbar spine.

The shape of the disc corresponds to that of the body to which it is attached, adhering to the bodies by the cartilaginous end plate. The end plate consists of thin layers of cartilage covering the inferior and superior surfaces of the vertebral bodies. The cartilaginous end plates are approximately 1 mm thick and allow fluid to move between the disc and the vertebral body. The discs are primarily avascular, with only the periphery receiving a blood supply. The remainder of the disc receives nutrition by diffusion, primarily through the cartilaginous end plate. Until the age of 8, the intervertebral discs have some vascularity; however, this vascularity decreases with age.

Usually, the intervertebral disc has no nerve supply, although the peripheral posterior aspect of the annulus fibrosus may be innervated by a few nerve fibers from the sinuvertebral nerve.[4, 5] The lateral aspects of the disc are innervated peripherally by the branches of the anterior rami and gray rami communicantes. The pain-sensitive structures around the intervertebral disc are the anterior longitudinal ligament, posterior longitudinal ligament, vertebral body, nerve root, and cartilage of the facet joint.

With the movement of fluid vertically through the cartilaginous end plate, the pressure on the disc is decreased as an individual approaches the natural lordotic posture in the lumbar spine. Direct vertical pressure on the disc can cause the disc to push fluid into the vertebral body. If the pressure is great enough, defects may occur in the cartilaginous end plate, resulting in *Schmorl's nodes*, which are herniations of the nucleus pulposus into the vertebral body. An adult is usually 1 to 2 cm taller in the morning than in the evening. This change is due to the fluid movement in and out of the disc during the day through the cartilaginous end plate. This fluid shift acts as a safety valve to protect the disc.

If there is an injury to the disc, four problems can result. There may be a *protrusion of the disc*, in which the disc bulges posteriorly without rupturing the annulus fibrosus. In the case of a *disc prolapse*, only the outermost fibers of the annulus fibrosus contain the nucleus. A *disc extrusion* means that the annulus fibrosus is perforated and discal material (part of nucleus pulposus) moves into the epidural space. The fourth problem is a *sequestrated disc*, or a formation of discal fragments from the annulus fibrosus and nucleus pulposus outside the disc proper (Fig. 8–2).[6]

Within the lumbar spine, different postures can increase the pressure on the intervertebral disc (Fig. 8–3). This information is based on the work of Nachemson and coworkers,[7, 8] who performed studies of intradiscal pressure changes in the L3 disc with changes in posture. In regard to these figures, the pressure in the standing position is classified as the norm, and the values given are increases above this norm that occur with the change in posture. For example, the following actions increase the pressure in the L3 intervertebral disc by the following amounts:

1. Coughing or straining, 5 to 35 per cent.
2. Laughing, 40 to 50 per cent.

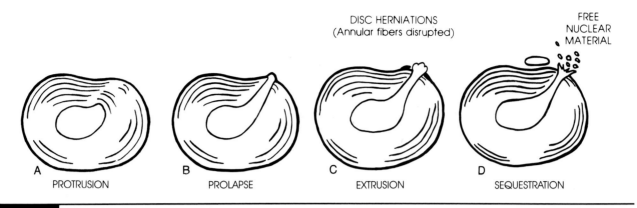

DISC HERNIATIONS
(Annular fibers disrupted)

FREE
NUCLEAR
MATERIAL

A PROTRUSION B PROLAPSE C EXTRUSION D SEQUESTRATION

FIGURE 8–2. *Types of disc herniations. (Modified from MacNab, I.: Backache. Baltimore, Williams & Wilkins, 1977, p. 94.)*

3. Walking, 15 per cent.
4. Side bending, 25 per cent.
5. Small jumps, 40 per cent.
6. Bending forward, 150 per cent.
7. Rotation, 20 per cent.
8. Lifting a 20-kg weight with the back straight and knees bent, 73 per cent.
9. Lifting a 20-kg weight with the back bent and knees straight, 169 per cent.

In general, the L5–S1 segment is the most common site of problems in the vertebral column because this joint bears more weight than any other vertebral joint. The center of gravity passes directly through this vertebra, which is of benefit because it may decrease the shearing stresses to this segment. There is a transition from the mobile segment, L5, to the stable or fixed segment of the sacrum, which can increase the stress on this area. Because the angle between L5 and S1 is greater than those between the other vertebrae, it has a greater chance of having stress applied to it. Another factor that increases the amount of stress on this area is the relatively greater amount of movement that occurs at this level compared with movement at other levels of the lumbar spine.

PATIENT HISTORY

In addition to the general questions asked in Chapter 1, the following information should be determined:

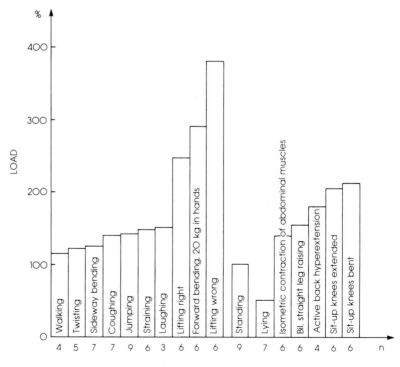

FIGURE 8–3. *Mean change in load on L3 disc compared with upright standing. (From Nachemson, A., and C. Elfstrom: Scand. J. Rehabil. Med. [Suppl. 1] 31:1970)*

TABLE 8–1. Some Implications of Painful Reactions*

Activity	Reaction of Pain	Possible Structural and Pathological Implications
Lying sleeping	↓	Decreased compressive forces—low intradiscal pressures Absence of forces produced by muscle activity
	↑	Change of position—noxious mechanical stress Decreased mechanoreceptor input Motor segment "relaxed" into a position compromising affected structure Poor external support (bed) Nonmusculoskeletal cause
First rising (stiffness)	↑	Nocturnal imbibition of fluid, disc volume greatest Mechanical inflammatory component Prolonged stiffness, active inflammatory disease (e.g., ankylosing spondylitis)
Sitting	↑	Compressive forces High intradiscal pressure
With extension	↓	Intradiscal pressure reduced Decreased paraspinal muscle activity
	↑	Greater compromise of structures of lateral and central canals Compressive forces on lower apophyseal joints
With flexion	↓	Little compressive load on lower apophyseal joints Greater volume lateral and central canals Reduced disc bulge posteriorly
	↑	Very high intradiscal pressures Increased compressive loads upper and mid apophyseal joints
Prolonged sitting	↑	Gradual creep of tissues
Sitting to standing	↑	Creep, time for reversal, difficulty in straightening up Extension of spine, increase disc bulge posteriorly

Walking	↑	Shock loads greater than body weight
		Compressive loads (vertical creep)
		Leg pain
		   Neurological claudication
		   Vascular claudication

Driving	↑	Sitting: compressive forces Vibration: vibro creep repetitive loading, decreased hysteresis loading, decreased hysteresis Increased dural tension sitting with legs extended Short hamstrings: pulls lumbar spine into greater flexion
Coughing, sneezing, straining	↑	Increased pressure subarachnoid space (increased blood flow, Batson's plexus, compromises space in lateral and central canal) Increased intradiscal pressure Mechanical "jarring" of sudden uncontrolled movement

*From Jull, G. A.: Examination of the lumbar spine. In Grieve, G. P. (ed.): Modern Manual Therapy of the Vertebral Column. Edinburgh, Churchill Livingstone, 1986, p. 553.

1. What is the patient's usual activity or pastime?

2. What kind of activity originally caused the back pain? Often, lifting is a common cause of low back pain (Tables 8–1 and 8–2). This fact is not surprising when one considers the forces exerted on the lumbar spine and disc. For example, a 77-kg man lifting a 91-kg weight approximately 36 cm from the intervertebral disc exerts a force of 940 kg on that disc. The force exerted on the disc can be roughly calculated as approximately 10-fold the weight being lifted. Pressure on the intervertebral discs varies depending on the position of the person. From the work of Nachemson and coworkers[7, 8] it has been shown that pressure on the disc can be decreased by increasing the *supported* inclination of the back rest (e.g., an angle of 130° decreases the pressure on the disc by 50 per cent). Using the arms for support can also decrease the pressure on the disc. When one is standing, the disc pressure is approximately 35 per cent of the pressure that occurs in the relaxed sitting position. The examiner should also keep in mind that stress on the lower back tends to be 15 to 20 per cent higher in men than in women because men are taller and their weight is distributed higher in the body.

3. Where are the sites and boundaries of pain? Have the patient point to the location(s).

4. Is there any radiation of pain? It is helpful for the examiner to remember this and correlate it with dermatome findings when evaluating sensation.

5. Is the pain deep? Superficial? Shooting? Burning? Aching?

6. Is there paresthesia (pins and needles) or anesthesia? Asensation or lack of sensation may be experienced if there is pressure on a nerve root.

TABLE 8–2. Some Mechanisms of Musculoskeletal Pain*

Behavior of Pain	Possible Mechanisms
Constant ache	Inflammatory process venous hypertension
Pain on movement	Noxious mechanical stimulus (stretch, pressure, crush)
Pain accumulates with activity	Repeated mechanical stress Inflammatory process Degenerative disc—hysteresis decreased, less protection from repetitive loading
Pain increases with sustained postures	Fatigue in muscle support Gradual creep of tissues may stress affected part of motor unit
Latent nerve root pain	Movement has produced an acute and temporary neurapraxia

*From Jull, G. A.: Examination of the lumbar spine. *In* Grieve, G. P. (ed.): Modern Manual Therapy of the Vertebral Column. Edinburgh, Churchill-Livingstone, 1986, p. 553.

Paresthesia occurs if pressure is relieved from a nerve trunk. Does the patient experience any paresthesia or tingling and numbness in the extremities, perineal (saddle) area, or pelvic area? Abnormal sensations in the perineal (saddle) area often have associated micturition (urination) problems. The examiner must remember that the adult spinal cord ends at the bottom of the L1 vertebra and becomes the cauda equina within the spinal column. The nerve roots extend in such a way that it is rare for the disc to pinch on the nerve root of the same level. For example, the L5 nerve root is more likely to be compressed by the L4 intervertebral disc than by the L5 intervertebral disc (Fig. 8–4). Seldom is the nerve root compressed by the disc at the same level except when the protrusion is more lateral.

7. Which activities aggravate the pain? Is there anything in the patient's lifestyle that increases the pain?

8. Which activities ease the pain?

9. Is the pain improving? Worsening? Staying the same?

10. What about the patient's sleeping position? Is there any problem sleeping? What type of mattress is used (hard, soft)?

11. Does the patient have any difficulty with micturition? If so, the examiner should proceed with caution because the condition may involve more than the lumbar spine. Conversely, this symptom may result from a disc protrusion or spinal stenosis with minimal or no back pain or sciatica. A disc derangement may cause total urinary retention; chronic, long-standing partial retention; vesicular irritability; or the loss of desire or awareness of the necessity to void.

12. Is there any increase in pain with coughing? Sneezing? Deep breathing? Laughing? All of these actions increase the *intrathecal pressure* (the pressure inside the covering of the spinal cord).

13. Are there any postures or actions that specifically increase or decrease the pain or cause difficulty?[9, 10] For example, if sitting increases the pain and other symptoms, the examiner could suspect that sustained flexion is causing mechanical deformation of the spine. If sitting decreases the pain and other symptoms, sustained flexion is decreasing the mechanical deformation. If standing increases the pain and other symptoms, the examiner might suspect that extension, especially relaxed standing, is

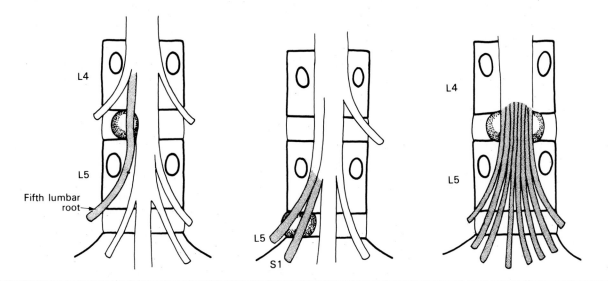

FIGURE 8–4. *Possible effects of disc herniation. (A) Herniation of the disc between L4 and L5 will compress the fifth lumbar root. (B) Large herniation of the L5–S1 disc will compromise not only the nerve root crossing it (first sacral nerve root) but also the nerve root emerging through the same foramen (fifth lumbar nerve root). (C) Massive central sequestration of the disc at the L4–L5 level will involve all of the nerve roots in the cauda equina and may result in bowel and bladder paralysis. (From MacNab, I.: Backache. Baltimore, Williams & Wilkins, 1977, pp. 96–97.)*

the cause. If walking increases the pain and other symptoms, extension is probably causing the mechanical deformation because walking accentuates extension. If lying (especially prone) increases the pain and other symptoms, extension may be the cause. Persistent pain or progressive increase in pain while the patient is in the supine position would lead the examiner to suspect neurogenic or space-occupying lesions, such as infection or tumor. It must be remembered that pain may radiate to the lumbar spine from a pathological condition in other areas as well as from direct mechanical problems. For example, tumors of the pancreas refer pain to the low back. Stiffness and/or pain after rest may be indicative of ankylosing spondylitis or Scheuermann's disease. Pain from mechanical breakdown tends to increase with activity and decrease with rest. Discogenic pain increases if a patient maintains one posture (especially flexion) for a long period. Pain arising from the spine almost always is influenced by posture and movement.

14. Is the pain altered by changing posture?[10] For example, does the pain increase or decrease when the patient goes from a standing to a sitting position? The normal lumbosacral angle while standing is 140°, the normal sacral angle is 30° (Fig. 8–5), and the normal pelvic angle is 30°. The pelvis is the key to proper back posture. For the pelvis to "sit" properly on the femora, the abdominal, hip flexor, hip extensor, and back extensor muscles must be strong, supple, and balanced. Any deviation in the normal alignment should be noted and recorded.

15. Is the pain worse in the morning? Evening? As the day progresses? Is the pain better as the day progresses? For example, osteoarthritis of the facet joints leads to morning stiffness, which in turn is relieved by activity.

16. Which movements hurt? Which movements are stiff? The examiner must help the patient differentiate between true pain and discomfort that is due to stretching. *Postural*, or *static*, *muscles* tend to respond to pathology with tightness in the form of spasm or adaptive shortening; *dynamic*, or *phasic*, *muscles* tend to respond with atrophy. For example, the iliopsoas muscle will adaptively shorten, but the abdominal muscles will weaken in certain pathological conditions. Does the patient describe a painful arc of movement on forward or side flexion? If so, it may indicate a disc protrusion with a nerve root riding over the bulge.[10]

17. Is the patient receiving any medication? For example, long-term use of steroid therapy can lead to osteoporosis.

18. What is the patient's sex? Lower back pain has a higher incidence in females. Female patients should be asked about any changes that occur with menstruation, such as altered pain patterns, irregular menses, and swelling of the abdomen or breasts. Knowledge of the most recent pelvic examination is also useful.

19. What is the patient's occupation? Back pain tends to be more prevalent in individuals with strenuous occupations. For example, truck drivers and warehouse workers have a very high incidence of back injury.

OBSERVATION

The patient must be suitably undressed. Males must wear only shorts, and females must wear only a bra and shorts. When doing the observation, the examiner should note the willingness of the patient to move and the pattern of movement. The patient should be observed first standing and then sitting. The examiner should note the following:

Body Type (see Fig. 15–18). There are three general body types:

1. *Ectomorphic.* Thin body build, characterized by relative prominence of structures developed from the embryonic ectoderm.

2. *Mesomorphic.* Muscular or sturdy body build, characterized by relative prominence of structures developed from the embryonic mesoderm.

3. *Endomorphic.* Heavy (fat) body build, characterized by relative prominence of structures developed from the embryonic endoderm.

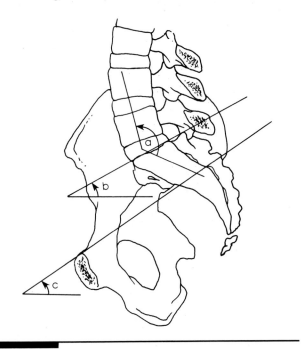

FIGURE 8–5. *Angles of the spine and sacrum. a = Lumbosacral angle (normal = 140°); b = sacral angle (normal = 30°); c = pelvic angle (normal = 30°).*

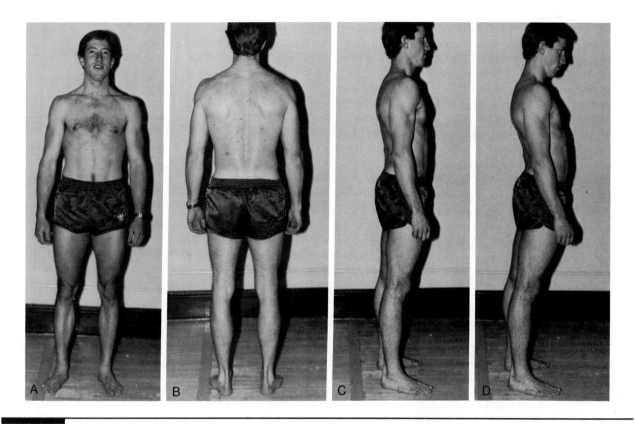

FIGURE 8–6. *Views of the patient in the standing position.* (A) *Anterior view.* (B) *Posterior view.* (C) *Lateral view.* (D) *Lateral view with excessive lordosis.*

Gait. Does the gait appear to be normal when the patient walks into the area, or is it altered in some way? If it is altered, the examiner must take time to find out whether the problem is in the limb or whether the gait is altered to relieve symptoms elsewhere.

Attitude. Is the patient tense? Bored? Lethargic? What is the appearance of the individual? Healthy looking? Emaciated? Overweight?

Total Spinal Posture. The patient should be examined in the habitual relaxed posture that is usually adopted. The patient should be observed anteriorly, laterally, and posteriorly (Fig. 8–6). Anteriorly, the head should be straight "on the shoulders" and the nose in line with the manubrium sternum and xiphisternum or umbilicus. The shoulders and clavicles should be level and equal, although the dominant side may be slightly lower. The waist angles should be equal. The arbitrary "high" points on both iliac crests should be the same height. If they are not, the possibility of unequal leg length should be considered. The difference in height would indicate a functional limb length discrepancy. This discrepancy could be due to altered bone length, altered mechanics (e.g., pronated foot on one side), or joint dysfunction (Table 8–3). The anterior superior iliac spines should be level on each side. The patella should point straight ahead. The lower limbs should be straight and not in genu varum or genu valgum. The heads of the fibulae should be level. The medial malleoli should be level, as should be the lateral malleoli. The medial longitudinal arches of the feet should be evident, and the feet should angle out equally. The arms should be an equal distance from the trunk and equally medially or laterally rotated. Any protrusion or depression of the sternum, ribs, or costocartilage as well as any bowing of bones should be noted. The bony or soft-tissue contours should be equal on both sides.

TABLE 8–3. Functional Limb Length Difference*

Joint	Functional Lengthening	Functional Shortening
Foot	Supination	Pronation
Knee	Extension	Flexion
Hip	Lowering Extension External rotation	Lifting Flexion Internal rotation
Sacroiliac	Anterior rotation	Posterior rotation

*From Wallace, L. A.: Lower quarter pain: Mechanical evaluation and treatment. *In* Grieve, G. P. (ed.): Modern Manual Therapy of the Vertebral Column. Edinburgh, Churchill Livingstone, 1986, p. 467.

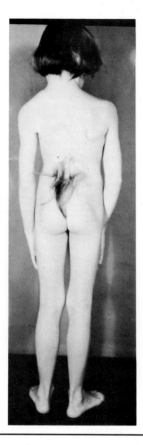

FIGURE 8–7. *Congenital scoliosis and a diastematomyelia in a 9-year-old girl. This type of hairy patch strongly indicates a congenital maldevelopment of the neural axis. (From Rothman, R. H., and F. A. Simeone: The Spine. Philadelphia, W. B. Saunders Co., 1982, p. 371.)*

From the side, the examiner should look at the head to ensure that the ear lobe is in line with the tip of the shoulder (acromion process) and the arbitrary high point of the iliac crest. Each segment of the spine should have a normal curve. Are any of the curves exaggerated or decreased? Is lordosis present? Kyphosis? Do the shoulders droop forward? Are the knees straight, flexed, or in recurvatum (hyperextended)?

From behind, the examiner should note the level of the shoulders, spines of the scapula, and inferior angles; any deformities (such as a Sprengel's deformity) should also be noted. Any lateral spinal curve (scoliosis) should be noted (Fig. 8–7). The waist angles should be equal from the posterior aspect as they were from the anterior aspect. The posterior superior iliac spines should be level. The examiner should note how the posterior superior iliac spine relates to the anterior superior iliac spine (higher or lower?). The gluteal folds and knee joints should be level. The Achilles tendons and heels should appear to be straight. The examiner should note whether there is any protrusion of the ribs or bowing of bones. Does the pelvic angle appear to be normal? Any deviation in the normal spinal postural alignment should be noted and recorded. The various possible sources of pathology are discussed in Chapter 15, "Assessment of Posture."

Markings. A "faun's beard" (tuft of hair) may indicate a spina bifida occulta or diastematomyelia (Fig. 8–7).[11] Café au lait spots may indicate neuro-

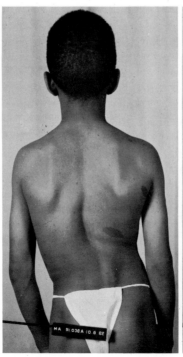
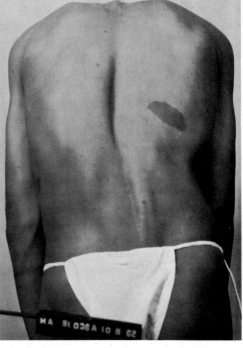

FIGURE 8–8. *Neurofibromatosis with scoliosis. Note the café-au-lait spots on the right side of the trunk. (From Tachdjian, M. O.: Pediatric Orthopedics. Philadelphia, W. B. Saunders Co., 1990, p. 1290.)*

fibromatosis or collagen disease (Fig. 8–8). Unusual skin markings or the presence of skin lesions in the midline may lead the examiner to consider the possibility of underlying neural and mesodermal anomalies.

Step Deformity. A step deformity in the lumbar spine may indicate a spondylolisthesis.

EXAMINATION

The examiner must remember that a complete examination of the lumbar spine and lower limbs is to be performed. Many of the symptoms that occur in the lower limb may originate in the lumbar spine. Unless there is a history of definitive trauma to a peripheral joint, a screening examination must accompany assessment of that joint to rule out problems within the lumbar spine. It is often helpful at this stage to ask the patient to demonstrate the movement(s) that produce or have produced the pain. If the patient is asked to do this, time must be allowed for symptoms to disappear before the remainder of the examination is carried out.

Active Movements

Active movements are performed with the patient standing (Fig. 8–9). The examiner is looking for differences in range of movement and the patient's willingness to do the movement. The range of motion taking place during the active movement is normally the summation of the movements of the entire lumbar spine, not just movement at one level. The most painful movements are done last.

While the patient is doing the active movements, the examiner must remember to look for limitation of movement and its possible causes, such as pain, spasm, stiffness, or blocking. As the patient reaches the full range of active movement, passive overpressure may be applied—but only if the active movement appears to be full and painfree. The overpressure must be applied with extreme care because the upper body weight is already being applied to the lumbar joints by virtue of their position and gravity. If the patient reports that a sustained position increases the symptoms, then the examiner should consider having the patient maintain the position (e.g., flexion) at the end of the range of motion for 10 to 20 seconds to see if symptoms increase.

The greatest motion in the lumbar spine occurs between L4 and L5 and between L5 and S1. There is considerable individual variability in the range of motion of the lumbar spine (Fig. 8–10).[12–16] In reality, little obvious movement occurs in the lumbar spine as a result of the shape of the facet joints, tightness of the ligaments, intervertebral discs, and size of the vertebral bodies. The following active movements are carried out in the lumbar spine:

1. Forward flexion (40 to 60°).
2. Extension (20 to 35°).
3. Lateral flexion (left and right) (15 to 20°).
4. Rotation (left and right) (3 to 18°).

For *flexion* (forward bending), the maximum of range of motion is 40 to 60°. The examiner must ensure that the movement is occurring in the lumbar spine and not in the hips or thoracic spine. It must be remembered that an individual can touch the toes even if no movement occurs in the spine. On forward flexion, the lumbar curve should normally go from its normal lordotic curvature to at least a straight or slightly flexed curve (Fig. 8–11). If it does not do this, there is probably some hypomobility in the lumbar spine. As with the thoracic spine, the examiner may use a tape measure to obtain the distance of the increase in spacing of the spinous processes on forward flexion. Normally, the measurement should increase 7 to 8 cm if it is taken between the T12 spinous process and S1 (see Figs. 8–9A and 8–9B). The examiner should note how far forward the patient is able to bend (i.e., to midthigh, knees, midtibia, or floor) and compare this finding with the straight leg raising tests, since straight leg raising, especially bilaterally, is essentially the same, except that it is a movement occurring from below upward instead of from above downward.

Extension (backward bending) is normally limited to 20 to 35° in the lumbar spine. While performing the movement, the patient is asked to place the hands in the small of the back to help stabilize the back. Bourdillon and Day[17] advocate doing this movement in the prone lying position to hyperextend the spine. They called the resulting position the *Sphinx position.* The patient hyperextends the spine by resting on the elbows with the hands holding the chin (Fig. 8–12) and allowing the abdominal wall to relax. The position is held for 10 to 20 seconds.

Lateral flexion is approximately 15 to 20° in the lumbar spine. The patient is asked to run the hand down the side of the leg and not to bend forward or backward while performing the movement. The examiner can then "eyeball" the movement and compare the movement to the left with that to the right. One may also measure the distance from the fingertips to the floor on both sides and note any differences. As the patient side flexes, the examiner should watch the lumbar curve. (Normally, the lumbar curve should form a smooth curve on side flexion, and there should be no obvious angulation

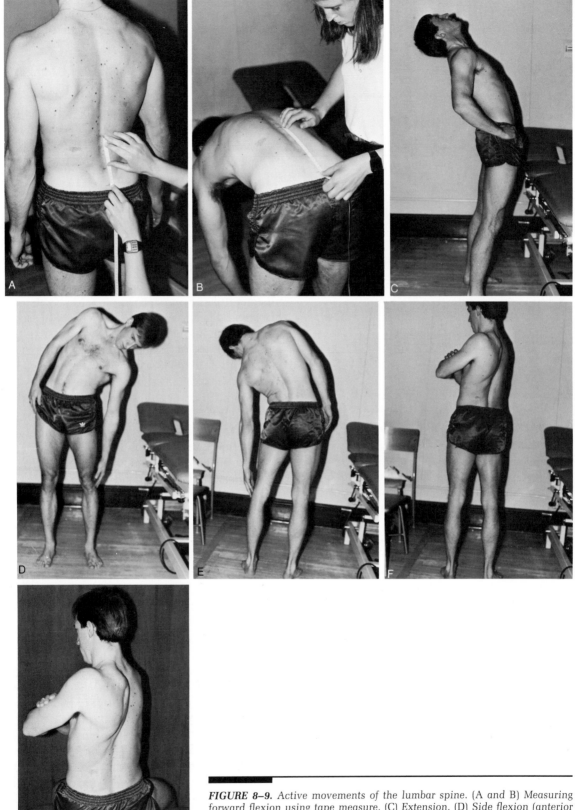

FIGURE 8–9. Active movements of the lumbar spine. (A and B) Measuring forward flexion using tape measure. (C) Extension. (D) Side flexion (anterior view). (E) Side flexion (posterior view). (F) Rotation (standing). (G) Rotation (sitting).

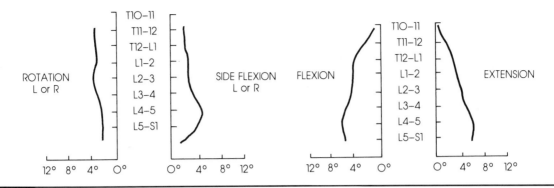

FIGURE 8–10. *Average range of motion in the lumbar spine. (Adapted from Grieve, G. P.: Common Vertebral Joint Problems. Edinburgh, Churchill Livingstone, 1981.)*

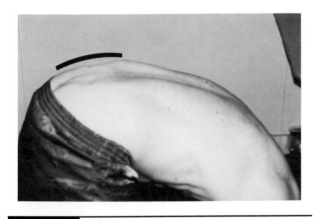

FIGURE 8–11. *On forward flexion, the lumbar curve should normally flatten or go into slight flexion, as shown.*

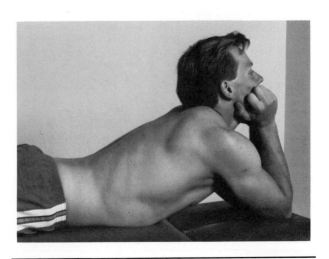

FIGURE 8–12. The Sphinx position.

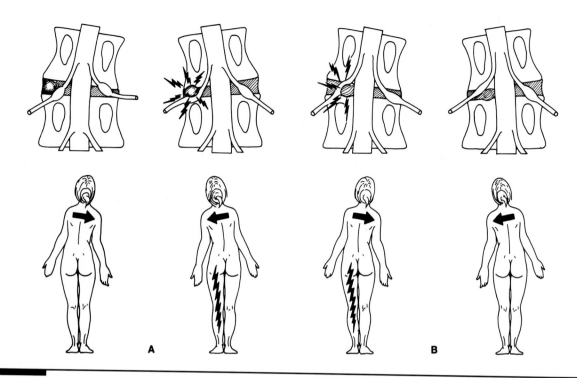

FIGURE 8–13. *Patients with herniated disc disease may sometimes list to one side. This is a voluntary or involuntary mechanism to alleviate nerve root irritation. The list in some patients is toward the side of the sciatica; in others, it is toward the opposite side. A reasonable hypothesis suggests that when the herniation is lateral to the nerve root (A), the list is to the side opposite the sciatica because a list to the same side would elicit pain. Conversely, when the herniation is medial to the nerve root (B), the list is toward the side of the sciatica because tilting away would irritate the root and cause pain. (From White, A. A., and M. M. Panjabi: Clinical Biomechanics of the Spine, 2nd ed. Philadelphia, J. B. Lippincott, 1990, p. 415.)*

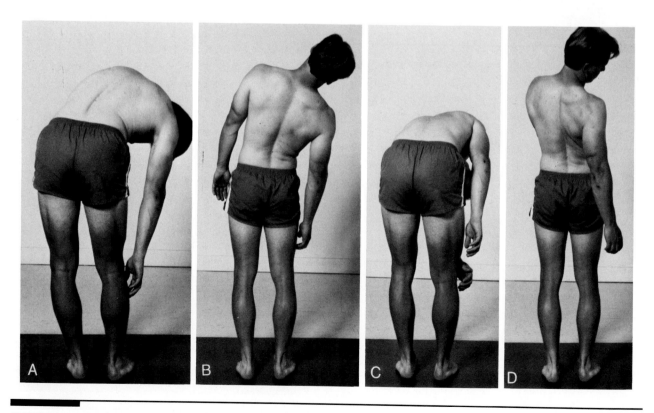

FIGURE 8–14. *Combined active movements. (A) Lateral flexion in flexion. (B) Lateral flexion in extension. (C) Rotation and flexion. (D) Rotation and extension.*

at only one level.) If angulation does occur, it may indicate hypomobility or hypermobility at one level of the lumbar spine.

Rotation in the lumbar spine is normally 3 to 18° to the left and right and is accomplished by a shearing movement of the lumbar vertebrae on each other. Although the patient is usually in the standing position, it may be done sitting to eliminate pelvic and hip movement. If the patient stands, the examiner must take care to watch for this accessory movement and try to eliminate it as much as possible by stabilizing the pelvis.

If a movement such as side flexion toward the painful side increases the symptoms, (1) the lesion is intra-articular because the muscles and ligaments on that side are relaxed, or (2) a disc protrusion, if present, is lateral to the nerve root, increasing the pain. If a movement such as side flexion away from the painful side alters the symptoms, (1) the lesion may be articular or muscular in origin, or (2) a disc protrusion, if present, is medial to the nerve root (Fig. 8–13).

McKenzie[9] advocates repeating the active movements, especially flexion and extension, 10 times to see whether the movement increases or decreases the symptoms. He also advocates a side gliding movement in which the head and feet remain in position and the patient shifts the pelvis to the left and to the right.

If the examiner finds that side flexion and rotation have been equally limited followed by extension, a capsular pattern may be suspected. A capsular pattern in one lumbar segment, however, may be difficult to detect.

Because back injuries rarely occur during a "pure" movement (e.g., flexion, extension, side flexion, or rotation), it has been advocated that combined movements of the spine should be included in the examination.[18] Thus, the examiner may want to test the following more habitual movements:

1. Lateral flexion in flexion.
2. Lateral flexion in extension.
3. Flexion and rotation.
4. Extension and rotation.

These combined movements (Fig. 8–14) may cause signs and symptoms different from those of "pure" movements and are definitely indicated if the patient has shown that a combined movement is what causes the symptoms.

While the patient is standing, a "quick test" may be done (Fig. 8–15). The patient squats down as far as possible, bounces two or three times, and returns to the standing position. This action will quickly test the ankles, knees, and hips for any pathological condition. If the patient can fully squat and bounce without any signs and symptoms, these joints are in

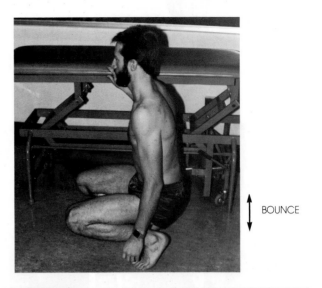

BOUNCE

FIGURE 8–15. *Quick test.*

all probability free of pathology related to the complaint. It must be remembered that this test should be used only with caution and should not be done with patients suspected of having arthritis in the lower limb joints, pregnant patients, or older individuals who exhibit weakness and hypomobility. If this test is negative, there is no need to test the peripheral joints with the patient in the lying position.

The patient is then asked to balance on one leg and to go up and down on the toes four or five times. While the patient does this, the examiner should watch for a Trendelenburg sign (Fig. 8–16). A positive sign may be due to a weak gluteus medius muscle or a coxa vara. If the patient is unable to complete the movement by going up and down on the toes, the examiner might suspect an S1 nerve root lesion. Both legs are tested.

McKenzie advocates doing flexion movement in the supine lying position as well.[9] In the standing position, flexion will take place from above downward so that pain at the end of the range of motion indicates that L5–S1 is affected. When the patient is in the supine lying position, with the knees being lifted to the chest, flexion takes place from below upward so that pain at the beginning of movement indicates that L5–S1 is affected. It must also be remembered that greater stretch is placed on L5–S1 when the patient is in the lying position.

During the observation stage of the assessment, the examiner will have noted any changes in functional limb length. Wallace[19] developed a method for measuring functional leg length. The patient is first assessed in a relaxed stance. In this position, the examiner palpates the anterior superior iliac spine (ASIS) and the posterior superior iliac spine,

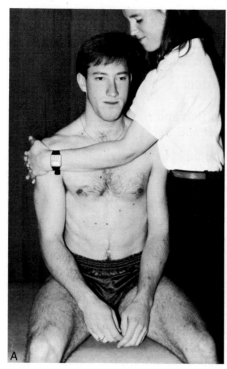
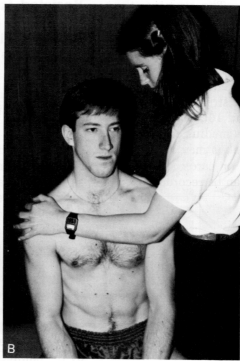

FIGURE 8–19. Positioning for resisted isometric movements of the lumbar spine. (A) Flexion, extension, and side flexion. (B) Rotation to right.

approximately 40 to 55 per cent of their body weight depending on the speed tested.[20]

Functional Assessment

Injury to the lumbar spine can greatly affect the patient's ability to function. Activities such as stand-

ing, walking, bending, lifting, traveling, socializing, dressing, and sexual intercourse are affected. Lehmann et al.[21] developed a rating scale for lumbar dysfunction (Fig. 8–20) that includes assessment criteria, physician criteria, and, equally important, patient criteria for determining the degree of dysfunction. These criteria can be determined during the normal assessment of the patient.

TABLE 8–4. Muscles of the Lumbar Spine: Their Action and Innervation

Action	Muscles Involved	Innervation
Forward flexion	1. Psoas major	L1–L3
	2. Rectus abdominis	T6–T12
	3. External abdominal oblique	T7–T12
	4. Internal abdominal oblique	T7–T12, L1
	5. Transversus abdominis	T7–T12, L1
Extension	1. Latissimus dorsi	Thoracodorsal (C6–C8)
	2. Erector spinae	L1–L3
	3. Transversospinalis	L1–L5
	4. Interspinales	L1–L5
	5. Quadratus lumborum	T12, L1–L4
Side flexion	1. Latissimus dorsi	Thoracodorsal (C6–C8)
	2. Erector spinae	L1–L3
	3. Transversospinalis	L1–L5
	4. Intertransversarii	L1–L5
	5. Quadratus lumborum	T12, L1–L4
	6. Psoas major	L1–L3
	7. External abdominal oblique	T7–T12
Rotation*	—	—

*Very little rotation occurs in the lumbar spine because of the shape of the facet joints. Any rotation would be due to a shearing movement. If shear does occur, the transversospinal muscles would be responsible for the movement.

A. Physical criteria   ———
B. Patient's perception   ———
C. Physician's perception   ———
    TOTAL   ———

A. PHYSICAL CRITERIA (Max: 30)
  1. Range of motion—Total flexion and   ———
     extension in degrees
     Points (1 point for every 10 degrees—   ———
     15 points maximum)
  2. Trunk strength—Total flexion and ex-   ———
     tension in kilograms
     Points (1 point for every 8 kg, Male
     patients—15 points maximum)
     Points (1 point for every 4 kg, Female
     patients—15 points maximum)

B. PATIENT'S PERCEPTION (Max: 40)
  1. Average pain (visual-analog scale)   (15) ———
  2. How disabled: ———
     No disability, able to work full-time   (10)
     Able to work full-time but at a lower   (8)
     level
     Able to work part-time but at usual   (6)
     level
     Able to work only part-time but at   (4)
     lower level
     Not able to work at all   (0)
  3. Activities you can perform—1 point   ———
     for each **Yes** answer

C. PHYSICIAN'S PERCEPTION (Max: 30)
  1. How much pain would you expect for   ———
     this patient at this time? (visual-ana-
     log scale)
  2. At the present time, what is the de-   ———
     gree of impairment?
     None   (10)
     Mild but should not affect most activ-   (8)
     ities
     Moderate, cannot perform some stren-   (6)
     uous activities
     Only light activities, cannot perform   (2)
     any strenuous activities
     Severely limited, cannot perform most   (0)
     light activities or some activities of
     daily living
  3. Current drugs and daily doses (quan-   ———
     tity)
     Analgesics (occasional use = less
     than 5 times per week)
     Major narcotic, regular use   (0)
     Major narcotic, occasional use   (2)
     Minor narcotic, regular use   (4)
     Minor narcotic, occasional use   (6)
     Nonnarcotic, regular use   (8)
     Nonnarcotic, occasional use   (10)
TOTAL   ———

FIGURE 8–20. *Functional rating scale for the lumbar spine. (Modified from Lehmann, T. R., et al.: Spine 8:309, 1983.)*

Peripheral Joints

Once the resisted isometric movements have been completed, if the examiner did not use the "quick test" for peripheral joints or is unsure of the findings, the peripheral joints should be quickly scanned to rule out obvious pathology in the extremities. Any deviation from normal could lead the examiner to do a detailed examination of that joint. The following joints are scanned.[22]

Sacroiliac Joints. With the patient standing, the examiner palpates the PSIS on one side with one thumb and one of the sacral spines with the other thumb. The patient then flexes the hip on that side, and the examiner notes whether the PSIS drops as it normally should on the movement or whether it elevates, indicating fixation of the sacroiliac joint on that side (Fig. 8–21). The examiner then compares the other side. The examiner next places one thumb on one of the patient's ischial tuberosities and one thumb on the sacral apex. The patient is then asked to flex the hip on that side again. If the movement is normal, the thumb on the ischial tuberosity will move laterally. If the sacroiliac joint on that side is fixed, the thumb will move up. The other side is then tested for comparison.

Hip Joints. These joints are actively moved through as full a range of motion of flexion, extension, abduction, adduction, and medial and lateral rotation as possible. Any pattern of restriction or pain should be noted. As the patient flexes the hip, the examiner may palpate the ilium, sacrum, and lumbar spine to determine when during flexion movement begins at the sacroiliac joint on that side and at the lumbar spine. The two sides should be compared.

Knee Joints. The patient actively moves the knee joints through as full a range of flexion and extension as possible. Any restriction of movement or abnormal signs and symptoms should be noted.

Foot and Ankle Joints. Plantar flexion, dorsiflexion, supination, and pronation of the foot and ankle as well as flexion and extension of the toes are actively performed through a full range of motion. Again, any alteration in signs and symptoms should be noted.

Myotomes

Having completed the scanning examination of the peripheral joints, the examiner next tests muscle power and possible neurological weakness (Table 8–5).[22]

With the patient lying supine, the myotomes are tested by assessing the following resisted isometric movements (Fig. 8–22):

1. Hip flexion tests the L2 myotome.
2. Knee extension tests the L3 myotome.
3. Ankle dorsiflexion tests the L4 myotome.
4. Toe extension tests the L5 myotome.
5. Ankle plantar flexion tests the S1 myotome.
6. Ankle eversion tests the S1 myotome.

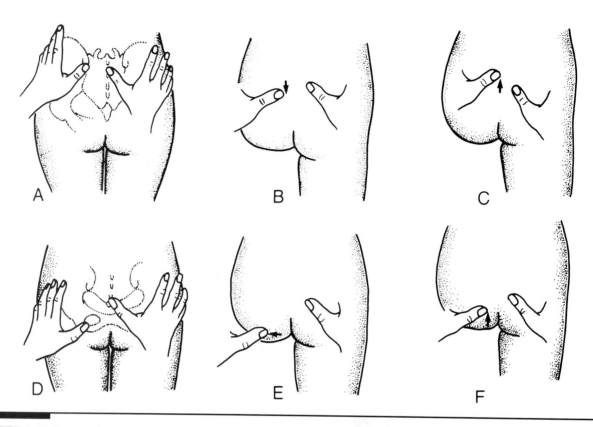

FIGURE 8–21. Tests to demonstrate left sacroiliac fixation. Tests for upper part of joint in (A), (B), and (C) and for lower part in (D), (E), and (F). (A) Examiner places the left thumb on the posterior superior iliac spine and the right thumb over one of the sacral spinous processes. (B) When movement is normal, the examiner's left thumb moves downward as the patient raises the left leg. (C) When the joint is fixed, the examiner's left thumb moves upward as the patient raises the left leg. (D) The examiner places the left thumb over the ischial tuberosity and the right thumb over the apex of the sacrum. (E) When movement is normal, the examiner's left thumb moves laterally as the patient raises the left leg. (F) When the joint is fixed, the examiner's left thumb moves slightly upward as the patient raises the left leg. (From Kirkaldy-Willis, W. H.: Managing Low Back Pain. New York, Churchill Livingstone, 1983, p. 94.)

TABLE 8–5. Lumbar Root Syndromes

Root	Dermatome	Muscle Weakness	Reflexes Affected	Paresthesias
L1	Back, over trochanter, groin	None	None	Groin, after holding posture, which causes pain
L2	Back, front of thigh to knee	Psoas, hip adductors	None	Occasionally front of thigh
L3	Back, upper buttock, front of thigh and knee, medial lower leg	Psoas, quadriceps—thigh wasting	Knee jerk sluggish, PKB positive, pain on full SLR	Inner knee, anterior lower leg
L4	Inner buttock, outer thigh, inside of leg, dorsum of foot, big toe	Tibialis anterior, extensor hallucis	SLR limited, neck-flexion pain, weak or a bent knee jerk; side flexion limited	Medial aspect of calf and ankle
L5	Buttock, back and side of thigh, lateral aspect of leg, dorsum of foot, inner half of sole and first, second, and third toes	Extensor hallucis, peroneal, gluteus medius, ankle dorsiflexor, hamstrings—calf wasting	SLR limited to one side, neck-flexion pain, ankle jerk decreased, crossed-leg raising—pain	Lateral aspect of leg, medial three toes
S1	Buttock, back of thigh, and lower leg	Calf and hamstrings, wasting of gluteals, peroneals, plantar flexors	SLR limited	Lateral two toes, lateral foot, lateral leg to knee, plantar aspect of foot
S2	Same as S1	Same as S1 except peroneals	Same as S1	Lateral leg, knee, heel
S3	Groin, inner thigh to knee	None	None	None
S4	Perineum, genitals, lower sacrum	Bladder, rectum	None	Saddle area, genitals, anus, impotence

Note: Manipulation and traction are contraindicated if S4 or massive posterior displacement causes bilateral sciatica and S3 pain. PKB = Prone knee bendings; SLR = straight leg raise.

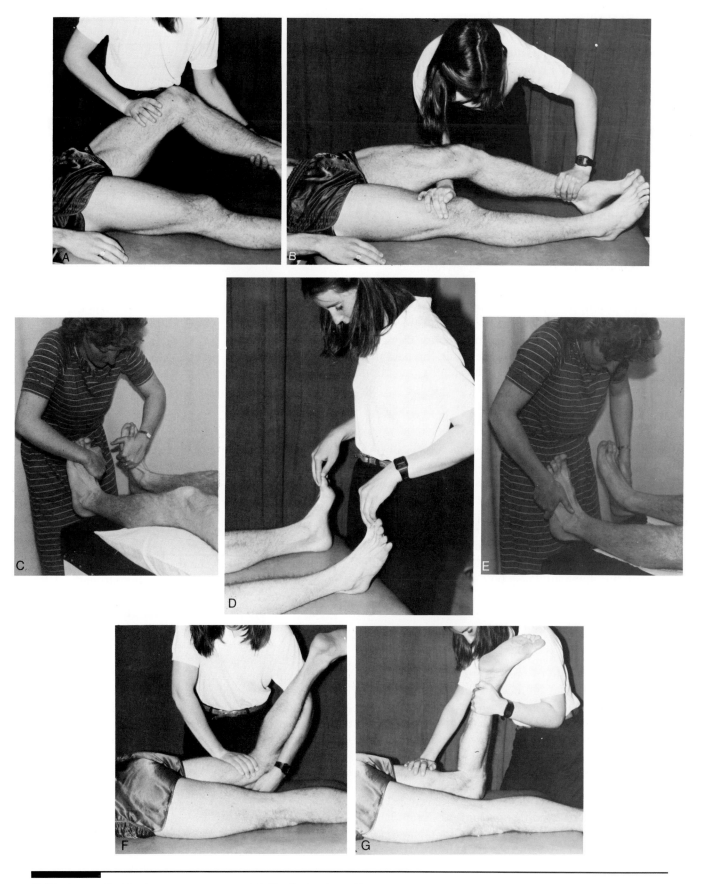

FIGURE 8–22. Positioning to test myotomes. (A) Hip flexion (L2). (B) Knee extension (L3). (C) Foot dorsiflexion (L4). (D) Extension of big toe (L5). (E) Ankle eversion (S1). (F) Hip extension (S1). (G) Knee flexion (S1–S2).

It should be remembered that the examiner has previously tested the S1 myotome with the patient standing and has tested for the positive Trendelenburg sign; thus, these movements are repeated here only if the examiner is unsure of the result and wants to test again. The ankle movements should be tested with the knee flexed approximately 30°, especially if the patient complains of sciatic pain. The extended knee will increase the stretch on the sciatic nerve and may result in false signs, such as weakness that is due to pain rather than weakness that is due to pressure on the nerve root.

With the patient lying prone, the following resisted isometric movements may be tested:

1. Hip extension tests the S1 myotome.
2. Knee flexion tests the S1–S2 myotomes.

If the patient is in extreme pain, these last myotomes should be tested only after all tests with the patient in the supine position have been completed. This action will cut down on the amount of movement the patient has to do, decreasing the patient's discomfort. Ideally, all tests in the standing position should be performed, followed by tests in the sitting, supine, side lying, and prone positions. This procedure is shown in the précis at the end of the chapter.

When testing myotomes (Table 8–6), the examiner should place the test joint(s) in a neutral or resting position and then apply a resisted isometric pressure. The contraction should be held for at least 5 seconds to show any weakness. When feasible, the examiner should test the two sides simultaneously to provide a comparison. The simultaneous bilateral comparison is not possible for movements involving the hip and knee joints, so both sides must be done individually. The examiner should not apply pressure over the joints because this action may mask symptoms or the true problem.

Hip flexion (L2 myotome) is tested by flexing the patient's hip to 30 to 40°. The examiner then applies a resisted force into extension proximal to the knee while ensuring that the heel of the patient's foot is not resting on the examining table. The other side is then tested for comparison. To prevent excessive stress on the lumbar spine, the examiner must ensure that the patient does not increase the lumbar lordosis while doing the test.

To test *knee extension* or the L3 myotome, the examiner flexes the patient's knee to 25 to 35° and then applies a resisted flexion force at the midshaft of the tibia. The other side is tested for comparison.

Ankle dorsiflexion (L4 myotome) is tested by asking the patient to place the feet at 90° relative to the leg. The examiner applies a resisted force to the

TABLE 8–6. Myotomes of the Lower Limb

Nerve Root	Test Action	Muscles
L1–L2	Hip flexion	Psoas, iliacus, sartorius, gracilis, pectineus, adductor longus, adductor brevis
L3	Knee extension	Quadriceps, adductor longus, magnus, and brevis
L4	Ankle dorsiflexion	Tibialis anterior, quadriceps, tensor fasciae latae, adductor magnus, obturator externus, tibialis posterior
L5	Toe extension	Extensor hallucis longus, extensor digitorum longus, gluteus medius and minimus, obturator internus, semimembranosus, semitendinosus, peroneus tertius, popliteus
S1	Ankle plantar flexion Ankle eversion Hip extension Knee flexion	Gastrocnemius, soleus, gluteus maximus, obturator internus, piriformis, biceps femoris, semitendinosus, popliteus, peroneus longus and brevis, extensor digitorum brevis
S2	Knee flexion	Biceps femoris, piriformis, soleus, gastrocnemius, flexor digitorum longus, flexor hallucis longus, intrinsic foot muscles
S3		Intrinsic foot muscles (except abductor hallucis), flexor hallucis brevis, flexor digitorum brevis, extensor digitorum brevis

dorsum of each foot and compares the two sides. *Ankle plantar flexion* (S1 myotome) is compared in a similar fashion, but the resistance is applied to the sole of the foot. As a result of the strength of the plantar flexor muscles, it is better to test this myotome with the patient standing. The patient slowly moves up and down on the toes of each foot in turn, and the examiner compares the differences as previously described. *Ankle eversion* (S1 myotome) is tested with the patient in the supine lying position, and the examiner applies a force into inversion.

Toe extension (L5 myotome) is tested with the patient holding both large toes in a neutral position. The examiner applies resistance to the nails of both toes and compares the two sides. It is imperative that the resistance is isometric so that the amount of force in this case is less than that applied during knee extension, as an example.

Hip extension (S1 myotome) is tested with the patient lying prone. The knee is flexed to 90°. The examiner then lifts the patient's thigh slightly off the examining table while stabilizing the leg. A downward force is applied to the patient's posterior thigh with one hand while the other hand ensures that the patient's thigh is not resting on the table.

Knee flexion (S1–S2 myotomes) is tested in the same position with the knee flexed to 90°. An extension isometric force is applied just above the ankle. Although it is possible to test both knee flexors at the same time, it is not advisable to do this because the stress on the lumbar spine may be too great.

Special Tests

When the examiner performs special tests in the lumbar assessment, the straight leg raising test, the prone knee bending test, and the slump test should always be done. The other tests need be done only if the examiner feels they are relevant or will confirm a diagnosis.

Tests for Neurological Dysfunction

Straight Leg Raising Test. Also known as *La-sègue's test* (Fig. 8–23), the straight leg raising test is done by the examiner with the patient completely relaxed.[23–30] It is a passive test, and each leg is tested individually. With the patient in the supine position, the hip medially rotated and adducted, and the knee extended, the examiner flexes the hip until the patient complains of pain or tightness. The examiner then slowly and carefully drops the leg back slightly until there is no pain or tightness. The patient is then asked to flex the neck so the chin is on the chest; in some cases, if the patient has limited neck movement, the examiner may dorsiflex the patient's foot, or both actions may be done simultaneously. The neck flexion movement has also been called *Hyndman's sign, Brudzinski's sign, Lidner's sign,* and the *Soto-Hall test.* The ankle dorsiflexion movement has also been called the *Braggard's test.* Pain that increases with neck flexion, ankle dorsiflexion, or both indicates stretching of the dura mater of the spinal cord. Pain that does not increase with neck flexion may indicate a lesion in the hamstring area (tight hamstrings) or the lumbosacral or sacroiliac joints. *Sicard's test* involves straight leg raising and then extension of the big toe instead of foot dorsiflexion. *Turyn's test* involves only extension of the big toe.[31] A *unilateral straight leg raise* is full at 70°; that is, the nerve roots (sciatic nerve) are completely stretched, primarily the L5, S1, and S2 nerve roots, having an excursion of approximately 2 to 6 mm.[28] Thus, pain after 70° is probably joint pain from the lumbar area or sacroiliac joints (Fig. 8–24). The examiner should compare the two legs for any differences.

The examiner should then test both legs simulta-

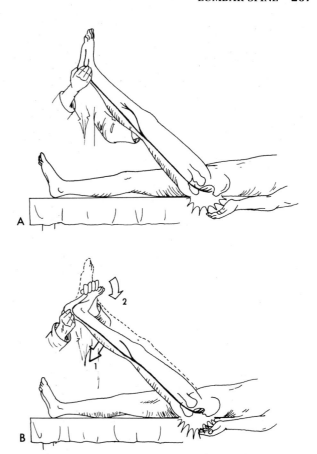

FIGURE 8–23. *Straight leg raising. (A) Radicular symptoms are precipitated on the left with the straight leg raised. (B) The leg is lowered slowly until pain is relieved. The foot is then dorsiflexed, causing a return of symptoms; this indicates a positive test. (From Reilly, B. M.: Practical Strategies in Outpatient Medicine. Philadelphia, W. B. Saunders Co., 1991, p. 912.)*

neously *(bilateral straight leg raise)*, as in Figure 8–25. This test must be done with care because the examiner is lifting the weight of both lower limbs. With the patient relaxed in the supine position and knees extended, the examiner lifts both of the patient's legs by flexing the hips until the patient complains of pain or tightness. If the test causes pain before 70°, the lesion is probably in the sacroiliac joints; if the test causes pain after 70°, the lesion is probably in the lumbar spine.

When doing the unilateral straight leg raising test, 80 to 90° of hip flexion is normal. If one leg is lifted and the patient complains of pain on the opposite side, it is an indication of a space-occupying lesion (e.g., a herniated disc). This finding indicates pain when testing the opposite (good) leg, showing a positive test, and may be called the *well leg raising test of Fajersztajn* (Fig. 8–26), a *prostrate leg raising test, sciatic phenomenon, Lhermitt's test,* or the *cross-over sign.*[28, 32, 33] It is usually indicative of a rather large intervertebral disc protrusion, usually

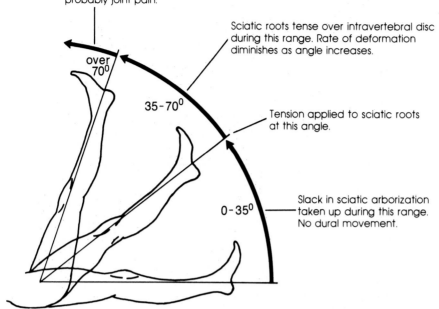

Practically no further deformation of roots occurs during further straight leg raising. Pain is probably joint pain.

Sciatic roots tense over intravertebral disc during this range. Rate of deformation diminishes as angle increases.

over 70°

35-70°

Tension applied to sciatic roots at this angle.

0-35°

Slack in sciatic arborization taken up during this range. No dural movement.

FIGURE 8-24. *Dynamics of single straight leg raising test. (Modified from Fahrni, W. H.: Observations on straight leg raising with special reference to nerve root adhesions. Can. J. Surg. 9:44, 1966.)*

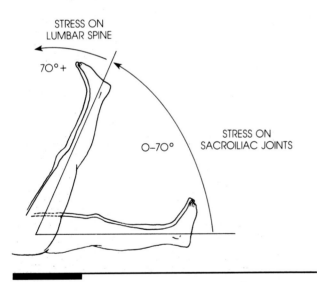

STRESS ON LUMBAR SPINE

70°+

0-70°

STRESS ON SACROILIAC JOINTS

FIGURE 8-25. *Dynamics of the bilateral straight leg raise.*

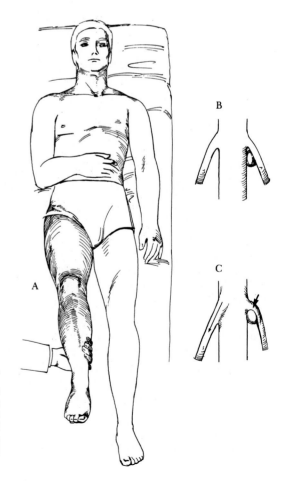

FIGURE 8-26. *Well leg raising test of Fajersztajn. (A) Movement of nerve roots occurs when the leg on the opposite side is raised. (B) Position of disc and nerve root before opposite leg is lifted. (C) When the leg is raised on the unaffected side, the roots on the opposite side slide slightly downward and toward the midline. In the presence of a disc lesion, this movement increases the root tension. (From DePalma, A. F., and R. H. Rothman: The Intervertebral Disc. Philadelphia, W. B. Saunders Co., 1970.)*

medial to the nerve root.[28] The test causes stretching of the ipsilateral as well as the contralateral nerve root, pulling laterally on the dural sac.

During the unilateral straight leg raising test, tension develops in a sequential manner. It first develops in the greater sciatic foramen, followed by tension over the ala of the sacrum. Next, as the nerve crosses over the pedicle, tension develops in this area. Finally, tension occurs in the intervertebral foramen. The test will cause traction on the sciatic nerve, lumbosacral nerve roots, and dura mater. Adhesions within these areas may result from herniation of the intervertebral disc or extradural or meningeal irritation. Pain comes from the dura mater, nerve root, adventitial sheath of the epidural veins, or synovial facet joints. The test is positive if pain extends from the back down into the leg in the sciatic nerve distribution.

A *central protrusion* of an intervertebral disc will lead to pain primarily in the back; a *protrusion in the intermediate area* will cause pain in the posterior aspect at the lower limb and low back; and a *lateral protrusion* will cause posterior leg pain primarily.

Prone Knee Bending (Nachlas) Test. The patient lies prone while the examiner passively flexes the knee as far as possible so that the patient's heel rests against the buttock.[34] At the same time, the examiner should ensure that the patient's hip is not rotated. If the examiner is unable to flex the patient's knee past 90° because of a pathological condition, the test may be done by passive extension of the hip while the knee is flexed as much as possible. Unilateral pain in the lumbar area may indicate an L2 or L3 nerve root lesion (Fig. 8–27). The test also stretches

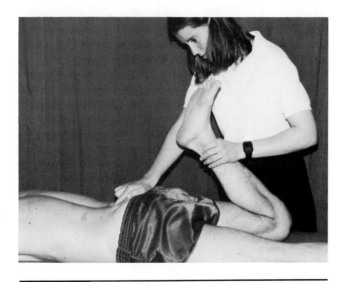

FIGURE 8–27. *Prone knee bending test. Examiner is pointing to where one would expect pain in the lumbar spine with a positive test.*

the femoral nerve. Pain in the anterior thigh indicates tight quadriceps muscles. If the rectus femoris is tight, the examiner should remember that taking the heel to the buttocks may cause anterior torsion to the ilium, which could lead to sacroiliac or lumbar pain. The flexed knee position should be maintained for 45 to 60 seconds.

Slump Test. The patient is seated on the edge of the examining table with the legs supported, the hips in neutral position (i.e., no rotation or abduction/adduction), and the hands behind the back (Fig. 8–28). The patient is asked to "slump" the back into full thoracic and lumbar flexion. The examiner maintains the patient's chin in the neutral position to prevent neck and head flexion. The examiner then uses one arm to apply overpressure and maintain flexion of the thoracic and lumbar spines. While this position is held, the patient is asked to actively flex the cervical spine and head as far as possible (i.e., chin to chest). The examiner then applies overpressure to maintain flexion of all three parts of the spine (cervical, thoracic, and lumbar) using the hand of the same arm to maintain overpressure in the cervical spine. With the other hand, the examiner holds the patient's foot in maximum dorsiflexion. While the examiner holds these positions, the patient is asked to actively straighten the knee as much as possible. The test is repeated with the other leg and then with both legs together. If the patient is unable to fully extend the knee because of pain, the examiner releases the overpressure to the cervical spine and the patient actively extends the neck. If the knee extends further, the symptoms decrease with neck extension, or the positioning of the patient increases the patient's symptoms, then the test is considered positive for increased tension in the neuromeningeal tract.[35–37]

Kernig/Brudzinski Test. The patient is supine with the hands cupped behind the head (Fig. 8–29).[38–41] The patient is instructed to flex the head onto the chest. The extended leg is raised actively by flexing the hip until pain is felt. The patient then flexes the knee, and the pain will disappear. The mechanics of the Kernig/Brudzinski test are similar to those of the straight leg raising test except that the movements are done actively by the patient. Pain is a positive sign and may indicate meningeal irritation, nerve root involvement, or dural irritation. The neck flexion aspect of the test was originally described by Brudzinski, and the hip flexion component was described by Kernig. The two parts of the test may be done individually, in which case they are described as the test of the original author (i.e., Brudzinski's sign or Kernig's sign).

Naffziger's Test. The patient lies supine while the examiner gently compresses the jugular veins (which lie beside the carotid artery) for approxi-

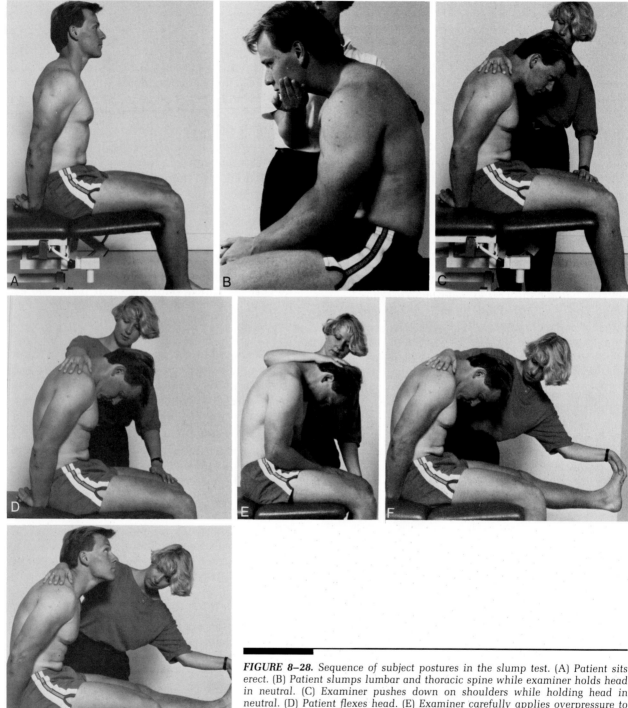

FIGURE 8–28. Sequence of subject postures in the slump test. (A) Patient sits erect. (B) Patient slumps lumbar and thoracic spine while examiner holds head in neutral. (C) Examiner pushes down on shoulders while holding head in neutral. (D) Patient flexes head. (E) Examiner carefully applies overpressure to cervical spine. (F) Examiner extends patient's knee and dorsiflexes foot. (G) Patient extends head.

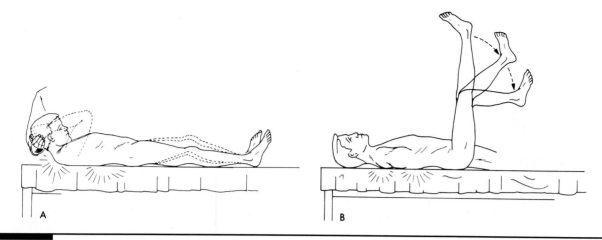

FIGURE 8–29. Brudzinski's (A) and Kernig's (B) parts of the Brudzinski/Kernig test. (A) The patient lies supine. The head is elevated from the table. The patient complains of neck and low back discomfort and attempts to relieve the meningeal irritation by involuntary flexion of the knees and hips. (B) The patient lies supine with the hip and knee flexed. Complaints of pain in the lower back, neck, and/or head are suggestive of meningeal irritation. Knee flexion relieves pain. (Modified from Reilly, B. M.: Practical Strategies in Outpatient Medicine. Philadelphia, W. B. Saunders Co., 1991, p. 95.)

mately 10 seconds (Fig. 8–30). The patient's face will flush. The patient is then asked to cough. If coughing causes pain in the low back, the spinal theca is being compressed, leading to an increase in intrathecal pressure. (The theca is the covering [pia mater, arachnoid mater, and dura mater] around the spinal cord.)

Valsalva Maneuver. The seated patient is asked to take a breath, hold it, and then bear down as if evacuating the bowels (Fig. 8–31). If pain increases, it is an indication of increased intrathecal pressure. The symptoms may be accentuated by having the patient first flex the hip to a position just short of causing pain.[28]

Femoral Nerve Traction Test. The patient lies on the unaffected side with the unaffected limb flexed slightly at the hip and knee (Fig. 8–32).[42] The patient's back should be straight, not hyperextended. The patient's head should be slightly flexed. The examiner grasps the patient's affected or painful limb and extends the knee while gently extending

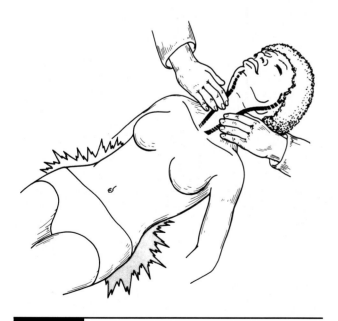

FIGURE 8–30. Naffziger's test. This test may be done while the patient is standing or lying down. The test is based on the hypothesis that bilateral jugular compression increases cerebral spinal fluid pressure. The pressure increase in the subarachnoid space in the root canal may cause back or leg pain by irritating a local mechanical or inflammatory condition. (From White, A. A., and M. M. Panjabi: Clinical Biomechanics of the Spine, 2nd ed. Philadelphia, J. B. Lippincott, 1990, p. 416.)

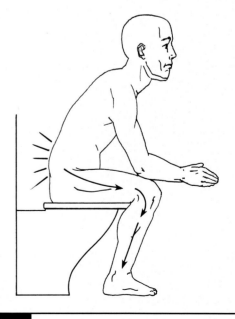

FIGURE 8–31. The Valsalva maneuver. Increased intrathecal pressure leads to symptoms in the sciatic nerve distribution in a positive test.

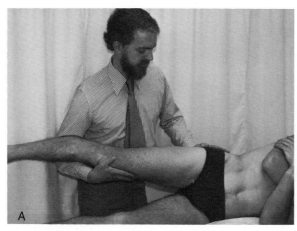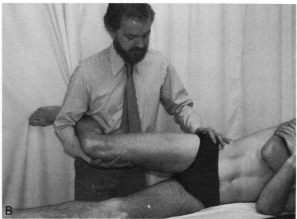

FIGURE 8–32. Femoral nerve traction test. (A) Step 1: Hip and knee extended. (B) Step 2: Hip extended and knee flexed.

the hip approximately 15°. The patient's knee is then flexed on the affected side; this movement further stretches the femoral nerve. Pain will radiate down the anterior thigh if the test is positive.

This is a traction test for the nerve roots at the midlumbar area (L2–L4). As with the straight leg raising test, there may also be a contralateral positive test. Pain in the groin and hip that radiates along the anterior medial thigh indicates an L3 nerve root problem; pain extending to the midtibia indicates an L4 nerve root problem.

"Bowstring" Test (Cram Test or Popliteal Pressure Sign). The examiner carries out a straight leg raising test, and pain results (Fig. 8–33).[6, 43] The knee is slightly flexed (20°), reducing the symptoms; the thigh remains in the same position. Thumb or finger pressure is then applied to the popliteal area to reestablish the painful radicular symptoms. The test is an indication for tension or pressure on the sciatic nerve. The test may also be done in the sitting

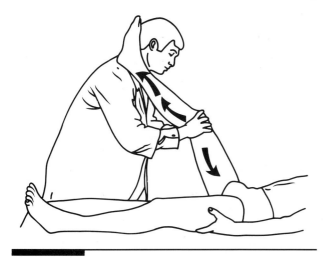

FIGURE 8–33. Bowstring sign. (From MacNab, I.: Backache. Baltimore, Williams & Wilkins, 1977, p. 175.)

position with the examiner passively extending the knee to produce pain. The knee is then slightly flexed to reduce symptoms, and pressure is again applied in the popliteal space. In this case, the test is called the *sciatic tension test.*[60]

Sitting Root Test. The patient sits with a flexed neck. The knee is actively extended while the hip remains flexed at 90°. Increased pain indicates tension on the sciatic nerve. This test is sometimes used to catch the patient unaware. In this case, the examiner passively extends the knee while pretending to examine the foot. Patients with true sciatic pain will arch backwards and complain of pain into the buttock, posterior thigh, and calf when the leg is straightened, indicating a positive test.[44] *Bechterewis test*[32] follows a similar pattern. The patient is asked to extend one knee at a time. If no symptoms result, the patient is asked to extend both legs simultaneously. A positive response is indicated by symptoms in the back or leg.[45]

Sciatic Tension Test. The patient is instructed to sit with the back straight without twisting and is then told not to move but to support or brace the body with the arms.[40] The knee of the affected limb is passively extended to the point of pain. It is then lowered slightly below the point of pain and held clasped between the examiner's knees while the examiner presses the fingers of both hands into the popliteal space. Pain resulting from these maneuvers indicates a positive test and pressure or tension on the sciatic nerve. The test is similar to the bowstring test.

Flip Sign. While the patient is sitting, the examiner extends the patient's knee and looks for symptoms. The patient is then placed supine, and a unilateral straight leg raising test is performed. For the sign to be positive, both tests must cause pain in the sciatic nerve distribution. If only one test is positive, the examiner should be suspicious of problems in the lower lumbar spine. This is a combination of the classic *Lasègue test* and the sitting root test.

Babinski Test. The examiner runs a pointed object along the plantar aspect of the patient's foot.[46] A positive Babinski test suggests an upper motor neuron lesion and is demonstrated by extension of the big toe and abduction (splaying) of the other toes. In an infant up to a few weeks old, a positive test is normal. The test is often performed to determine pathological reflexes.

Oppenheim Test. The examiner runs a fingernail along the crest of the patient's tibia.[46] A negative Oppenheim test is indicated by no reaction or no pain. A positive test is indicated by a positive Babinski sign and suggests an upper motor neuron lesion.

Gluteal Skyline Test. The patient is relaxed in a prone position with the head straight and arms by the sides.[47] The examiner stands at the patient's feet and observes the buttocks from the level of the buttocks. The affected gluteus maximus muscle will be flat as a result of atrophy. The patient is asked to contract the gluteal muscles. The affected side may show less contraction, or it may be atonic and remain flat. If this occurs, the test is positive and may indicate damage to the inferior gluteal nerve or pressure on the L5, S1, and/or S2 nerve roots.

Tests for Joint Dysfunction

Schober Test. The Schober test may be used to measure the amount of flexion occurring in the lumbar spine. A point is marked midway between the PSISs ("dimples of the pelvis"), which is the level of S2; then, points 5 cm below and 10 cm above that level are marked. The distance between the three points is measured, the patient is asked to flex forward, and the distance is remeasured. The difference between the two measurements is an indication of the amount of flexion occurring in the lumbar spine. Little[48] reported a modification of the Schober test to measure extension as well. After completing the flexion movement, the patient extends the spine, and the distance between the marks is noted. Little also advocated using four marking points (one below the "dimples" and three above), all 10 cm apart.

Yeoman's Test. The patient lies prone while the examiner stabilizes the pelvis and extends each of the patient's hips in turn with the knees extended. The examiner then extends each of the patient's legs in turn with the knee flexed. In both cases, the patient remains passive. A positive test is indicated by pain in the lumbar spine during both parts of the test.

Milgram's Test. The patient lies supine and simultaneously actively lifts both legs off the examining table 5 to 10 cm and holds this position for 30 seconds. The test is positive if the limbs or affected limb cannot be held for 30 seconds or symptoms are reproduced in the affected limb.[32, 45] This test should always be performed with caution because of the high stress load placed on the lumbar spine when doing the test.

McKenzie's Side Glide Test. The patient stands with the examiner standing to one side. The examiner grasps the patient's pelvis with both hands and places a shoulder against the patient's lower thorax. Using the shoulder as a "block," the examiner pulls the pelvis toward the examiner's body (Fig. 8–34). The position is held for 10 to 15 seconds and repeated on the opposite side.[9, 45] Note that if the patient has an evident scoliosis, the side to which the scoliosis curves should normally be tested first. A positive test is indicated by increased symptoms on the affected side. It will also indicate whether the symptoms are actually causing the scoliosis.

One-Leg Standing (Stork Standing) Lumbar Extension Test. The patient stands on one leg and extends the spine while balancing on the leg (Fig.

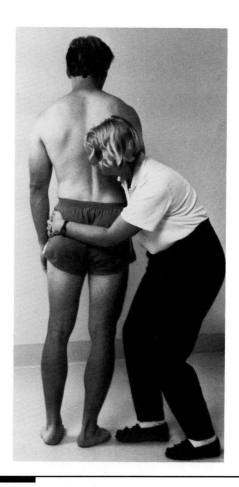

FIGURE 8–34. McKenzie's side glide test.

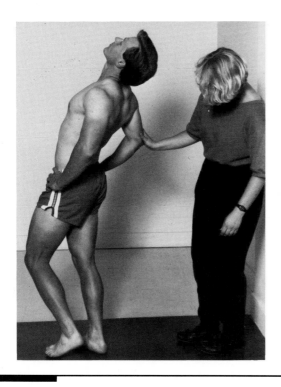

FIGURE 8–35. One-leg standing lumbar extension test.

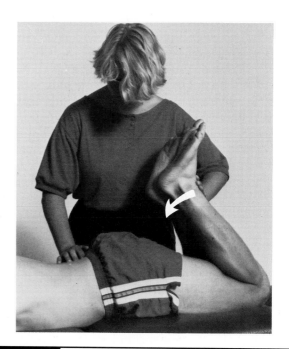

FIGURE 8–36. Pheasant test.

8–35). The test is repeated with the patient standing on the opposite leg. A positive test is indicated by pain in the back and is associated with a pars interarticularis stress fracture. If the stress fracture is unilateral, standing on the ipsilateral leg will cause more pain.[49, 50]

Pheasant Test. The patient lies prone. With one hand, the examiner gently applies pressure to the posterior aspect of the lumbar spine. With the other hand, the examiner passively flexes the patient's knees until the heels touch the buttocks (Fig. 8–36). If pain is produced in the leg by this hyperextension of the spine, the test is considered positive and indicates an unstable spinal segment.[51]

Quadrant Test. The patient stands with the examiner standing behind. The patient extends the spine while the examiner controls the movement by holding the patient's shoulder and using the examiner's shoulders to hold the occiput and take the weight of the head. Overpressure is applied in extension while the patient side flexes and rotates to the side of pain. The movement is continued until the limit of range is reached or symptoms are produced (Fig. 8–37). This position causes maximum narrowing of the intervertebral foramen. The test is positive if symptoms are produced.[52] Cipriano[31] describes a similar test as *Kemp's test.*

Segmental Instability Test. The patient lies prone with the body on the examining table and the legs over the edge resting on the floor (Fig. 8–38). The

examiner applies pressure to the posterior aspect of the lumbar spine while the patient rests in this position. The patient then lifts the legs off the floor, and the examiner again applies posterior compression to the lumbar spine. If pain is elicited in the resting position only, the test is positive because the muscle action is masking the instability.[53]

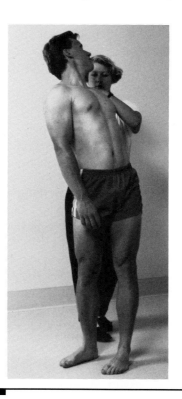

FIGURE 8–37. Quadrant test for the lumbar spine.

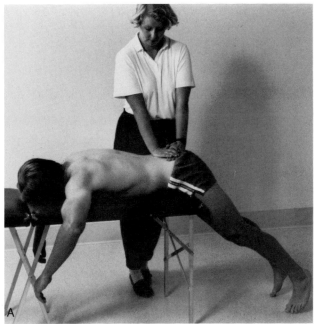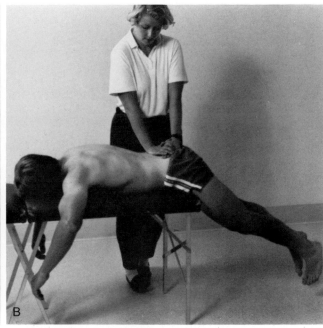

FIGURE 8–38. Segmental instability test. (A) Toes on floor. (B) Feet lifted off floor.

Tests for Muscle Dysfunction

Beevor's Sign. The patient lies supine. The patient flexes the head against resistance, coughs, or attempts to sit up with the hands resting behind the head.[32, 54] The sign is positive if the umbilicus does not remain in a straight line when the abdominals contract, indicating pathology in the abdominal muscles (i.e., paralysis).

Tests for Intermittent Claudication

Stoop Test. The stoop test is done to assess neurogenic intermittent claudication to determine whether a relationship exists among neurogenic symptoms, posture, and walking.[55] When the patient with neurogenic intermittent claudication walks briskly for 1 minute, pain will ensue in the buttock and lower limb within a distance of 50 m. To relieve the pain, the patient flexes forward. These symptoms may also be relieved when the patient is sitting and forward flexing. If flexion does not relieve the symptoms, the test is negative. Extension may also be used to bring the symptoms back.

Bicycle Test of van Gelderen.[56] The patient is seated on an exercise bicycle and is asked to pedal against resistance. The patient starts pedaling while leaning backward to accentuate the lumbar lordosis (Fig. 8–39). If pain into the buttock and posterior thigh occurs, followed by tingling in the affected lower extremity, the first part of the test is positive. The patient is then asked to lean forward while continuing to pedal. If the pain subsides over a short period of time, the second part of the test is positive; if the patient sits upright again, the pain returns. The test is used to determine if the patient has neurogenic intermittent claudication.

Tests for Malingering

Hoover Test. The patient lies supine. The examiner places one hand under each calcaneus while the patient's legs remain relaxed on the examining table (Fig. 8–40).[57–59] The patient is then asked to lift one leg off the table, keeping the knees straight, as in an active straight leg raise. If the patient does not lift the leg or the examiner does not feel pressure under the opposite calcaneus, the patient is probably not really trying or may be a malingerer. However, if the lifted limb is weaker, pressure under the normal heel will increase because of the increased effort to lift the weak leg. The two sides are compared for differences.

Burn's Test. The patient is asked to kneel on a chair and then bend forward to touch the floor with the fingers (Fig. 8–41). The test is positive for malingering if the patient is unable to perform the test or the patient overbalances.[45]

Other Tests

Sign of the Buttock. The patient lies supine,[22] and the examiner performs a passive unilateral straight leg raising test. If there is unilateral restriction, the

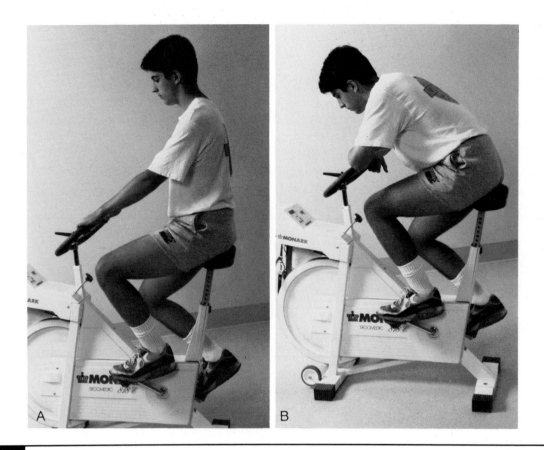

FIGURE 8–39. Bicycle test of van Gelderen. (A) Part one of test—sitting erect. (B) Part two of test—sitting flexed.

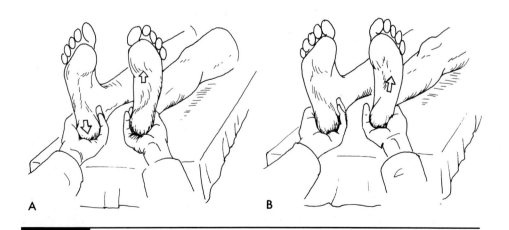

FIGURE 8–40. The Hoover test. (A) Normally, attempts to elevate one leg will be accompanied by downward pressure by the opposite leg. (B) When the "weak" leg attempts to elevate but the opposite (asymptomatic) leg does not "help," at least some of the weakness is probably feigned. (From Reilly, B. M.: Practical Strategies in Outpatient Medicine. Philadelphia, W. B. Saunders Co., 1991, p. 946.)

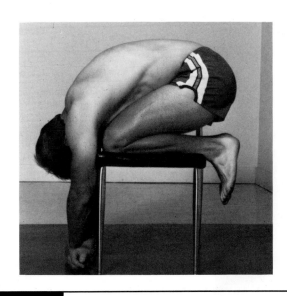

FIGURE 8–41. Burn's test.

examiner then flexes the knee to see whether hip flexion increases. If the problem is in the lumbar spine, hip flexion will increase. This finding indicates a negative sign of the buttock test. If hip flexion does not increase when the knee is flexed, it is a positive sign of the buttock test and indicates disease in the buttock, such as a bursitis, tumor, or abscess. The patient should also exhibit a noncapsular pattern of the hip.

Reflexes and Cutaneous Distribution

After the special tests, the following reflexes should be checked for differences between the two sides (Fig. 8–42):

1. Patellar (L3–L4).
2. Medial hamstrings (L5–S1).
3. Lateral hamstrings (S1–S2).

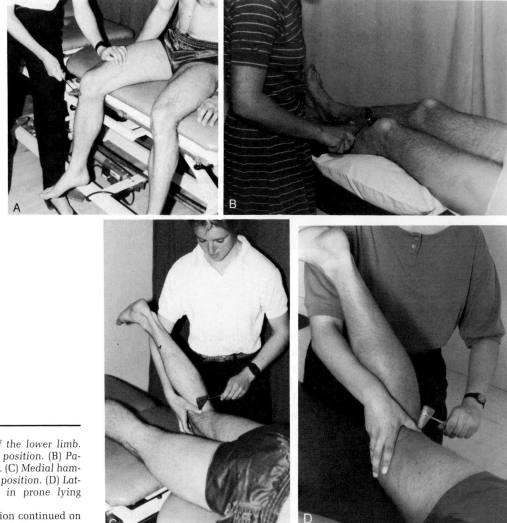

FIGURE 8–42. Reflexes of the lower limb. (A) Patellar (L3) in sitting position. (B) Patellar (L3) in lying position. (C) Medial hamstrings (L5) in prone lying position. (D) Lateral hamstrings (S1, S2) in prone lying position.

Illustration continued on following page

TABLE 8–8. Differential Diagnosis of Intermittent Claudication

	Vascular	**Neurogenic**
Pain	Related to exercise; occurs at various sites simultaneously	Related to exercise; sensations spread from area to area
Pulse	Absent after exercise	Present after exercise
Protein content of cerebrospinal fluid	Normal	Raised
Sensory change	Variable	Follows more specific dermatomes

One must remember that neurogenic intermittent claudication may cause the reflexes to be absent soon after exercise (Table 8–8).[61, 62] If neurogenic intermittent claudication is suspected, it is necessary to do the reflexes immediately because reflexes may return within 1 to 3 minutes after stopping the activity.

Another reflex that may be tested is the *superficial cremasteric reflex*, which occurs in males only (Fig. 8–44). The patient lies supine while the examiner strokes the inner side of the upper thigh with a pointed object. The test is negative if the scrotal sac on the tested side pulls up. Absence or reduction of both superficial reflexes suggests an upper motor neuron lesion. A unilateral absence suggests a lower motor neuron lesion between L1 and L2. Absences have increased significance if they are associated with increased deep tendon reflexes.[63]

Two other superficial reflexes are the *superficial abdominal reflex* (Fig. 8–45) and the *superficial anal reflex*. To test the superficial abdominal reflex, the examiner uses a pointed object to stroke each quadrant of the abdomen of the supine patient in a triangular fashion around the umbilicus. Absence of the reflex indicates an upper motor neuron lesion, whereas unilateral absence indicates a lower motor neuron lesion from T7 to L2, depending on where the absence is noted as a result of the segmental innervation.

The examiner tests the superficial anal reflex by touching the perianal skin. A normal result is shown by contraction of the anal sphincter muscles (S2–S4).

Finally, the examiner should perform one or more of the pathological reflex tests used to determine upper motor lesions or pyramidal tract disease, such as the Babinski or Oppenheim tests, which were described previously. The presence of these reflexes indicates the possible presence of disease, whereas their absence reflects the normal situation.

Joint Play Movements

The joint play movements have special importance in the lumbar spine because they are used to deter-

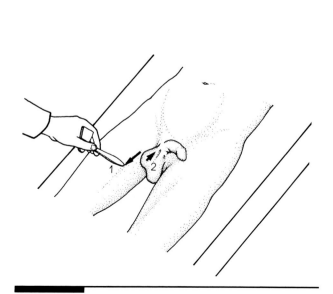

FIGURE 8–44. *Cremasteric reflex.*

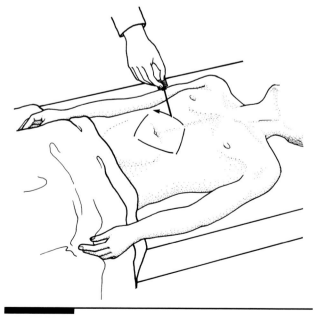

FIGURE 8–45. *Superficial abdominal reflex.*

mine the end feel of joint movement as well as the presence of joint play. The following joint play movements should be performed, with any decreased range of motion, pain, or difference in end feel noted:

1. Forward flexion, extension, and side flexion.
2. Posteroanterior central vertebral pressure.
3. Posteroanterior unilateral vertebral pressure.
4. Transverse vertebral pressure.

Flexion, Extension, and Side Flexion

Flexion is accomplished with the patient in the side lying position. The examiner flexes both of the patient's hips to the chest with the knees bent (Fig. 8–46A). While palpating between the spinous processes of the lumbar vertebrae with one hand (one finger on the spinous process, one finger above, and one finger below the process), the examiner passively flexes and releases the patient's hips; the examiner's body weight is used to cause the movement. The examiner should feel the spinous processes "gap" or move apart on flexion. If this gapping does not occur between two spinous processes or if it is excessive relative to the other gapping movements, the segment is hypomobile or hypermobile, respectively.

Extension and side flexion are tested in a similar fashion, except that the movement is passive extension or passive side flexion rather than passive flexion.

Central, Unilateral, and Transverse Vertebral Pressures (PACVP, PAUVP, and TVP)

To perform the last three joint play movements, the patient lies prone.[64] The lumbar spinous processes are palpated beginning at L5 and working up to L1.

The examiner positions the hands, fingers, and thumbs as shown in Figure 8–46B to perform posteroanterior central vertebral pressure. Pressure is applied through the thumbs, with the vertebrae being pushed anteriorly. The examiner must take care to apply the pressure slowly and carefully so that the "feel" of movement can be recognized. In reality, the movement is minimal. This "springing test" may be repeated several times to determine the quality of the movement.

To perform posteroanterior unilateral vertebral pressure, the examiner moves the fingers laterally away from the tip of the spinous process so the thumbs rest on the lamina or transverse process of the lumbar vertebra (Fig. 8–46C). The same anterior springing pressure is applied as in the central pressure technique. The two sides should be evaluated and compared.

To perform transverse vertebral pressure, the examiner's fingers are placed along the side of the spinous process of the lumbar spine (Fig. 8–46D). The examiner then applies a transverse springing pressure to the side of the spinous process, feeling for the quality of movement. Pressure should be applied to both sides of the spinous process to compare the quality of movement.

Palpation

If the examiner, having completed the scanning examination of the lumbar spine, decides that the problem is in another joint, palpation should not be done until the joint is completely examined. However, when palpating the lumbar spine, any tenderness, altered temperature, muscle spasm, or other signs and symptoms that may indicate the source of pathology should be noted. If the problem is suspected to be in the lumbar spine area, palpation should be carried out in a systematic fashion, starting on the anterior aspect and working around to the posterior aspect.

Anterior Aspect

With the patient lying supine, the following structures are anteriorly palpated (Fig. 8–47):

Umbilicus. The umbilicus lies at the level of the L3–L4 disc space and is the point of intersection of the "lines" that divide the abdomen into quadrants. It is also the point at which the aorta divides into the common iliac arteries. With some individuals, the examiner may be able to palpate the anterior aspects of L4, L5, and S1 vertebrae along with the discs and anterior longitudinal ligament. The abdomen may also be carefully palpated for symptoms arising from internal organs. For example, the appendix is palpated in the right lower quadrant and the liver is palpated in the right upper quadrant; the kidneys are located in the left and right upper quadrants; and the spleen is found in the left upper quadrant.

Inguinal Area. The inguinal area is located between the ASIS and the symphysis pubis. The examiner should carefully palpate for symptoms of a hernia, abscess, infection (lymph nodes), or other pathological conditions in the area.

Iliac Crest. The examiner palpates the iliac crest from the ASIS posteriorly, looking for any symptoms (e.g., hip pointer or apophysitis).

Symphysis Pubis. The symphysis pubis is palpated with the examiner using both thumbs. Standing at the patient's side, the examiner pushes both thumbs down onto the symphysis pubis so that the thumbs rest on the superior aspect of the pubis

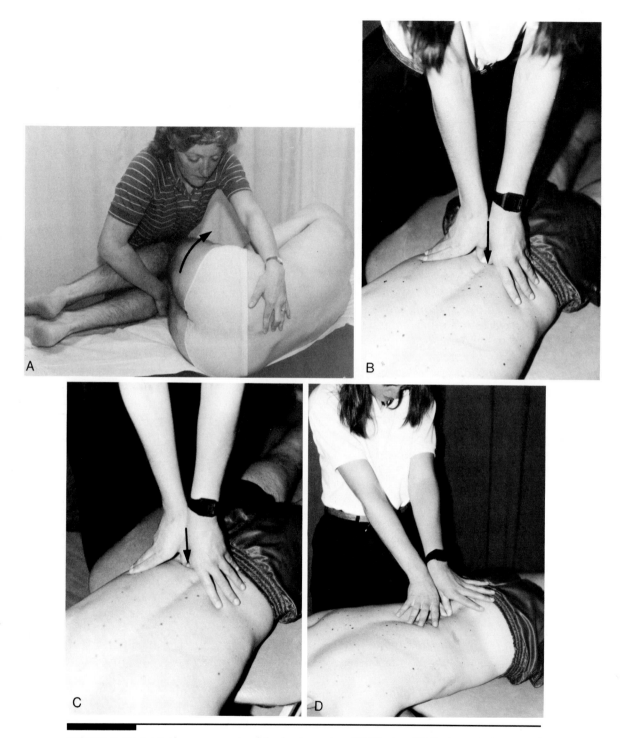

FIGURE 8–46. *Joint play movements of the lumbar spine.* (A) Flexion. (B) Posteroanterior central vertebral pressure. (C) Posteroanterior unilateral vertebral pressure. (D) Transverse vertebral pressure.

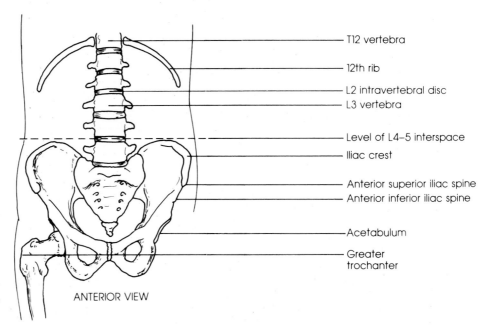

FIGURE 8–47. Bony landmarks of the lumbar spine.

bones (see Fig. 9–4). In this way, one can ensure that the two pubic bones are level at any joint. The symphysis pubis may also be palpated for any tenderness (e.g., osteitis pubis).

Posterior Aspect

The patient is then asked to lie prone, and the following structures are posteriorly palpated (Fig. 8–48):

Spinous Process of the Lumbar Spine. The examiner palpates a point in the midline, which is on a line joining the high point of the two iliac crests. This point is the L4–L5 interspace. Moving down to the first hard mass, the fingers will rest on the spinous process of L5. Moving toward the head, the interspaces and spinous processes of the remaining lumbar vertebrae can be palpated. In addition to looking for tenderness, muscle spasm, and other signs of pathology, the examiner should watch for signs of a spondylolisthesis, which is most likely to occur at L4–L5 or L5–S1. A visible or palpable dip from one spinous process to another may be evident, depending on the type of spondylolisthesis present. Absence of a spinous process may be seen in spina bifida. If the examiner moves laterally 2 to 3 cm from the spinous processes, the fingers will rest over the lumbar facet joints. These joints should also be palpated for signs of pathology. Because of the depth of these joints, the examiner may have difficulty palpating them. However, pathology in this area will

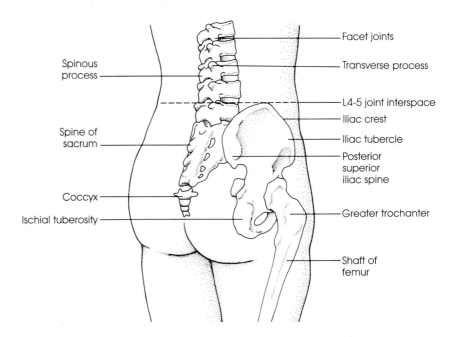

FIGURE 8–48. Palpation of the posterior lumbar spine.

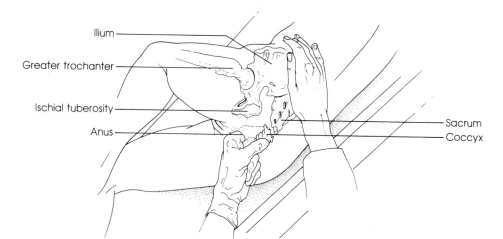

Ilium

Greater trochanter

Ischial tuberosity

Anus

Sacrum
Coccyx

FIGURE 8–49. *Palpation of the coccyx.*

result in spasm of the overlying paraspinal muscles, which should be palpated at the same time.

Sacrum, Sacral Hiatus, and Coccyx. If the examiner returns to the spinous process of L5 and moves caudally, the fingers will rest on the sacrum. Like the lumbar spine, the sacrum has spinous processes, but they are much harder to distinguish because there is no interposing soft-tissue spaces between them. The S2 spinous process is at the level of a line joining the two PSISs ("posterior dimples"). Moving distally, the examiner's fingers may palpate the sacral hiatus, which is the caudal portion of the sacral canal. It has an inverted "U" shape and lies approximately 5 cm above the tip of the coccyx. The two bony prominences on either side of the hiatus are called the *sacral cornua* (see Fig. 9–25). As the examiner's fingers move further distally, they will eventually rest on the posterior aspect of the coccyx. Proper palpation of the coccyx requires a rectal examination using a surgical rubber glove (Fig. 8–49). The index finger is lubricated and inserted into the anus while the patient's sphincter muscles are relaxed. The finger is inserted as far as possible and then rotated so that the pulpy surface rests against the anterior surface of the coccyx. The examiner then places the thumb of the same hand against the posterior aspect of the sacrum. In this way, the coccyx can be moved back and forth. Any major tenderness (e.g., coccydynia) should be noted.

Iliac Crest, Ischial Tuberosity, and Sciatic Nerve. Beginning at the PSISs, the examiner moves along the iliac crest, palpating for signs of pathology. Then, moving slightly distally, the examiner palpates the gluteal muscles for spasm, tenderness, or the presence of abnormal nodules. Just under the gluteal folds, the examiner should palpate the ischial tuberosities on both sides for any abnormality. As the examiner moves laterally, the greater trochanter of the femur is palpated. It is often easier to palpate if the hip is flexed to 90°. Palpating midway between

the ischial tuberosity and the greater trochanter, the examiner may be able to palpate the sciatic nerve. Deep to the gluteal muscles, the piriformis muscle should also be palpated for potential pathology. This muscle is in a line dividing the PSIS of the pelvis/greater trochanter of the femur and the ASIS of the pelvis/ischial tuberosity of the pelvis.

Radiographic Examination[65–72]

Anteroposterior View. With this view (Fig. 8–50), the examiner should note the following:

1. Shape of the vertebrae.
2. Any wedging of the vertebrae, possibly resulting from fracture (Fig. 8–51).
3. Disc spaces. Do they appear normal, or are there height decreases, as are seen in spondylosis?
4. Any vertebral deformity, such as a hemivertebra or other anomalies (Figs. 8–52, 8–53, 8–54, and 8–55).
5. The presence of a bamboo spine, as seen in ankylosing spondylosis.
6. Any evidence of lumbarization of S1, in which case S1 becomes mobile, making S1–S2 the first mobile segment rather than L5–S1. Lumbarization is seen in 2 to 8 per cent of the population (Fig. 8–56).
7. Any evidence of sacralization of L5, in which case L5 becomes fused to the sacrum or pelvis, making the L4–L5 level the first mobile segment rather than L5–S1. This anomaly is seen in 3 to 6 per cent of the population (Fig. 8–57).
8. Any evidence of spina bifida occulta, seen in 6 to 10 per cent of the population (Fig. 8–54).

Lateral View. With this view (Fig. 8–58), the examiner should note the following:

1. Any evidence of spondylolysis or spondylolisthesis, which is seen in 2 to 4 per cent of the

Text continued on page 292

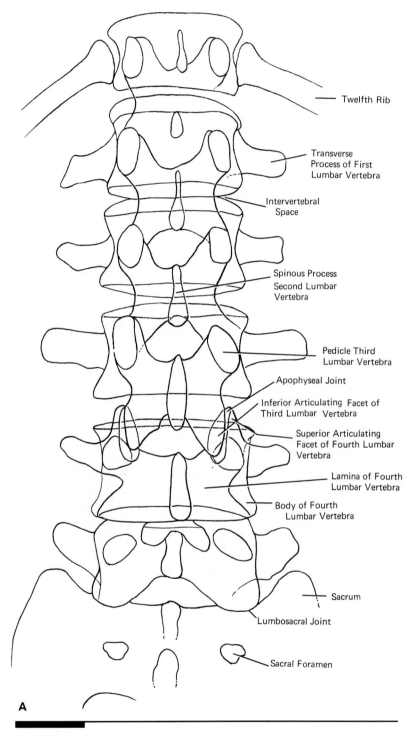

Twelfth Rib

Transverse Process of First Lumbar Vertebra

Intervertebral Space

Spinous Process Second Lumbar Vertebra

Pedicle Third Lumbar Vertebra

Apophyseal Joint

Inferior Articulating Facet of Third Lumbar Vertebra

Superior Articulating Facet of Fourth Lumbar Vertebra

Lamina of Fourth Lumbar Vertebra

Body of Fourth Lumbar Vertebra

Sacrum

Lumbosacral Joint

Sacral Foramen

A

FIGURE 8–50. *Anteroposterior radiograph of the lumbar spine. (A) Film tracing.*
Illustration continued on following page

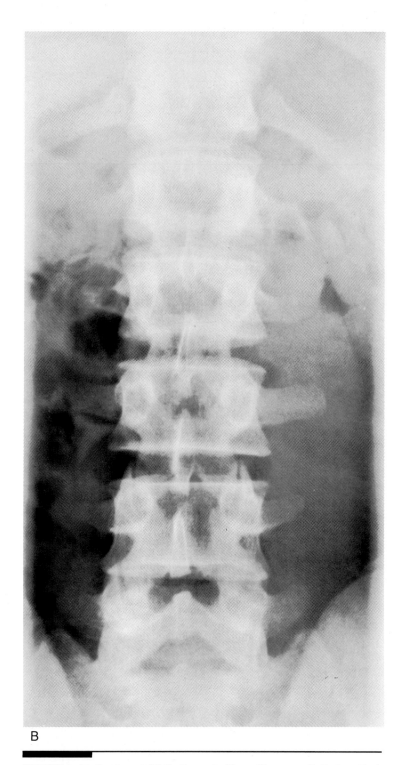

B

FIGURE 8–50. Continued (B) Radiograph. (From Finneson, B. E.: Low Back Pain. Philadelphia, J. B. Lippincott, 1973, pp. 52–53.)

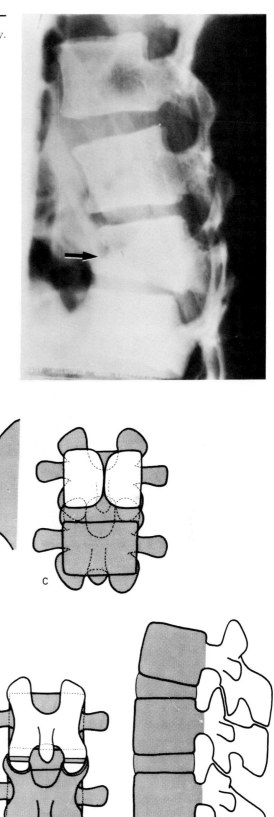

FIGURE 8–51. Wedging of a vertebral body.

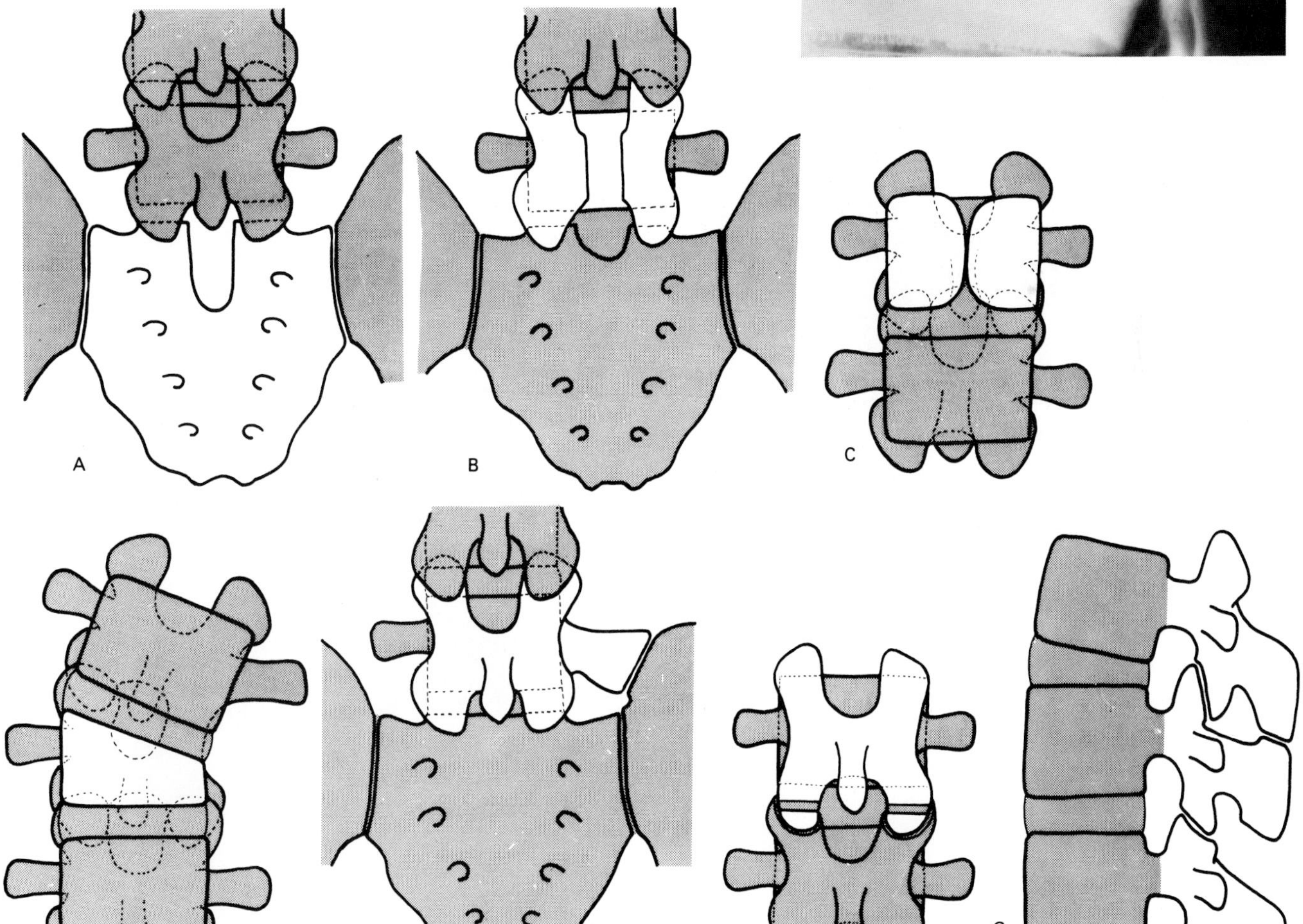

FIGURE 8–52. Diagrammatic representation of the x-ray appearance of common anatomic anomalies in the lumbosacral spine. (A) Spina bifida occulta, S1. (B) Spina bifida, L5. (C) Anterior spina bifida ("butterfly vertebra"). (D) Hemivertebra. (E) Iliotransverse joint. (F) Ossicles of Oppenheimer. These are free ossicles seen at the tip of the inferior articular facets and usually found at the level of L3. (G) "Kissing" spinous processes. (From MacNab, I.: Backache. Baltimore, Williams & Wilkins, 1977, pp. 14–15.)

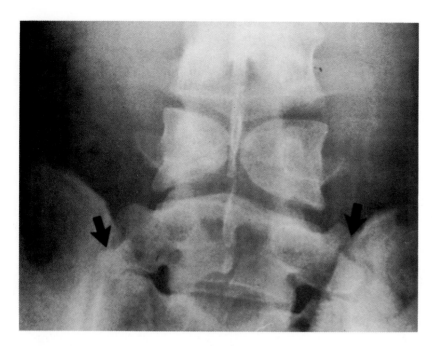

FIGURE 8–53. *Butterfly vertebra. Also note transitional segments (large arrows). (Modified from Jaeger, S. A.: Atlas of Radiographic Positioning—Normal Anatomy and Developmental Variants. Norwalk, Conn., Appleton & Lange, 1988, p. 333.)*

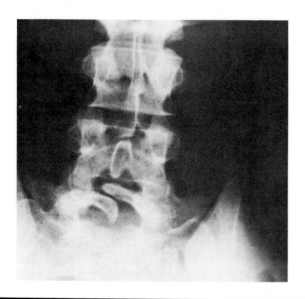

FIGURE 8–54. *Spina bifida occulta. (From Jaeger, S. A.: Atlas of Radiographic Positioning—Normal Anatomy and Developmental Variants. Norwalk, Conn., Appleton & Lange, 1988, p. 317.)*

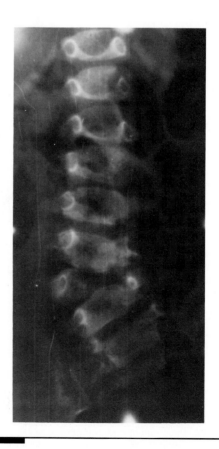

FIGURE 8–55. *Hemivertebra shown on an anteroposterior radiograph.*

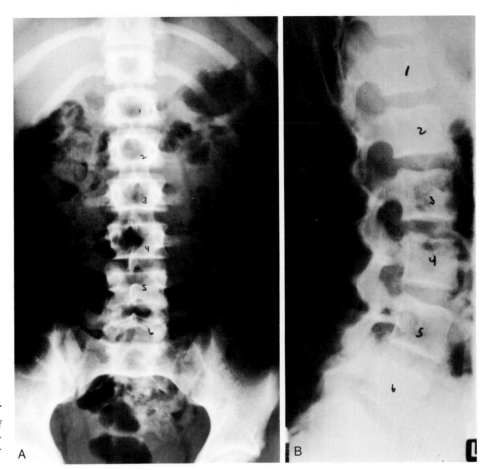

FIGURE 8–56. Lumbarization of the S1 vertebra seen on anteroposterior (A) and lateral (B) radiographs.

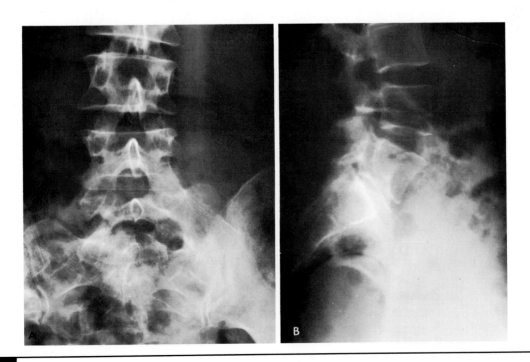

FIGURE 8–57. Unilateral sacralization of the fifth lumbar vertebra. (A) Note the massive formation of sacral ala on the left side with relatively normal transverse process on the right (anteroposterior view). (B) Lateral view showing the very narrow disc space and the massive arches. (From O'Donoghue, D. H.: Treatment of Injuries to Athletes, 4th ed. Philadelphia, W. B. Saunders Co., 1984, p. 403.)

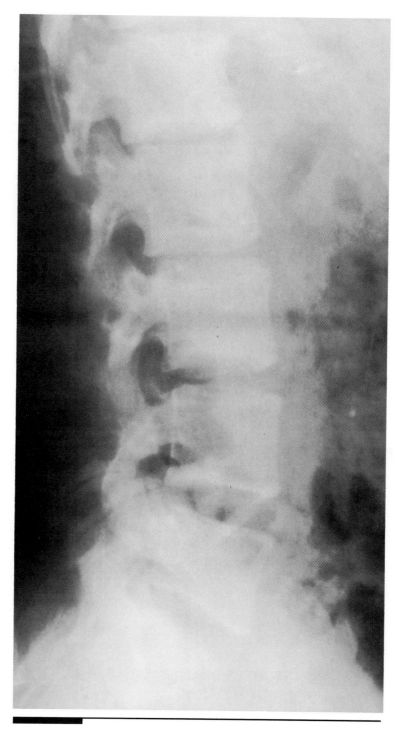

FIGURE 8–58. *Lateral radiograph of the lumbar spine.* (A) *Film tracing.*

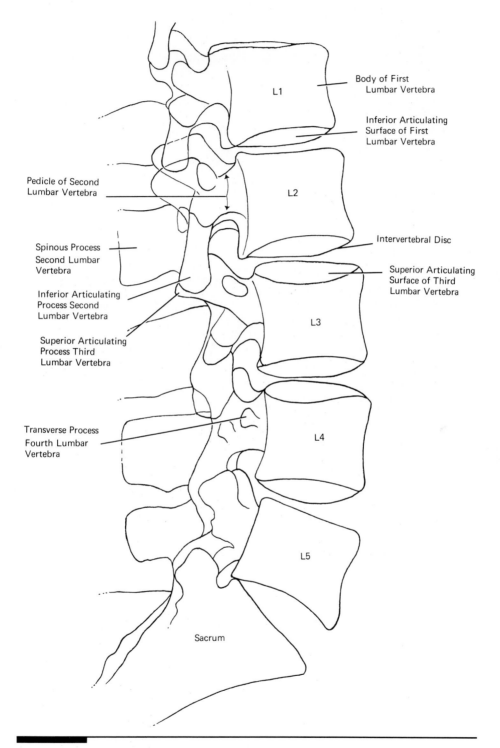

Body of First
Lumbar Vertebra

Inferior Articulating
Surface of First
Lumbar Vertebra

Pedicle of Second
Lumbar Vertebra

Intervertebral Disc

Spinous Process
Second Lumbar
Vertebra

Superior Articulating
Surface of Third
Lumbar Vertebra

Inferior Articulating
Process Second
Lumbar Vertebra

Superior Articulating
Process Third
Lumbar Vertebra

Transverse Process
Fourth Lumbar
Vertebra

Sacrum

L1

L2

L3

L4

L5

FIGURE 8–58. Continued (B) Radiograph. *(From Finneson, B. E.: Low Back Pain. Philadelphia, J. B. Lippincott, 1973, pp. 54–55.)*

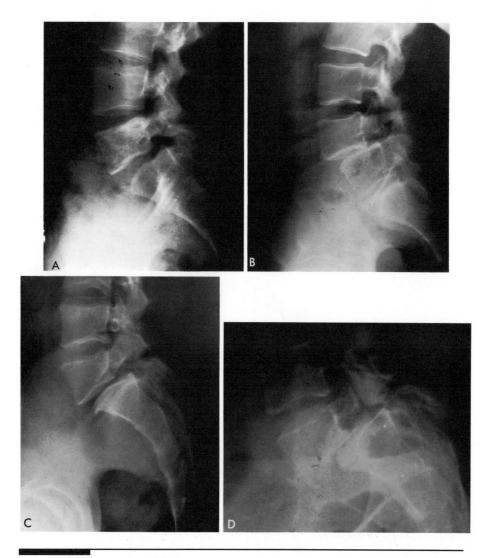

FIGURE 8–59. *Spondylolisthesis. (A) Grade 1. The arch defect in L5 with mild forward displacement of L5 on S1. Backache but no gross disability. (B) Grade 2. Note more forward slipping between L4 and L5 with collapse of the intervertebral disc. Definite symptomatic back with restriction of motion, muscle spasm, and curtailment of activities. (C) Grade 3. More extensive slipping combined with a wide separation at the arch defect and degenerative changes of the disc. Grossly symptomatic. (D) Grade 4. Vertebrae slipped forward more than halfway. Severe disability. (From O'Donoghue, D. H.: Treatment of Injuries to Athletes, 4th ed. Philadelphia, W. B. Saunders Co., 1984, p. 402.)*

population (Fig. 8–59). The degree of slipping can be graded as shown in Figure 8–60.

2. A normal lordosis.

3. Any wedging of the vertebrae.

4. Normal disc spacing.

5. Any osteophyte formation or traction spurs (Fig. 8–61).[72] Traction spurs indicate an unstable lumbar intervertebral segment. A traction spur occurs approximately 1 mm from the disc border; an osteophyte occurs at the discal border with the vertebral body.

Oblique View. With the oblique view (Fig. 8–62), the examiner should look for any evidence of spondylolisthesis (sometimes referred to as a "Scotty dog decapitated") or spondylolysis (sometimes referred to as a "Scotty dog with a collar") (Fig. 8–63).

Myelogram. A myelogram can confirm the presence of a protruding intervertebral disc, a tumor, or spinal stenosis (Figs. 8–64, 8–65, and 8–66). The examiner must be careful of the side effects of myelograms, which include headache, stiffness, low back pain, cramps, and paresthesia in the lower limbs. Although side effects do occur, no permanent injury has been noted.

CT Scan. A CT scan may be used to delineate a fracture or show the presence of spinal stenosis caused by protrusion or a tumor (Figs. 8–67, 8–68, and 8–69). It is a technique that provides an axial projection of the spine, showing the anatomy of not only the spine but also the paravertebral muscles, vascular structures, and organs of the body cavity. In doing so, it shows more precisely the relationship

Text continued on page 303

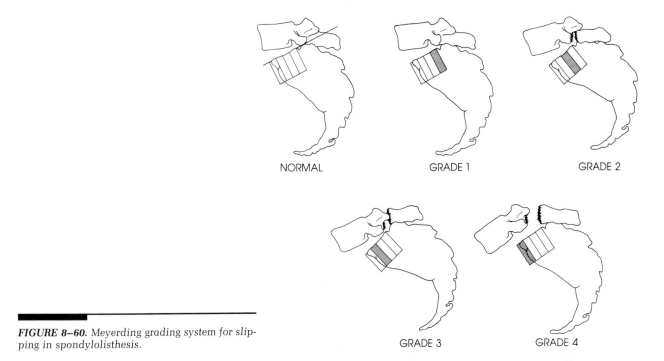

NORMAL GRADE 1 GRADE 2

GRADE 3 GRADE 4

FIGURE 8–60. Meyerding grading system for slipping in spondylolisthesis.

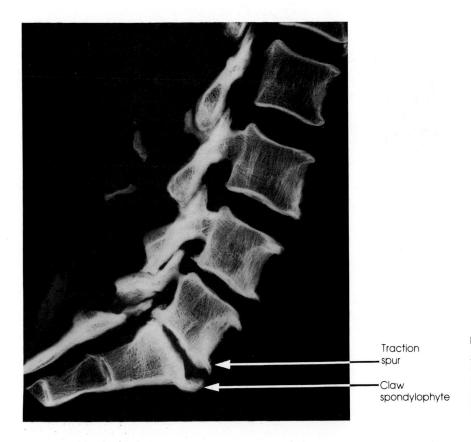

Traction spur

Claw spondylophyte

FIGURE 8–61. Lateral radiograph of a thin-slice pathological section of lumbar spine. Note traction spur and claw spondylophyte. (From Rothman, R. H., and F. A. Simeone: The Spine. Philadelphia, W. B. Saunders Co., 1982, p. 512.)

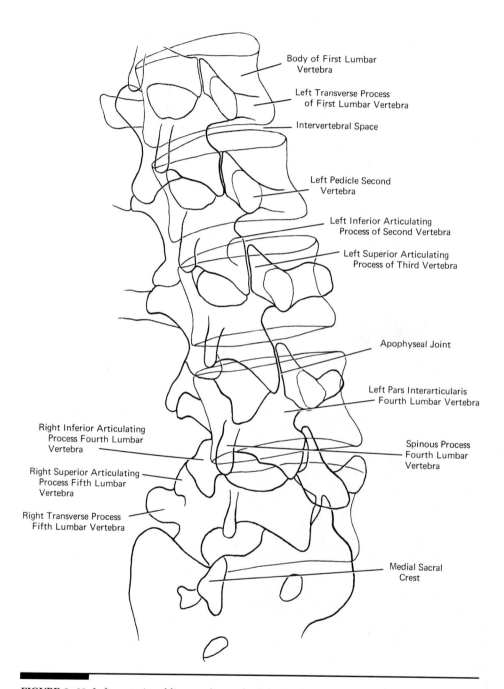

Body of First Lumbar
Vertebra

Left Transverse Process
of First Lumbar Vertebra

Intervertebral Space

Left Pedicle Second
Vertebra

Left Inferior Articulating
Process of Second Vertebra

Left Superior Articulating
Process of Third Vertebra

Apophyseal Joint

Left Pars Interarticularis
Fourth Lumbar Vertebra

Spinous Process
Fourth Lumbar
Vertebra

Right Inferior Articulating
Process Fourth Lumbar
Vertebra

Right Superior Articulating
Process Fifth Lumbar
Vertebra

Right Transverse Process
Fifth Lumbar Vertebra

Medial Sacral
Crest

FIGURE 8–62. Left posterior oblique radiograph of the lumbar spine. (A) Film tracing.

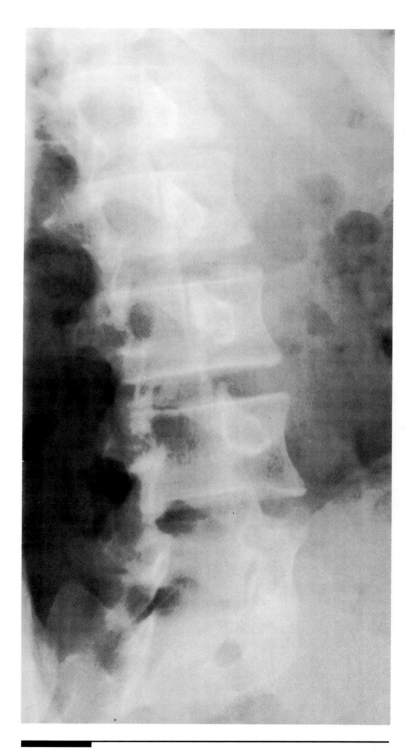

FIGURE 8–62. Continued (B) *Radiograph. (From Finneson, B. E.: Low Back Pain. Philadelphia, J. B. Lippincott, 1973, pp. 56–57.)*

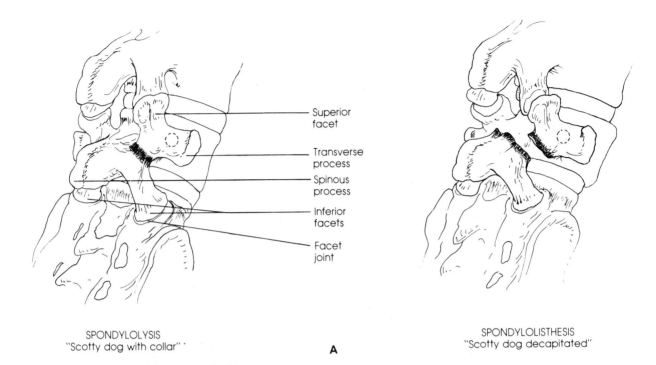

Superior facet

Transverse process

Spinous process

Inferior facets

Facet joint

SPONDYLOLYSIS
"Scotty dog with collar"

A

SPONDYLOLISTHESIS
"Scotty dog decapitated"

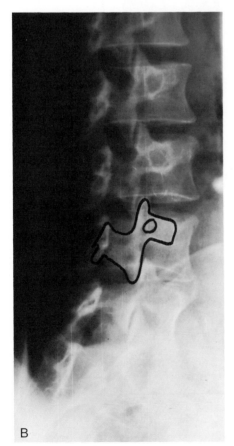

FIGURE 8–63. (A) Diagrammatic representation (posterior oblique view) illustrating spondylolysis and spondylolisthesis. (B) Posterior oblique film showing "Scotty dog."

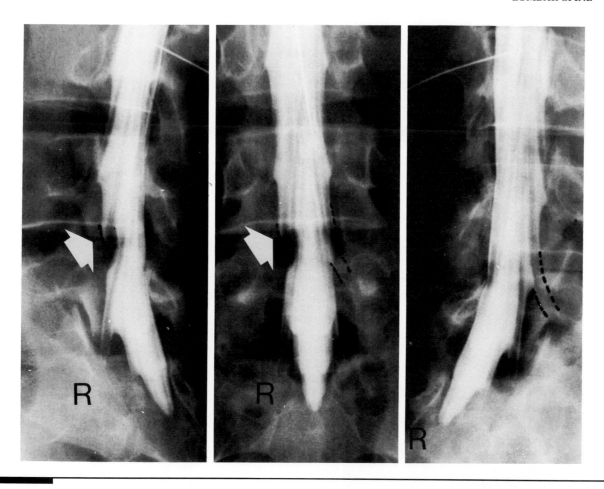

FIGURE 8–64. Metrizamide myelogram illustrating herniated disc at L4–L5 on the right. Note amputation of the nerve root sleeve and indentation of the dural sac. (From Rothman, R. H., and F. A. Simeone: The Spine. Philadelphia, W. B. Saunders Co., 1982, p. 550.)

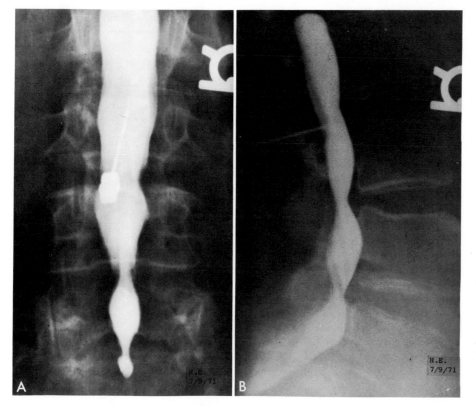

FIGURE 8–65. Oil myelograms show the characteristic appearance of chronic disc degeneration and spinal stenosis with diffuse posterior bulging of the annulus and osteophyte formation. (A) There is symmetric wasting of the dye column in the anteroposterior view. Note the hourglass configuration. (B) Indentation of the dye column of the annulus anteriorly and the buckled ligamentum flavum and facet joints posteriorly (lateral view). (From Rothman, R. H., and F. A. Simeone: The Spine. Philadelphia, W. B. Saunders Co., 1982, p. 553.)

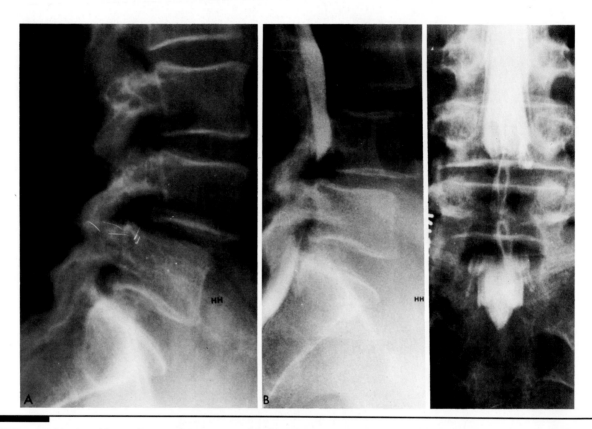

FIGURE 8–66. Metrizamide myelogram shows stenotic block at the L4–L5 level as a result of degenerative spondylolisthesis and spinal stenosis at the L4–L5 level. (A) Note the 4-mm anterior migration of L4 on L5 caused by the degenerative spondylolisthesis. (B) The extensive block on the myelogram is due to spinal stenosis. (From Rothman, R. H., and F. A. Simeone: The Spine. Philadelphia, W. B. Saunders Co., 1982, p. 553.)

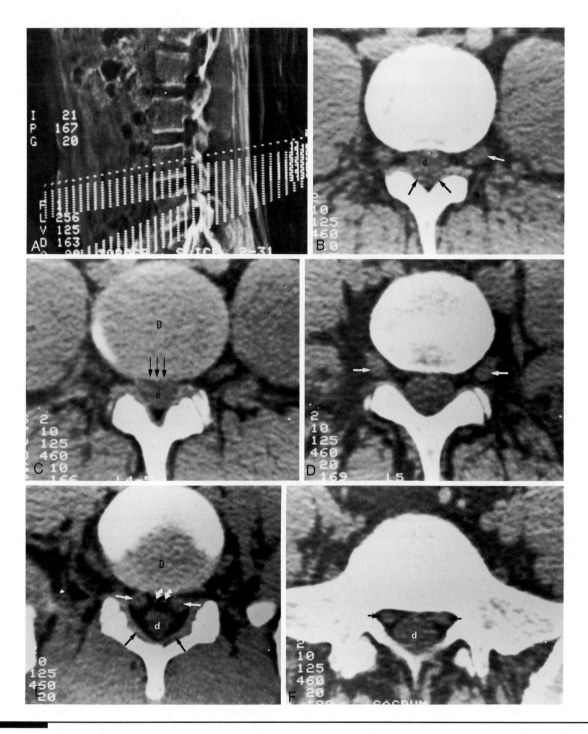

FIGURE 8–67. *Normal disc anatomy on CT. (A) Scout view. The chosen sections (dashed lines) can be planned and angled along the plane of the discs. (B) CT scan through the L4 vertebral body shows the neural foramina and the L4 nerve root ganglia (white arrow on left ganglion). The dural sac (d) and ligamenta flava (black arrows) are shown. (C) CT scan through the L4–L5 disc (D) shows very little fat between the posterior margin of the disc (arrows) and the dural sac (d). The nerve roots are not clearly seen. (D) CT scan through the L5 vertebral body and foramina shows the L5 nerve root ganglia (arrows). (E) CT scan through the L5–S1 disc (D) space shows the L5 nerve roots (straight white arrows), the dural sac (d), and the ligamenta flava (black arrows). Small epidural veins are noted (curved arrows). (F) At the S1 level, the S1 nerve roots (arrows) and dural sac (d) are clearly visualized. (From Weismann, B. N. W., and C. B. Sledge: Orthopedic Radiology. Philadelphia, W. B. Saunders Co., 1986, p. 306.)*

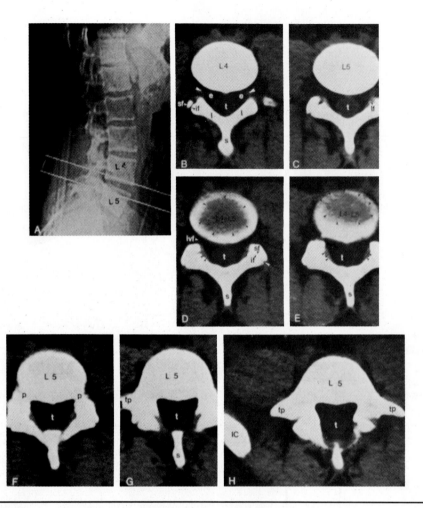

FIGURE 8–68. Soft-tissue detail of the L4–L5 intervertebral disc space. (A) Lateral digital scout view obtained through the lumbosacral spine. The upper and lower scan limits through the L4–L5 region are designated with an electronic cursor. Scan collimation is 5 mm thick; incrementation is 3 mm (2-mm overlap). (B) Axial CT section of L4. The L4 root ganglia and spinal nerves are seen within the intervertebral foramina (white arrowheads) surrounded by abundant epidural fat (e). The thecal sac (t) is bounded anterolaterally by fat in the lateral recess. The posterior arch of L4 consists of inferior facets (if), laminae (l), and spinous process (s). The superior facet of L5 (sf) is just visible. (C) The next lower axial section demonstrates the L4–L5 facet articulations. The ligamentum flavum (lf) is contiguous with the facet joint capsule. Again, the thecal sac (t) is readily apparent; it is slightly higher in density than the adjacent epidural fat. Note that without subarachnoid contrast media, the intrathecal contents cannot be discerned. (D) Axial CT section at the L4–L5 disc space. The disc (multiple black arrowheads) is a region of central hypodensity surrounded by the cortical margin of L4. The posterior arch of L4 projects below the disc level. The intervertebral foramina (ivf) have begun to close. The cartilaginous articular surfaces (white arrowhead) between superior (sf) and inferior (if) facets are poorly demonstrated with these window settings. The ligamentum flavum (double black arrowheads) is noted medial to the facet joints (t = thecal sac; s = spinous process.) (E) The next inferior CT section demonstrates the disc (multiple arrowheads) positioned somewhat more anteriorly, marginated posteriorly at this level by the posterosuperior cortical rim of the L5 body. The ligamentum flavum (double arrowheads) normally maintains a flat medial surface adjacent to the thecal sac (t). The posterior arch of L4 and its spinous process (s) are still in view. (F) Axial CT section through the L5 body at the level of the pedicles (p). The canal now completely encloses the thecal sac (t). (G) Immediately below, only the spinous process (s) of the posterior arch of L4 is visible. The transverse process (tp) of L5 is noted (t = thecal sac). (H) At the level of the iliac crest (IC), the posterior arch of L5 (small arrowheads) has just begun to form. The transverse processes (tp) are quite large at this level (t = thecal sac). (From LeMasters, D. L., and R. L. Dowart: High-resolution, cross-sectional computed tomography of the normal spine. Orthop. Clin. North Am. 16:359, 1985.)

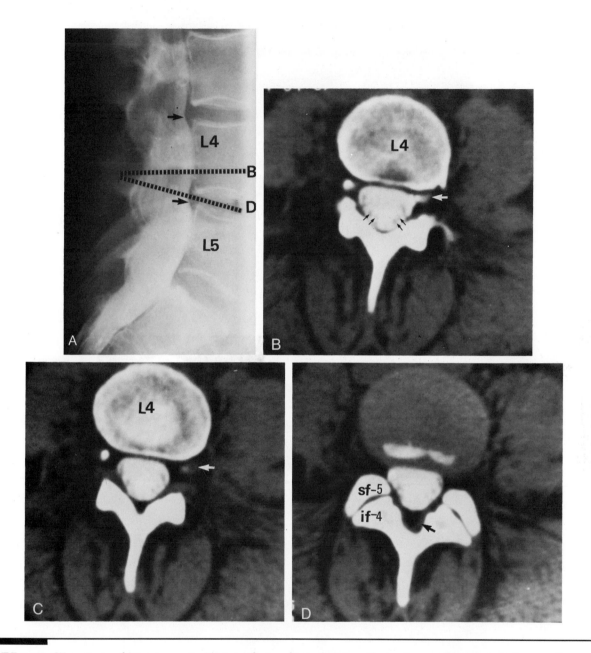

FIGURE 8–69. CT anatomy of L4 nerve roots. (A) Lateral view during metrizamide myelogram shows indentations on the anterior aspect of the contrast column (arrows) at L3–L4 and L4–L5 resulting from bulging intervertebral discs. The levels for subsequent CTs B and D are marked. (B) CT section through the L4 vertebra and L4–L5 foramina 1 hour after a metrizamide myelogram shows contrast agent filling the left axillary pouch (white arrow) and the right nerve root sleeve. Small arrows indicate the filling defects produced by the remaining nerve roots. (C) CT section slightly more distal than B shows the L4 nerve root ganglia (left ganglion indicated by arrow). (D) Section through the L4–L5 disc and the posterior inferior body of L4 shows an abnormally bulging disc without compression of the subarachnoid space. The ligamentum flavum on the left (arrow), the superior facet of L5 (sf-5), and the inferior facet of L4 (if-4) are indicated. (From Weismann, B. N. W., and C. B. Sledge: Orthopedic Radiology. Philadelphia, W. B. Saunders Co., 1986, p. 284.)

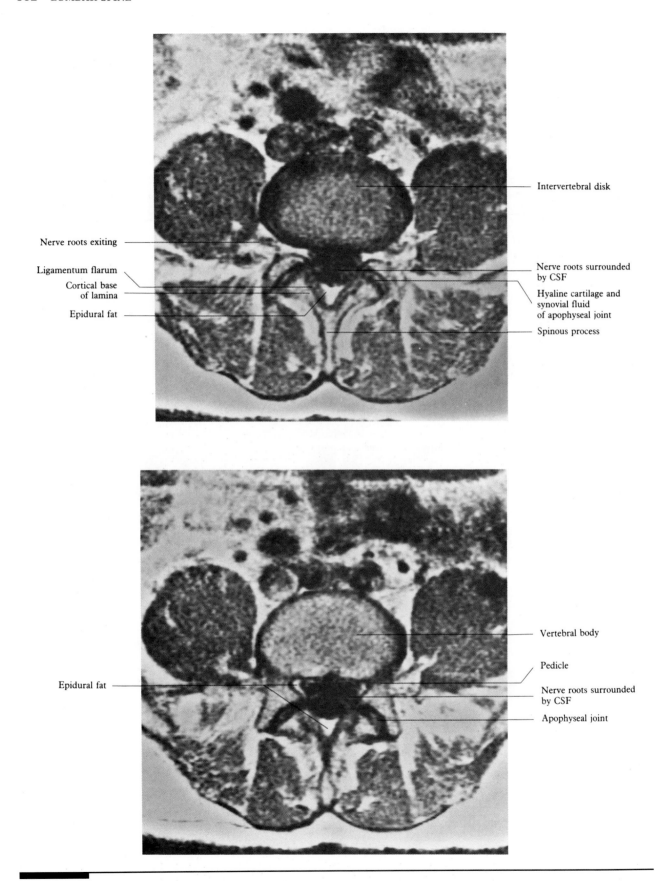

FIGURE 8–70. MRI of normal lumbar spine. (A) Level of neural canal. (B) Level of pedicle (CSF = cerebrospinal fluid). (From Bassett, L. W., et al.: MRI Atlas of the Musculoskeletal System. London, Martin Dunitz, 1989, p. 40.)

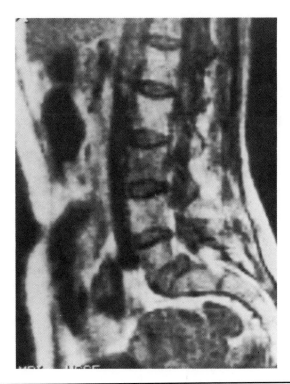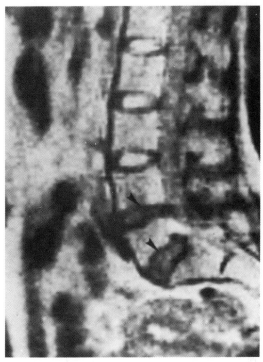

FIGURE 8–71. *Disc degeneration. (A) T1-weighted image. There is little difference in intensity between the intervertebral discs. A grade 1 spondylolisthesis is present at L5–S1. (B) T2-weighted image. The L4–L5 and L5–S1 discs (arrowheads) are darker than the other, normal discs. A degenerating disc dehydrates, which shortens the T2 and consequently decreases the signal intensity on a T2-weighted image. (From Gillespy, T., et al.: MRI Atlas of the Lumbar Spine: The Lumbar Spine and Back Pain. Edinburgh, Churchill Livingstone, 1987, p. 292.)*

among the intervertebral disc, spinal canal, facet joints, and intervertebral foramen. It may be used in conjunction with a water-soluble contrast medium (computer-assisted myelography) to further delineate the structures.

MRI. This noninvasive technique can be used in several planes (transaxial, coronal, or sagittal) to delineate bony and soft tissues. The delineation of soft tissues is much greater with MRI than with CT scans. For example, with MRI, the nucleus pulposus and the annulus fibrosis are easier to differentiate because of their different water contents, making it the preferred imaging for disc disease (Figs. 8–70 and 8–71).

PRÉCIS OF THE LUMBAR SPINE ASSESSMENT*

History (sitting)
Observation (standing)
Examination

*The précis is shown in an order that will limit the amount of moving that the patient has to do but ensure that all necessary structures are tested.

Active movements (standing)
   Forward flexion
   Extension
   Side flexion (left and right)
   Rotation (left and right)
   Quick test
   Trendelenburg and S1 nerve root test
Passive movements (only with care and caution)
Peripheral joint scan (standing)
   Sacroiliac joints
Resisted isometric movements (sitting)
   Forward flexion
   Extension
   Side flexion (left and right)
   Rotation (left and right)
Peripheral joint scan (supine lying)
   Hip joints (flexion, abduction, adduction, and medial and lateral rotation)
   Knee joints (flexion and extension)
   Ankle joints (dorsiflexion and plantar flexion)
   Foot joints (supination, pronation)
   Toe joints (flexion, extension)
Myotomes (supine lying)
   Hip flexion (L2)
   Knee extension (L3)
   Ankle dorsiflexion (L4)
   Toe extension (L5)
   Ankle eversion and/or plantar flexion (S1)
Special tests (supine lying)
Reflexes and cutaneous distribution (anterior and side aspects)

Palpation (supine lying)
Joint play movements
    Flexion (side lying)
    Posteroanterior central vertebral pressure (prone lying)
    Posteroanterior unilateral vertebral pressure (prone lying)
    Transverse vertebral pressure (prone lying)
Peripheral joint scan (prone lying)
    Hip joints (extension, medial, and lateral rotation)
Myotomes (prone lying)
    Hip extension (S1)
    Knee flexion (S1–S2)
Special tests (prone lying)
Reflexes and cutaneous distribution (prone lying) (posterior aspect)
Palpation (prone lying)
Radiographic examination

After any examination, the patient should always be warned of the possibility of exacerbation of symptoms as a result of the assessment.

CASE STUDIES

When doing these case studies, the examiner should list the appropriate questions to be asked and why they are being asked, what to look for and why, and what things should be tested and why. Depending on the answers of the patient (and the examiner should consider different responses), several possible causes of the patient's problem may become evident (examples given in parentheses). If so, a differential diagnosis chart should be made up. The examiner can then decide how different diagnoses may affect the treatment plan.

1. A 23-year-old man comes to you complaining of a low backache. He works as a dishwasher, and although the pain has been present for 5 months, he has not missed any work. The pain gets worse as the day progresses and is relieved by rest. X-rays reveal some sclerosis in the area of the sacroiliac joints. Describe your assessment plan for this patient (ankylosing spondylitis versus lumbar sprain).

2. A 36-year-old woman comes to you complaining of a chronic backache of 6 months' duration. The pain has been gradually increasing in severity and is worse at rest and in the morning on arising from bed. When present, the pain is centered in her low back and radiates into her buttocks and posterior left thigh. Describe your assessment plan for this patient (lumbar strain versus lumbar disc lesion).

3. A 13-year-old female gymnast comes to you complaining of low back pain. The pain increases when she extends the spine. Typical for most gymnasts, she is hypermobile in most of her joints. Describe your assessment plan for this patient (spondylolisthesis versus lumbar sprain).

4. A 56-year-old male steel worker comes to you complaining of low back pain that was brought on when he slipped on ice and twisted his trunk while trying to avoid falling. The injury occurred 2 days ago, and he has right-sided sciatica. X-rays show some lipping at L4–L5 and L5–S1 with slight narrowing of the L5 disc. He has difficulty bending forward. Describe your assessment plan for this patient (lumbar spondylosis versus acute lumbar disc herniation).

5. A 28-year-old man had a laminectomy for a herniated L5 disc 2 days ago. He is still an inpatient. Describe your assessment plan for this patient.

6. An 18-year-old female synchronized swimmer was "boosting" another swimmer out of the water and felt a sharp pain in her back. She found that she could no longer swim because of the pain. She demonstrated paresthesia on the dorsum of the foot and lateral aspect of the leg. Describe your assessment plan for this patient (acute disc herniation versus lumbar strain).

7. A 32-year-old man comes to you complaining of back pain and stiffness, especially with activity. He has a desk job and has no history of unusual activity. Describe your assessment plan for this patient (chronic lumbar sprain versus congenital dysfunction).

8. A 39-year-old male electrician comes to you complaining of back pain after a motor vehicle accident in which he was hit from behind while stopped for a red light. The accident occurred 3 days ago. Describe your assessment program for this patient (lumbar sprain versus lumbar spondylosis).

9. A 26-year-old woman comes to you complaining of low back pain. She appears to have a functional leg length difference. Describe your assessment plan for this patient (lumbar sprain versus congenital anomaly).

REFERENCES

CITED REFERENCES

1. Kramer, J.: Intervertebral Disk Diseases: Causes, Diagnosis, Treatment and Prophylaxis. Chicago, Year Book Medical Publishers, 1981.
2. Farfan, H. F.: Mechanical Disorders of the Low Back. Philadelphia, Lea & Febiger, 1973.
3. Coventry, M. B., R. K. Ghormley, and J. W. Kernohan: The intervertebral disc: Its microscopic anatomy and pathology. Part I—anatomy, development and physiology; Part II—changes in the intervertebral disc concomitant with age; Part III—pathological changes in the intervertebral disc. J. Bone Joint Surg. 27:105 (Part I), 233 (Part II), 460 (Part III), 1945.
4. Bogduk, N.: The innervation of the lumbar spine. Spine 8:286, 1983.
5. Edgar, M. A., and J. A. Ghadially: Innervation of the lumbar spine. Clin. Orthop. Relat. Res. 115:35, 1976.
6. Macnab, I.: Backache. Baltimore, Williams & Wilkins, 1977.
7. Nachemson, A., and J. M. Morris: In vivo measurements of intradiscal pressure. J. Bone Joint Surg. 46A:1077, 1964.
8. Nachemson, A., and C. Elfstrom: Intravital dynamic pressure measurements in lumbar discs. Scand. J. Rehabil. Med. (Suppl. 1), 1970.
9. McKenzie, R. A.: The Lumbar Spine: Mechanical Diagnosis and Therapy. Waikanae, New Zealand, Spinal Publications Ltd., 1981.
10. Stoddard, A.: Manual of Osteopathic Practice. New York, Harper & Row, 1970.
11. Matson, D. D., R. P. Woods, J. B. Campbell, and F. D. Ingraham: Diastematomyelia (congenital clefts of the spinal cord). Pediatrics 6:98, 1950.
12. Allbrook, D.: Movements of the lumbar spinal column. J. Bone Joint Surg. 39B:339, 1957.
13. Moll, J. M. H., and V. Wright: Normal range of spinal mobility: An objective clinical study. Ann. Rheum. Dis. 30:381, 1971.

14. Moll, J., and V. Wright: Measurement of spinal movement. In Jayson, M. (ed.): The Lumbar Spine and Back Pain. New York, Grune & Stratton, Inc., 1976.

15. Pennal, G. F., G. S. Conn, G. McDonald, et al.: Motion studies of the lumbar spine. J. Bone Joint Surg. 54B:442, 1972.

16. Tanz, S. S.: Motion of the lumbar spine: A roentgenologic study. Am. J. Roentgenol. 69:399, 1953.

17. Bourdillon, J. F., and E. A. Day: Spinal Manipulation. London, Wm. Heinemann Medical Books, 1987.

18. Edwards, B. C.: Clinical assessment: The use of combined movements in assessment and treatment. In Twomey, L. T., and J. R. Taylor (eds.): Physical Therapy of the Low Back. Clinics in Physical Therapy. Edinburgh, Churchill Livingstone, 1987.

19. Wallace, L. A.: Limb length difference and back pain. In Grieve, G. P. (ed.): Modern Manual Therapy of the Vertebral Column. Edinburgh, Churchill Livingstone, 1986.

20. Smith, S. S., T. G. Mayer, R. J. Gatchel, and T. J. Becker: Quantification of lumbar function: Isometric and multispeed isokinetic trunk strength measures in sagittal and axial planes in normal subjects. Spine 10:757, 1985.

21. Lehmann, T. R., R. A. Brand, and T. W. O. Gorman: A low-back rating scale. Spine 8:308, 1983.

22. Cyriax, J.: Textbook for Orthopaedic Medicine, vol. I: Diagnosis of Soft Tissue Lesions. London, Bailliere Tindall, 1975.

23. Breig, A., and J. D. G. Troup: Biomechanical considerations in straight-leg-raising test: Cadaveric and clinical studies of the effects of medical hip rotation. Spine 4:242, 1979.

24. Charnley, J.: Orthopedic signs in the diagnosis of disc protrusion with special reference to the straight-leg-raising test. Lancet 1:156, 1951.

25. Edgar, M. A., and W. M. Park: Induced pain patterns on passive straight-leg-raising in lower lumbar disc protrusion. J. Bone Joint Surg. 56B:658, 1974.

26. Fahrni, W. H.: Observations on straight-leg-raising with special reference to nerve root adhesions. Can. J. Surg. 9:44, 1966.

27. Goddard, B. S., and J. D. Reid: Movements induced by straight-leg-raising in the lumbo-sacral roots, nerves, and plexus and in the intrapelvic section of the sciatic nerve. J. Neurol. Neurosurg. Psychiatry 28:12, 1965.

28. Scham, S. M., and T. K. F. Taylor: Tension signs in lumbar disc prolapse. Clin. Orthop. Relat. Res. 75:195, 1971.

29. Urban, L. M.: The straight-leg-raising test: A review. J. Orthop. Sports Phys. Ther. 2:117, 1981.

30. Wilkins, R. H., and I. A. Brody: Lasègue's sign. Arch. Neurol. 21:219, 1969.

31. Cipriano, J. J.: Photographic Manual of Regional Orthopedic Tests. Baltimore, Williams & Wilkins, 1985.

32. Hudgins, W. R.: The crossed-straight-leg-raising test. N. Engl. J. Med. 297:1127, 1977.

33. Woodhall, R., and G. J. Hayes: The well-leg-raising test of Fajersztajn in the diagnosis of ruptured lumbar intervertebral disc. J. Bone Joint Surg. 32A:786, 1950.

34. Herron, L. D., and H. C. Pheasant: Prone knee—flexion provocative testing for lumbar disc protrusion. Spine 5:65, 1980.

35. Maitland, G. D.: The slump test: Examination and treatment. Aust. J. Physiother. 31:215, 1985.

36. Philip, K., P. Lew, and T. A. Matyas: The inter-therapist reliability of the slump test. Aust. J. Physiother. 35:89, 1989.

37. Maitland, G. D.: Negative disc exploration: Positive canal signs. Aust. J. Physiother. 25:129, 1979.

38. Wartenberg, R.: The signs of Brudzinski and of Kernig. J. Pediatr. 37:679, 1950.

39. Brody, I. A., and R. H. Williams: The signs of Kernig and Brudzinski. Arch. Neurol. 21:215, 1969.

40. Brudzinski, J.: A new sign of the lower extremities in meningitis of children (neck sign). Arch. Neurol. 21:217, 1969.

41. Kernig, W.: Concerning a little noted sign of meningitis. Arch. Neurol. 21:216, 1969.

42. Dyck, P.: The femoral nerve traction test with lumbar disc protrusion. Surg. Neurol. 6:163, 1976.

43. Cram, R. H.: A sign of sciatic nerve root pressure. J. Bone Joint Surg. 35B:192, 1953.

44. Spengler, D. M.: Low Back Pain—Assessment and Management. Orlando, Fla., Grune & Stratton, 1982.

45. Palmer, M. L., and M. Epler: Clinical Assessment Procedures in Physical Therapy. Philadelphia, J. B. Lippincott, 1990.

46. Dommisse, G. F., and L. Grobler: Arteries and veins of the lumbar nerve roots and cauda equina. Clin. Orthop. Relat. Res. 115:22, 1976.

47. Katznelson, A., J. Nerubay, and A. Level: Gluteal skyline (G. S. L.): A search for an objective sign in the diagnosis of disc lesions of the lower lumbar spine. Spine 7:74, 1982.

48. Little, H.: The Neck and Back: The Rheumatological Physical Examination. Orlando, Fla., Grune & Stratton, 1986.

49. Garrick, J. G., and D. R. Webb: Sports Injuries: Diagnosis and Management. Philadelphia, W. B. Saunders, 1990.

50. Jackson, D. W., and J. V. Ciullo: Injuries of the spine in the skeletally immature athlete. In Nicholas, J. A., and E. B. Hershman (eds.): The Lower Extremity and Spine in Sports Medicine, Vol. 2. St. Louis, C. V. Mosby Co., 1986.

51. Kirkaldy-Willis, W. H.: Managing Low Back Pain. Edinburgh, Churchill Livingstone, 1983.

52. Corrigan, B., and G. D. Maitland: Practical Orthopedic Medicine. London, Butterworths, 1985.

53. Wadsworth, C. T., R. F. DeFabio, and D. Johnson: The spine. In: Manual Examination and Treatment of the Spine and Extremities. Baltimore, Williams & Wilkins, 1988.

54. Post, M.: Physical Examination of the Musculoskeletal System. Chicago, Year Book Medical Pub., 1987.

55. Dyck, P.: The stoop-test in lumbar entrapment radiculopathy. Spine 4:89, 1979.

56. Dyck, P., and J. B. Doyle: "Bicycle test" of van Gelderen in diagnosis of intermittent caudo equina compression syndrome. J. Neurosurg. 46:667–670, 1977.

57. Archibald, K. C., and F. Wiechec: A reappraisal of Hoover's test. Arch. Phys. Med. Rehabil. 51:234, 1970.

58. Arieff, A. J., E. I. Tigay, J. F. Kurtz, and W. A. Larmon: The Hoover sign: An objective sign of pain and/or weakness in the back or lower extremities. Arch. Neurol. 5:673, 1961.

59. Hoover, C. F.: A new sign for the detection of malingering and functional paresis of the lower extremities. J.A.M.A. 51:746, 1908.

60. Deyerle, W. M., and V. R. May: Sciatic tension test. South. Med. J. 49:999, 1956.

61. Dyck, P., H. C. Pheasant, J. B. Doyle, and J. J. Reider: Intermittent cauda equina compression syndrome. Spine 2:75, 1977.

62. Joffe, R., A. Appleby, and V. Arjona: Intermittent ischemia of the cauda equina due to stenosis of the lumbar canal. J. Neurol. Neurosurg. Psychiatry 29:315, 1966.

63. Hoppenfeld, S.: Physical Examination of the Spine and Extremities. New York, Appleton-Century-Crofts, 1976.

64. Maitland, G. D.: Examination of the lumbar spine. Aust. J. Physther. 17:5, 1971.

65. Fullenlove, T. M., and A. J. Williams: Comparative roentgen findings in symptomatic and asymptomatic back. Radiology 68:572, 1957.

66. Gillespie, H. W.: The significance of congenital lumbosacral abnormalities. Br. J. Radiol. 22:270, 1949.

67. Magora, A., and A. Schwartz: Relation between the low back pain syndrome and x-ray findings. Scand. J. Rehabil. Med. 10:135, 1978.

68. Southworth, J. D., and S. R. Bersack: Anomalies of the lumbosacral vertebrae in five hundred and fifty individuals without symptoms referable to the low back. Am. J. Roentgenol. 64:624, 1950.

69. Tulsi, R. S.: Sacral arch defect and low backache. Australas. Radiol. 18:43, 1974.

70. Willis, T. A.: An analysis of vertebral anomalies. Am. J. Surg. 6:163, 1929.

71. Willis, T. A.: Lumbosacral anomalies. J. Bone Joint Surg. 41A:935, 1959.

72. Macnab, I.: The traction spur: An indicator of segmental instability. J. Bone Joint Surg. 53A:663, 1971.

GENERAL REFERENCES

Adams, M. A., and W. C. Hutton: The mechanical function of the lumbar apophyseal joints. Spine 8:327, 1983.

Anderson, B. J. G., R. Ortengen, A. L. Nachemson, et al.: The sitting posture: An electromyographic and discometric study. Orthop. Clin. North Am. 6:105, 1975.

Barasch, E., and R. DeMaro: Typical MRI findings in sports medicine evaluation for degenerative joint disease. J Orthop. Sports Phys. Ther. 10:290, 1989.

Bassett, L. W., R. H. Gold, and L. L. Seeger: MRI Atlas of the Musculoskeletal System. London, Martin Dunitz Ltd., 1989.

Brown, L.: Treatment and examination of the spine by combined movements. Physiotherapy 76:66, 1990.

Brown, M. D.: Diagnosis of pain syndromes of the spine. Orthop. Clin. North Am. 6:233, 1975.

Cacayorin, E. D., L. Hockhauser, and G. R. Petro: Lumbar and thoracic spine pain in the athlete: Radiographic evaluation. Clin. Sports Med. 6:767, 1987.

Carmichael, S. W., and S. L. Buckart: Clinical anatomy of the lumbosacral complex. Phys. Ther. 59:966, 1979.

Chadwick, P. R.: Examination, assessment and treatment of the lumbar spine. Physiotherapy 70:2, 1984.

Crock, H. V.: Normal and pathological anatomy of the lumbar spinal nerve root canals. J. Bone Joint Surg. 63B:487, 1981.

Crock, H. V., and H. Yoshizawa: The blood supply of the lumbar vertebral column. Clin. Orthop. Relat. Res. 115:6, 1976.

Crouch, J. E.: Functional Human Anatomy. Philadelphia, Lea & Febiger, 1972.

Crow, N. E.: The "normal" lumbosacral spine. Radiology 72:97, 1959.

Cyriax, J.: Examination of the spinal column. Physiotherapy 56:206, 1970.

Davies, E. M.: Backache and its treatment by active exercise. Physiotherapy 49:81, 1963.

Davis, P. R.: The mechanics and movements of the back in working situations. Physiotherapy 53:44, 1967.

Dixon, A. St.: Diagnosis of low back pain: Sorting the complainers. In Jayson, M. (ed.): The Lumbar Spine and Back Pain. New York, Grune & Stratton, Inc., 1976.

Dohrmann, G. J., and W. J. Nowack: The upgoing great toe: Optimal method of elicitation. Lancet 1:339, 1973.

Dommisse, G. F., and L. Grobler: Arteries and veins of the nerve roots and cauda equina. Clin. Orthop. Relat. Res. 115:22, 1976.

Edgelow, P. I.: Physical examination of the lumbosacral complex. Phys. Ther. 59:974, 1979.

Fairbank, J. C. T., H. Hall, P. F. van Akkerveeken, B. L. Rydevik, D. L. Spencer, and S. Haldeman. Diagnoses and neuromechanisms—History taking and physical examination. In Weinstein, J. N., and S. W. Wiesel (eds.): The Lumbar Spine. Philadelphia, W. B. Saunders Co., 1990.

Finneson, B. E.: Low Back Pain, 2nd ed. Philadelphia, J. B. Lippincott Co., 1981.

Floman, Y., S. W. Wiesel, and R. H. Rothman: Cauda equina syndrome presenting as a herniated lumbar disc. Clin. Orthop. Relat. Res. 147:234, 1980.

Forrester, D. M., and J. C. Brown: The Radiology of Joint Disease. Philadelphia, W. B. Saunders Co., 1987.

Forst, J. J.: Contribution to the clinical study of sciatica. Arch. Neurol. 21:220, 1969.

Friberg, O.: Clinical symptoms and biomechanics of lumbar spine and hip joint in leg length inequality. Spine 8:643, 1983.

Gartland, J. J.: Fundamentals of Orthopedics. Philadelphia, W. B. Saunders Co., 1979.

Golub, B. S., and B. Silverman: Transforaminal ligaments of the lumbar spine. J. Bone Joint Surg. 51A:947, 1969.

Gould, J. A.: The Spine: Orthopedic and Sports Physical Therapy. St. Louis, C. V. Mosby Co., 1990.

Grieve, G. P.: Common Vertebral Joint Problems. New York, Churchill Livingstone, 1981.

Grieve, G. P.: Mobilization of the Spine. New York, Churchill Livingstone, 1979.

Gutrecht, J. A., P. A. Espinosa, and P. J. Dyck: Early descriptions of common neurologic signs. Mayo Clin. Proc. 43:807, 1968.

Hall, G. W.: Neurologic signs and their discoveries. J.A.M.A. 95:703, 1930.

Helfet, A. J., and Lee, D. M.: Disorders of the Lumbar Spine. Philadelphia, J. B. Lippincott Co., 1978.

Hirsch, C., R. O. Ingelmark, and M. Miller: The anatomical bases for low back pain. Acta Orthop. Scand. 33:1, 1963.

Hollinshead, W. H., and D. B. Jenkins: Functional Anatomy of the Limbs and Back. Philadelphia, W. B. Saunders Co., 1981.

Jackson, H. C., R. K. Winkelmann, and W. H. Bickel: Nerve endings in the human lumbar spinal column and related structures. J. Bone Joint Surg. 48A:1272, 1966.

Jaeger, S. A.: Atlas of Radiographic Positioning—Normal Anatomy and Developmental Variants. Norwalk, Conn., Appleton and Lange, 1988.

Jayson, M.: The Lumbar Spine and Back Pain. New York, Grune & Stratton, 1987.

Jensen, G. M.: Biomechanics of the lumbar intervertebral disk: A review. Phys. Ther. 60:765, 1980.

Jonck, L. M.: The mechanical disturbances resulting from lumbar disc space narrowing. J. Bone Joint Surg. 43:362, 1961.

Jull, G. A.: Examination of the lumbar spine. In Grieve, G. P. (ed.): Modern Manual Therapy of the Vertebral Column. Edinburgh, Churchill Livingstone, 1986.

Kapandji, L. A.: The Physiology of Joints, Vol. 3: The Trunk and Vertebral Column. New York, Churchill Livingstone, 1974.

Keim, H. A.: Low back pain. Clin. Symp. 26:2, 1974.

Keim, H. A.: The Adolescent Spine. New York, Springer-Verlag, 1982.

Kirkaldy-Willis, W. H.: Diagnosis and treatment of lumbar spinal stenosis. American Academy of Orthopedic Surgeons Symposium on the Lumbar Spine. St. Louis, C. V. Mosby Co., 1976.

Kirkaldy-Willis, W. H.: Managing Low Back Pain. New York, Churchill Livingstone, 1983.

Kirkaldy-Willis, W. H.: The relationship of structural pathology to the nerve root. Spine 9:49, 1984.

Koreska, J., D. Robertson, R. H. Mills, D. A. Gibson, and A. M. Albisser: Biomechanics of the lumbar spine and its clinical significance. Orthop. Clin. North Am. 8:121, 1977.

Lamb, D. W.: The neurology of spinal pain. Phys. Ther. 59:971, 1979.

Lucas, D. B.: Mechanics of the spine. Hospital for Joint Diseases (New York Bulletin) 31:115, 1970.

Maigne, R.: Orthopaedic Medicine: A New Approach to Vertebral Manipulation. Springfield, Ill., Charles C Thomas, 1972.

Maitland, G. D.: The Maitland concept: Assessment, examination, and treatment by passive movement. In Twomey, L. T., and J. R. Taylor (eds.): Physical Therapy of the Low Back. Clinics in Physical Therapy. Edinburgh, Churchill Livingstone, 1987.

McCall, I. W.: Radiologic assessment of back pain. Semin. Orthop. 1:71, 1986.

McRae, R.: Clinical Orthopaedic Examination. New York, Churchill Livingstone, 1976.

Mitchell, F. L., P. S. Moran, and N. A. Pruzzo: An Evaluation and Treatment Manual of Osteopathic Muscle Energy Procedures. Valley Park, Mo., Mitchell, Moran and Pruzzo, 1979.

Morris, J. M.: Biomechanics of the spine. Arch. Surg. 107:418, 1973.

Murphy, R. W.: Nerve roots and spinal nerves in degenerative disc disease. Clin. Orthop. Relat. Res. 129:46, 1977.

Nachemson, A.: Towards a better understanding of low back pain: A review of the mechanics of the lumbar disc. Rheumatol. Rehabil. 14:129, 1975.

O'Donoghue, D. H.: Treatment of Injuries to Athletes, 4th ed. Philadelphia, W. B. Saunders Co., 1984.

Paris, S. V.: Anatomy as related to function and pain. Orthop. Clin. North Am. 14:475, 1983.

Porterfield, J. A., and C. DeRosa: Mechanical Low Back Pain: Perspectives in Functional Anatomy. Philadelphia, W. B. Saunders Co., 1991.

Ramsey, R. H.: The anatomy of the ligamentum flava. Clin. Orthop. Relat. Res. 44:129, 1966.

Rauschnig, W., K. B. Heithoff, D. W. Stoller, H. K. Genant, I. A. F. Stokes, R. P. Jackson, and R. R. Jacobs: Radiology. In Weinstein, J. N., and S. W. Wiesel (eds.): The Lumbar Spine. Philadelphia, W. B. Saunders Co., 1990.

Reilly, B. M.: Practical Strategies in Outpatient Medicine. Philadelphia, W. B. Saunders Co., 1984.

Rose, K., and P. Balasubramaniam: Nerve root canals in the lumbar spine. Spine 9:16, 1984.

Rothman, R. H., and F. A. Simeone: The Spine. Philadelphia, W. B. Saunders Co., 1982.

Rydevik, B., M. D. Brown, and G. Lundberg: Pathoanatomy and pathophysiology of nerve root compression. Spine 9:7, 1984.

Seimen, L. P.: Low Back Pain: Clinical Diagnosis and Management. Norwalk, Conn., Appleton-Century-Crofts, 1983.

Selby, D. K.: When to operate and what to operate on. Orthop. Clin. North Am. 14:577, 1983.

Snook, S. H.: Low back pain in industry. American Academy of Orthopaedic Surgeons Symposium on Idiopathic Low Back Pain, St. Louis, C. V. Mosby Co., 1982, pp. 23–38.

Tachdjian, M. O.: Pediatric Orthopedics. Philadelphia, W. B. Saunders Co., 1972.

Waddell, G.: Clinical assessment of lumbar impairment. Clin. Orthop. Relat. Res. 221:110, 1987.

Waddell, G., and C. J. Main: Assessment of severity in low back disorders. Spine 9:204, 1984.

Weissman, B. N. W., and C. B. Sledge: Orthopedic Radiology. Philadelphia, W. B. Saunders Co., 1986.

White, A. A., and M. M. Panjabi: Clinical Biomechanics of the Spine. Philadelphia, J. B. Lippincott Co., 1978.

Wiesel, S. W., P. Bernini, and R. H. Rothman: The Aging Lumbar Spine. Philadelphia, W. B. Saunders Co., 1982.

Williams, P. L., and Warwick, R. (eds.): Gray's Anatomy, 36th British ed. Philadelphia, W. B. Saunders Co., 1980.

Yong-Hing, K., and W. H. Kirkaldy-Willis: The pathophysiology of degenerative disease of the lumbar spine. Orthop. Clin. North Am. 14:491, 1983.

CHAPTER 9

Pelvic Joints

The *sacroiliac joints* form the "key" of the arch between the two pelvic bones; with the *symphysis pubis*, they help to transfer the weight from the spine to the lower limbs. This triad of joints also acts as a buffer to decrease the force of jars and bumps to the spine and upper body from the lower limbs' contact with the ground. Because of this shock-absorbing function, the structure of the sacroiliac and symphysis pubis joints is different from that of most joints that are assessed. Assessment of the sacroiliac joints and symphysis pubis should be included in the examination of the lumbar spine and/or hips if there is no direct trauma to either one of these joints. Normally, a comprehensive examination is not made of the sacroiliac joints until examination of the lumbar spine and/or hip has been completed. If both of these joints are examined and the problem appears to still be present and remains undiagnosed, an examination of the pelvic joints should be initiated.

APPLIED ANATOMY

The sacroiliac joints are part *synovial* and part *syndesmosis*. A syndesmosis is a type of fibrous joint in which the intervening fibrous connective tissue forms an interosseous membrane or ligament. The synovial portion of the joint is C-shaped with the convex iliac surface of the "C" facing anteriorly and inferiorly. Kapandji[1] states that the greater or more acute the angle of the "C," the more stable the joint and the less the likelihood of a lesion to the joint. The sacral surface is slightly concave.

The size, shape, and roughness of the articular surfaces vary greatly among individuals. In the child, these surfaces are smooth. In the adult, they become irregular depressions and elevations that fit into one another; by so doing, they restrict movement at the joint and add strength to the joint for transferring weight from the lower limb to the spine.

The articular surface of the ilium is covered with fibrocartilage; the articular surface of the sacrum is covered with hyaline cartilage that is three-fold thicker than that of the ilium. In older persons, part of the joint surfaces may be obliterated by adhesions.

Although the sacroiliac joints are relatively mobile in young people, they become progressively stiffer with age. In some cases, ankylosis results. It must be remembered that the movements occurring in the sacroiliac and symphysis pubis joints are slight compared with the movements occurring in the spinal joints.

The symphysis pubis is a cartilaginous joint. There is a disc of fibrocartilage between the two joint surfaces called the *interpubic disc.*

The sacroiliac joints and symphysis pubis have no muscles that control their movements directly. However, they are influenced by the action of the muscles moving the lumbar spine and hip because many of these muscles attach to the sacrum and pelvis.

The *sacrococcygeal joint* is usually a fused line (symphysis) united by a fibrocartilaginous disc. It is found between the apex of the sacrum and the base of the coccyx. Occasionally, the joint is freely movable and synovial. With advanced age, the joint may fuse and be obliterated.

PATIENT HISTORY

In addition to the general questions asked in Chapter 1, the following information should be determined:

1. What is the patient's usual activity or pastime?
2. Where is the pain, and does it radiate? With a lesion of the sacroiliac joint, pain tends to be unilateral and can be referred to the posterior thigh, iliac fossa, and buttock on the affected side.
3. When does the pain occur? Pain that is due to sacroiliac joint problems is usually felt when turning

in bed, getting out of a bed, or stepping up with the affected leg. Often, the pain is constant and unrelated to position. Symphysis pubis pain tends to be localized and increases with any movement involving the adductor or rectus abdominus muscles.

4. Does the patient have or feel any weakness in the lower limb? Neurological deficit in the limbs can be present if the sacroiliac joint is affected.

5. Has there been a recent pregnancy? Sprain of the sacroiliac ligaments can be the result of increased laxity of the ligaments caused by hormonal changes. It may take 3 or 4 months or longer for the ligaments to return to their "normal" state after a pregnancy.

6. Has the patient experienced any recent falls, twists, or strains? These movements increase the chance of sacroiliac joint sprains.

7. What is the patient's habitual working stance? Is a great deal of sitting or twisting involved?

8. Is there any particular position or activity that aggravates the condition? Climbing or descending stairs, walking, and standing from a sitting position all stress the sacroiliac joint.

9. Does the patient have a past history of rheumatoid arthritis, Reiter's disease, or ankylosing spondylitis? Each of these conditions can involve the sacroiliac joints.

OBSERVATION

The patient must be suitably undressed. For the sacroiliac joints to be observed properly, the patient is often required to be nude from the mid-chest to the toes. If the patient wishes to wear shorts, they must be rolled down as far as possible so that the sacroiliac joints are visible. The patient stands and is viewed from the front, side, and back. The examiner should note the following:

1. Whether the posture and gait are normal. If *contranutation*[2] occurs at the sacroiliac joint (which indicates an anterior torsion of the joint on that side), the lower limb on that side will probably be medially rotated. Contranutation occurs when the anterior superior iliac spine (ASIS) is lower and the posterior superior iliac spine (PSIS) is higher on that particular side.[2] A painful sacroiliac joint may cause reflex inhibition of the gluteus medius, leading to a Trendelenburg gait or lurch. *Nutation*[2] is the backward rotation of the ilium on the sacrum (Fig. 9–1). If nutation occurs only on one side, the ASIS is higher and the PSIS is lower on that side.[2] Nutation occurs when a person goes into a "pelvic tilt" position. Contranutation occurs when a person goes into a "lordotic" or "anterior pelvic tilt" position.

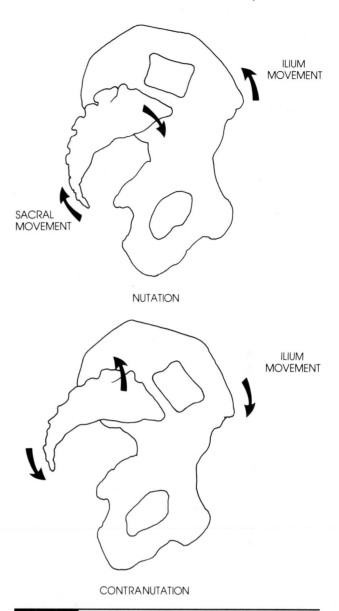

FIGURE 9–1. *Movements of nutation and contranutation.*

2. Whether the anterior superior iliac spines are level when viewed anteriorly (Fig. 9–2). On the affected side, they tend to be higher and slightly forward. The examiner must remember this difference, if present, when the patient is viewed from behind (Fig. 9–3). If the ASIS and PSIS on one side are higher than the ASIS and PSIS on the other side, this indicates an upslip of the ilium on the sacrum on the high side or a short leg.[3, 4] If the ASIS is higher on one side and the PSIS is lower at the same time, it indicates a torsion of the sacrum on that side.[3] This torsion may result in a spinal scoliosis and/or an altered functional leg length. The sacrum is lower on the pelvic side that has rotated backward. The most common rotation of the innominate bones is left posterior rotation. The posterior rotational

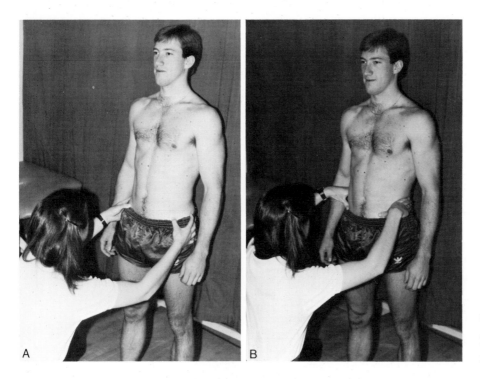

FIGURE 9–2. Anterior observation view. (A) *Level of anterior superior iliac spines.* (B) *Level of iliac crests.*

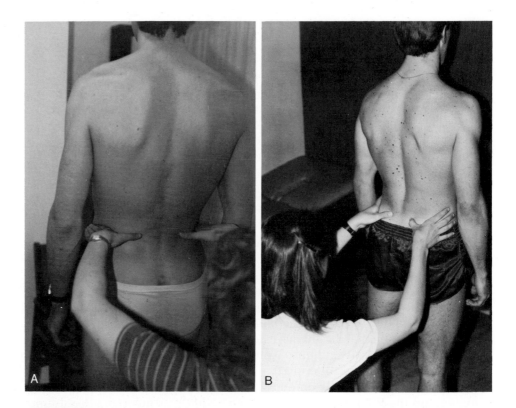

FIGURE 9–3. *Posterior observational view.* (A) *Level of iliac crests.* (B) *Level of posterior superior iliac spines.*

Illustration continued on opposite page

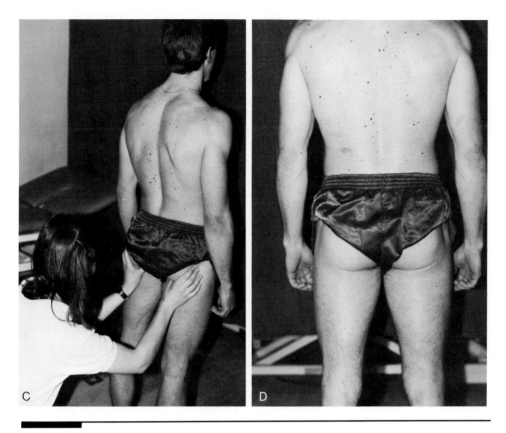

FIGURE 9–3 Continued (C) *Level of ischial tuberosities.* (D) *Level of gluteal folds.*

dysfunctions are usually the result of falling on an ischeal tuberosity, lifting when forward flexed with the knees straight, repeated standing on one leg, vertical thrusting onto an extended leg, or sustaining hyperflexion and abduction of hips. Anterior rotational dysfunction is seen most frequently in posterior horizontal thrust of the femur (dashboard injury), golf or baseball swing, or any forced anterior diagonal pattern.[4]

3. Whether both pubic bones are level at the

symphysis pubis. The examiner tests for level equality by placing one finger or thumb on the superior aspect of each pubic bone and comparing the heights (Fig. 9–4). If the ASIS on one side is higher, the pubic bone on that side is suspected to be higher and can be confirmed by this procedure, indicating a backward torsion problem on that side. This procedure is usually done with the patient lying supine.

4. Whether the patient stands with equal weight on both feet, favors one leg, or has a lateral pelvic

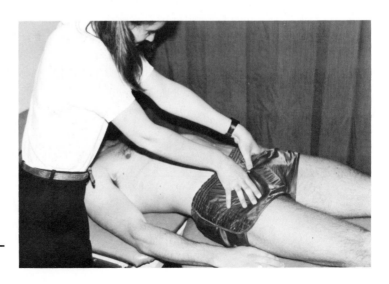

FIGURE 9–4. *Determining level of pubic bones.*

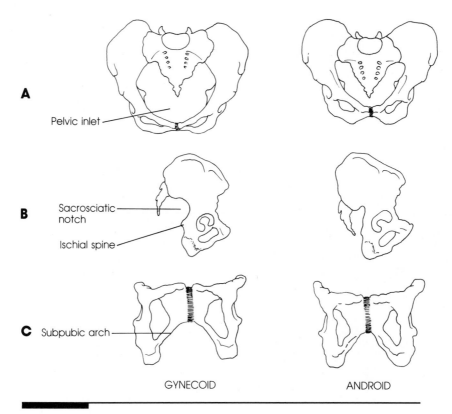

A

Pelvic inlet

B

Sacrosciatic notch

Ischial spine

C Subpubic arch

GYNECOID   ANDROID

FIGURE 9–5. Gynecoid (predominantly female) and android (primarily male) pelvises. (A) Anterosuperior view. (B) Lateral view. (C) Anterior view of the pubis and ischium.

tilt. This finding may indicate pathology or a short leg.

5. Whether the anterior superior iliac spines are equidistant from the center line of the body.

6. What type of pelvis the patient has. Gynecoid and android types are the most common (as described in Fig. 9–5 and Table 9–1).

7. Whether the sacrovertebral or lumbosacral angle is normal (140°).

8. Whether the pelvic angle or inclination is normal (30°).

9. Whether the sacral angle is normal (30°) (Fig. 9–6).

10. Whether the iliac crests are level. Leg length may alter the height.

TABLE 9–1. A Comparison of the Two Most Common Types of Pelvises Seen in Males and Females

Feature	Gynecoid	Android
Inlet	Round	Triangular
Sacrosciatic notch	Average size	Narrow
Sacrum	Average	Forward
Subpubic arch	Inclination well curved	Inclination straight

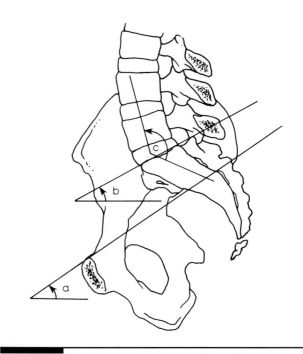

FIGURE 9–6. Angles of the pelvic joints. a, Pelvic angle (normal = 30°). b, Sacral angle (normal = 30°). c, Lumbosacral angle (normal = 140°).

11. Whether the posterior superior iliac spines are level.

12. Whether the buttock contours or gluteal folds are normal. The painful side will often be flatter if there is loss of tone in the gluteus maximus muscle.

13. Whether there is any unilateral or bilateral spasm of the erector spinae muscles.

14. Whether the ischial tuberosities are level. If one tuberosity is higher, it may indicate an upslip of the ilium on the sacrum on that side.[3]

15. Whether there is excessive lumbar lordosis. Forward or backward sacral torsion may increase or decrease the lordosis.

16. Whether the posterior superior iliac spines are equidistant from the center line of the body.

17. Whether the sacral sulci are equal. If one is deeper, it may indicate a sacral torsion.

18. Whether the feet face forward to the same degree. Often, the affected limb will be medially rotated. With spasm of the piriformis muscle, the limb would be laterally rotated on the affected side.

EXAMINATION

When assessing the pelvic joints, the examiner should first assess the lumbar spine and hip unless the history definitely indicates one of the pelvic joints.

The lumbar spine and hip can, and frequently do, refer pain to the sacroiliac joint area. Because the sacroiliac joints are in part a syndesmosis, movement at these joints is minimal compared with that of the other peripheral joints. It should also be remembered that any condition that alters the position of the sacrum relative to the ilium will cause a corresponding change in the position of the symphysis pubis.

Active Movements

Unlike other peripheral joints, the sacroiliac joints do not have muscles that directly control their movement. However, because contraction of the muscles of the other joints may stress these joints or the symphysis pubis, the examiner must be careful during the active or resisted isometric movements of other joints and be sure to ask the patient about the exact location of the pain on each movement. For example, resisted abduction of the hip can cause pain in the sacroiliac joint on the same side if it is injured because the gluteus medius muscle pulls the ilium away from the sacrum when it contracts strongly. In addition, side flexion to the

same side increases the shearing stress to the sacroiliac joint on that side.

The sacroiliac joints move in a "nodding" fashion of anteroposterior rotation. The sacrum moves forward on the ilia when one changes from a standing to a lying position or flexes the trunk. The opposite occurs for movements in the opposite direction. Normally, the posterior superior iliac spines approximate when one stands and separate when one lies prone. When one stands on one leg, the pubic bone on the supported side moves forward in relation to the pubic bone on the opposite side as a result of rotation at the sacroiliac joint.

The examiner looks for unequal movement, loss of movement (hypomobility), tissue contracture, tenderness, inflammation, or hypermobility. The following active movements should be carried out with the patient standing:

1. Forward flexion of the spine (40 to 60°).
2. Extension of the spine (20 to 35°).
3. Rotation of the spine (left and right) (3 to 18°).
4. Side flexion of the spine (left and right) (15 to 20°).
5. Flexion of the hip (110 to 120°).
6. Abduction of the hip (30 to 50°).
7. Adduction of the hip (30°).
8. Extension of the hip (0 to 15°).
9. Medial rotation of the hip (30 to 40°).
10. Lateral rotation of the hip (40 to 60°).

The movements of the spine put a stress on the sacroiliac joints as well as the lumbar and lumbosacral joints. Forward flexion movement while standing tests the movement of the ilia on the sacrum.

The hip movements performed are also affected by sacroiliac lesions. As the patient flexes each hip maximally, the examiner should observe the range of motion present, the pain produced, and the movement of the posterior superior iliac spines. The examiner first notes whether the posterior superior iliac spines are level before the patient flexes the hip (Fig. 9–7A). Normally, flexion of the hip with the knee flexed to 90° causes the sacroiliac joint on that side to drop or move caudally relative to the other sacroiliac joint. If this drop does not occur, it may indicate hypomobility on the flexed side. The examiner can also test this movement by placing one thumb over the PSIS and the other thumb over the spinous process of S2.

After the test, the examiner places one thumb over the lowest sacral spinous process palpable and the other thumb over the PSIS. The patient is again asked to flex the hip with the knee flexed as far as possible (Fig. 9–7B). The examiner should normally note a downward movement of the thumb over the PSIS relative to the other thumb in the normal

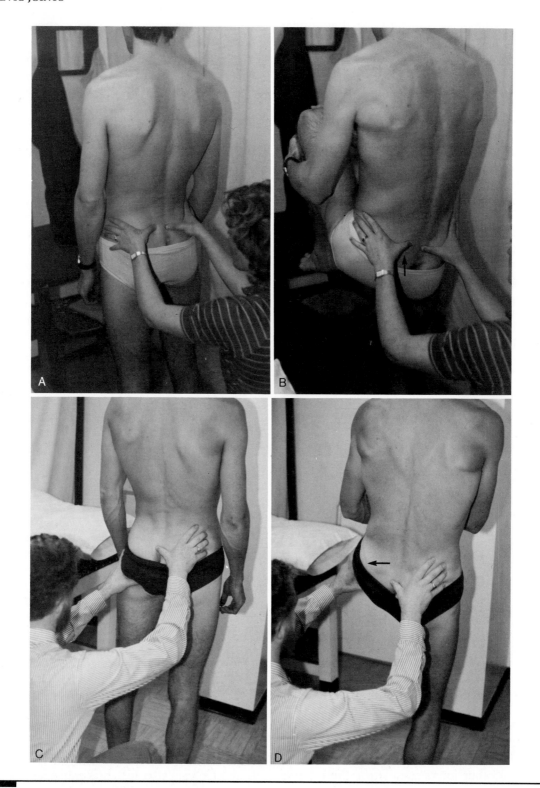

FIGURE 9–7. *Active movements demonstrating how to show hypomobility of the sacroiliac joints. (A) Starting position for sacral spine and posterior superior iliac spine. (B) Hip flexion (tight sacroiliac joint illustrated; ilium does not drop). (C) Starting position for sacral spine and ischial tuberosity. (D) Hip flexion. Ischial tuberosity moves laterally, as one would normally expect.*

sacroiliac joint. In the hypomobile sacroiliac joint, this thumb would remain in the same position relative to the other thumb or would move up cranially. The two sides are compared. The examiner

then leaves the one thumb over the sacral spinous process and moves the other thumb over the ischial tuberosity (Fig. 9–7C). The patient is again asked to flex the hip as far as possible. In the normal sacro-

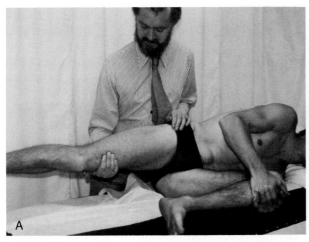
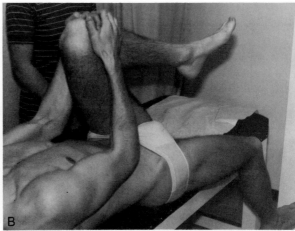

FIGURE 9–16. Gaenslen's test. (A) Method 1. Examiner extends test leg. (B) Method 2. Test leg is extended over the edge of the table.

rotate forward, usually before the knee reaches 90° flexion.[6, 7]

Tests for Sacroiliac Joint Involvement

Piedallu's Sign. The patient is asked to sit on a hard, flat surface (Fig. 9–15). This position keeps the muscles (e.g., the hamstrings) from affecting the pelvic flexion symmetry and increases the stability of the ilia. In effect, it is a test of the sacrum on the ilia. The examiner palpates the posterior superior iliac spines and compares their heights. If one PSIS, usually the painful one, is lower than the other, the patient is asked to forward flex while remaining seated. If the lower PSIS becomes the higher one on forward flexion, the test is positive; it is that side that is affected. Because the affected joint does not move properly and is hypomobile, it goes from a low to a high position. It indicates an abnormality in the torsion movement at the sacroiliac joint.

Gaenslen's Test. The patient lies on the side with the upper leg hyperextended at the hip (Fig. 9–16). The patient holds the lower leg flexed against the chest. The examiner stabilizes the pelvis while extending the hip of the uppermost leg, which is the test leg. Pain indicates a positive test. The pain may be due to an ipsilateral sacroiliac joint lesion, hip pathology, or an L4 nerve root lesion.

Gaenslen's test is sometimes done with the patient supine, but this position may limit the amount of hyperextension available. The patient is positioned so that the test hip extends beyond the edge of the table. The patient draws both legs up onto the chest and then slowly lowers the test leg down into extension. The other leg is tested in a similar fashion for comparison. Pain in the sacroiliac joints is indicative of a positive test.

Laguere's Sign. The patient lies supine (Fig. 9–17). The examiner then flexes, abducts, and laterally rotates the patient's hip, applying an overpressure at the end of the range of motion. The examiner must stabilize the pelvis on the opposite side by holding the opposite ASIS down. Pain in the sacroiliac joint on that side constitutes a positive test. This test should be performed with caution for patients with hip pathology because hip pain may ensue.

Gillet's (Sacral Fixation) Test.[4] While the patient stands, the examiner palpates the posterior superior iliac spines. The patient is then asked to stand on one leg while pulling the opposite knee up toward the chest. The test is repeated with the other leg. If the sacroiliac joint on the side on which the knee is

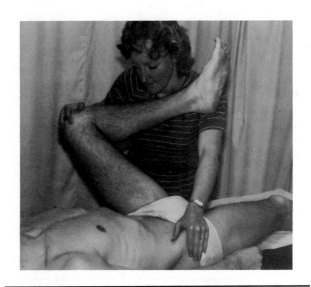

FIGURE 9–17. Laguere's sign.

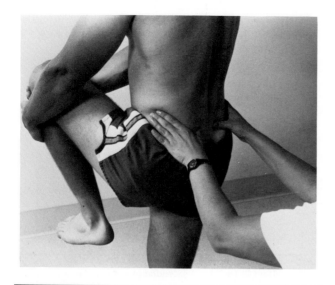

FIGURE 9–18. Gillet's (sacral fixation) test.

flexed moves minimally, the joint is hypomobile, or "blocked," indicating a positive test. On the normal side, the test PSIS will move down or inferiorly (Fig. 9–18).

Supine-to-Sit Test. The patient lies supine with the legs straight. The patient is asked to sit up, and the examiner observes if one leg moves up (proximally) farther than the other leg (Figs. 9–19 and 9–20). If one leg moves up farther than the other, there is a functional leg length difference resulting from a pelvic dysfunction due to pelvic torsion.[6, 8]

Goldthwait's Test. The patient lies supine. The examiner places one hand under the lumbar spine so that each finger is in an interspinous space (i.e., L5–S1, L4–L5, L3–L4, and L2–L3 interspaces). The examiner uses the other hand to perform straight leg raising. If pain is elicited before movement occurs at the interspaces, the problem is in the sacroiliac joint. Pain during interspace movement indicates a lumbar spine dysfunction. As with the straight leg raising test, pain may be referred along the course of the sciatic nerve.[7]

Yeoman's Test. The patient lies prone. The examiner flexes the patient's knee to 90° and extends the hip (Fig. 9–21). Pain localized to the sacroiliac joint indicates pathology in the anterior sacroiliac ligaments. Lumbar pain indicates lumbar involvement.[7]

Flamingo Test or Maneuver. The patient is standing and is asked to stand on one leg (Fig. 9–22).

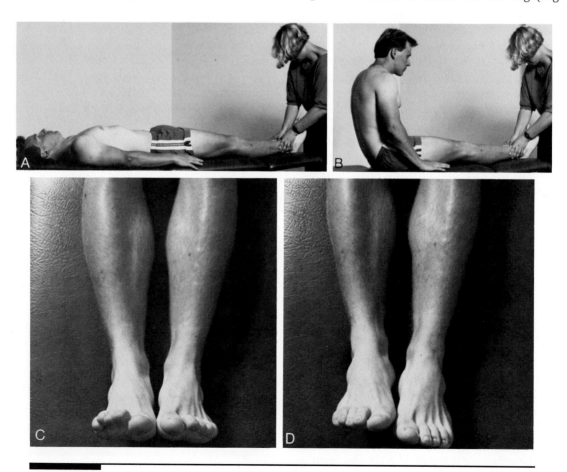

FIGURE 9–19. Supine-to-sit test for functional leg length discrepancy. (A) Initial position. (B) Final position. (C) Symmetric leg lengths. (D) Asymmetric leg lengths.

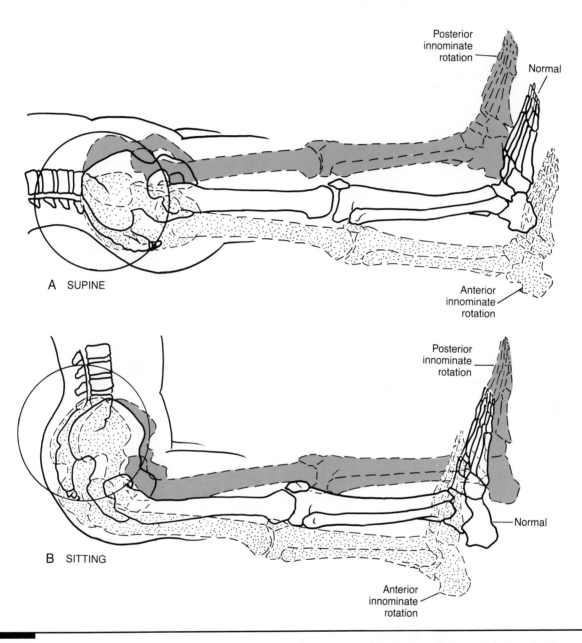

FIGURE 9–20. Supine-to-sit test. Leg length reversal: supine (A) versus sitting (B). If the lower limb on the affected side appears longer when a patient lies supine but shorter when sitting, the test is positive, implicating anterior innomination rotation on the affected side. (Adapted from Wadsworth, C. T. (ed.): Manual Examination and Treatment of the Spine and Extremities. Baltimore, Williams & Wilkins, 1988 p. 82.)

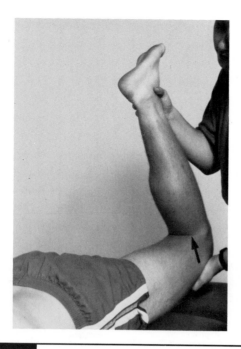

FIGURE 9–21. Yeoman's test.

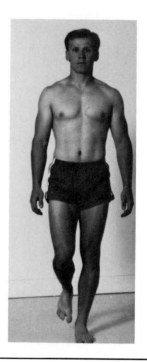

FIGURE 9–22. Flamingo test.

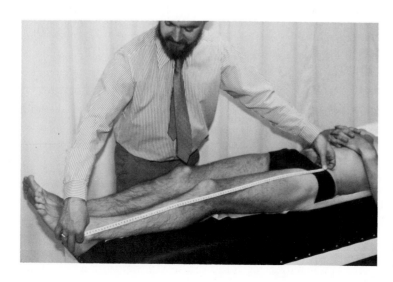

FIGURE 9–23. Measuring leg length.

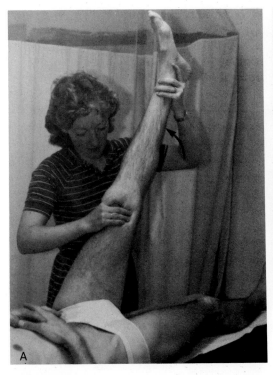
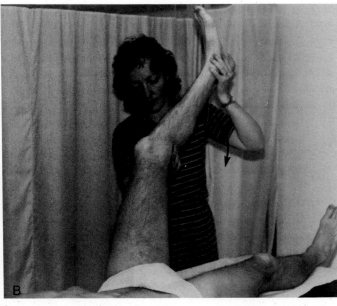

FIGURE 9–24. Sign of the buttock test. (A) Step 1. Flex hip with knee straight until resistance or pain is felt. (B) Step 2. Once resistance or pain is felt, flex knee to see if further hip flexion can be achieved.

Pain in the symphysis pubis or sacroiliac joint indicates a positive test for lesions in whichever structure is painful. The stress may be increased by having the patient hop on one leg. This position is also used for a stress x-ray of the symphysis pubis.

Tests for Limb Length

Leg Length Test. The leg length test, described in detail in Chapter 10, should always be performed if the examiner suspects a sacroiliac joint lesion. Nutation (backward rotation) of the ilium on the sacrum will result in a decrease in leg length, as will contranutation (anterior rotation) on the opposite side. If the iliac bone on one side of the symphysis pubis is lower, the leg on that side will usually be shorter. True leg length is measured by having the patient in a supine position with the anterior superior iliac spines level and the patient's lower limbs perpendicular to the line joining the anterior superior iliac spines (Fig. 9–23). Using a flexible tape measure, the examiner obtains the distance from the ASIS to the medial or lateral malleolus on the same side. The measurement is repeated on the other side, and the results are compared. A difference of 1 to 1.3 cm is considered normal.

Functional Limb Length Test.[9] The patient stands relaxed while the examiner palpates the anterior superior iliac spines and the posterior superior iliac spines, noting any asymmetry. The patient is then placed in the correct stance (subtalar joint neutral, knees fully extended, and toes facing straight ahead), and the anterior superior iliac spines and posterior superior iliac spines are palpated, with the examiner noting whether the asymmetry has been corrected. If the asymmetry has been corrected, there is a functional limb length difference, and the test is considered positive.

Other Tests

Sign of the Buttock Test. With the patient supine, the examiner performs a passive unilateral straight leg raising test as done previously (Fig. 9–24). If restriction is found on one side, the examiner flexes the patient's knee to see whether flexion of the hip increases. If the problem is in the lumbar spine, hip flexion will increase. This finding indicates a negative sign of the buttock test. If hip flexion does not increase when the knee is flexed, it is a positive sign of the buttock test and indicates pathology in the buttock such as a bursitis, tumor, or abscess. The patient would also exhibit a noncapsular pattern of the hip.

Trendelenburg's Test or Sign. The patient is standing (Fig. 9–25) and is asked to stand or balance first on one leg and then on the other leg. While the patient is balancing on one leg, the examiner watches the movement of the pelvis. If the pelvis on the side of the nonstance leg rises, the test is considered negative. If the pelvis on the side of the nonstance leg falls, the test is considered positive

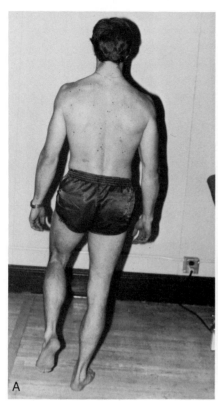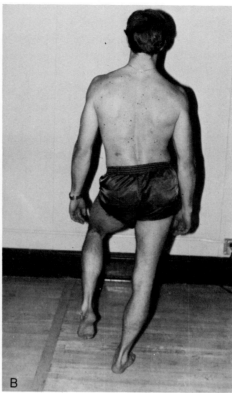

FIGURE 9–25. Trendelenburg test. (A) Negative. (B) Positive.

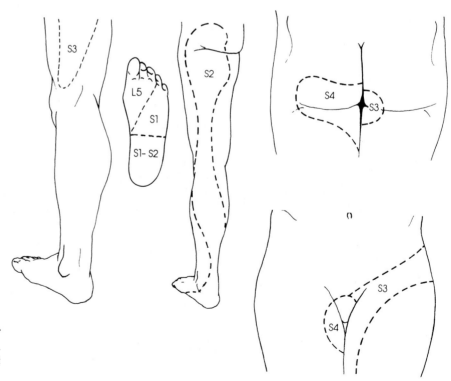

FIGURE 9–26. Posterior sacral dermatomes. Representation in the lower right is an anterior view.

and is an indication of weakness or instability of the hip abductor muscles, primarily the gluteus medius on the stance side.

Reflexes and Cutaneous Distribution

There are no reflexes to test for the pelvic joints. However, the examiner must be aware of the dermatomes from the sacral nerve roots (Fig. 9–26). Pain may be referred to the sacroiliac joints from the lumbar spine and the hip (Fig. 9–27). In addition, the sacroiliac joint may refer pain to these same structures or along the courses of the superior gluteal and obturator nerves.

Joint Play Movements

The joint play movements are minimal for the sacroiliac joints and are similar to the passive movements in that they are stress tests. The following joint play movements are performed (Fig. 9–28):

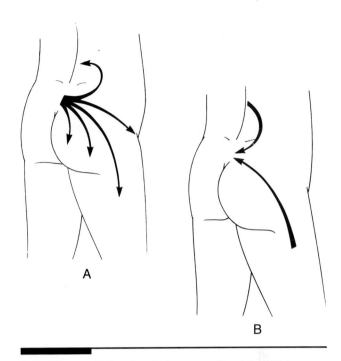

FIGURE 9–27. Referred pain from sacroiliac joint (A) to sacroiliac joint (B).

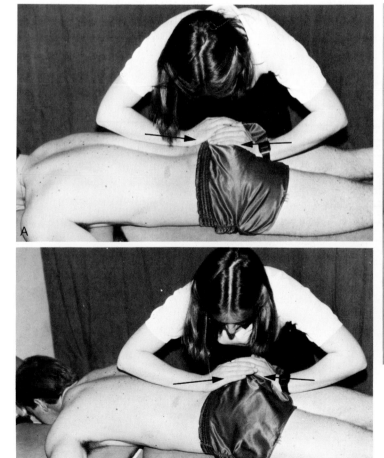

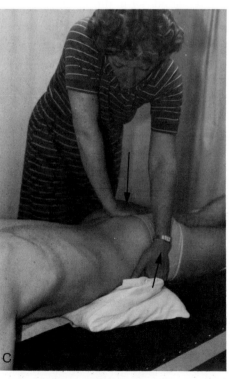

FIGURE 9–28. Joint play movements of the sacroiliac joints. (A) Cephalad movement of sacrum/caudal movement of ilium. (B) Cephalad movement of ilium/caudal movement of sacrum. (C) Anterior movement of sacrum on ilium (left side demonstrated).

1. Cephalad movement of the sacrum/caudal movement of the ilium (left and right).
2. Cephalad movement of the ilium/caudal movement of the sacrum (left and right).
3. Anterior movement of the sacrum on the ilium.

To test all of the movements, the patient is in the prone position. For the first and second joint play movements, the examiner places the heel of one hand over the iliac crest and the heel of the other hand over the apex of the sacrum. The ilium is pushed down or caudally with one hand while the sacrum is pushed up or cephalad with the other hand. The test is repeated for the other ilium (Fig. 9–28A). The examiner should "feel" only minimal movement and no pain if the joint is normal. In an affected sacroiliac joint, there is usually pain over the joint and little or no movement. This positioning tests for cephalad movement of the sacrum and caudal movement of the ilium.

To test caudal movement of the sacrum and cephalad movement of the ilium, the examiner places the heel of one hand over the base of the sacrum and the heel of the other hand over the ischial tuberosity (Fig. 9–28B). The examiner then pushes the pelvis cephalad and the sacrum caudally. The test is repeated with the other half of the pelvis being moved. The movement and amount of pain are compared.

The anterior movement of the sacrum on the ilium is tested with the patient lying prone (Fig. 9–28C). The examiner places the heel of one hand over the sacrum and places the other hand under the iliac crest in the area of the ASIS on one side. The hand is then pushed down on the sacrum while the other hand lifts up. The process is repeated on the other side, and the results are compared.

Palpation

Because many structures are included in the assessment of the pelvic joints, palpation of this area is extensive, beginning on the anterior aspect and concluding posteriorly. While palpating, the examiner should note any tenderness, muscle spasm, or other signs that may indicate the source of pathology.

Anterior Aspect

The following structures should be carefully and thoroughly palpated (Fig. 9–29).

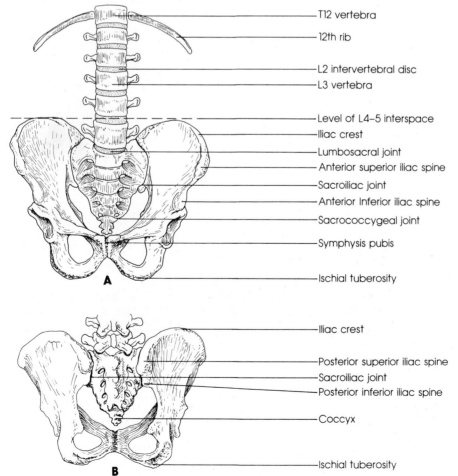

- T12 vertebra
- 12th rib
- L2 intervertebral disc
- L3 vertebra
- Level of L4–5 interspace
- Iliac crest
- Lumbosacral joint
- Anterior superior iliac spine
- Sacroiliac joint
- Anterior inferior iliac spine
- Sacrococcygeal joint
- Symphysis pubis
- Ischial tuberosity

- Iliac crest
- Posterior superior iliac spine
- Sacroiliac joint
- Posterior inferior iliac spine
- Coccyx
- Ischial tuberosity

FIGURE 9–29. Landmarks of the sacroiliac joints and symphysis pubis. (A) Anterior view. (B) Posterior view.

Iliac Crest and Anterior Superior Iliac Spine.
The palpating fingers are placed on the iliac crests on both sides and gently moved anteriorly until each ASIS is reached. The inguinal ligament attaches to the ASIS and runs downward and medially to the symphysis pubis.

McBurney's Point and Baer's Point. The examiner may then draw an imaginary line from the right ASIS to the umbilicus. *McBurney's point* lies along this line approximately one third the distance from the ASIS and is especially tender in the presence of acute appendicitis. *Baer's point* is located in the right iliac fossa anterior to the right sacroiliac joint and slightly medial to McBurney's point. It is tender in the presence of infection or when there are sprains of the right sacroiliac ligament and indicates spasm and tenderness of the iliacus muscle.

Lymph Nodes, Symphysis Pubis (Pubic Tubercles), Greater Trochanter of the Femur, Trochanteric Bursa, Femoral Triangle, and Surrounding Musculature. The examiner then returns to the ASIS and gently palpates the length of the inguinal ligament, feeling for any tenderness or swelling of the *lymph nodes* or possible inguinal hernia. At the distal end of the inguinal ligament, the examiner will come to the *pubic tubercles,* which should be palpated for tenderness or signs of pathology.

The examiner then places the thumbs over the pubic tubercles and moves the fingers laterally until the bony *greater trochanter of the femur* is felt. The trochanters are usually level. The *trochanteric bursa* lies over the greater trochanter and is palpable only if it is swollen.

Returning to the ASIS, the examiner can move on to palpate the *femoral triangle,* which has as its boundaries the inguinal ligament superiorly, the adductor longus muscle medially, and the sartorius muscle laterally. It is in the superior aspect of the triangle that the examiner palpates for swollen lymph nodes. The femoral pulse can be palpated deeper in the triangle. Although almost impossible to palpate, the femoral nerve lies lateral to the artery, whereas the femoral vein lies medial to it. The psoas bursa may also be palpated within the femoral triangle but only if it is swollen. Before moving on to the posterior structures, the examiner should determine whether the adjacent *musculature*—the abductor, flexor, and adductor muscles—shows any indication of pathology.

Posterior Aspect

To complete the posterior palpation, the patient lies in the prone position. The following structures should be palpated.

Iliac Crest and Posterior Superior Iliac Spine. Again, the examiner places the fingers on the iliac crest and moves posteriorly until they rest on the PSIS, which is at the level of the S2 spinous process. On many individuals, "dimples" indicate the position of the PSIS.

Ischial Tuberosity. If the examiner then moves distally from the PSIS and down to the level of the gluteal folds, the ischial tuberosities may be palpated. It is important that they be palpated because the hamstring muscles attach here and the bony prominences are what one "sits on."

Sacral Sulcus and Sacroiliac Joints. Returning to the PSIS as a starting point, the examiner should palpate slightly below it on the sacrum adjacent to the ilium. (This area is sometimes referred to as the *sacral sulcus.*) The depth on the right side should be compared with that on the left side. If one side is deeper than the other, sacral torsion or rotation on the ilium around the horizontal plane is indicated.

If the examiner then moves slightly medially and distal to the PSIS, the fingers will rest adjacent to the *sacroiliac joints.* To palpate these joints, the patient's knee is flexed to 90° and the hip is passively medially rotated while the examiner palpates the sacroiliac joint on the same side (Fig. 9–30). This procedure is identical to the prone gapping test previously described in "Passive Movements." The procedure is repeated on the other side, and the two are compared.

Sacrum, Lumbosacral Joint, Coccyx, Sacral Hiatus, Sacral Cornua, and Sacrotuberous and Sacrospinous Ligaments. The examiner again returns to the PSIS and moves to the midline of the *sacrum,* where the S2 spinous process can be palpated.

Moving superiorly two spinous processes, the fingers now rest on the spinous process of L5. As a check, the examiner may look to see if the fingers rest just below a horizontal line drawn from the

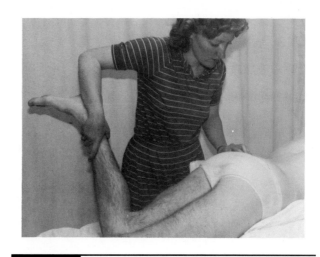

FIGURE 9–30. *Palpation of the left sacroiliac joint.*

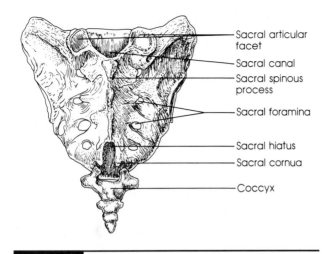

FIGURE 9–31. *Posterior view of the sacrum and coccyx.*

high point of the iliac crests. This horizontal line will normally pass through the interspace between L4 and L5. Having found the L5 spinous process, the examiner then palpates between the spinous processes of L5 and S1, feeling for signs of pathology at the *lumbosacral joint.* Moving laterally approximately 2 to 3 cm, the fingers will lie over the lumbosacral facet joints, which are not palpable. However, the overlying structures may be palpated for tenderness or spasm, which may indicate pathology of these joints or related structures. In a similar fashion, the spinous processes and facet joints of the other lumbar spines and intervening structures can be palpated.

The examiner then returns to the S2 spinous process or tubercle. Carefully palpating further distally, just before the coccyx, the examiner may be able to palpate the *sacral hiatus* lying in the midline. If the fingers are moved slightly laterally, the *sacral cornua,* which constitute the distal aspect of the sacrum, may be palpated (Fig. 9–31).

To palpate the *coccyx* properly, the examiner performs a rectal examination (Fig. 9–32). A rubber glove is put on, and the index finger is lubricated. The index finger is then carefully pushed into the rectum as the patient relaxes the sphincter muscles. The index finger then palpates the anterior surface of the coccyx while the thumb of the same hand palpates its posterior aspect. While holding the coccyx between the finger and thumb, the examiner is able to move it back and forth, rocking it at the sacrococcygeal joint. Normally, this action should not cause pain.

The examiner then returns to the PSIS. Moving straight down or distally from the PSIS, the fingers will follow the path of the *sacrotuberous ligament,* which should be palpated for tenderness. Slightly more than halfway between the PSIS and ischial tuberosity and slightly medially, the examiner will pass over the *sacrospinous ligament,* which is deep to the sacrotuberous ligament. Tenderness in this area may indicate pathology of this ligament.

Radiographic Examination

With the *anteroposterior view* (Figs. 9–33 and 9–34), the examiner should look for or note the following:

1. Ankylosis of sacroiliac joints (e.g., ankylosing spondylitis) (Fig. 9–35).
2. Possible displacement of one sacroiliac joint and/or the symphysis pubis (Fig. 9–36).
3. Demineralization, sclerosis, or periosteal reaction of one or both pubic bones at the symphysis pubis (e.g., osteitis pubis) (Fig. 9–37).
4. Any fracture.
5. Relation of the sacrum to the ilium.

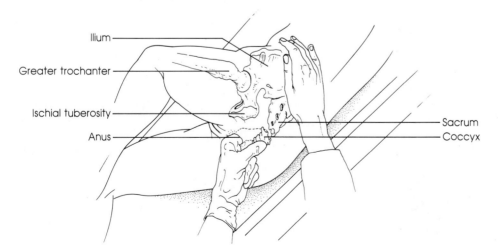

FIGURE 9–32. *Palpation of the coccyx.*

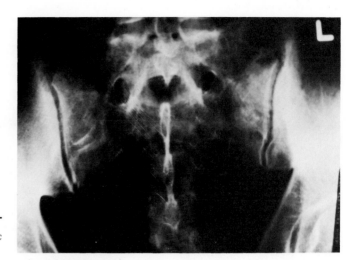

FIGURE 9–33. Anteroposterior radiograph of the sacroiliac joint.

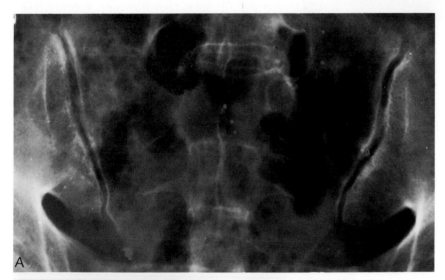

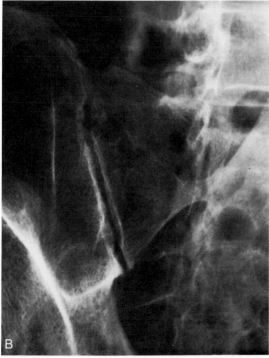

FIGURE 9–34. Normal sacroiliac joints. Angled (A) and oblique (B) views show normally maintained cortices and cartilage spaces. (From Weissman, B. N. W., and C. B. Sledge: Orthopedic Radiology. Philadelphia, W. B. Saunders Co., 1986, p. 347.)

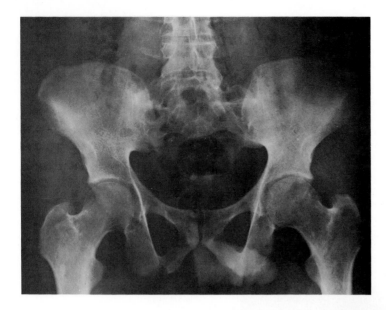

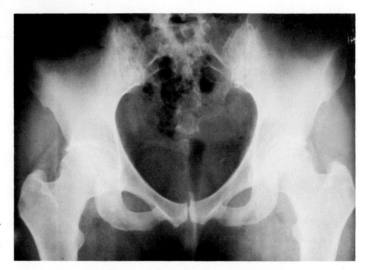

FIGURE 9–35. Fusion of sacroiliac joint spaces in the late stage of sacroiliitis of ankylosing spondylitis. The sclerosis has resorbed, and there is slight narrowing of the left hip joint. (From Rothman, R. H., and F. A. Simeone: The Spine. Philadelphia, W. B. Saunders Co., 1982, p. 921.)

FIGURE 9–36. Anteroposterior radiograph of the pelvis. Note higher left pubic bone.

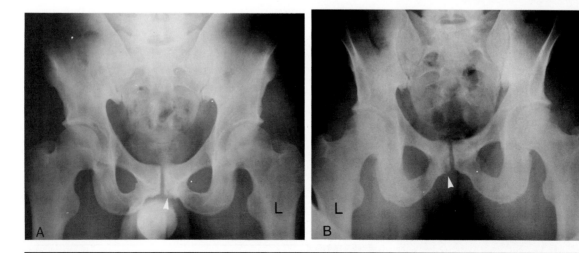

FIGURE 9–37. Osteitis pubis. (A) Anteroposterior view of pelvis showing well-concealed bony lesion at inferior corner of left pubis at the symphysis. (B) Posteroanterior view of pelvis; bony fragment is well delineated in this view. (From Wiley, J. J.: Traumatic osteitis pubis: The gracilis syndrome. Am. J. Sports Med. 11:361, 1983 Copyright.)

PRÉCIS OF THE PELVIC JOINTS ASSESSMENT*

History (sitting)
Observation (standing)
Examination
    Active movements (standing)
        Flexion of the spine
        Extension of the spine
        Rotation of the spine (left and right)
        Side flexion of the spine (left and right)
        Flexion of the hip
        Abduction of the hip
        Adduction of the hip
        Extension of the hip
        Medial rotation of the hip
        Lateral rotation of the hip
    Special tests (standing)
    Special tests (sitting)
    Passive movements (supine)
        Gapping test
        "Squish" test
        Rocking ("knee-to-shoulder") test
        Sacral apex pressure test
    Resisted isometric movements (supine)
        Forward flexion of the spine
        Flexion of the hip
        Abduction of the hip
        Adduction of the hip
        Extension of the hip
    Special tests (supine)
    Passive movements (side lying) (approximation test)
    Reflexes and cutaneous distribution (supine, then prone)
    Passive movements (prone) (sacral apex pressure test)
    Special tests (prone)
    Joint play movements (prone)
        Cephalad movement of the sacrum/caudal movement of the ilium
        Cephalad movement of the ilium/caudal movement of the sacrum
    Palpation (prone, then supine)
    Radiographic examination

As previously stated, assessment of the sacroiliac joints and symphysis pubis is done only after an assessment of the lumbar spine and hips unless there has been specific trauma to the sacroiliac joints or symphysis pubis. Thus, completing the examination of the sacroiliac joints and symphysis pubis may involve only passive movements, special tests, joint play movements, and palpation because the other tests would have been completed when assessing the other joints.

After any examination, the patient should always be warned of the possibility of exacerbation of symptoms as a result of the assessment.

---

*The précis is shown in an order that will limit the amount of moving or changing position that the patient has to do but ensure that all necessary structures are tested.

CASE STUDIES

When doing these case studies, the examiner should list the appropriate questions to be asked and why they are being asked, what to look for and why, and what things should be tested and why. Depending on the answers of the patient (and the examiner should consider different responses), several possible causes of the patient's problem may become evident (examples given in parentheses). If so, a differential diagnosis chart should be made up. The examiner can then decide how different diagnoses may affect the treatment plan.

1. A 26-year-old male soccer player presents complaining of lower abdominal pain that is referred into the right groin. Sit-ups are painful, and he experiences pain when he kicks the ball. Describe your assessment plan for this patient (abdominal strain versus osteitis pubis).

2. A 35-year-old man presents complaining of "back pain." He complains that his back is stiff and sore when he gets up in the morning and that the stiffness remains for most of the day. Sclerosis of the sacroiliac is evident on x-ray. Describe your assessment plan for this patient (ankylosing spondylitis versus osteoarthritis of the sacroiliac joints).

3. An 18-year-old female figure skater presents complaining of back pain that increases when she is skating; it is prominent on one leg. The ASIS and PSIS are higher on the right side. Describe your assessment plan for this patient (sacroiliac dysfunction versus short leg syndrome).

REFERENCES

CITED REFERENCES

1. Kapandji, L. A.: The Physiology of the Joints, vol. III: The Trunk and Vertebral Column. New York, Churchill Livingstone, 1974.
2. Maigne, R.: Orthopaedic Medicine: A New Approach to Vertebral Manipulation. Springfield, Ill., Charles C Thomas, 1972.
3. Mitchell, F. L., P. S. Moran, and N. A. Pruzzo: An Evaluation and Treatment Manual of Osteopathic Muscle Energy Procedures. Valley Park, Mo., Mitchell, Moran and Pruzzo, 1979.
4. Woerman, A. L.: Evaluation and treatment of dysfunction in the lumbar-pelvic-hip complex. In Donatelli, R., and M. J. Wooden (eds.): Orthopedic Physical Therapy. Edinburgh, Churchill Livingstone, 1989.
5. Lee, D.: The Pelvic Girdle. Edinburgh, Churchill Livingstone, 1989.
6. Porterfield, J. A., and C. DeRosa: Mechanical Low Back Pain—Perspectives in Functional Anatomy. Philadelphia, W. B. Saunders Co., 1991.
7. Cipriano, J. J.: Photographic Manual of Regional Orthopedic Tests. Baltimore, Williams & Wilkins, 1985.
8. Palmer, M. C., and M. Epler: Clinical Assessment Procedures in Physical Therapy. Philadelphia, J. B. Lippincott, 1990.
9. Wallace, L. A.: Limb length difference and back pain. In Grieve, G. P. (ed.): Modern Manual Therapy of the Vertebral Column. Edinburgh, Churchill Livingstone, 1986.

GENERAL REFERENCES

Alderink, G. J.: The sacroiliac joint: Review of anatomy, mechanics, and function. J Orthop Sports Phys Therap 13:71, 1991.

Bourdillon, J. F.: Spinal Manipulation, 3rd ed. New York, Appleton-Century-Crofts, 1982.

Bowen, V., and J. D. Cassidy: Macroscopic and microscopic anatomy of the sacroiliac joint from embryonic life until the eighth decade. Spine 6:620, 1981.

Brooke, R.: The sacro-iliac joint. J. Anat. 58:299, 1924.

Cohen, A. S., J. M. McNeill, E. Calkins, et al.: The "normal" sacroiliac joint. Analysis of 88 sacroiliac roentgenograms. Am. J. Roentgenol. 100:559, 1967.

Cyriax, J.: Textbook of Orthopaedic Medicine, vol. 1: Diagnosis of Soft Tissue Lesions. London, Bailliere Tindall, 1975.

Finneson, B. E.: Low Back Pain. Philadelphia, J. B. Lippincott Co., 1981.

Forrester, D. M., and J. C. Brown: The Radiology of Joint Disease. Philadelphia, W. B. Saunders Co., 1987.

Frigerio, N. A., R. R. Stowe, and J. W. Howe: Movement of the sacroiliac joint. Clin. Orthop. Relat. Res. 100:370, 1974.

Gray, H.: Sacro-iliac joint pain: The finer anatomy. New International Clinics 2:54, 1938.

Grieve, G. P.: Mobilization of the Spine. New York, Churchill Livingstone, 1979.

Grieve, G. P.: The sacro-iliac joint. Physiotherapy, 62:382, 1976.

Grieve, G. P.: Common Vertebral Joint Problems. New York, Churchill Livingstone, 1981.

Hanson, P. G., M. Angevine, and J. H. Juhl: Osteitis pubis in sports activities. Phys Sports Med 6:111, 1978.

Hollinshead, W. H., and D. R. Jenkins: Functional Anatomy of the Limbs and the Trunk and Vertebral Column. New York, Churchill Livingstone, 1981.

Kirkaldy-Willis, W. H.: Managing Low Back Pain. New York, Churchill Livingstone, 1983.

Klinefelter, F. W.: Osteitis pubis. Am. J. Roentgenol. 63:368, 1950.

Macnab, I.: Backache. Baltimore, Williams & Wilkins, 1977.

McGillivray, D.: The pelvic girdle. In Little, H. (ed.): Rheumatological Physical Examination. Orlando, Grune and Stratton Inc., 1986.

McRae, R.: Clinical Orthopedic Examination. New York, Churchill Livingstone, 1976.

Nicholas, J. A.: Football injuries. In Nicholas, J. A., and E. B. Hershman (eds.): The Lower Extremity and Spine in Sports Medicine, vol. II. St. Louis, C. V. Mosby Co., 1986.

Pitkin, H. C., and H. C. Pheasant: Sacrathrogenetic telalgia: A study of referred pain. J. Bone Joint Surg. 18:111, 1936.

Porterfield, J. A., and C. DeRosa: The sacroiliac joint. In Gould, J. A. (ed.): Orthopedic and Sports Physical Therapy. St. Louis, C. V. Mosby Co., 1990.

Post, M.: Examination of the thoracic and lumbar spine. In Post, M. (ed.): Physical Examination of the Musculoskeletal System. Chicago, Year Book Medical Pub., 1987.

Reilly, B. M.: Practical Strategies in Outpatient Medicine. Philadelphia, W. B. Saunders Co., 1984.

Rothman, R. H., and F. A. Simeone: The Spine. Philadelphia, W. B. Saunders Co., 1982.

Rudge, S. R., A. J. Swannell, D. H. Rose, and J. H. Todd: The clinical assessment of sacro-iliac joint involvement in ankylosing spondylitis. Rheumatol. Rehabil. 51:15, 1982.

Stoddard, A.: Manual of Osteopathic Practice. New York, Harper & Row, 1970.

Stoddard, A.: Manual of Osteopathic Technique. Atlantic Highlands, N. J., Humanities Press, 1969.

Wadsworth, C. T., R. P. DiFabio, and D. Johnson: The spine. In Wadsworth, C. T. (ed.): Manual Examination and Treatment of the Spine and Extremities. Baltimore, Williams & Wilkins, 1988.

Weissman, B. N. W., and C. B. Sledge: Orthopedic Radiology. Philadelphia, W. B. Saunders Co., 1986.

Wells, P. E.: The examination of the pelvic joints. In Grieve, G. P. (ed.): Modern Manual Therapy of the Vertebral Column. Edinburgh, Churchill Livingstone, 1986.

Wiley, J. J.: Traumatic osteitis pubis: The gracilis syndrome. Am. J. Sports Med. 11:360, 1983.

Williams, P. L., and R. Warwick (eds.): Gray's Anatomy, 36th British ed. Philadelphia, W. B. Saunders Co., 1980.

Willis, T. A.: Lumbosacral anomalies. J. Bone Joint Surg. 41A:935, 1959.

CHAPTER 10 Hip

The hip joint is one of the largest and most stable joints in the body. If it is injured or exhibits pathology, the lesion is usually immediately perceptible during walking. Because pain from the hip can be referred to the sacroiliac joint or the lumbar spine, it is imperative, unless there is evidence of direct trauma to the hip, that these joints be examined along with the hip.

APPLIED ANATOMY

The hip joint is a multiaxial ball-and-socket joint that has maximum stability because of the deep insertion of the head of the femur into the acetabulum. It has a strong capsule and very strong muscles that control its actions. The acetabulum is formed by fusion of the ilium, ischium, and pubis and is deepened by a labrum. The acetabulum opens outward, forward, and downward. It is half of a sphere, and the femoral head is two thirds of a sphere.

The joint has three degrees of freedom. The *resting position* of the hip is 30° of flexion, 30° of abduction, and slight lateral rotation. The *capsular pattern* of the hip is flexion, abduction, and medial rotation. These three movements will always be affected the most in a capsular pattern, but the order may be altered. For example, medial rotation may be most limited, followed by flexion and abduction. The *close packed position* of the joint is maximum extension, medial rotation, and abduction.

Under low loads, the joint surfaces are incongruous; under heavy loads, they become congruous, providing maximum surface contact. The maximum contact brings the load per unit area down to a tolerable level. Examples of the forces involved in the hip are as follows:

1. Standing—one third of the body weight.
2. Standing on one limb—2.4 to 2.6 times the body weight.
3. Walking—1.3 to 5.8 times the body weight.
4. Walking up stairs—3 times the body weight.
5. Running—4.5 times the body weight.

PATIENT HISTORY

In addition to the general history questions presented in Chapter 1, the following information should be determined:

1. What is the patient's usual activity or pastime?
2. Is there any history of trauma to the joint?
3. What are the details of the present pain and other symptoms? Hip pain is felt mainly in the groin and frontal or medial side of the thigh. In this position, the pain may simulate L4 nerve root pain; therefore, the back should also be examined for problems. Hip pain may also be referred to the knee or back and may increase on walking. Snapping heard in the hip is sometimes due to the slipping of the iliopsoas tendon over the osseous ridge of the lesser trochanter. This condition is sometimes referred to as the *snapping hip syndrome.*
4. Is the condition improving? Worsening? Staying the same?
5. Does any type of activity ease the pain or make it worse?
6. What is the age of the patient? Different conditions occur in different age groups, and range of motion decreases with age. For example, congenital hip dysplasia is seen in infancy, primarily in girls; Legg-Calvé-Perthes disease is more frequent in boys 3 to 12 years old; and elderly women are more prone to osteoporotic femoral neck fractures.
7. Are there any movements that the patient feels are weak or abnormal? For example, in *piriformis syndrome*, the sciatic nerve may be compressed, the piriformis muscle is tender, and hip abduction and lateral rotation are weak.

OBSERVATION

When the patient comes into the assessment area, the gait should be observed. If the hip is affected, the weight will be lowered carefully on the affected side and the knee will bend slightly to absorb the shock. The length of the step on the affected side will be shorter so that weight can be taken off the leg quickly. If the hip is stiff, the entire trunk and affected leg swing forward together. It is also important to watch for "balance" of the pelvis on the hip. If there is an imbalance of the flexors or extensors in the sagittal plane, the forward-backward motion of the trunk will be altered to help maintain balance. For example, a bilateral hip flexion contracture causes the lumbar spine to extend to a greater degree (increased lordosis) as a compensating mechanism. Weak extensors will cause the patient to move the trunk backward to maintain balance and avoid falling as a result of the unopposed action of the flexors. If the lateral rotators are significantly stronger than the medial rotators (lateral rotators are normally stronger than the medial rotators), excessive toe-out can result. In addition, the patellae may have a "frog eyes" appearance (turn out). Contracture of either of the rotators may lead to a "pivoting" at the hip during gait.[1] The different types of gait are discussed in greater detail in Chapter 14.

If the patient uses a cane, it should be held in the hand opposite the affected side to negate some of the force of gravity on the affected hip. The use of a cane can decrease the load on the hip as much as 40 per cent.[2]

The patient should be standing and suitably undressed for the examiner to do a proper observation. The following are viewed from the front, side, and behind:

1. Posture. The examiner should watch for pelvic obliquity caused by, for example, unequal leg length, muscle contractures, or scoliosis.

2. Whether the patient can and/or will stand on both legs. Two bathroom scales may be used to indicate asymmetry of weight bearing.

3. Balance. It is important to check the patient's proprioceptive control in the joints being assessed. This control may be done by asking the patient to balance first on one leg (the good one) and then the other leg—first with the eyes open, and then with the eyes closed. Differences should be noted through comparison. Loss of proprioceptive control is especially obvious when the patient's eyes are closed. The use of the stork standing test[1] (Fig. 10–1) has also been advocated for testing proprioception. With both methods, the examiner should watch for a positive Trendelenburg sign, which would negate the proprioceptive tests.

4. Whether the limb positions are equal and symmetric. The position of the limb may indicate the type of injury. With traumatic posterior hip dislocation, the limb is shortened, adducted, and medially rotated, and the greater trochanter is prominent. With an anterior hip dislocation, the limb is ab-

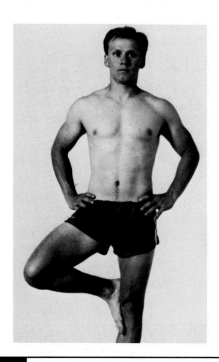

FIGURE 10–1. Stork standing test.

ducted and laterally rotated and may appear cyanotic or swollen owing to pressure in the femoral triangle. With intertrochanteric fractures, the limb is shortened and laterally rotated.

5. Any obvious shortening of a leg.
6. Color and texture of the skin.
7. Any scars or sinuses.
8. The patient's willingness to move.

Anterior View. The examiner should note any abnormality of the bony and soft-tissue contours. With many individuals, differences in these contours may be difficult to detect because of muscle bulk and other soft-tissue deposition. The examiner must therefore look closely. The same is true for swelling. Swelling in the hip joint itself is virtually impossible to detect by observation, and swelling resulting from a psoas or trochanteric bursitis may be easily missed if the examiner is not careful.

Lateral View. When the patient is viewed from the side, the contour of the buttock should be observed for any abnormality. In addition, a hip flexion deformity is best observed from this position. The examiner should take the time to compare the two sides to note any subtle differences.

Posterior View. The position of the hip and the effect, if any, of this position on the spine should be noted. For example, a hip flexion contracture may lead to an increased lumbar lordosis. Any differences in bony and soft-tissue contours should again be noted.

EXAMINATION

When doing an examination of the hip, the examiner must keep in mind that pain may be referred to the hip from the sacroiliac joints and lumbar spine, and vice versa. Thus, the examination may be an extensive one. If there is any doubt as to the location of the lesion, an assessment of the lumbar spine and sacroiliac joints should be performed. It is only through a careful examination of the three areas that the examiner is able to discern the location of the lesion.

As with any examination, the examiner should compare one side of the body with the other, noting any differences. This comparison is necessary because of the individual differences among normal people.

Active Movements

The active movements are done in such a way that the most painful ones are done last. To keep movement of the patient to a minimum, some movements are tested with the patient in the supine position, and others are tested using the prone position. For ease of description, the movements will be described together. When examining the patient, however, the examiner should follow the order as stated in the précis at the end of the chapter.

The following movements should be actively completed in the hip region (Fig. 10–2):

1. Flexion (110 to 120°).
2. Extension (10 to 15°).
3. Abduction (30 to 50°).
4. Adduction (30°).
5. Lateral rotation (40 to 60°).
6. Medial rotation (30 to 40°).

Flexion of the hip normally ranges from 110 to 120° with the knee flexed. The patient's knee is flexed during the test to prevent hamstring tightness from limiting movement.

Extension of the hip normally ranges from 0 to 15°. The patient is in the prone position, and the examiner must ensure that only hip movement is occurring. Patients will have a tendency to extend the lumbar spine, giving the appearance of increased hip extension. This lumbar extension should not be allowed to occur.

Hip abduction normally ranges from 30 to 50° and is tested with the patient in the supine position. Before asking the patient to do the abduction or adduction movement, the examiner should ensure that the patient's pelvis is "balanced"—with the anterior superior iliac spines (ASIS) level and the legs perpendicular to a line joining the two anterior superior iliac spines. The patient is then asked to abduct one leg at a time without pelvic motion. Pelvic motion is detected by palpation of the ASIS and by telling the patient to stop the movement as soon as the ASIS on either side starts to move. When the patient abducts the leg, the opposite ASIS will move first; with an adduction contracture, this will occur earlier in the range of movement.

Hip adduction is normally 30° and is measured from the same starting position. The patient is asked to adduct one leg over the other resting leg while the examiner ensures that the pelvis does not move. An alternate method is for the patient to flex the opposite hip and hold the limb in flexion with the arms. The patient then adducts the test leg. This method is useful only for thin patients. When the patient adducts the leg, the ASIS on the same side will move first. This movement will occur earlier in the range of motion with an abduction contracture. Adduction may also be measured by asking the patient to abduct one leg and leave it abducted. The other leg is then tested for the amount of adduction present. The advantage of this method is that the test leg does not have to be flexed to clear the other leg before doing the adduction movement.

Rotation movements may be performed with the patient supine or prone. Medial rotation normally ranges from 30 to 40°, and lateral rotation normally ranges from 40 to 60°. In the supine position, the patient simply rotates the straight leg on a balanced pelvis. Turning the foot or leg outward tests lateral rotation; turning the foot or leg inward tests medial rotation. In another supine test (Fig. 10–2E), the patient is asked to flex both the hip and knee to 90°. When using this method, however, one must recognize that having the patient rotate the leg out tests medial rotation, whereas having the patient rotate the leg in tests lateral rotation. With the patient prone, the pelvis is balanced by aligning the legs at right angles to a line joining the posterior superior iliac spines (PSIS). The patient then flexes the knee to 90°. Again, medial rotation is being tested when the leg is rotated outward, and lateral rotation is being tested when the leg is rotated inward (Fig. 10–2F). Usually, one of the last two methods is used to measure hip rotation because it is easier to measure the angle when performing the test.

Passive Movements

If the range of movement was not full and the examiner was unable to test end feel during the active movements, passive movements should be performed to determine the end feel and passive range of motion. The passive movements are the same as the active movements. All the movements except extension can be tested with the patient in the supine lying position.

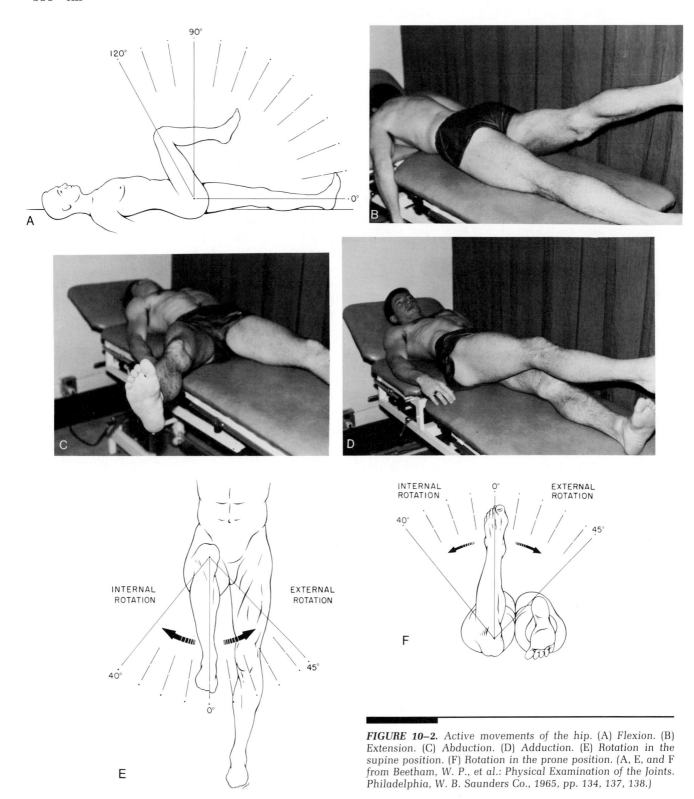

FIGURE 10–2. Active movements of the hip. (A) Flexion. (B) Extension. (C) Abduction. (D) Adduction. (E) Rotation in the supine position. (F) Rotation in the prone position. (A, E, and F from Beetham, W. P., et al.: Physical Examination of the Joints. Philadelphia, W. B. Saunders Co., 1965, pp. 134, 137, 138.)

The capsular pattern of the hip is flexion, abduction, and medial rotation. These movements are always the ones most limited in a capsular pattern, although the order of restriction may vary. For example, medial rotation may be most limited, followed by flexion and abduction. The hip joint is the only joint to exhibit this altered pattern of the same movements.

The normal end feels the examiner should find on passive movements of the hip are as follows:

1. Flexion—tissue approximation or tissue stretch.
2. Extension—tissue stretch.
3. Abduction—tissue stretch.
4. Adduction—tissue approximation or tissue stretch.

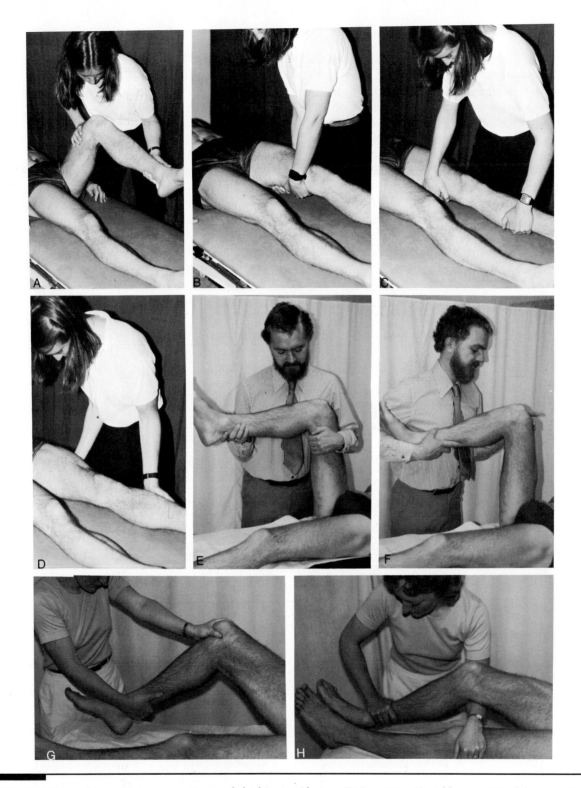

FIGURE 10–3. *Resisted isometric movements around the hip.* (A) *Flexion.* (B) *Extension.* (C) *Adduction.* (D) *Abduction.* (E) *Medial rotation.* (F) *Lateral rotation.* (G) *Knee flexion.* (H) *Knee extension.*

5. Medial rotation—tissue stretch.
6. Lateral rotation—tissue stretch.

Intra-abdominal inflammation in the lower pelvis, as in the case of an abscess, may elicit pain on passive medial and lateral rotation of the hip when the patient is supine with the hip and knee at 90°.

During hip movements, the pelvis should not move. Groin discomfort and a limited range of mo-tion on medial rotation are good indications of hip problems.

Resisted Isometric Movements

The resisted isometric movements are done with the patient in the supine position (Fig. 10–3). Because the hip muscles are very strong, the examiner should position the patient's hip properly and say to the patient, "Don't let me move your hip," to ensure that the movement is isometric. By carefully noting which movements cause pain or show weakness when the tests are done isometrically, the examiner should be able to determine which muscle, if any, is at fault. For example, the gluteus maximus is the only muscle that is involved in all of the following movements: extension, adduction, and lateral rotation. As with active movements, the most painful movements are performed last.

The movements tested isometrically are as follows:

1. Flexion of the hip.
2. Extension of the hip.
3. Abduction of the hip.
4. Adduction of the hip.
5. Medial rotation of the hip.
6. Lateral rotation of the hip.
7. Flexion of the knee.
8. Extension of the knee.

Resisted isometric flexion and extension of the knee must be performed because there are two joint muscles (hamstrings and rectus femoris) that act over the knee as well as the hip. The examiner must be aware that intra-abdominal inflammation in the

TABLE 10–1. Muscles of the Hip: Their Action, Innervation, and Nerve Root Deviation

Action	Muscle Involved	Innervation	Nerve Root Deviation
Flexion of hip	1. Psoas	L1–L3	L1–L3
	2. Iliacus	Femoral	L2–L3
	3. Rectus femoris	Femoral	L2–L4
	4. Sartorius	Femoral	L2–L3
	5. Pectineus	Femoral	L2–L3
	6. Adductor longus	Obturator	L2–L4
	7. Adductor brevis	Obturator	L2–L3, L5
	8. Gracilis	Obturator	L2–L3
Extension of hip	1. Biceps femoris	Sciatic	L5, S1–S2
	2. Semimembranosus	Sciatic	L5, S1–S2
	3. Semitendinosus	Sciatic	L5, S1–S2
	4. Gluteus maximus	Inferior gluteal	L5, S1–S2
	5. Gluteus medius (posterior part)	Superior gluteal	L5, S1
	6. Adductor magnus (ischio-condylar part)	Sciatic	L2–L4
Abduction of hip	1. Tensor fasciae latae	Superior gluteal	L4–L5
	2. Gluteus minimus	Superior gluteal	L5, S1
	3. Gluteus medius	Superior gluteal	L5, S1
	4. Gluteus maximus	Inferior gluteal	L5, S1–S2
	5. Sartorius	Femoral	L2–L3
Adduction of hip	1. Adductor longus	Obturator	L2–L4
	2. Adductor brevis	Obturator	L2–L4
	3. Adductor magnus (ischio-femoral portion)	Obturator	L2–L4
	4. Gracilis	Obturator	L2–L3
	5. Pectineus	Femoral	L2–L3
Medial rotation of hip	1. Adductor longus	Obturator	L2–L4
	2. Adductor brevis	Obturator	L2–L4
	3. Adductor magnus	Obturator and sciatic	L2–L4
	4. Gluteus medius (anterior part)	Superior gluteal	L5, S1
	5. Gluteus minimus (anterior part)	Superior gluteal	L5, S1
	6. Tensor fasciae latae	Superior gluteal	L4–L5
	7. Pectineus	Femoral	L2–L3
	8. Gracilis	Obturator	L2–L3
Lateral rotation of hip	1. Gluteus maximus	Inferior gluteal	L5, S1–S2
	2. Obturator internus	N. to obturator internus	L5, S1
	3. Obturator externus	Obturator	L3–L4
	4. Quadratus femoris	N. to quadratus femoris	L5, S1
	5. Piriformis	L5, S1–S2	L5, S1–S2
	6. Gemellus superior	N. to obturator internus	L5, S1
	7. Gemellus inferior	N. to quadratus femoris	L5, S1
	8. Sartorius	Femoral	L2–L3
	9. Gluteus medius (posterior part)	Superior gluteal	L5, S1

area of the psoas muscle may elicit pain on resisted hip flexion. The pain from intra-abdominal inflammation will not present in a subacute infection or with a rigid abdominal wall. Refer to Table 10–1 for the muscles that act on the hip.

Functional Assessment

Hip motion is necessary for more activities than just ambulation. In fact, more hip motion is required for daily living activities than is required for gait. Activities such as shoe tying, sitting, getting up from a chair, and picking things up from the floor all require a greater range of motion. Table 10–2 illustrates the ranges of motion necessary for various activities. Ideally, the patient should have functional ranges of 120° of flexion, 20° of abduction, and 20° of lateral rotation.

There are several scales with which to rate hip function. These rating methods are primarily based on pain, mobility, and gait. Tables 10–3 through 10–7 illustrate three different rating scales. D'Aubigne and Postel (Tables 10–3 through 10–5) developed one of the first hip rating scales based on pain, mobility, and ability to walk. The Harris hip rating scale (Table 10–6) is useful for rating hips before and after surgery. This scale is most often used because it emphasizes pain and function. The Iowa scale (Table 10–7) provides a single rating figure. Table 10–8 gives a functional strength and endurance testing scheme for the hip.

If the patient is able to perform normal active movements with little difficulty, the examiner may use a series of *functional tests* to determine if in-

TABLE 10–2. Range of Motion Necessary at the Hip for Selected Activities

Activity	Average Range of Motion Necessary
Shoe tying	120° of flexion
Sitting (average seat height)	112° of flexion
Stooping	125° of flexion
Squatting	115° of flexion/20° of abduction/20° of medial rotation
Ascending stairs (average stair height)	67° of flexion
Descending stairs (average stair height)	36° of flexion
Putting foot on opposite thigh	120° of flexion/20° of abduction/20° of lateral rotation
Putting on trousers	90° of flexion

creased intensity of activity produces pain or other symptoms. The functional activities in order of sequence are as follows:

1. Squatting.
2. Going up and down stairs one at a time.
3. Crossing the legs so that the ankle of one foot rests on the knee of the opposite leg.
4. Going up and down stairs two or more at a time.
5. Running straight ahead.
6. Running and twisting.
7. Jumping.

These tests must be geared to the individual patient. Older individuals should not be expected to perform the last four activities unless they have been doing these movements or similar ones in the recent past.

TABLE 10–3. Method of Grading Functional Value of Hip*

Grade	Pain	Mobility	Ability to Walk
0	Pain is intense and permanent	Ankylosis with bad position of the hip	None
1	Pain is severe, even at night	No movement; pain or slight deformity	Only with crutches
2	Pain is severe when walking; prevents any activity	Flexion less than 40°	Only with canes
3	Pain is tolerable with limited activity	Flexion between 40° and 60°	With one cane, for less than 1 hour; very difficult without a cane
4	Pain is mild when walking; it disappears with rest	Flexion between 60° and 80°; patient can reach own foot	A long time with a cane; a short time without cane and with limp
5	Pain is mild and inconstant; normal activity	Flexion between 80° and 90°; abduction at least 15°	Without cane but with slight limp
6	No pain	Flexion more than 90°; abduction to 30°	Normal

*Values used in conjunction with Table 10–4.
From D'Aubigne, R. M., and M. Postel: J. Bone Joint Surg. *36A*:451–457, 1954.

TABLE 10–7. Iowa Functional Hip Evaluation

Chart 1	Chart 2

Chart 1

Date _____

Name _____ Age _____

100-Point Scale for Hip Evaluation

Total points _____

Function (35 points)
Does most of housework or job that
requires moving about 5
Dresses unaided (includes tying shoes and
putting on socks) 5
Walks enough to be independent 5
Sits with difficulty at table or toilet 4
Picks up objects from floor by squatting 3
Bathes without help 3
Negotiates stairs foot over foot 3
Carries objects comparable to suitcase 2
Gets into car or public conveyance unaided and rides
comfortably 2
Drives a car 1
_____

Freedom From Pain (35 points) (circle 1 only)
No pain 35
Pain only with fatigue 30
Pain only with weight-bearing 20
Pain at rest but not with weight-bearing 15
Pain sitting or in bed 10
Continuous pain 0
_____

Gait (10 points) (circle 1 only)
No limp; no support 10
No limp using cane 8
Abductor limp 8
Short leg limp 8
Needs two canes 6
Needs two crutches 4
Cannot walk 0
_____

Absence of Deformity (10 points)
No fixed flexion over 30° 3
No fixed adduction over 10° 3
No fixed rotation over 10° 2
Not over 1″ shortening (ASIS-MM)* 2
_____

Range of Motion (10 points)
Flexion-extension (normal 140°) .... ___°
Abduction-adduction (normal 80°) .... ___°
External-internal rotation (normal 80°) .... ___°
　　　　Total degrees .... ___°
　　　　Points (1 point/30°) .... ___°
_____

Muscle Strength (no points)
Straight leg raising:
Less than gravity _____Gravity _____
Gravity + resistance _____
Abduction:
Less than gravity _____Gravity _____
Gravity + resistance _____
Extension:
Less than gravity _____Gravity _____
Gravity + resistance _____
　　　TOTAL (100 points maximum) _____

Chart 2

Name _____ Diagnosis _____
Age _____ Sex _____ Date of operation _____
Date of follow-up _____
Previous surgery: Date _____ Type _____
Subsequent surgery: Date _____ Type _____

Pain　　　　　　　　　　　　　　　　　　40%
　None 40
　Pain with fatigue 35
　Pain with weight-bearing:
　　Mild 30
　　Moderate 20
　　Severe 10
　Persistence with non–weight-bearing .... 10 (less than above)
　Continuous pain 0

Ability to Function　　　　　　　　　　　30%
　Work and household duties:
　　Full day, usual occupation 10
　　Modified work or duties 6
　　Severe restriction of work or duties 2
　Walking tolerances:
　　Long distances 10
　　Short distances 6
　　Two blocks or less 1
　Self-reliance:
　　Dresses self unaided 3
　　Help with shoes and socks 2
　　Sit at table and toilet 3
　Stairs:
　　Normal 2
　　One at a time 1
　　Gets into car or public conveyance without
　　　difficulty 2

Gait　　　　　　　　　　　　　　　　　　15%
　No limp, no support 15
　No limp, with cane 12
　Limp, mild, without cane 12
　Limp, mild, with cane 9
　Limp, moderate, without cane or crutch 9
　Limp, moderate, with cane or crutch 6
　Limp, severe, without cane or crutch 3
　Limp, severe, with cane or crutch 2
　Two canes or crutches 1

Anatomic Assessment　　　　　　　　　　15%
　A. Motion:
　　Flexion—up to 80° in range 0–100° × 0.1 ... 8
　　Abduction—up to 20° in range 0–30° × 0.1 .. 2
　B. Shortening:
　　None—½″ 3
　　½″–1″ 2
　　1″–2″ 1
　C. Trendelenburg—absent 2
　　　　　　　　　　　　　　　　　　　100%

Modified from Larson, C. B.: Clin. Orthop. *31*: 85–93, 1963.
*ASIS-MM = anterior superior iliac spine—medial malleolus.

TABLE 10–8. Functional Strength Testing of the Hip*

Starting Position	Action	Functional Test
Standing	Lift foot onto 20-cm step and return (hip flexion-extension)	5 to 6 Repetitions: Functional 3 to 4 Repetitions: Functionally fair 1 to 2 Repetitions: Functionally poor 0 Repetitions: Nonfunctional
Standing	Sit in chair and return to standing (hip extension-flexion)	5 to 6 Repetitions: Functional 3 to 4 Repetitions: Functionally fair 1 to 2 Repetitions: Functionally poor 0 Repetitions: Nonfunctional
Standing	Lift leg to balance on one leg keeping pelvis straight (hip abduction)	Hold 1 to 1.5 minutes: Functional Hold 30 to 59 seconds: Functionally fair Hold 1 to 29 seconds: Functionally poor Cannot hold: Nonfunctional
Standing	Walk sideways 6 m (hip adduction)	6 to 8 m one way: Functional 3 to 6 m one way: Functionally fair 1 to 3 m one way: Functionally poor 0 m: Nonfunctional
Standing	Test leg off floor (patient may hold onto something for balance) medially rotate non–weight-bearing hip	10 to 12 Repetitions: Functional 5 to 9 Repetitions: Functionally fair 1 to 4 Repetitions: Functionally poor 0 Repetitions: Nonfunctional
Standing	Test leg off floor (patient may hold onto something for balance) laterally rotate non–weight-bearing hip	10 to 12 Repetitions: Functional 5 to 9 Repetitions: Functionally fair 1 to 4 Repetitions: Functionally poor 0 Repetitions: Nonfunctional

*Adapted from Palmer, M. L., and M. Epler: Clinical Assessment Procedures in Physical Therapy. Philadelphia, J. B. Lippincott, 1990, p. 251–254.

Special Tests

Only those tests that the examiner feels are necessary should be performed. However, when assessing the hip, Patrick's test, Trendelenburg's test, and one of the leg length tests are usually performed. Other tests are done primarily to confirm a diagnosis or determine pathology.

Tests for Hip Pathology

Patrick's Test (Faber or Figure-4 Test). The patient lies supine, and the examiner places the patient's test leg so that the foot of the test leg is on top of the knee of the opposite leg (Fig. 10–4). The examiner then slowly lowers the test leg in abduction toward the examining table. A negative test is indicated by the test leg's falling to the table or at least being parallel with the opposite leg. A positive test is indicated by the test leg's remaining above the opposite straight leg. If positive, the test indicates that the hip joint may be affected, there may be iliopsoas spasm, or the sacroiliac joint may be affected. *Faber* (which stands for *f*lexion, *ab*duction, and *e*xternal *r*otation) is the position of the hip when the patient begins the test.

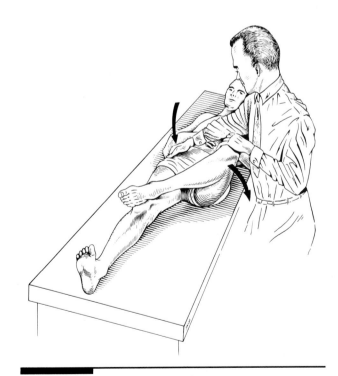

FIGURE 10–4. *Patrick's test (Faber or Figure-4 test) for the detection of limitation of motion in the hip. (From Beetham, W. P., et al.: Physical Examination of the Joints. Philadelphia, W. B. Saunders Co., 1965, p. 139.)*

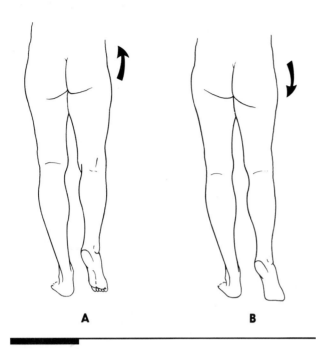

FIGURE 10–5. Trendelenburg sign. (A) Negative test. (B) Positive test.

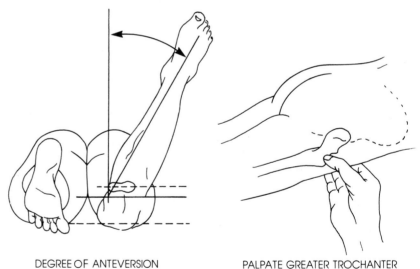

FIGURE 10–6. Craig's test for femoral anteversion.

DEGREE OF ANTEVERSION

PALPATE GREATER TROCHANTER PARALLEL TO TABLE

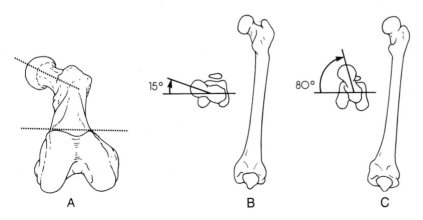

FIGURE 10–7. Anteversion of the hip. (A) Femoral anteversion angle. (From the American Orthopaedic Association: Manual of Orthopaedic Surgery. Chicago, 1979, p. 45.) (B) Normal angle. (C) Excessive angle.

Trendelenburg's Test. This test assesses the stability of the hip and the ability of the hip abductors to stabilize the pelvis on the femur. The patient is asked to stand on one lower limb. Normally, the pelvis on the opposite side should rise; this finding indicates a negative test (Fig. 10–5). If the pelvis on the opposite side drops when the patient is asked to stand on the affected leg, a positive test is indicated. The test should always be performed on the normal side first so that the patient understands what to do. If the pelvis drops on the opposite side, it indicates a weak gluteus medius or an unstable hip on the affected side (for example, as a result of hip dislocation).

Craig's Test. Craig's test measures femoral anteversion or forward torsion of the femur (Fig. 10–6). Anteversion of the hip is the angle made by the femoral neck with the femoral condyles (Fig. 10–7). It is the degree of forward projection of the femoral neck from the coronal plane of the shaft (Fig. 10–8), and it decreases with age. For example, at birth, the mean angle is approximately 30°; in the adult, the mean angle is 8 to 15° (Fig. 10–9). Increased anteversion will lead to squinting patellae and toeing-in. Excessive anteversion is twice as common in girls as in boys. A common clinical finding of excessive anteversion is excessive medial hip rotation (more than 60°) and decreased lateral rotation. In *retroversion*, the plane of the femoral neck rotates backward in relation to the coronal condylar plane.[3–6]

For Craig's test, the patient lies prone with the knee flexed to 90°. The examiner palpates the posterior aspect of the greater trochanter of the femur. The hip is then passively medially and laterally rotated until the greater trochanter is parallel with the examining table or reaches its most lateral position. The degree of anteversion can then be estimated, based on the angle of the lower leg with the vertical. The test is also called the *Ryder method* for measuring anteversion or retroversion.

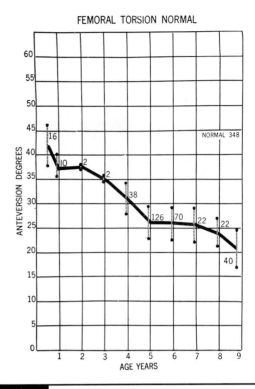

FEMORAL TORSION NORMAL

FIGURE 10–9. *The degree of normal femoral torsion in relation to age. Solid lines represent the mean; vertical lines represent the standard deviation. (From Crane, L.: J. Bone Joint Surg. 41A:423, 1959.)*

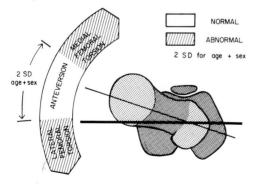

FIGURE 10–8. *Axial view of right femur showing approximately normal angle of anteversion and torsional deformity beyond. (From Staheli, L. T.: Orthop. Clin. North Am. 11:40, 1980.)*

Torque Test. The patient lies supine close to the edge of the examining table with the femur of the test leg extended over the edge of the table. The test leg is extended until the pelvis begins to move. The examiner uses one hand to medially rotate the femur to the end of range and the other hand to apply a slow posterolateral pressure along the line of the neck of femur for 20 seconds to stress the capsular ligaments and test the stability of the hip joint (Fig. 10–10).[7]

Nélaton's Line. Nélaton's line is an imaginary line drawn from the ischial tuberosity of the pelvis to the ASIS of the pelvis on the same side (Fig. 10–11).[3] If the greater trochanter of the femur is palpated well above the line, it is an indication of a dislocated hip or coxa vara. The two sides should be compared.

Bryant's Triangle. With the patient lying supine, the examiner drops an imaginary perpendicular line from the ASIS of the pelvis to the examining table.[5] A second imaginary line is projected up from the tip of the greater trochanter of the femur to meet the first line at a right angle (Fig. 10–12). This line is measured, and the two sides are compared for coxa vara, dislocated hip, and so on. This measurement can be done with radiographs, in which case the lines may be drawn on the radiograph.

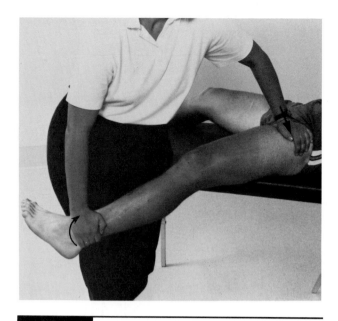

FIGURE 10–10. Torque test.

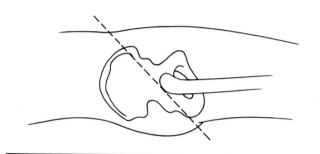

FIGURE 10–11. Nélaton's line.

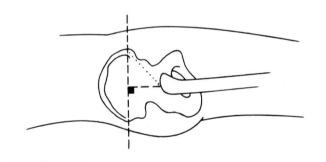

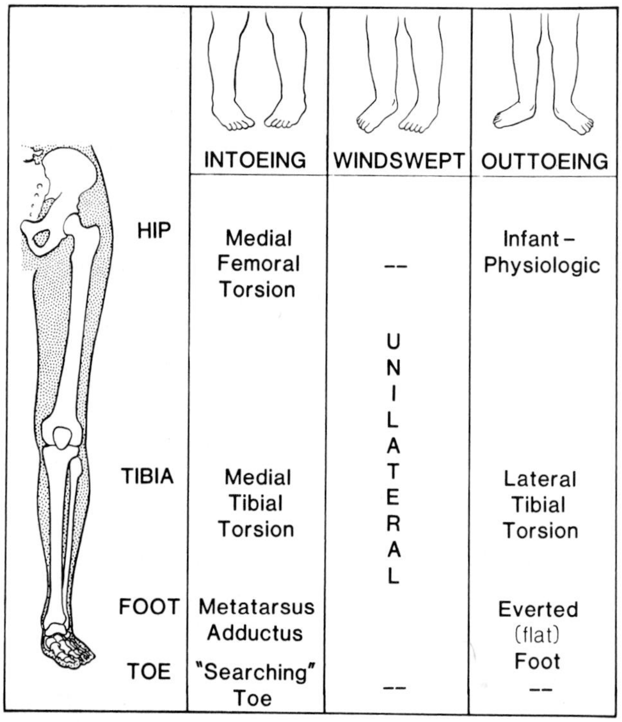

FIGURE 10–12. Bryant's triangle.

		INTOEING	WINDSWEPT	OUTTOEING
HIP		Medial Femoral Torsion	--	Infant– Physiologic
TIBIA		Medial Tibial Torsion	U N I L A T E R A L	Lateral Tibial Torsion
FOOT		Metatarsus Adductus		Everted (flat) Foot
TOE		"Searching" Toe	--	--

FIGURE 10–13. Rotational deformities in the lower limb. (From Staheli, L. T.: Paediatr. Clin. North Am. 33:1373–1383, 1986.)

Rotational Deformities. Rotational deformities can occur anywhere between the hip and the foot (Fig. 10–13). Many of these deformities are hereditary. The patient lies supine with the lower limbs straight while the examiner looks at the patellae.[4] If the patellae face in ("squinting" patellae), it is an indication of medial rotation of the femur or lateral rotation of the tibia. If the patellae face up, out, and away from each other ("frog eyes" or "grasshopper eyes"), it is an indication of lateral rotation of the femur or medial rotation of the tibia. If the tibia is affected, the feet will face in ("pigeon toes") for medial rotation and face out more than 10° for excessive lateral rotation of the tibia (Fig. 10–14).

Normally, the feet angle out 5 to 10° (Fick angle) for better balance.

Pediatric Tests for Hip Pathology

Ortolani's Sign. The Ortolani test can determine whether an infant has a congenital dislocation of the hip (Fig. 10–15A and B).[4] With the infant supine, the examiner flexes the hips and grasps the legs so that the thumbs are against the insides of the knees and thighs and the fingers are placed along the outsides of the thighs to the buttocks. With gentle traction, the thighs are abducted, and pressure is applied against the greater trochanters of the

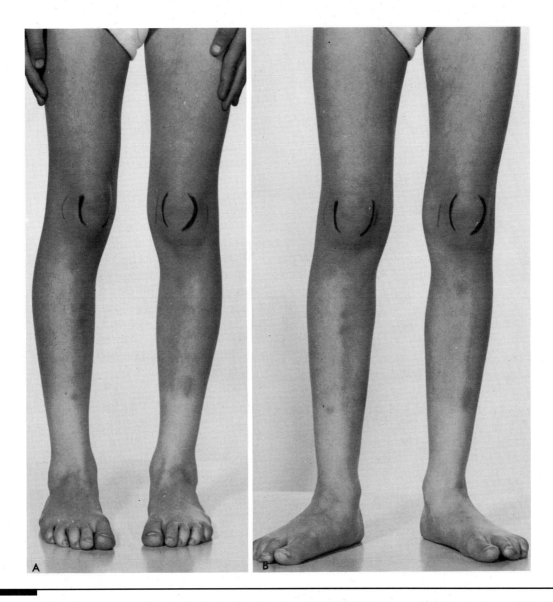

FIGURE 10–14. *Clinical appearance of excessive femoral torsion in a girl. (A) With the knees in full extension and the feet aligned (pointing straight forward), the legs appear bowed and the patellae face inward (squinting patella). (B) Upon lateral rotation of the hips so that the patellae are facing to the front, the feet and legs point outward and the bowleg appearance is corrected. (From Tachdjian, M. O.: Pediatric Orthopedics. Philadelphia, W. B. Saunders Co., 1990, p. 2802.)*

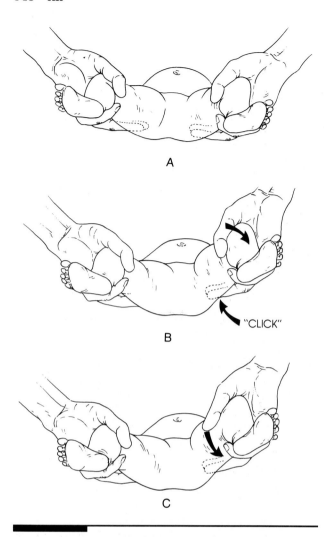

A

B

"CLICK"

C

FIGURE 10–15. *Ortolani's sign and Barlow's test. In the newborn, the two hips can be equally flexed, abducted, and externally rotated without producing a "click." (A) Normal. (B) Ortolani's sign or first part of Barlow's test. (C) Second part of Barlow's test.*

femora. Resistance will begin to be felt to abduction and lateral rotation at approximately 30 to 40°. The examiner may feel a "click," "clunk," or "jerk," which indicates a positive test and that the hip has reduced; in addition, increased abduction of the hip will be obtained. The femoral head has slipped over the acetabular ridge into the acetabulum, and normal abduction of 70 to 90° can be obtained.

This test is valid only for the first few weeks after birth and only for dislocated and lax hips, not for dislocations that are difficult to reduce. The examiner should take care to feel the quality of the click. Soft clicks may occur without dislocation and are thought to be due to the iliofemoral ligament's clicking over the anterior surface of the head of the femur as it is laterally rotated. Soft clicking usually occurs without the prior resistance that is seen with dislocations. By repeated rotation of the hip, the exact location of the click can be palpated. However,

Ortolani's test should not be repeated too often because it could lead to damage of the articular cartilage of the femoral head.

Barlow's Test. Barlow's test is a modification of Ortolani's test[4] (Fig. 10–15A, B, and C). The infant lies supine with the legs facing the examiner. The hips are flexed to 90°, and the knees are fully flexed. Each hip is evaluated individually while the examiner's other hand steadies the opposite femur and the pelvis. The examiner's middle finger of each hand is placed over the greater trochanter, and the thumb is placed adjacent to the inner side of the knee and thigh opposite the lesser trochanter. The hip is taken into abduction while the examiner's middle finger applies forward pressure behind the greater trochanter. If the femoral head slips forward into the acetabulum with a click, clunk, or jerk, the test is positive, indicating that the hip was dislocated. This part of the test is identical to Ortolani's test. The examiner then uses the thumb to apply pressure backward and outward on the inner thigh. If the femoral head slips out over the posterior lip of the acetabulum and then reduces again when pressure is removed, the hip is classified as "unstable." The hip is not dislocated but is dislocatable. The procedure is repeated for the other hip.

This test may be used for infants up to 6 months of age. It should not be repeated too often because it may result in a dislocated hip as well as articular damage to the head of the femur.

Galeazzi's Sign (Allis' Test). The Galeazzi test is good only for assessing unilateral congenital dislocation of the hip and may be used in children from 3 to 18 months of age. The child lies supine with the knees flexed and the hips flexed to 90°. A positive test is indicated by one knee being higher than the other (Fig. 10–16).

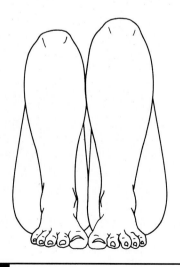

FIGURE 10–16. *Galeazzi's sign (Allis' test).*

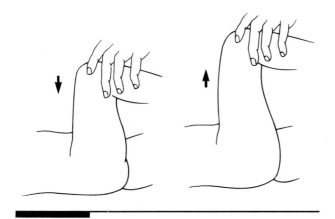

FIGURE 10–17. Telescoping of the hip.

Telescoping Sign. The telescoping sign is evident in a child with a dislocated hip. The child lies in the supine position. The examiner flexes the knee and hip to 90°. The femur is pushed down onto the examining table. The femur and leg are then lifted up and away from the table (Fig. 10–17). With the normal hip, little movement occurs with this action. With the dislocated hip, however, there will be a lot of relative movement. This excessive movement is called *telescoping*, or *pistoning*.

Tests for Leg Length

True Leg Length. Before any measuring is done, the examiner must set the pelvis square, level, or balanced with the lower limbs.[8–10] The legs should be 15 to 20 cm apart and parallel to each other (Fig. 10–18). If the legs are not placed in proper relation to the pelvis, apparent shortening of the limb may occur. The lower limbs must be placed in comparable positions relative to the pelvis, because abduction of the hip brings the medial malleolus closer to

the ASIS on that side and adduction of the hip takes the medial malleolus further from the ASIS on that side. If one hip is fixed in abduction or adduction as a result of contracture or some other cause, the normal hip should be adducted or abducted an equal amount to ensure accurate leg length measurement.

In North America, leg length measurement is usually taken from the ASIS to the medial malleolus; however, these values may be altered by muscle wasting or obesity. Measuring to the lateral malleolus is less likely to be affected by the muscle bulk. To obtain the leg length, the examiner measures from the ASIS to the lateral malleolus. The flat metal end of the tape measure is placed immediately distal to the ASIS and pushed up against it. The thumb then presses the tape end firmly against the bone, rigidly fixing the tape measure against the bone. The index finger of the other hand is placed immediately distal to the lateral malleolus and pushed against it. The thumbnail is brought down against the tip of the index finger so that the tape measure is pinched between them. A slight difference (as much as 1 to 1.5 cm) is considered normal; however, this difference can still cause symptoms.

The *Weber-Barstow maneuver* may also be used to measure leg length asymmetry. The patient lies supine with the hips and knees flexed (Fig. 10–19). The examiner stands at the patient's feet and palpates the distal aspect of the medial malleoli with the thumbs. The patient then lifts the pelvis from the examining table and returns to the starting position. Next, the examiner passively extends the patient's legs and compares the positions of the malleoli using the borders of the thumbs. Different levels indicate asymmetry.[11]

If one leg is shorter than the other (Fig. 10–20), the examiner can determine where the difference is by measuring the following:

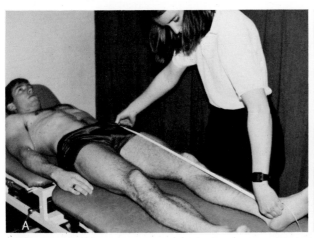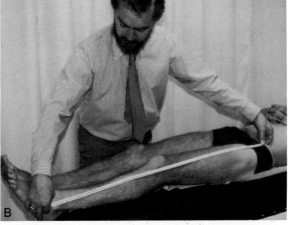

FIGURE 10–18. Measuring true leg length. (A) Measuring to the medial malleolus. (B) Measuring to the lateral malleolus.

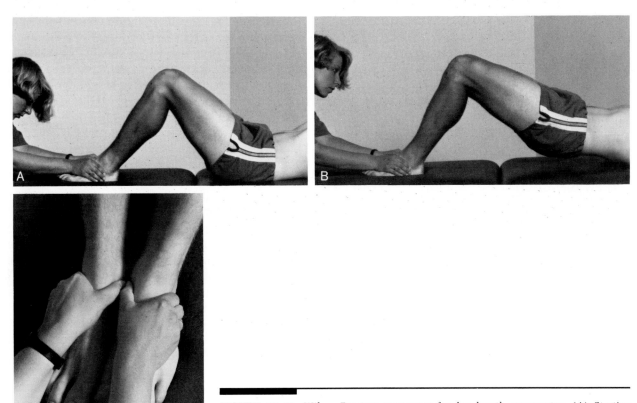

FIGURE 10–19. Wilson-Barstow maneuver for leg length asymmetry. (A) Starting position. (B) Patient lifts hips off bed. (C) Comparing height of medial malleoli.

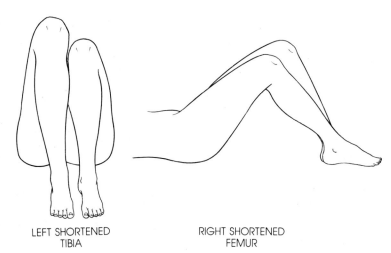

FIGURE 10–20. Leg length discrepancy.

LEFT SHORTENED TIBIA

RIGHT SHORTENED FEMUR

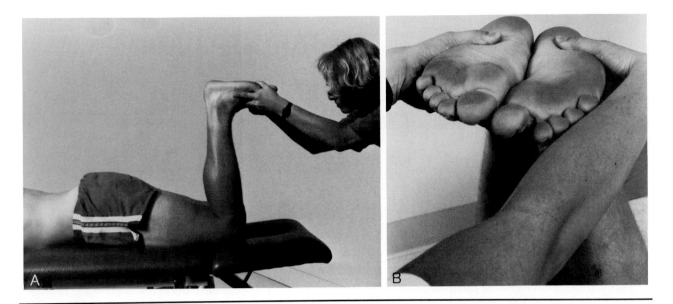

FIGURE 10–21. *Prone knee flexion test for tibial shortening. The prone knee flexion test is completed as the examiner (A) passively flexes the patient's knees to 90° and (B) sights through the plane of the heel pads to see whether a change in position has occurred.*

1. From the iliac crest to the greater trochanter of the femur (for coxa vara or coxa valga).
2. From the greater trochanter of the femur to the knee joint line on the lateral aspect (for femoral shaft shortening).
3. From the knee joint line on the medial side to the medial malleolus (for tibial shaft shortening).

The relative length of the tibia may also be tested with the patient lying prone. The examiner places the thumbs transversely across the soles of the feet just in front of the heels. The knees are flexed 90°,

and the relative heights of the thumbs are noted. Care must be taken to ensure that the legs are perpendicular to the examining table[11] (Fig. 10–21).

Apparent or functional shortening (Fig. 10–22) of the leg is evident if the patient has a lateral pelvic tilt when the measurement is taken. When measuring apparent leg length shortening, the examiner obtains the distance from the tip of the xiphi sternum or umbilicus to the medial malleolus. Values obtained by these measurements may be affected by muscle wasting, obesity, and asymmetric position of the xiphi sternum or umbilicus.

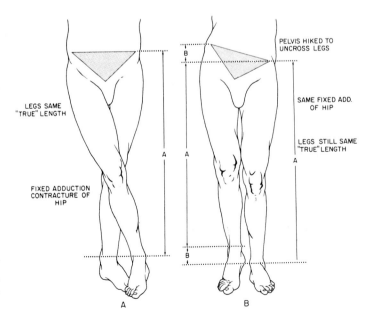

FIGURE 10–22. *Functional shortening. (From the American Orthopaedic Association: Manual of Orthopaedic Surgery. Chicago, 1972, p. 45.)*

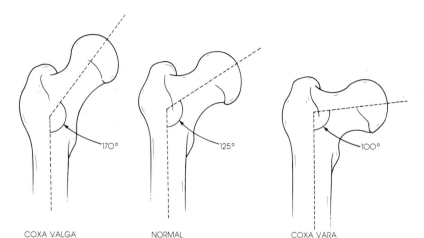

COXA VALGA   NORMAL   COXA VARA

FIGURE 10–23. Neck-shaft angles of the femur in adults.

The neck-shaft angle of the femur (Fig. 10–23) is normally from 150 to 160° at birth and decreases to from 120 to 135° in the adult (Fig. 10–24). If this angle is less than 120° in an adult, it is known as *coxa vara*; if it is more than 135° in the adult, it is known as *coxa valga*.

Standing (Functional) Leg Length. The patient is first assessed while in a relaxed stance. In this position, the examiner palpates the ASIS and the PSIS, noting any asymmetry. The examiner then places the patient in a symmetric stance ensuring that the subtalar joint is in neutral position (see Chapter 12), the toes are facing straight ahead, and the knees are extended. The ASIS and PSIS are again assessed for asymmetry. If differences are still noted, the examiner should check for structural leg length differences, sacroiliac joint dysfunction, and weak gluteus medius or quadratus lumborum.

Tests for Muscle Tightness on Pathology

Sign of the Buttock. The patient lies supine and the examiner performs a straight leg raising test. If there is limitation on the straight leg raise, the examiner then flexes the patient's knee to see if further hip flexion can be obtained. If hip flexion does not increase, the lesion is in the buttock and not in the hip, sciatic nerve, or hamstring muscles. There may also be some limited trunk flexion. Causes of a positive test include bursitis, a neoplasm, or an abscess in the buttock.

Thomas Test. The Thomas test is used to assess a hip flexion contracture, the most common contracture of the hip. The patient lies supine while the examiner checks for excessive lordosis, which is usually present with tight hip flexors. The examiner flexes one of the patient's hips, bringing the knee to the chest to flatten out the lumbar spine, and the patient holds the flexed hip against the chest. If there is no flexion contracture, the hip being tested (the straight leg) will remain on the examining table. If a contracture is present, the patient's straight leg will rise off the table (Fig. 10–25). The angle of contracture can be measured. If the lower limb is pushed down onto the table, the patient may exhibit an increased lordosis; again, this result indicates a positive test.

Rectus Femoris Contracture Test (Method 1). The patient lies supine with the knees bent over the end or edge of the examining table. The patient flexes one knee onto the chest and holds it (Fig. 10–26). The angle of the test knee should remain at 90°

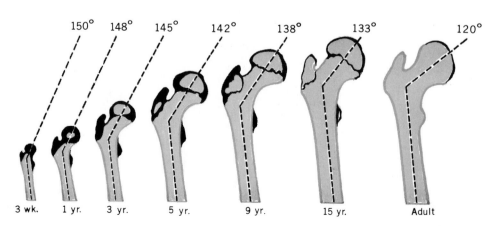

3 wk.   1 yr.   3 yr.   5 yr.   9 yr.   15 yr.   Adult

150°   148°   145°   142°   138°   133°   120°

FIGURE 10–24. Mean angle of the femoral neck-shaft in different age groups. (Modified from von Lanz, T., and W. Wachsmuth: Praktische Anatomie. Berlin, Julius Springer, 1938, p. 143.)

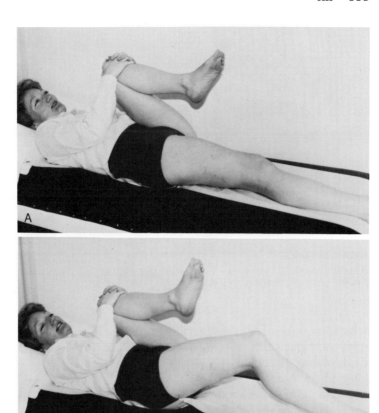

FIGURE 10–25. Thomas test. (A) Negative test. (B) Positive test.

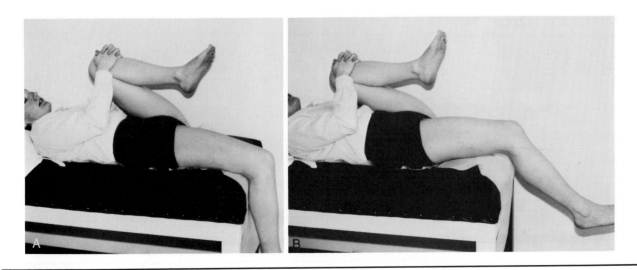

FIGURE 10–26. Rectus femoris contracture. (A) The movement leg is brought to the chest. The test leg remains bent over the end of the examining table, indicating a negative test. (B) The right knee extends, indicating a positive test.

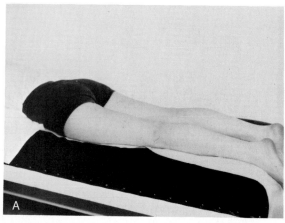
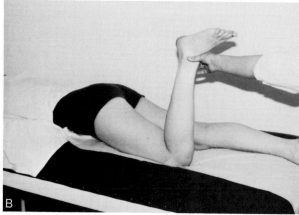

FIGURE 10–27. *Ely's test for a tight rectus femoris. (A) Position for the test. (B) Posture test shown by hip flexion when the knee is flexed.*

when the opposite knee is flexed to the chest. If it does not (i.e., the test knee extends slightly), a contracture is probably present. The examiner may attempt to passively flex the knee to see whether it will remain at 90° of its own volition. The examiner should always palpate for muscle tightness when doing any contracture test. If there is no palpable tightness, the probable cause of restriction is tight joint structures (e.g., the capsule). The two sides should be tested and compared.

Ely's Test (Tight Rectus Femoris) (Method 2). The patient lies prone, and the examiner passively flexes the patient's knee (Fig. 10–27).[12] On flexion of the knee, the patient's hip on the same side will spontaneously flex, indicating that the rectus femoris muscle is tight on that side and that the test is

positive. The two sides should be tested and compared.

Ober's Test. Ober's test assesses tensor fasciae latae (iliotibial band) for contracture (Fig. 10–28).[13] The patient is in the side lying position with the lower leg flexed at the hip and knee for stability. The examiner then passively abducts and extends the patient's upper leg with the knee straight or flexed to 90°. The examiner slowly lowers the upper limb; if a contracture is present, the leg will remain abducted and will not fall to the table. When doing this test, it is important to extend the hip slightly so that the iliotibial band passes over the greater trochanter of the femur. To do this, the examiner stabilizes the pelvis at the same time to stop the pelvis from "falling backward." Ober originally de-

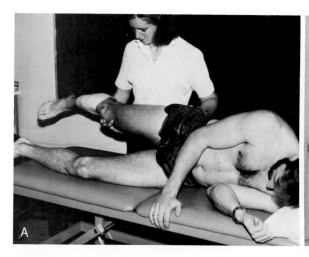
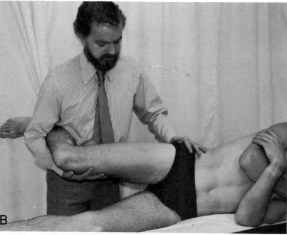

FIGURE 10–28. *Ober's test. (A) Knees straight. The hip is passively extended by the examiner to ensure that the tensor fasciae latae runs over the greater trochanter. A positive test is indicated when the leg remains abducted while the patient's muscles are relaxed. (B) Knee flexed.*

scribed the test with the knee flexed.[13] However, the iliotibial band has a greater stretch placed on it when the knee is extended.

Adduction Contracture Test. The patient lies supine with the anterior superior iliac spines level. If a contracture is present, the affected leg will form an angle of less than 90° with the line joining the two anterior superior iliac spines. If the examiner then attempts to "balance" the lower limb with the pelvis, the pelvis will shift up on the affected side or down on the unaffected side, and balancing will not be possible. This type of contracture can lead to functional shortening of the limb rather than true shortening.

In individuals, especially children, with adductor spasticity, abduction is performed quickly by the examiner. The patient is supine. If there is a "grab" or kicking in of the stretch reflex at less than 30°, the test for adductor spasticity is positive. The test should be repeated with the knee flexed to rule out medial hamstring contracture.[14]

Abduction Contracture Test. The patient lies supine with the anterior superior iliac spines level. If a contracture is present, the affected leg will form an angle of more than 90° with a line joining each ASIS. If the examiner then attempts to balance the lower limb with the pelvis, the pelvis will shift down on the affected side or up on the unaffected side, and balancing will not be possible. This type of contracture can lead to functional lengthening of the limb rather than true lengthening.

Noble Compression Test. This test is used to determine whether iliotibial band friction syndrome exists near the knee (Fig. 10–29).[15] The patient lies supine and the knee is flexed to 90° accompanied by hip flexion. The examiner then applies pressure with the thumb to the lateral femoral epicondyle or 1 to 2 cm proximal to it. While the pressure is maintained, the patient slowly extends the knee. At approximately 30° of flexion (0° being a straight leg), if the patient complains of severe pain over the lateral femoral condyle, a positive test is indicated.

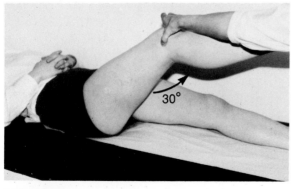

FIGURE 10–29. *Noble compression test for iliotibial band friction syndrome. The patient extends the knee. The examiner is indicating where pain will be felt.*

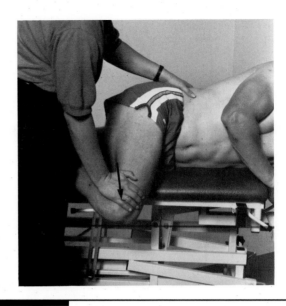

FIGURE 10–30. *Piriformis test.*

The patient will say it is the same pain that accompanies the patient's activity (e.g., running).

Piriformis Test. The patient is in the side lying position with the test leg uppermost. The patient flexes the test hip to 60° with the knee flexed. The examiner stabilizes the hip with one hand and applies a downward pressure to the knee (Fig. 10–30). If the piriformis muscle is tight, pain will be elicited in the muscle. If the piriformis muscle is pinching the sciatic nerve, pain will result in the buttock, and sciatica may be experienced by the patient.[1, 7] Resisted external rotation with the muscle on stretch (hip internally rotated) can cause the same sciatica.[16]

Hamstrings Contracture Test (Method 1). The patient is instructed to sit with one knee flexed against the chest to stabilize the pelvis and with the other knee extended (Fig. 10–31). The patient then attempts to flex the trunk and touch the toes of the extended lower limb (test leg) with the fingers. The test is repeated on the other side. A comparison is made between the two sides. Normally, an individual should be able to at least touch the toes while keeping the knee extended. If the patient is unable to so, it is an indication of tight hamstrings on the straight leg.

Tripod Sign (Hamstrings Contracture—Method 2). The patient is seated with both knees flexed to 90° over the edge of the examining table (Fig. 10–32).[17] The examiner then passively extends one knee. If the hamstring muscles on that side are tight, the patient will extent the trunk to relieve the tension in the hamstring muscles. The leg is returned to its starting position, and the other leg is tested. A comparison is made of the two legs. Extension of the spine is indicative of a positive test. The exam-

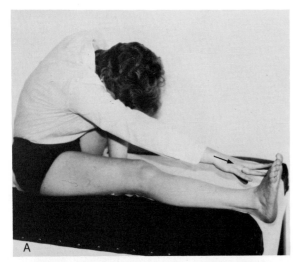

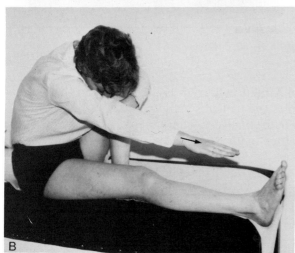

FIGURE 10–31. *Test for hamstring tightness (method 1). (A) Negative test. (B) Positive test.*

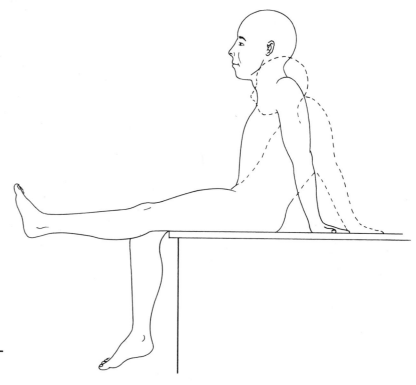

FIGURE 10–32. Tripod sign.

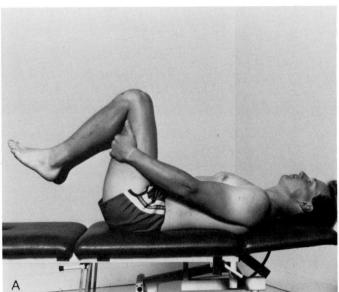 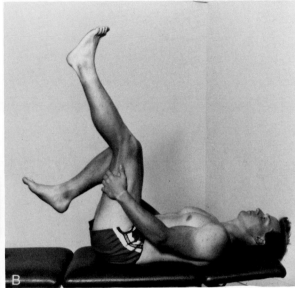

FIGURE 10–33. The 90–90 straight leg raise.

iner must be aware that nerve root problems (stretching of the sciatic nerve) can cause a similar positive sign.

90–90 Straight Leg Raising Test (Hamstrings Contracture—Method 3). The patient flexes the hip to 90° while the knee is bent. The patient then grasps behind the knee with both hands to stabilize the hips at 90° of flexion. The patient actively extends each knee in turn as much as possible. For normal flexibility in the hamstrings, knee extension should be within 20° of full extension (Fig. 10–33).[1, 18]

Reflexes and Cutaneous Distribution

There are no reflexes around the hip that can be easily evaluated. However, the examiner should assess the normal dermatome patterns of the nerve roots (Fig. 10–34) as well as the cutaneous distribution of the peripheral nerves (Fig. 10–35). For example, in a condition called *meralgia paresthetica*, there is pressure placed on the lateral cutaneous nerve of the thigh, running in the fascia near the ASIS as it passes under the inguinal ligament. There will be an alteration in sensation and possibly painful skin in the area supplied by the nerve. (Because dermatomes vary from person to person, the accompanying diagrams are estimations only.) Testing for altered sensation is performed by running the relaxed hands and fingers of the examiner over the pelvis and legs anteriorly, posteriorly, and laterally. Any difference in sensation should be noted and can be mapped out more exactly using a pinwheel, pin, cotton batten, and/or brush.

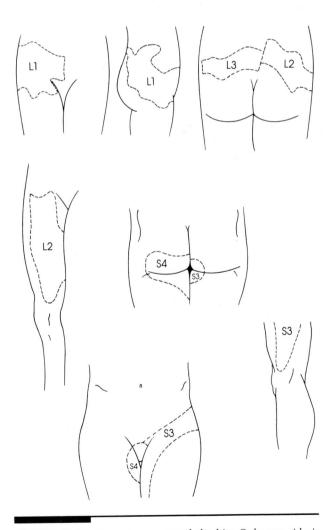

FIGURE 10–34. Dermatomes around the hip. Only one side is illustrated.

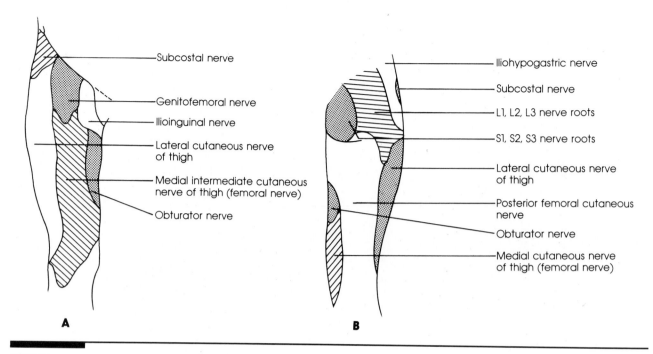

FIGURE 10–35. *Sensory distribution of peripheral nerves around the hip. (A) Anterior view. (B) Posterior view.*

True hip pain is usually referred to the groin, but it may also be referred to the ankle, knee, lumbar spine, and sacroiliac joints (Fig. 10–36). Similarly, the knee, sacroiliac joints, and lumbar spine may refer pain to the hip.

Joint Play Movements

The joint play movements are completed with the patient in the supine position. The examiner should

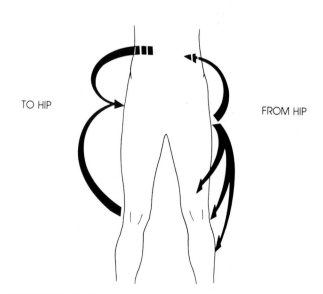

FIGURE 10–36. *Referred pain around the hip.*

attempt to compare the amounts of available movement of the two sides. Small differences may be difficult to detect because of the large muscle bulk in the area.

The joint play movements performed at the hip are shown in Figure 10–37:

1. Caudal glide of the femur (long leg traction or long-axis extension).
2. Compression.
3. Lateral distraction.
4. Quadrant test.[19]

Caudal Glide

The examiner places both hands around the patient's leg slightly above the ankle. The examiner then leans back, applying a long-axis extension to the entire lower limb. Part of the movement will occur in the knee. If one suspects some pathology in the knee or the knee is stiff, both hands should be placed around the thigh just proximal to the knee, and traction force should again be applied (Fig. 10–37A). The first method enables the examiner to apply a greater force. During the movement, any telescoping or excessive movement occurring in the hip should be noted.

Compression

The examiner places the patient's knee in the resting position and then applies a compressive force to the

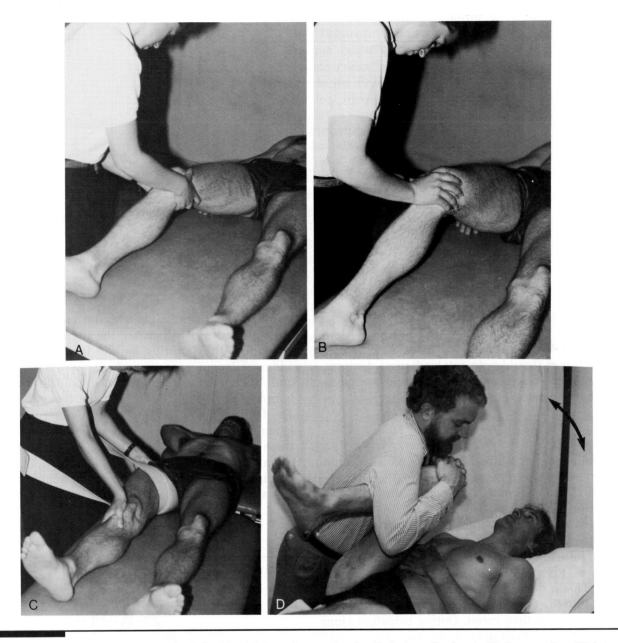

FIGURE 10–37. *Joint play movements of the hip. (A) Long leg traction (applied above the knee). (B) Compression. (C) Lateral distraction. (D) Quadrant test.*

hip through the longitudinal axis of the femur by pushing through the femoral condyles.

Lateral Distraction

The examiner applies the lateral distraction force to the hip by placing a wide strap around the leg as high up in the groin as possible. The strap is then wrapped around the examiner's buttocks. The examiner leans back, using the buttocks to apply the distractive force to the hip. The proximal hand is used to palpate hip movement, while the distal hand prevents abduction of the leg and, hence, torque to the hip.

Quadrant (Scouring) Test

The examiner flexes and adducts the patient's hip so that the hip faces the patient's opposite shoulder and resistance to the movement is felt. While slight resistance is being maintained, the patient's hip is taken into abduction while maintaining flexion in an arc of movement. As the movement is performed, the examiner should look for any irregularity in the movement (e.g., "bumps"), pain, or patient apprehension, which may give an indication of where the pathology is occurring in the hip.[19]

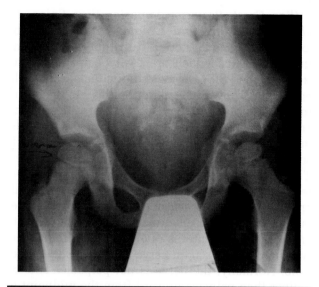

FIGURE 10–42. Legg-Calvé-Perthes disease of the left hip.

2. Presence of any bone disease (i.e., Legg-Calvé-Perthes disease, bony cysts, or tumors) (Fig. 10–42).

3. Neck-shaft angle. The examiner should note whether the angle is normal or whether the patient exhibits a coxa vara or coxa valga.

4. Shape of the femoral head.

5. Presence of osteophytes.

6. Whether *Shenton's line* is normal. Normally, Shenton's line is curved, drawn along the medial curved edge of the femur and continuing upward in a smooth arc along the inferior edge of the pubis (Fig. 10–43). If the head of the femur is dislocated or fractured, two lines form two separate arcs, indicating a broken line. A broken Shenton's line is diagnostic.

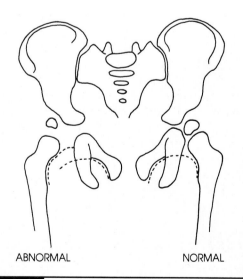

ABNORMAL   NORMAL

FIGURE 10–43. Shenton's line.

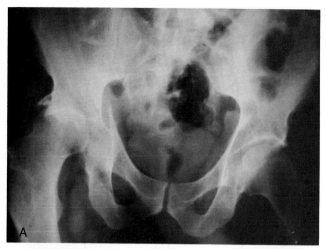

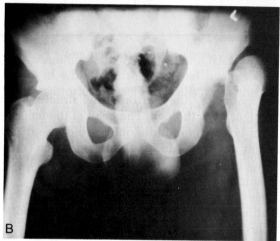

FIGURE 10–44. Trauma to the hip. (A) Fractured right acetabulum. (B) Dislocated left femur.

7. Any evidence of fracture or dislocation (Fig. 10–44). Is the pelvic ring intact, or has it been disrupted? Disruption of the pelvic ring indicates severe injury.

8. Pelvic distortion.

9. Whether Hilgenreiner's and Perkin's lines are within normal limits. *Hilgenreiner's line* is horizontal, drawn between the inferior parts of the ilium. *Perkin's line* is vertical, drawn through the upper outer point of the acetabulum (Fig. 10–45). Normally, the developing femoral head or ossification center of the femoral head lies in the inner distal quadrant formed by the two lines. If the ossification center lies in the upper outer quadrant, the finding is indicative of a dislocation. In the newborn, the ossification center is not visible (Fig. 10–46).

10. Whether the femoral head and acetabulum are normal on both sides. In congenital dislocation of the hip, both structures may show dysplasia, and the acetabular index on the affected side may be more than the normal 30°. The *acetabular index* is

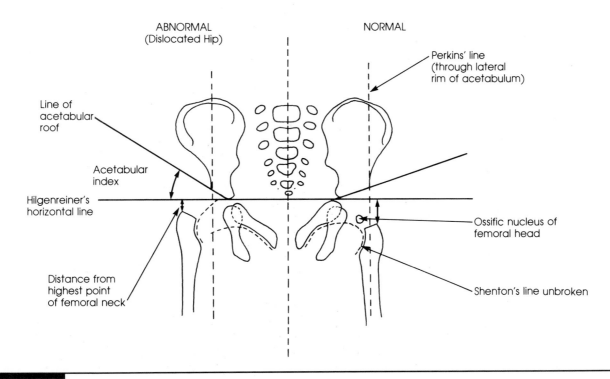

ABNORMAL
(Dislocated Hip)

NORMAL

Perkins' line
(through lateral
rim of acetabulum)

Line of
acetabular
roof

Acetabular
index

Hilgenreiner's
horizontal line

Ossific nucleus of
femoral head

Distance from
highest point
of femoral neck

Shenton's line unbroken

FIGURE 10–45. *Radiologic findings in congenital dislocation of the hip compared with normal findings in a 12- to 15-month-old child. Acetabular index: normal = 30°, in newborn = 27.5°. If the ossific nucleus of the femoral head is present, it should sit in the inner lower quadrant.*

determined by first drawing Hilgenreiner's line. An intersecting line is drawn from the lateral to the medial edge of the acetabulum, and the angle formed by the two lines is called the acetabular index, or *Hilgenreiner's angle* (Table 10–9). The greater the slope angle, the less stable the femoral head in the acetabulum.

11. "Sagging rope" sign. With Legg-Calvé-Perthes disease, only the head of the femur is affected. If avascular necrosis of a developing femoral head occurs, the *sagging rope sign* may be seen (Fig. 10–47). The sign indicates damage to the growth plate with marked metaphyseal reaction. Its presence indicates a severe disease process.

12. "Teardrop" sign. Migration of the femoral head upward in relation to the pelvis due to degeneration, as seen in osteoarthritis, may be detected by the *teardrop sign* (Fig. 10–48). The teardrop is visible at the base of the pubic bone, extending vertically downward to terminate in a round teardrop, or head. The x-ray beam must be centered relative to the pelvis. A line is drawn between the two teardrops and extended to the femoral heads on both sides. The examiner can then measure from the teardrop to the femoral head. A difference of more than 10 mm between the two sides indicates significant migration of the head of the femur. Serial films or films taken over a period of time will often show a progression of the migration.

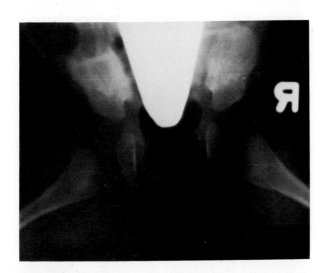

FIGURE 10–46. *Radiograph of the hip in the newborn. Ossification of the femoral head has not yet developed.*

TABLE 10–9. Average Values of Hilgenreiner Angle (Acetabular Index)

	Newborn	6 Months Old	1 Year Old
Male	26°	20°	20°
Female	28°	22°	20°

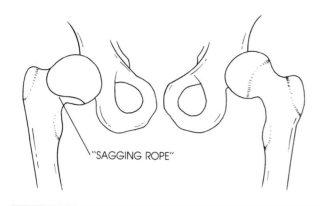

FIGURE 10–47. ''Sagging rope'' sign.

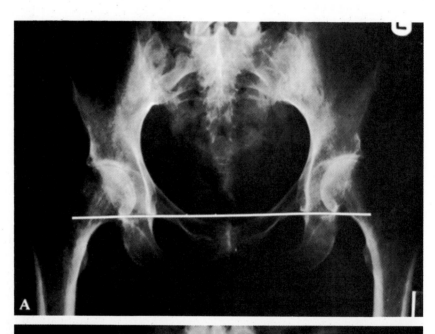

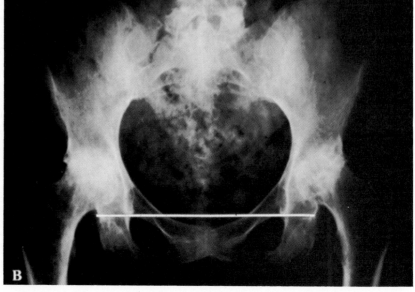

FIGURE 10–48. ''Teardrop'' sign. (A) A line has been drawn between the tips of the two ''teardrops'' and extended into the femoral neck. Osteoarthritis of both hip joints appears to be equal, with equivalent narrowing of the joint space, but the left hip is already at a slightly higher level than the right in relation to the line. (B) Later, both hips have gradually moved upward as a result of loss of the bone at the apex of each femoral head. The left hip is now at a higher level than the right, confirming the original observation that the process of destruction in the left hip was ahead of that in the right. (From Greubel-Lee, D. M.: Disorders of the Hip. Philadelphia, J. B. Lippincott, 1983, p. 61, p. 146.)

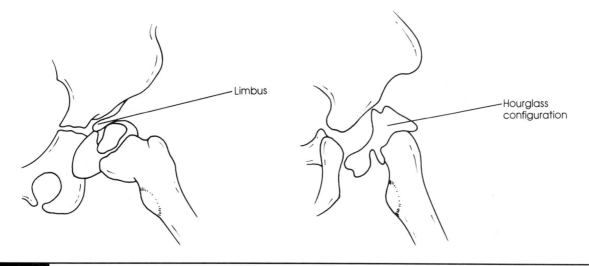

FIGURE 10–49. Drawings of arthrograms in congenital dislocation of the hip.

Lateral View

The examiner looks for any pelvic distortion or any slipping of the femoral head, as might be seen in slipped capital femoral epiphysis. The lateral view will be the first in which slipping may be seen.

Arthrogram

Although arthrograms are not routinely done on the hip, they may be done if the hip will not reduce after a dislocation (Fig. 10–49). The arthrogram will indicate a possible *inverted limbus* (infolding of a meniscus-like structure) or it may indicate an hourglass configuration from a contracted capsule. A normal hip arthrogram is shown in Figure 10–50.

CT Scan. CT scanning is useful in assessing abnormalities of the hip. For example, it can be used to measure anteversion and retroversion, and it can show the size and shape of the acetabulum and femoral head as well as the congruity and position

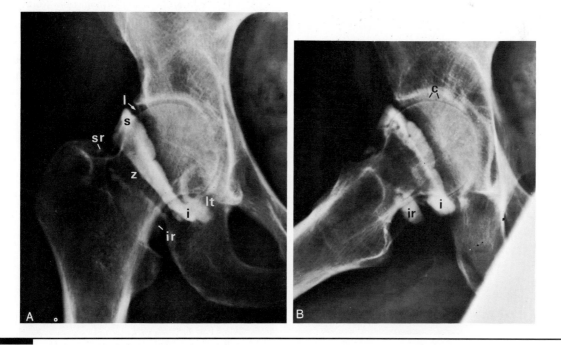

FIGURE 10–50. Normal hip arthrogram. Normal examination after intra-articular injection of approximately 6 ml of contrast medium. (A) Anteroposterior and (B) frog lateral views. c = contrast agent outlining articular cartilage (recess capitus); i = inferior articular recess; ir = recess colli inferior; l = acetabular labrum; lt = defect in contrast from transverse ligament; s = superior articular recess; sr = recess colli superior; z = zona orbicularis (impression on the intra-articular contrast by the iliofemoral ischiofemoral ligaments of the hip joint capsule). (From Weissman, B. N. W., and C. B. Sledge: Orthopedic Radiology. Philadelphia, W. B. Saunders Co., 1986, p. 396.)

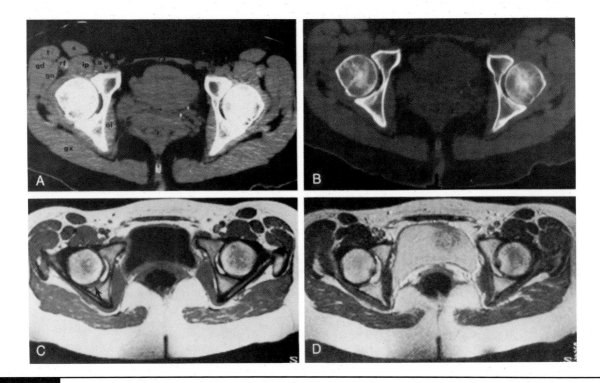

FIGURE 10–51. (A) Normal CT image at the level of the midacetabulum obtained with soft-tissue window settings shows the homogenous, intermediate signal of musculature. a = common femoral artery; gd = gluteus medius; gn = gluteus minimus; gx = gluteus maximus; ip = iliopsoas; oi = obturator internus; ra = rectus abdominis; rf = rectus femoris; s = sartorius; t = tensor fascia lata; v = common femoral vein. (B) Axial CT at bone window settings reveals improved delineation of cortical and medullary osseous details. Note anterior and posterior semilunar acetabular articular surfaces and the central nonarticular acetabular fossa. (C) Normal midacetabular T1-weighted axial 0.4-T MRI (TR, 600 msec; TE, 20 msec) of a different patient shows a normal, high-signal-intensity image of muscle and the absence of signal in the cortical bone. The thin articular hyaline cartilage is of intermediate signal intensity (arrow). (D) T2-weighted MRI (TR, 2,000 msec; TE, 80 msec) shows decreasing high-signal intensity in fatty marrow and subcutaneous tissue with increased signal intensity in the fluid filled urinary bladder. (From Pitt, M. J., et al.: Orthop. Clin. North Am. 21:553, 1990.)

of the femoral head relative to the acetabulum (Figs. 10–51 and 10–52). In newborns, the limited ossification limits its use.

MRI. MRI is a useful technique to study the hip because it is able to show soft tissue as well as osseous tissue (Fig. 10–53). This ability makes it an excellent technique to use for congenital abnormalities.

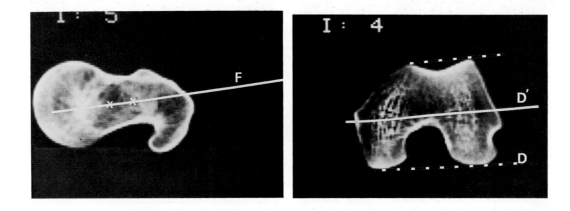

FIGURE 10–52. CT for determining femoral anteversion (using a femoral specimen). The diacondylar line (D) is drawn along the condyles, although Hernandez and coworkers construct it (D') midway between the anterior and posterior femoral surfaces (dashed lines). The axis of the femoral neck (F) is shown. The angle between the femoral neck axis (F) and the diacondylar line is the angle of anteversion. In this case, there are 2° of retroversion. (From Weissman, B. N. W., and C. B. Sledge: Orthopedic Radiology. Philadelphia, W. B. Saunders Co., 1986, p. 399.)

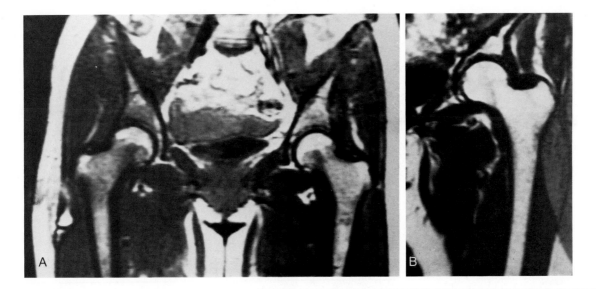

FIGURE 10–53. (A) Normal MRI scan of a young adult. Spin-echo T1-weighted image 600/25. Notice the bright signal of fat in the region of the femoral epiphysis and the greater trochanter. The intermediate signal intensity in the femoral neck represents hemopoietic marrow. (B) Normal elderly woman with same imaging sequence shows replacment of hemopoietic marrow in the femoral neck by fatty marrow. (From Dalinka, M. K., and L. M. Neustadter: Radiology of the hip. In Steinberg, M. E. [ed.]: The Hip and Its Disorders. Philadelphia, W. B. Saunders Co., 1991, p. 68.)

"Head at Risk" Signs

With Legg-Calvé-Perthes disease, the examiner should note the radiologic head at risk signs on an anteroposterior film:

1. Cage's sign. This is a small osteoporotic seg-

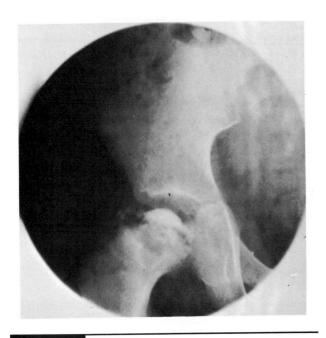

FIGURE 10–54. All of the signs of the "head at risk" are present: lateral subluxation, abnormal direction of the growth plates, Cage's sign, lateral calcification, and irregularity of the epiphysis. (From Greubel-Lee, D. M.: Disorders of the Hip. Philadelphia, J. B. Lippincott, 1983, p. 146.)

ment on the lateral side of the epiphysis that appears to be translucent (Fig. 10–54).
2. Calcification lateral to the epiphysis (if collapse is occurring).
3. Lateral subluxation of the head (an increase in the inferomedial joint space).
4. Angle of the epiphyseal line (horizontal in this case).
5. Metaphyseal reaction.

Patients who exhibit three or more head at risk signs have a poor prognosis, and surgery is usually performed.

Signs of a Slipped Capital Femoral Epiphysis

With a slipped capital femoral epiphysis (Fig. 10–55), the following x-ray signs may be noted:

1. The epiphyseal line may widen.
2. Lipping or stepping may be seen, as occurs on lateral films.
3. The superior femoral neck line does not transect the overhanging ossified epiphysis as it does in the normal hip.
4. Shenton's line does not describe a continuous arc. (The line is also broken if the hip is dislocated or subluxed.)

In addition to a slipped capital femoral epiphysis causing a coxa vara, fractures and congenital malformations may lead to the same deformity (Figs. 10–56 and 10–57).

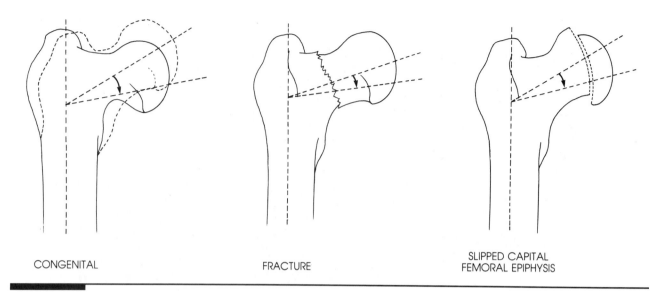

CONGENITAL   FRACTURE   SLIPPED CAPITAL
                                                          FEMORAL EPIPHYSIS

FIGURE 10–55. Some causes of coxa vara.

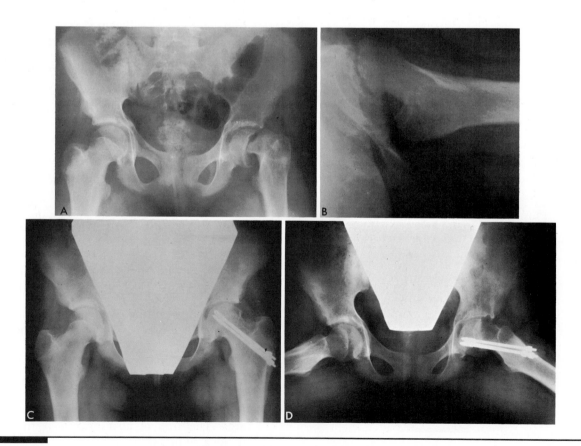

FIGURE 10–56. Acute slipped femoral epiphysis in a 14-year-old boy. After a fall, the patient complained of severe pain in the left groin and anterior thigh and was unable to bear weight on the left lower limb. (A and B) Preoperative roentgenograms show the severe slip on the left. The patient was placed in bilateral split Russell traction with internal rotation straps on the left thigh and leg. Gradually, within a period of 3 to 4 days, the slip was reduced. (C and D) Postoperative roentgenograms approximately 6 months later show closure of epiphyseal plate and normal position of femoral head. The hip had full range of motion. (From Tachdjian, M. O.: Pediatric Orthopedics. Philadelphia, W. B. Saunders Co., 1972, p. 470.)

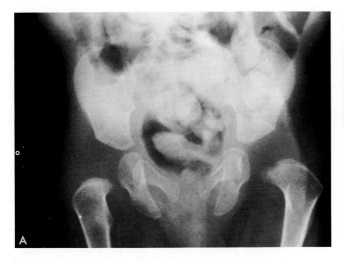

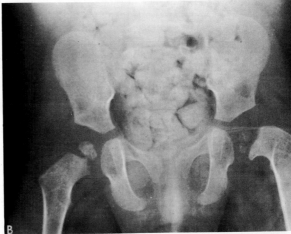

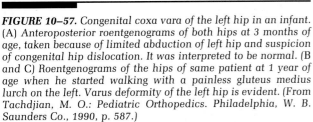

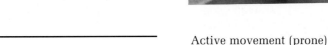

FIGURE 10–57. Congenital coxa vara of the left hip in an infant. (A) Anteroposterior roentgenograms of both hips at 3 months of age, taken because of limited abduction of left hip and suspicion of congenital hip dislocation. It was interpreted to be normal. (B and C) Roentgenograms of the hips of same patient at 1 year of age when he started walking with a painless gluteus medius lurch on the left. Varus deformity of the left hip is evident. (From Tachdjian, M. O.: Pediatric Orthopedics. Philadelphia, W. B. Saunders Co., 1990, p. 587.)

PRÉCIS OF THE HIP ASSESSMENT*

History
Observation
Examination
  Active movements (supine)
    Hip flexion
    Hip abduction
    Hip adduction
    Hip lateral rotation
    Hip medial rotation
  Passive movements (supine) (as in active movements, if necessary)
  Resisted isometric movements (supine)
    Hip flexion
    Hip extension
    Hip adduction
    Hip abduction
    Hip medial rotation
    Hip lateral rotation
    Knee flexion
    Knee extension
  Special tests (supine)
  Reflexes and cutaneous sensation (supine)
  Joint play movements (supine)
    Caudal glide
    Compression
    Lateral distraction
    Quadrant test
  Palpation (supine)

  Active movement (prone)
    Hip extension
  Passive movement (prone)
    Hip extension
  Resisted isometric movements (prone)
    Hip medial rotation (if not previously done)
    Hip lateral rotation (if not previously done)
    Knee flexion (if not previously done)
    Knee extension (if not previously done)
  Special tests (prone and side lying)
  Reflexes and cutaneous sensation (prone)
  Palpation (prone)
  Radiographic examination

When the rest of the examination is completed, the examiner can ask the patient to perform the appropriate functional tests.

After any examination, the patient should always be warned of the possibility of exacerbation of symptoms as a result of assessment.

---

*The précis is shown in an order that will limit the amount of moving that the patient has to do but ensure that all necessary structures are tested.

CASE STUDIES

When doing these case studies, the examiner should list the appropriate questions to be asked and why they are *being asked, what to look for and why, and what things should be tested and why. Depending on the answers of the patient (and the examiner should consider different responses), several possible causes of the patient's problem may become evident (examples are given in parentheses). If so, a differential diagnosis chart should be made up. The examiner can then decide how different diagnoses may affect the treatment plan.*

1. A 7-year-old boy is brought by his parents for assessment . He walks with a limp and has done so during the past 5 weeks at irregular times, the limp becoming more pronounced when the boy becomes tired. The boy also complains of a painful left knee. Describe your assessment plan for this patient (Legg-Calvé-Perthes disease versus slipped capital femoral epiphysis).

2. A 71-year-old woman had an Austin Moore prosthesis inserted into the left hip 1 day ago. The prosthesis has relieved the pain she had in her hip. X-rays reveal that the prosthesis is solid. The surgeon has asked you to get the patient up and moving. Before doing this, however, you must do a bedside assessment. Outline how you would do the assessment.

3. A 14-year-old boy was well until he fell from a chair onto his buttocks. He did not appear hurt, but 1 week later his parents brought him in for assessment because of a limp and pain in his right thigh and knee. The teenager is a tall, thin boy who prefers to walk with the right foot laterally rotated. Design your assessment plan for this patient (slipped capital femoral epiphysis versus ischial bursitis).

4. A 3-week-old girl is referred to you to fit with a Pavlik harness for congenital dislocation of the hip. Before you can fit the harness, you must do an assessment. Design your assessment plan for this patient.

5. A 55-year-old man presents complaining of hip and back pain. There is some sciatica with pain into the groin. The pain is especially bad when he walks. He has a desk job but has been very active throughout his life. Describe your assessment plan for this patient (piriformis syndrome versus lumbar spondylosis).

6. A 35-year-old woman presents complaining of lateral hip pain. She states she was in a motor vehicle accident 2 weeks ago in which she was hit from the passenger side (she was driving) and her car was pushed against a telephone pole. She was wearing a seat belt. Describe your assessment plan for this patient (trochanteric bursitis versus muscle contusion).

7. An 18-year-old man was surfing when he was thrown by a wave and hurt his hip. The hip is medially rotated and shortened. He has some sciatic pain. Describe your assessment plan for this patient (posterior hip dislocation versus trochanteric fracture).

8. A 23-year-old female diver comes to you complaining of hip pain. She says it bothers her when she does any quick flexion of the hip. Describe your assessment plan for this patient (psoas bursitis versus psoas strain).

REFERENCES

CITED REFERENCES

1. Saudek, C. E.: The hip. In Gould, J. A. (ed.): Orthopedic and Sports Physical Therapy. St. Louis, C. V. Mosby Co., 1990.
2. Brand, R. A., and R. D. Crowninshield: The effect of cane use on hip contact force. Clin. Orthop. Relat. Res. 147:181, 1980.
3. Adams, M. C.: Outline of Orthopaedics. London, E & S Livingstone, 1968.
4. Tachdjian, M. O.: Pediatric Orthopedics. Philadelphia, W. B. Saunders Co., 1972.
5. Crane, L.: Femoral torsion and its relation to toeing-in and toeing-out. J. Bone Joint Surg. 41A:421, 1959.
6. Staheli, L. T.: Medial femoral torsion. Orthop. Clin. North Am. 11:39, 1980.
7. Lee, D.: The Pelvic Girdle. Edinburgh, Churchill Livingstone, 1989.
8. Clarke, G. R.: Unequal leg length: An accurate method of detection and some clinical results. Rheumatol. Phys. Med. 11:385, 1972.
9. Fisk, J. W., and M. L. Balgent: Clinical and radiological assessment of leg length. N. Z. Med. J. 81:477, 1975.
10. Woerman, A. L., and S. A. Binder-Macleod: Leg-length discrepancy assessment: Accuracy and precision in five clinical methods of evaluation. J. Orthop. Sports Phys. Ther. 5:230, 1984.
11. Woerman, A. L.: Evaluation and treatment of dysfunction in the lumbar-pelvic-hip complex. In Donatelli, R., and M. J. Wooden (eds.): Orthopedic Physical Therapy. Edinburgh, Churchill Livingstone, 1989.
12. Gruebel-Lee, D. M.: Disorders of the Hip. Philadelphia, J. B. Lippincott Co., 1983.
13. Ober, F. B.: The role of the iliotibial and fascia lata as a factor in the causation of low-back disabilities and sciatica. J. Bone Joint Surg. 18:105, 1936.
14. Crawford, A. H.: Neurologic disorders. In Steinberg, M. E. (ed.): The Hip and Its Disorders. Philadelphia, W. B. Saunders Co., 1991.
15. Noble, H. B., M. R. Hajek, and M. Porter: Diagnosis and treatment of iliotibial band tightness in runners. Physician Sportsmedicine 10:67, 1982.
16. Garrick, J. G., and D. R. Webb: Sports Injuries: Diagnosis and Treatment. Philadelphia, W. B. Saunders Co., 1990.
17. American Orthopaedic Association: Manual of Orthopaedic Surgery. Chicago, 1972.
18. Palmer, M. L., and M. Epler: Clinical Assessment Procedures in Physical Therapy. Philadelphia, J. B. Lippincott, 1990.
19. Maitland, G. D.: The Peripheral Joints: Examination and Recording Guide. Adelaide, Australia, Virgo Press, 1973.

GENERAL REFERENCES

Andersson, G.: Hip assessment: A comparison of nine different methods. J. Bone Joint Surg. 54B:621, 1972.
Bassett, L. W., R. H. Gold, and L. L. Seeger: MRI Atlas of the Musculoskeletal System. London, Martin Dunitz Ltd., 1989.
Beetham, W. P., H. F. Polley, C. H. Slocumb, and W. F. Weaver: Physical Examination of the Joints. Philadelphia, W. B. Saunders Co., 1965.
Bertol, P., M. F. Macnicol, and G. P. Mitchell: Radiographic features of neonatal congenital dislocation of the hip. J. Bone Joint Surg. 64B:176, 1982.
Bos, C. F. A., J. L. Bloem, W. R. Obermann, and P. M. Roging: Magnetic resonance imaging in congenital dislocation of the hip. J. Bone Joint Surg. 70B:174, 1988.
Chung, S. M. K.: Hip Disorders in Infants and Children. Philadelphia, Lea & Febiger, 1981.
Clarke, G. R.: Unequal leg length: An accurate method of detection and some clinical results. Rheumatol. Phys. Med. 11:385, 1972.
Clarkson, H. M., and G. B. Gilewich: Musculoskeletal Assessment—Joint Range of Motion and Manual Muscle Strength. Baltimore, Williams & Wilkins, 1989.
Crock, H. V.: An atlas of the arterial supply of the head and neck of the femur in man. Clin. Orthop. Relat. Res. 152:17, 1980.
Crouch, J. E.: Functional Human Anatomy. Philadelphia, Lea & Febiger, 1973.
Cyriax, J.: Textbook of Orthopaedic Medicine, volume 1. Diagnosis of Soft Tissue Lesions. London, Bailliere Tindall, 1975.
Dalinka, M. K., and L. M. Neustadter: Radiology of the hip. In Steinberg, M. E. (ed.): The Hip and Its Disorders. Philadelphia, W. B. Saunders Co., 1991.
Debrunner, H. N.: Orthopaedic Diagnosis. London, E & S Longman Group Ltd., 1973.

Fisk, J. W., and M. L. Bargent: Clinical and radiological assessment of leg length. N. Z. Med. J. 81:477, 1975.

Forrester, D. M., and J. C. Brown: The Radiology of Joint Disease. Philadelphia, W. B. Saunders Co., 1987.

Friberg, O.: Clinical symptoms and biomechanics of lumbar spine and hip joint in leg length inequality. Spine 8:643, 1983.

Goddard, N. J., and P. T. Gosling: Intra-articular fluid pressure and pain in osteoarthritis of the hip. J. Bone Joint Surg. 70B:52, 1988.

Grieve, G. P.: The hip. Physiotherapy 57:212, 1971.

Harris, W. H.: Traumatic arthritis of the hip after dislocation and acetabular fracture: treatment by mold arthroplasty. J. Bone Joint Surg. 51A:737, 1969.

Hoaglund, F. T., A. C. Yau, and W. L. Wong: Osteoarthritis of the hip and other joints in southern Chinese in Hong Kong. J. Bone Joint Surg. 55A:545, 1973.

Hoaglund, F. T., and W. D. Low: Anatomy of the femoral neck and head, with comparative data from Caucasians and Hong Kong Chinese. Clin. Orthop. Relat. Res. 152:10, 1980.

Hollinshead, W. H., and D. B. Jenkins: Functional Anatomy of the Limbs and Back. Philadelphia, W. B. Saunders Co., 1969.

Hoppenfeld, S.: Physical Examination of the Spine and Extremities. New York, Appleton-Century-Crofts, 1976.

Hunt, G. C., W. A. Fromherz, J. Danoff, and T. Waggoner: Femoral transverse torque: An assessment method. J. Orthop. Sports Phys. Ther. 7:319, 1986.

Judge, R. D., G. D. Zuidema, and F. T. Fitzgerald: Clinical Diagnosis: A Physiological Approach. Boston, Little, Brown and Co., 1982.

Kaltenborn, F. M.: Mobilization of the Extremity. Oslo, Olaf Norlis Bokhandel, 1980.

Kapandji, I. A.: The Physiology of the Joints, vol. II. Lower Limb. New York, Churchill Livingstone, 1970.

Landon, G. C., and J. O. Galante: Physical examination of the hip joint. In Post, M. (ed.): Physical Examination of the Musculoskeletal System. Chicago, Year Book Medical Pub., 1987.

Larson, C. B.: Rating scale for hip disabilities. Clin. Orthop. Relat. Res. 31:85, 1963.

McGann, W. A.: History and physical examination. In Steinberg, M. E. (ed.): The Hip and Its Disorders. Philadelphia, W. B. Saunders Co., 1991.

McRae, R.: Clinical Orthopaedic Examination. New York, Churchill Livingstone, 1976.

Milch, H.: The measurement of hip motion in the sagittal and coronal planes. J. Bone Joint Surg. 41A:713, 1959.

Morscher, E., and G. Figner: Measurement of leg length. Prog. Ortho. Surg. 1:21, 1977.

Moseley, C. F.: The biomechanics of the pediatric hip. Orthop. Clin. North Am. 11:39, 1980.

Nichols, P. J. R., and N. T. J. Bailey: The accuracy of measuring leg length difference—an "observer error" experiment. Br. Med. J. 2:1247, 1955.

O'Donoghue, D. H.: Treatment of Injuries to Athletes, 4th ed. Philadelphia, W. B. Saunders Co., 1984.

Peterson, H. A., R. A. Klassen, R. A. McLeod, and A. D. Hoffman: The use of computerized tomography in dislocation of the hip and femoral neck anteversion in children. J. Bone Joint Surg. 63B:198, 1981.

Pitt, M. J., P. J. Lund, and D. P. Speer: Imaging of the pelvis and hip. Orthop. Clin. North Am. 21:545, 1990.

Radin, E. L.: Biomechanics of the hip. Clin. Orthop. Relat. Res. 152:28, 1980.

Rydell, N.: Biomechanics of the hip. Clin. Orthop. Relat. Res. 92:6, 1973.

Schaberg, J. E., M. C. Harper, and W. C. Allen: The snapping hip syndrome. Am. J. Sports Med. 12:361, 1984.

Staheli, L. T.: Torsional deformity. Paediatr. Clin. North Am. 33:1373, 1986.

Wadsworth, C. T.: Manual Examination and Treatment of the Spine and Extremities. Baltimore: Williams & Wilkins, 1988.

Weissman, B. N. W., and C. B. Sledge: Orthopedic Radiology. Philadelphia, W. B. Saunders Co., 1986.

Williams, P. L., and Warwick, P. (eds.): Gray's Anatomy, 36th British ed. Philadelphia, W. B. Saunders Co., 1980.

CHAPTER 11 Knee

The knee joint is particularly susceptible to traumatic injury because it is located at the ends of two long lever arms—the tibia and the femur. The joint depends on the ligaments and muscles that surround it for its strength and stability, not on its bony configuration.

Because the knee joint depends on its ligaments to such a great extent, it is imperative that the ligaments be tested during the examination of the knee. Thus, the assessment of the knee varies slightly from other assessments in that the ligamentous tests are not included under "Special Tests" but instead are listed in a separate section. This change ensures that the ligaments are always included in the examination of the knee.

The knee is a complicated area to assess, and the examiner must take time to ensure that all of the relevant structures are tested. It must also be remembered that because the lumbar spine, hip, and ankle may refer pain to the knee, these joints must be assessed if it appears that joints other than the knee may be involved.

APPLIED ANATOMY

The *tibiofemoral joint* is the largest joint in the body. It is a modified hinge joint having three rotational degrees of freedom. The *synovium* around the joint is extensive; it communicates with many of the bursae and pouches around the knee joint. Although the synovial membrane "encapsulates" the entire knee joint, its distribution within the knee is such that the *cruciate ligaments*, which run from the middle of the tibial plateau to the intercondylar area of the femur, are extrasynovial. ("Cruciate" means that the ligaments cross each other.)

The articular surfaces of the tibia and femur are not congruent, which enables the two bones to move different amounts guided by the muscles and ligaments. The two bones approach congruency in full extension, which is the close packed position. Kaltenborn[1] has stated that the close packed position includes full lateral rotation of the tibia. The lateral femoral condyle projects anteriorly more than the medial femoral condyle to help prevent lateral dislocation of the patella. In females, this enlargement is important because of the female's broader pelvis and increased inward angle of the femur, which allow the femoral condyles to be parallel with the ground (Fig. 11–1). The resting position of the joint is approximately 25° of flexion, and the capsular pattern is flexion more limited than extension.

The space between the two bones is partially filled by two menisci that are attached to the tibia to add congruency. The *medial meniscus* is a small part of a large circle (i.e., "C"-shaped) and is thicker posteriorly than anteriorly. The *lateral meniscus* is a large part of a small circle (i.e., "O"-shaped) and is generally of equal thickness throughout. Both menisci are thicker along the periphery and thinner along the inner margin.

During the movement from extension to flexion, both menisci move posteriorly, the lateral meniscus being displaced more than the medial meniscus. The menisci are avascular in their cartilaginous inner two thirds and are partly vascular and fibrous in their outer one third.[2] They are held in place by the coronary ligaments attaching to the tibia.

The menisci serve several functions in the knee. They aid in the lubrication and nutrition of the joint and act as shock absorbers, spreading the stress over the articular cartilage and decreasing cartilage wear. They make the joint surfaces more congruent and improve weight distribution by increasing the area of contact between the condyles. The menisci reduce friction during movement and aid the ligaments and capsule in preventing hyperextension. The menisci prevent the joint capsule from entering the joint and participate in the "locking" mechanism of the joint by directing the movement of the femoral articular condyles. Because most recent literature indicates that removal of the entire meniscus can lead to early

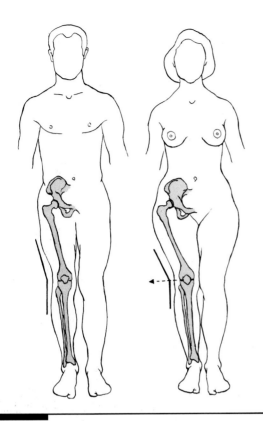

FIGURE 11–1. Q-angle differences in males and females. Note that because of the broader pelvis in the female, it is necessary for the femur to come inward at an increased angle to make the distal end of the condyles parallel with the ground. The quadriceps, patella, and patellar tendon form an angle centered at the patella. As the quadriceps contracts, the angle tends to straighten, which forces the patella laterally. (From O'Donoghue, D. H.: Treatment of Injuries to Athletes, 4th ed. Philadelphia, W. B. Saunders Co., 1984, p. 522.)

degeneration of the joint,[3, 4] most surgeons today remove only the torn portion of the meniscus.

Because the meniscus possesses no nerves, there is no pain when it is damaged unless the coronary ligaments have been damaged as well. Because the menisci are primarily avascular, especially in the inner two thirds, there is seldom bloody effusion in

injury; however, there may be synovial effusion. Their poor blood supply gives them a low regeneration potential.

The lateral meniscus is not as firmly attached to the tibia as the medial meniscus and thus is less prone to injury. The coronary ligaments tend to be longer on the lateral aspect, and the horns of the lateral meniscus are closer together. The lateral meniscus has an excursion of 10 mm, and the medial meniscus has an excursion of 2 mm.

The *patellofemoral joint* is a modified plane joint, the lateral articular surface of the patella being wider. The patella contains the thickest layer of cartilage in the body. It has five facets, or ridges—superior, inferior, lateral, medial, and odd. It is the "odd" facet that is most frequently the first part of the patella to be affected in chondromalacia patellae (i.e., premature degeneration of the patellar cartilage).

During the movement from flexion to extension, different parts of the patella articulate with the femoral condyles (Fig. 11–2).[5, 6] For example, the odd facet does not come into contact with the femoral condyles until at least 135° of flexion is reached. Incorrect alignment or malalignment of the patellar movement over the femoral condyles can lead to patellofemoral arthralgia. The capsule of this joint is continuous with the capsule of the tibiofemoral joint.

The *patella* improves the efficiency of extension during the last 30° of extension (i.e., 30° to 0° of extension with the straight leg being 0°) because it holds the quadriceps tendon away from the axis of movement. The patella also functions as a guide for the quadriceps tendon, decreases friction of the quadriceps mechanism, controls capsular tension in the knee, acts as a bony shield for the cartilage of the femoral condyles, and improves the aesthetic appearance of the knee. Loading of the patella will vary with activity. For example, in walking, the pressure exerted on the patella is one third body

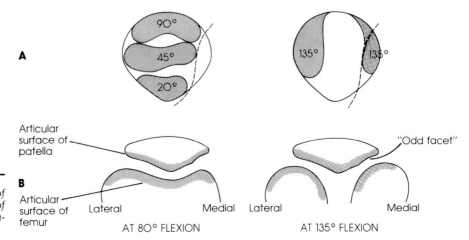

FIGURE 11–2. (A) Area of contact of the patella during different degrees of flexion. (B) Articulation between patella and femur.

weight. Climbing stairs increases the load to three times body weight, whereas squatting increases the load to seven times body weight.

The *superior tibiofibular joint* is a plane synovial joint between the tibia and the head of the fibula. Movement occurs in this joint with any activity involving the ankle. Hypomobility at this joint can lead to pain in the knee area on activity because the fibula can bear up to one sixth of the body weight. In approximately 10 per cent of the population, the capsule of this joint is continuous with that of the tibiofemoral joint.

PATIENT HISTORY

In addition to the general history questions outlined in Chapter 1, the following information should be determined:

1. What is the patient able or unable to do functionally? Is there disability on running, cutting, pivoting, twisting, climbing, or descending stairs?

2. Is there any pain? If so, where? What type is it? Is it diffuse? Aching? Retropatellar? Aching pain may indicate degenerative changes, whereas sharp, "catching" pain usually indicates a mechanical problem. Arthritic pain is more likely to be associated with stiffness in the morning and to ease with activity. Pain at rest is not usually mechanical in origin. Pain during activity is usually seen in struc-

tural abnormalities such as subluxation or patellar tracking disorders. Pain after activity is characteristic of inflammatory disorders such as synovial plica irritation or early tendinitis. Pain in the area of the knee is usually characteristic of contusions or partial tears of muscles or ligaments. Instability rather than pain tends to be the major presenting factor in complex ligament disruptions.

3. Is there any "clicking," or was there a "pop" when the injury occurred? A distinct pop may indicate an anterior cruciate ligament tear or osteochondral fracture.

4. Does the knee "give way," or catch? This finding usually indicates instability in the knee, meniscus pathology, or patellar subluxation if present when rotation or stopping is involved. Giving way when walking uphill or downhill is more likely the result of a retropatellar lesion.

5. Do certain positions or activities have an increased or decreased effect on the pain? Which activities produce pain? How much activity is needed to produce pain? Which positions or activities ease the pain? Does the pain go away when activity ceases? The examiner must take note of constant pain that is unrelated to activity, time, or posture because it is usually indicative of serious pathology such as a tumor.

6. Is the gait normal?

7. Has the knee been injured before, or does it have any feeling of weakness?

8. How did the accident occur? Was it the result of trauma, such as a direct or an indirect blow? Was

TABLE 11–1. Mechanisms of Injury to the Knee and Possible Structures Injured*

Mechanism of Injury	Structure Possibly Injured
Varus or valgus contact without rotation	1. Collateral ligament 2. Epiphyseal fracture 3. Patellar dislocation or subluxation
Varus or valgus contact with rotation	1. Collateral and cruciate ligaments 2. Collateral ligaments and patellar dislocation or subluxation 3. Meniscus tear
Blow to patellofemoral joint, or fall on flexed knee, foot dorsiflexed	Patellar articular injury or osteochondral fracture
Blow to tibial tubercle, or fall on flexed knee, foot plantar flexed	Posterior cruciate ligament
Anterior blow to tibia, resulting in knee hyperextension	1. Anterior cruciate ligament 2. Anterior and posterior cruciate ligament
Noncontact hyperextension	1. Anterior cruciate ligament 2. Posterior capsule
Noncontact deceleration	Anterior cruciate ligament
Noncontact deceleration, with tibial medial rotation or femoral lateral rotation on fixed tibia	Anterior cruciate ligament
Noncontact, quickly turning one way with tibia rotated in opposite direction	Patellar dislocation or subluxation
Noncontact, rotation with varus or valgus loading	Meniscus injury

the patient bearing weight at the time of injury? From which direction did the injuring force come (i.e., what is the mechanism of injury)? For example, meniscal injuries, especially those on the medial side, occur as a result of torsion injury that combines compression and rotation. Slowly developing forces tend to cause bony avulsions, whereas rapidly developing forces tend to tear ligaments. Table 11–1 lists typical mechanisms of injury to the knee and the structures injured. The lower limb may be viewed as an open (foot off the ground) or a closed (foot on the ground) kinetic chain. There is less chance of injury when the lower limb is an open kinetic chain. As a closed kinetic chain, the lower limb is an encapsulated system in which all parts work in concert. Thus, forces applied to one part of the chain must be absorbed by that part as well as other parts of the closed chain. If the forces are too great, injury results.

9. Is the joint swollen? Often there may be no swelling in the knee after severe injury. This lack of swelling occurs with a severe injury because the fluid extravasates into the soft tissues surrounding the joint; also, a number of structures around the knee joint are avascular and can be injured without bloody swelling occurring. Synovial swelling may occur 8 to 24 hours after the injury; swelling caused by blood will begin to occur almost immediately. Localized swelling may be due to an inflamed bursa (Fig. 11–3).

10. On movement, is there any grating or clicking in the knee? Grating or clicking may be due to

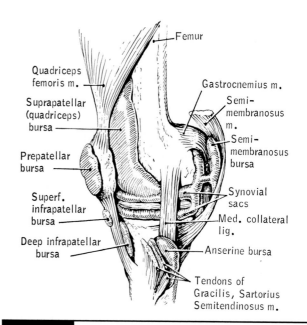

FIGURE 11–3. *The bursae around the knee (medial aspect). (From O'Donoghue, D. H.: Treatment of Injuries to Athletes, 4th ed. Philadelphia, W. B. Saunders Co., 1984, p. 466.)*

degeneration or to one structure snapping over another.

11. What type of shoes does the person wear? Shoes with negative heels (e.g., "earth" shoes) can often increase the incidence of chondromalacia patellae.

TABLE 11–1. Mechanisms of Injury to the Knee and Possible Structures Injured* *Continued*

Noncontact, compressive rotation	1. Meniscus injury 2. Osteochondral fracture
Hyperflexion	1. Meniscus (posterior horn) 2. Anterior cruciate ligament
Forced medial rotation	1. Meniscus injury (lateral meniscus)
Forced lateral rotation	1. Meniscus injury (medial meniscus) 2. Medial collateral ligament and possibly anterior cruciate ligament 3. Patellar dislocation
Flexion-varus-medial rotation	1. Anterolateral instability
Flexion-varus-lateral rotation	1. Anteromedial instability
Dashboard injury	1. Isolated posterior cruciate ligament 2. Posterior cruciate ligament and posterior capsule 3. Posterolateral instability 4. Posteromedial instability 5. Patellar fracture 6. Tibial fracture (proximal) 7. Tibial plateau fracture 8. Acetabular and pelvic fracture

*Adapted from Clancy, W. G.: Evaluation of acute knee injuries. American Association of Orthopedic Surgeons, Symposium on Sports Medicine: The Knee. St. Louis, C. V. Mosby, 1985, and Strobel, M., and H. W. Stedtfeld: Diagnostic Evaluation of the Knee. Berlin, Springer-Verlag, 1990.

If not, something must be limiting the movement (e.g., swelling, loose body, or meniscus).

Is there any apparent swelling in the knees? If there is intracapsular swelling, or at least sufficient swelling, the knee will assume a position of 15 to 25° of flexion, which provides the synovial cavity with the maximum capacity to hold fluid. This position is also called the *resting position* of the knee.

Is the swelling intracapsular or extracapsular? Intracapsular swelling is evident over the entire joint; extracapsular swelling tends to be more localized. An example of extracapsular swelling is shown in Figure 11–8, which illustrates *prepatellar bursitis*.

The examiner should ask the patient to contract the quadriceps muscles to see whether there is any visible wasting of the quadriceps muscles. The prominence of the vastus medialis is due to the obliquity of the distal fibers, the inferior position of its insertion, and the thinness of the fascial covering compared with the other quadriceps muscles.

The position of the patella should be noted. A "squinting" patella may be indicative of medial femoral or lateral tibial torsion (Fig. 11–9). Patients with abnormal torsion are prone to patellofemoral instability. Any bruising or discoloration around the knee should also be noted as well as any scars or sinuses indicating recent injury or surgery.

Lateral View, Standing

The examiner then views the patient from both sides for comparison. It should be noted whether *genu recurvatum* (hyperextended knee) is present and whether one or both patellae are higher (*patella alta*) or lower (*patella baja*) than normal (Fig. 11–

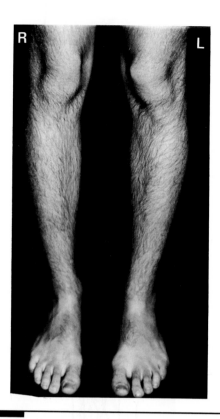

FIGURE 11–9. *"Squinting" patellae, especially prominent on the patient's left knee. Both patellae point inward in a medial fashion, a sign of excessive femoral anteversion or increased femoral torsion. (From Carson, W. A., et al.: Clin. Orthop. Relat. Res. 185:169, 1984.)*

10). With an abnormally high patella, a "camel sign" may be present (Fig. 11–11). Because of the high patella (one "hump"), the infrapatellar fat pad (second hump) becomes more prominent. This finding is especially noticeable in females. The patient should again extend the knees to see if the active range of motion is the same for both limbs. The examiner should note whether the patient stands "on the ligaments" with both legs completely extended or with the knees slightly flexed or unlocked. An individual with an excessive lordosis in the lumbar spine will often hyperextend the knees to compensate for the poor posture. This change may lead to posterior knee pain.

Posterior View, Standing

Next, the examiner views the patient from behind, looking for findings similar to those from the anterior aspect. In addition, one should look for abnormal swellings such as a popliteal (Baker's) cyst (i.e., herniation of synovial tissue through a weakening in the posterior capsule wall) (Fig. 11–12).

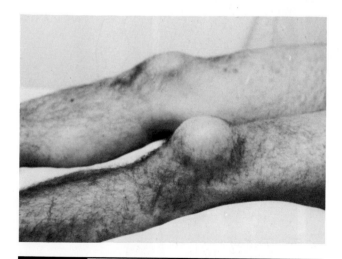

FIGURE 11–8. *Prepatellar bursitis.*

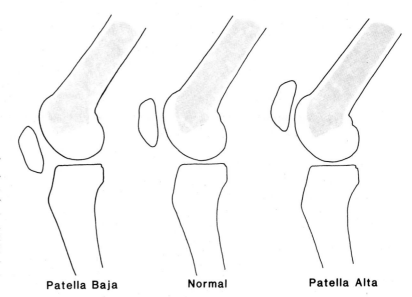

Patella Baja **Normal** **Patella Alta**

FIGURE 11–10. *The normal patellar posture for exerting deceleration forces in the functional position of 45° of knee flexion places the patellar articular surface squarely against the anterior femur. A lower posture represents patellar baja. A higher posture represents patella alta. Patella alta makes the patella less efficient in exerting normal forces. (From Hughston, J. C., et al.: Patellar Subluxation and Dislocation. Philadelphia, W. B. Saunders Co., 1984, p. 8.)*

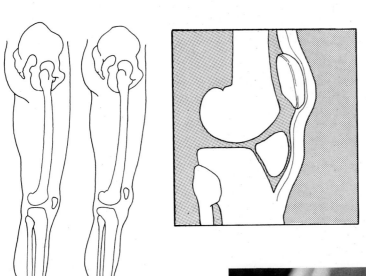

FIGURE 11–11. *"Camel" sign. Double hump seen from side caused by high-riding patella and uncovered infrapatellar fat pad. (From Hughston, J. C., et al.: Patellar Subluxation and Dislocation. Philadelphia, W. B. Saunders Co., 1984, p. 22.)*

FIGURE 11–12. *Popliteal (Baker's) cysts. (A) This 74-year-old man presented with the acute onset of calf pain and swelling without knee pain. The initial suspected diagnosis was popliteal thrombosis. A venogram was normal. An arthrogram reveals a collection of dye posterior to the joint space—the popliteal cysts (arrow). (From Reilly, B. M.: Practical Strategies in Outpatient Medicine. Philadelphia, W. B. Saunders Co., 1991, p. 1179.) (B) Schematic diagram of Baker's cyst.*

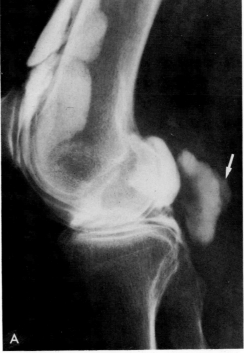

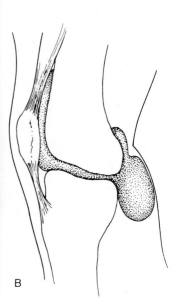

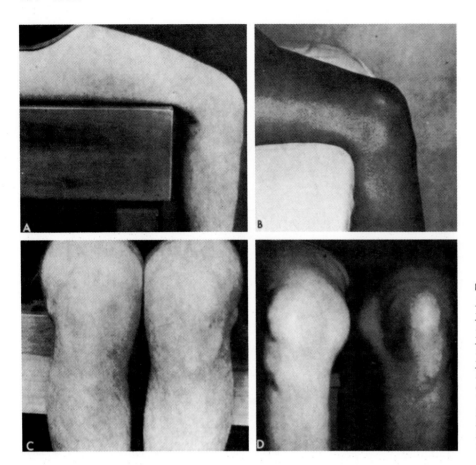

FIGURE 11–13. (A) Normal knee seen from side; patella faces straight ahead in line with femur. (B) Patella alta seen from side; patella points toward ceiling. (C) Normal patellae seen from front; patellae centered in outline of knees. (D) High and lateral posturing of patellae seen from front, giving "grasshopper eyes" or "frog eyes" appearance. (From Hughston, J. C., et al.: Patellar Subluxation and Dislocation. Philadelphia, W. B. Saunders Co., 1984, p. 23.)

Anterior and Lateral Views, Sitting

For the final part of the observation, the patient sits with the knees flexed to 90° and the feet either not bearing weight or dangling free. The patient is observed from the front and the side. In this position,

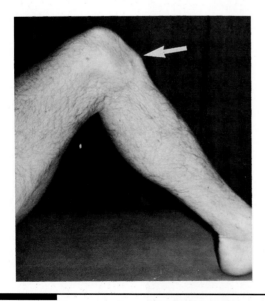

FIGURE 11–14. Osgood-Schlatter disease (enlarged tibial tuberosity).

the patella should face forward and should very nearly rest on the distal end of the femur. With patella alta, the patella will become more aligned with the anterior surface of the femur. If the patella is laterally displaced or laterally displaced with a patella alta, the patella will take on the appearance of "frog eyes" or "grasshopper eyes" (Fig. 11–13), meaning that the patellae face upward and outward, away from each other. Any bony enlargements such as those seen in Osgood-Schlatter disease (i.e., an enlarged tibial tubercle) should be noted (Fig. 11–14).

In the same position, any tibial torsion should be noted (Fig. 11–15).[7, 8] If there is tibial torsion, it is medial torsion that is associated with genu varum. Genu valgum is associated with lateral tibial torsion. Normally, the forefoot points straight forward or slightly laterally. With medial tibial torsion, the feet point toward each other, resulting in a "pigeon-toed" foot deformity. These deformities can be exacerbated by habitual postures. The positions illustrated in Figures 11–16 and 11–17A cause problems only if they are used habitually. Excessive tibial torsion can contribute to conditions such as chondromalacia patellae, patellofemoral instability, and fat pad entrapment. When standing, most people exhibit a lateral tibial torsion—the Fick angle (see Fig. 12–18)—which increases as the child grows.

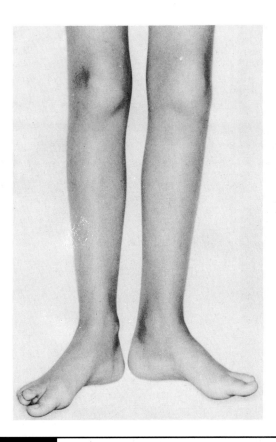

FIGURE 11–15. Exaggerated lateral tibial torsion. In stance, with the patellae facing straight forward, the feet point outward. (From Tachdjian, M. O.: Pediatric Orthopedics. Philadelphia, W. B. Saunders Co., 1990, p. 2816.)

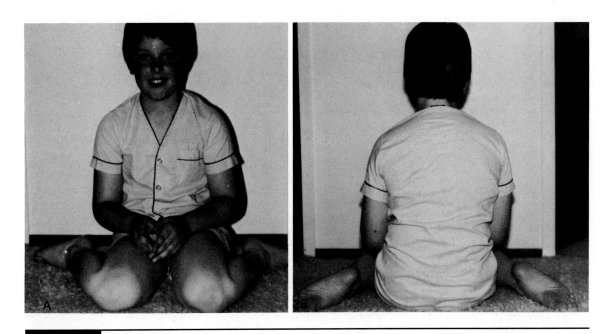

FIGURE 11–16. "Television" or "W" sitting position may lead to excessive lateral tibial torsion. (A) Anterior view. (B) Posterior view.

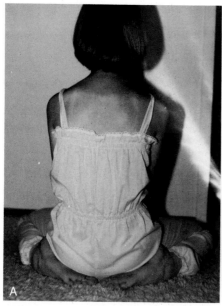
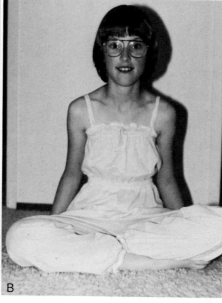

FIGURE 11–17. Medial tibial torsion. (A) Position to be avoided to prevent excessive medial tibial torsion. (B) Tailor position maintains normal medial tibial torsion.

This angle is approximately 5° in babies and as much as 18° in adults. To test for tibial torsion, the examiner aligns the patient's straight legs (knees extended) so that the patellae face straight ahead. The examiner then looks at the feet to determine their angle relative to the shaft of the tibia.

Femoral torsion, or anteversion (discussed in Chapter 10), can also affect the position of the patella relative to the femur and tibia.

EXAMINATION

Active Movements

Examination is performed initially with the patient sitting and then lying. During the active movements, the examiner should observe (1) the excursion of the patella to ensure that it tracks freely and smoothly; (2) the range of motion available; (3) whether pain occurs during the movement and, if so, where; and (4) what appears to be limiting the movement. The active movements may be done in the sitting or supine position, and, as always, the most painful movements should be done last (Fig. 11–18).

The active movements to be assessed for the knee are shown in Figure 11–19:

1. Flexion (0 to 135°).
2. Extension (0 to 15°).
3. Medial rotation of the tibia on the femur (20 to 30°).
4. Lateral rotation of the tibia on the femur (30 to 40°).

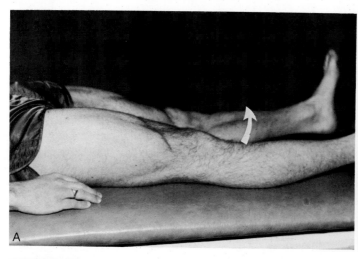
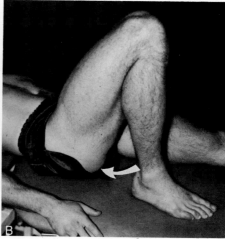

FIGURE 11–18. Active movements of the knee. (A) Extension. (B) Flexion.

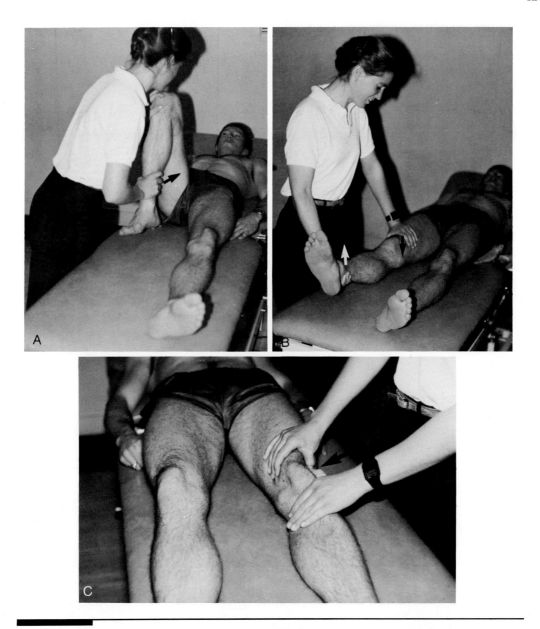

FIGURE 11–19. *Passive movements of the knee. (A) Flexion. (B) Extension. (C) Patella (medially shown).*

Full knee flexion is 135° (0° being straight knee). Active knee extension is approximately 0° but may be −15°, especially in women, who are more likely to have hyperextended knees (genu recurvatum). The knee extensor muscles develop the greatest force around the angle of 60°, and the knee flexor muscles develop their greatest force at the angles of 45° and 10°. To complete the last 15° of knee extension, a 60 per cent increase in force of the quadriceps muscles is required. The examiner should also watch for evidence of quadriceps lag, which is the result of the loss of mechanical advantage, muscle atrophy, decreasing power of the muscle as it shortens, adhesion formation, effusion, or reflex inhibition. The active medial rotation of the tibia on the femur should be 20 to 30°; active lateral rotation should be 30 to 40°.

Passive Movements

If, on active movements, the range of motion is full, overpressure may be gently applied to test the end feel of the various movements in the tibiofemoral joint. This action would preclude the need to do passive movements to the tibiofemoral joint. However, the examiner must do movements of the patella passively (see Fig. 11–19).

At the tibiofemoral joint, the end feel of flexion is tissue approximation; the end feel of extension and medial and lateral rotation of the tibia on the femur is tissue stretch. It must be remembered that during the passive movement, the examiner is also looking for a capsular pattern of the tibiofemoral joint. This pattern is more limitation of flexion than extension. Passive medial rotation of the tibia on the femur should be approximately 30° when the knee is flexed to 90°. Passive lateral rotation of the tibia on the femur at 90° of knee flexion should be 40°.

Passive medial and lateral movement of the patella is also carried out to determine its mobility and to compare it with the unaffected side. Normally, the patella should move half its width medially and laterally in extension. The side-to-side passive motion of the patella should also be tested in 45° of flexion, which is a more functional position and gives a better indication of functional instability of the patella.[9] The end feel of these movements is tissue stretch. Lateral displacement must be done with care, especially in patients who have experienced a dislocated patella.

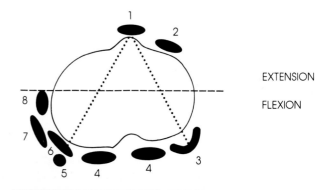

FIGURE 11–20. Movement diagram of the knee showing quadriceps hamstrings tripod. 1 = Patellar tendon (quadriceps); 2 = iliotibial band; 3 = biceps femoris; 4 = gastrocnemius; 5 = semitendinosus; 6 = semimembranosus; 7 = gracilis; 8 = sartorius.

The examiner must also ensure full and normal flexibility of the quadriceps, hamstring, and abductor and adductor muscles of the thigh as well as the gastrocnemius muscles (Fig. 11–20). Tightness of

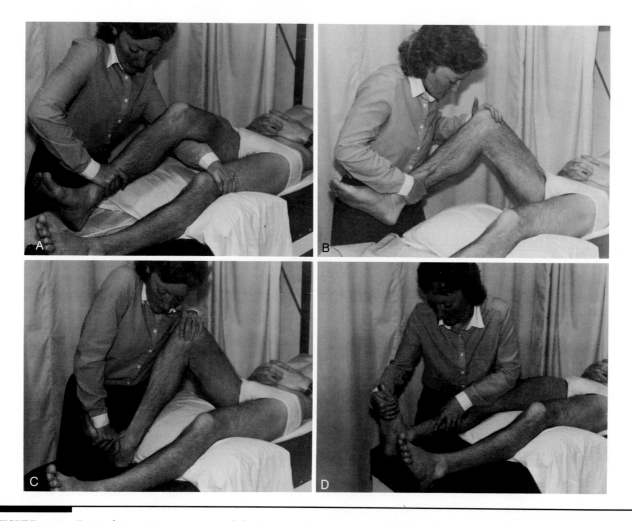

FIGURE 11–21. Resisted isometric movements of the knee. (A) Knee extension. (B) Knee flexion. (C) Ankle dorsiflexion. (D) Ankle plantar flexion.

any of these structures can alter gait and postural mechanics, which may lead to pathology. Tests for the hamstring, abductor, adductor, and rectus femoris muscles have been described in Chapter 10. A functional test for the quadriceps (described under "Special Tests" in this chapter) is a passive movement test (heel to buttock) for the femoral nerve. To test the gastrocnemius muscle, the examiner extends the patient's knee and, while holding it straight, dorsiflexes the patient's ankle. The examiner should be able to reach at least 90°, although 10 to 15° of dorsiflexion is more common.

Resisted Isometric Movements

For a proper test of the muscles, resisted and isometric movements must be done. The patient should be in the supine position and perform the following movements (Fig. 11–21):

1. Flexion of the knee.
2. Extension of the knee.
3. Ankle plantar flexion.
4. Ankle dorsiflexion.

Ideally, these tests are performed with the joint in its resting position. Segal and Jacob[10] suggest testing the quadriceps muscle at 0°, 30°, 60°, and 90° while observing any abnormal tibial movement (e.g., ligament instability) or excessive pain from patellar compression (e.g., chondromalacia patellae). Table 11–2 lists the muscles acting at the knee.

Although these movements are tested with the patient in the supine lying position, the hamstrings are usually tested with the patient prone. If the knee is flexed to 90° and the heel is turned out, the greatest stress is placed on the lateral hamstring muscle (biceps femoris) with resisted knee flexion. If the heel is turned in, the greatest stress is placed on the medial hamstring (semimembranosus and semitendinosus) muscles.

Kannus et al.[11] developed a scoring scale for measuring isokinetic and isometric strength (Table 11–3). The scale can be used to show improvement in strength over time. Depending on the speed, the hamstring-to-quadriceps ratio is normally approximately 50 to 60 per cent, with the higher percentage seen at slower test speeds.[12]

Functional Assessment

Instabilities produced on the examining table are easily produced functionally, especially in athletes who participate in activities such as vigorous cutting and jumping or rapid deceleration, which produce high physiological joint loads. Noyes et al.[13] developed the Cincinnati Rating System (Table 11–4), which deals with pain, swelling, stability, and activity level and is a good functional rating system for active individuals. The Knee Society[14] also has a rating scale (Table 11–5). The Knee Society advocates keeping knee rating and functional assessment separate. This knee-rating scale deals with pain,

TABLE 11–2. Muscles of the Knee: Their Actions, Nerve Supply, and Nerve Root Derivations

Action	Muscles Involved	Innervation	Nerve Root Derivation
Flexion of knee	1. Biceps femoris	Sciatic	L5, S1–S2
	2. Semimembranosus	Sciatic	L5, S1–S2
	3. Semitendinosus	Sciatic	L5, S1–S2
	4. Gracilis	Obturator	L2–L3
	5. Sartorius	Femoral	L2–L3
	6. Popliteus	Tibial	L4–L5, S1
	7. Gastrocnemius	Tibial	S1–S2
	8. Tensor fasciae latae (in 45 to 145° of flexion)	Superior gluteal	L4–L5
	9. Plantaris	Tibial	S1–S2
Extension of knee	1. Rectus femoris	Femoral	L2–L4
	2. Vastus medialis	Femoral	L2–L4
	3. Vastus intermedius	Femoral	L2–L4
	4. Vastus lateralis	Femoral	L2–L4
	5. Tensor fasciae latae (in 0 to 30° of flexion)	Superior gluteal	L4–L5
Medial rotation of flexed leg (non–weightbearing)	1. Popliteus	Tibial	L4–L5
	2. Semimembranosus	Sciatic	L5, S1–S2
	3. Semitendinosus	Sciatic	L5, S1–S2
	4. Sartorius	Femoral	L2–L3
	5. Gracilis	Obturator	L2–L3
Lateral rotation of flexed leg (non–weightbearing)	Biceps femoris	Sciatic	L5, S1–S2

TABLE 11–3. A Scoring Scale for Isokinetic and Isometric Strength Measurements of the Knee Joint*

	Peak Torque		Difference		
	Uninjured	*Injured*	*Absolute*	*Percent*	Score†
Isokinetic					
Extension 60°/sec	_____	_____	_____	_____	_____
Flexion 60°/sec	_____	_____	_____	_____	_____
Extension 180°/sec	_____	_____	_____	_____	_____
Flexion 180°/sec	_____	_____	_____	_____	_____
Isometric					
Extension 60°	_____	_____	_____	_____	_____
Flexion 60°	_____	_____	_____	_____	_____
Total score (maximum 100 points)					_____

†Scoring System
Isokinetic

17 points = per cent difference (uninjured − injured):	≤2%
15 points = per cent difference (uninjured − injured):	3 to 5%
13 points = per cent difference (uninjured − injured):	6 to 10%
9 points = per cent difference (uninjured − injured):	11 to 25%
5 points = per cent difference (uninjured − injured):	26 to 49%
0 points = per cent difference (uninjured − injured):	≥50%

Isometric

16 points = per cent difference (uninjured − injured):	≤2%
14 points = per cent difference (uninjured − injured):	3 to 5%
12 points = per cent difference (uninjured − injured):	6 to 10%
8 points = per cent difference (uninjured − injured):	11 to 25%
4 points = per cent difference (uninjured − injured):	26 to 49%
0 points = per cent difference (uninjured − injured):	≥50%

*Modified from Kannus, P., M. Jarvinea, and K. Latvala: Knee strength evaluation. Scand. J. Sport Sci. 9:9, 1987.

TABLE 11–4. Cincinnati Rating System*

Symptoms (50 points):

Left	Right			Left	Right	
☐	☐	20	**1. Pain** No pain, normal knee, performs 100%.	☐	☐	*Location of pain:* Medial (inner side)
☐	☐	16	Occasional pain with strenuous sports or heavy work, knee not entirely normal, some limitations, but minor and tolerable.	☐	☐	Anterior-patellar (front/knee cap)
				☐	☐	Posterior (back of knee)
☐	☐	12	Occasional pain with light recreational sports or moderate work activities, frequently brought on by vigorous activities, running, heavy labor, strenuous sports.	☐	☐	Diffuse (all over)
				☐	☐	Diffuse (all over)
☐	☐	8	Pain, usually brought on by sports, light recreational activities, or moderate work. Occasionally occurs with walking, standing, or light work.			*Pain occurs on:*
				☐	☐	Stairs
				☐	☐	Sitting
				☐	☐	Kneeling
				☐	☐	Standing
☐	☐	4	Pain is a significant problem with activities as simple as walking. Relieved by rest. Unable to do sports.			*Type of pain:*
				☐	☐	Sharp
				☐	☐	Aching
☐	☐	0	Pain present all the time, occurs with walking, standing and at nighttime. Not relieved with rest.	☐	☐	Throbbing
				☐	☐	Burning
☐	☐		I do not know what my pain level is. I have not tested my knee. **Intensity of pain:** ☐ Mild ☐ Moderate ☐ Severe **Frequency:** ☐ Intermittent ☐ Constant			
☐	☐	10	**2. Swelling** No swelling, normal knee, 100% activity.			
☐	☐	8	Occasional swelling with strenuous sports or heavy work. Some limitations but minor and tolerable.			
☐	☐	6	Occasional swelling with light recreational sports or moderate work activities, frequently brought on by vigorous activities, running, heavy labor, strenuous sports.			

*From Noyes, F. R., et al.: Functional disability in the anterior cruciate insufficient knee syndrome. Sports Med. 1:286–287, 1984.

TABLE 11–4. Cincinnati Rating System *Continued*

Symptoms (50 points):

Left	Right		
☐	☐	4	Swelling limits sports and moderate work. Occurs infrequently with simple walking activities or light work (about 3 times/year).
☐	☐	2	Swelling brought on by simple walking activities and light work. Relieved with rest.
☐	☐	0	Severe problem all of the time, with simple walking activities.
☐	☐		I do not know what my swelling level is. I have not tested my knee.
			If swelling occurs it is: (check one box on each line)
			Intensity: ☐ Mild ☐ Moderate ☐ Severe
			Frequency: ☐ Intermittent ☐ Constant

3. Giving-way.

Left	Right		
☐	☐	20	No giving-way, normal knee, performs 100%.
☐	☐	16	Occasional giving-way with strenuous sports or heavy work. Can participate in all sports but some guarding or limitations are still present.
☐	☐	12	Occasional giving-way with light recreational activities or moderate work. Able to compensate, limits vigorous activities; sports or heavy work; not able to cut or twist suddenly.
☐	☐	8	Giving-way limits sports and moderate work; occurs infrequently with walking or light work (about 3 times/year).
☐	☐	4	Giving-way with simple walking activities and light work. Occurs once per month. Requires guarding.
☐	☐	0	Severe problem with simple walking activities; cannot turn or twist while walking without giving-way.
☐	☐		I do not know my level of giving-way. I have not tested my knee.

4. Other Symptoms (unscored)

Left	Right	Knee stiffness			Kneecap grinding			Knee locking
☐	☐	None	☐	☐	None	☐	☐	None
☐	☐	Occasional	☐	☐	Mild	☐	☐	Occasional
☐	☐	Frequent	☐	☐	Moderate	☐	☐	Frequent
			☐	☐	Severe			

Function (50 points):

5. Overall activity level

Left	Right		
☐	☐	20	No limitation, normal knee, able to do everything including strenuous sports or heavy labor.
☐	☐	16	Perform sports including vigorous activities, but at a lower performance level, involves guarding or some limits to heavy labor.
☐	☐	12	Light recreational activities possible with rare symptoms, more strenuous activities cause problems. Active but in different sports, limited to moderate work.
☐	☐	8	No sports or recreational activities possible. Walking activities possible with rare symptoms, limited to light work.
☐	☐	4	Walking, activities of daily living cause moderate symptoms, frequent limitation.
☐	☐	0	Walking, activities of daily living cause severe problems, persistent symptoms.
☐	☐		I do not know what my real activity level is, I have not tested my knee, or I have given up strenuous sports.

6. Walking

Left	Right		
☐	☐	10	Normal, unlimited.
☐	☐	8	Slight/mild problem.
☐	☐	6	Moderate problem: smooth surface possible up to 800 m.
☐	☐	4	Severe problem: only 2–3 blocks possible.
☐	☐	2	Severe problem: requires cane, crutches.

7. Stairs

Left	Right		
☐	☐	10	Normal, unlimited.
☐	☐	8	Slight/mild problem.
☐	☐	6	Moderate problem: only 10–15 steps possible.
☐	☐	4	Severe problem: requires bannister, support.
☐	☐	2	Severe problem: only 1–5 steps possible.

8. Running activity

Left	Right		
☐	☐	5	Normal, unlimited: fully competitive, strenuous.
☐	☐	4	Slight/mild problem: run half-speed.
☐	☐	3	Moderate problem: only 2–4 km possible.
☐	☐	2	Severe problem: only 1–2 blocks possible.
☐	☐	1	Severe problem: only a few steps.

9. Jumping or twisting activities

Left	Right		
☐	☐	5	Normal, unlimited, fully competitive, strenuous.
☐	☐	4	Slight/mild problem: some guarding, but sports possible.
☐	☐	3	Moderate problem: gave up strenuous sports; recreational sports possible.
☐	☐	2	Severe problem: affects all sports, must constantly guard.
☐	☐	1	Severe problem: only light activity possible (golf, swimming).

Total: Left [＿＿＿] Right [＿＿＿] (Maximum: 100 points)

TABLE 11–5. Knee Society Knee Score

Patient category
A. Unilateral or bilateral (opposite knee successfully replaced)
B. Unilateral, other knee symptomatic
C. Multiple arthritis or medical infirmity

Pain	Points	Function	Points
None	50	Walking	50
Mild or occasional	45	Unlimited	40
Stairs only	40	>10 blocks	30
Walking and stairs	30	5–10 blocks	20
Moderate		<5 blocks	10
Occasional	20	Housebound	0
Continual	10	Unable	
Severe	0	Stairs	
		Normal up and down	50
Range of Motion		Normal up; down with rail	40
(5° = 1 point)	25	Up and down with rail	30
		Up with rail; unable down	15
Stability (maximum		Unable	0
movement in any position)			
		Subtotal	
Anteroposterior			
<5 mm	10	Deductions (minus)	
5–10 mm	5	Cane	5
10 mm	0	Two canes	10
Mediolateral		Crutches or walker	20
<5°	15		
6°–9°	10	**Total deductions**	
10°–14°	5		
15°	0		
		Function score	
Subtotal			
Deductions (minus)			
Flexion contracture			
5°–10°	2		
10°–15°	5		
16°–20°	10		
>20°	15		
Extension lag			
<10°	5		
10°–20°	10		
>20°	15		
Alignment			
5°–10°	0		
0°–4°	3 points each degree		
11°–15°	3 points each degree		
Other	20		
Total deductions			
Pain score (if total is a minus number, score is 0)			

Adapted from Insall, J. N. et al.: Rationale of the Knee Society clinical rating system. Clin. Orthop. Relat. Res. 248:14, 1989

range of motion, and stability on the one hand, giving positive points up to 100 and grouping deductions that can take away from the overall value. Function is dealt with separately on the scale. Kettelkamp and Thompson[15] developed a knee-rating scale that gives one overall score (Table 11–6). The most recent knee scale is the documentation form developed by the International Knee Documentation Committee (Table 11–7). Each of these knee-rating scales is slightly different. The scale that works best for the examiner and the examiner's clientele should be used.

Although full extension is usually preferable for everyday activities (e.g., standing, walking), full flexion (135°) is not necessary. However, approximately 117° of flexion is necessary for activities such as squatting to tie a shoelace or pull on a sock. Sitting in a chair requires approximately 90° of flexion, and climbing stairs (average height) requires approximately 80° of flexion.

TABLE 11–6. Knee Scoring Scale I

	Points R	Points L		Points R	Points L
Pain with Activity			*Flexion in Degrees*		
None	26 20	26 20	> 100°	2	2
Usually heavy activity	22 18	22 18	70°–99°	1	1
End of day—not limiting	18 15	18 15	<75°	0	0
End of day—limiting	14 12	14 12			
Few hours or few blocks	10 9		*Anterior Drawer*		
Less than 1 hr or 1 block	6 6	6 6	Negative	6 7	6 7
Every step	3 3	3 3	Slightly positive	4 5	4 5
Constant	0 0	0 0	Moderately positive	2 3	2 3
			Markedly positive	0 0	0 0
Shoes and Socks					
No trouble	6	6	*Rotational Instability*	4	4
Difficult	4	4	None	2	2
Sock, not shoe	2	2	Mild	1	1
Can't	0	0	Moderate	0	0
			Severe		
Stairs					
No trouble	22 19	22 19	*Lateral Ligament (30°)*	8 7	8 7
Slow alternating	14 13	14 13	Intact	6 5	6 5
One at a time	6 6	6 6	Mildly loose	4 3	4 3
Can't	0 0	0 0	Moderately loose	0 0	0 0
			Markedly loose		
Gait					
No limp	2	2	*Pain with Flexion and Extension*	6	6
Limp, 1 cane or 1 crutch	1	1	No	3	3
2 canes, 2 crutches	0	0	On flexion or extension	0	0
			On both		
Synovial Thickening					
None	4 6	4 6	*Pain on Rotation (90°)*		
Mild	2 4	2 4	No	8 6	8 6
Moderate	1 2	1 2	Either ext or int	4 3	4 3
Severe	0 0	0 0	Both	0 0	0 0
Flexion Contracture					
0 degrees	8	8	*Varus-Valgus (standing)*		
1–5	6	6	5°–9° valgus	1	1
6–10	4	4	Less than 5° and	0	0
11–15	2	2	more than 9°		
16–20	1	1			
>20	0	0	TOTAL POINTS (103)	____	____

From Kettlelkamp, D. B., and C. Thompson: Development of a knee scoring scale. Clin. Orthop. Relat. Res. 107:96, 1975

If the active, passive, and resisted isometric movements are performed with little difficulty, the examiner may put the patient through a series of *functional tests* to see if these sequential activities produce pain or other symptoms. The functional activities in order of sequence are as follows:

1. Squatting (both knees should flex symmetrically).
2. Squatting and then bouncing at the end of the squat (again, the two knees should act symmetrically).
3. Ascending and descending stairs.
4. Running straight ahead.
5. Running and twisting (figure-eight running).
6. Jumping.
7. Jumping and going into a full squat.

These functional activities, which are provided as examples, must be geared to the individual patient. Older individuals should not be expected to accomplish the last four movements unless they have, in the recent past, been doing these or similar activities. Functional strength tests for sedentary individuals are shown in Table 11–8.

Functional tests for active individuals are more demanding. Losee[16] mentioned several tests. For example, in the *deceleration test,* the patient is asked to run full speed and stop suddenly on command. The test is positive for rotary instability if the patient

TABLE 11–7. Knee Ligament Standard Evaluation Form*
(Proposed Field Trial by the International Knee Documentation Committee)

Patient Name _____ Date ____/____/____ Medical Record _____

Occupation _____ Sports 1st Choice _____ 2nd Choice _____

Age _____ Sex _____ Ht _____ Wt _____ Involved Knee: ☐ Right ☐ Left   Contralateral Normal: ☐ Yes ☐ No

Cause of Injury: ☐ ADL   Date of Injury ____/____/____   Procedure _____
                   ☐ Traffic
                   ☐ Contact Sport   Date of Index Operation ____/____/____   Post Op Dx _____
                   ☐ Noncontact Sport

ACTIVITY

		Pre-injury	Pre-Rx	Post-Rx
I.	Strenuous Activity jumping, pivoting, hard cutting (football, soccer)			
II.	Moderate Activity heavy manual work (skiing, tennis)			
III.	Light Activity (jogging, running)			
IV.	Sedentary Activity (housework, ADL)			

PREVIOUS SURGERY

Arthroscopy	Date	1 ____	2 ____	3 ____
Meniscectomy	Dx	1 ____	2 ____	3 ____
Stabilization	Procedure	1 ____	2 ____	3 ____

MENISCAL STATUS

	N1	1/3	2/3	Total
Med				
Lat				

TABLE 11–7. Knee Ligament Standard Evaluation Form*
(Proposed Field Trial by the International Knee Documentation Committee) *Continued*

SEVEN GROUPS	FOUR GRADES				*GROUP GRADE			
	A. Normal	B. Nearly Normal	C. Abnormal	D. Sev. Abnormal	A	B	C	D
1. PATIENT SUBJECTIVE ASSESSMENT How does your knee function?	☐ 0	☐ 1	☐ 2	☐ 3				
On a scale of 0 to 3, how does your knee affect your activity level?	☐ 0	☐ 1	☐ 2	☐ 3	☐	☐	☐	☐
2. SYMPTOMS (Grade at highest activity level with no significant symptoms. Exclude 0 to slight symptoms)	I. Strenuous Activity	II. Moderate Activity	III. Light Activity	IV. Sedentary Activity				
Pain	☐	☐	☐	☐				
Swelling	☐	☐	☐	☐				
Partial Giving Way	☐	☐	☐	☐				
Full Giving Way	☐	☐	☐	☐	☐	☐	☐	☐
3. RANGE OF MOTION Ext/Flex: Index side:___/___/___ Opposite side:___/___/___								
Lack of extension (from 0°)	☐ <3°	☐ 3 to 5°	☐ 6 to 10°	☐ >10°	☐	☐	☐	☐
Lack of flexion	☐ 0 to 5°	☐ 6 to 15°	☐ 16 to 25°	☐ <25°				
4. LIGAMENT EXAMINATION (manual, instrumented, x-ray) LACHMAN (25° flex)	☐ -1 to 2 mm	☐ 3 to 5 mm -1 to -3 stiff	☐ 6 to 10 mm < -3 stiff	☐ >10 mm				
Endpoint: firm/soft	☐ firm		☐ soft					
Total A.P. Transl. (70° flex)	☐ 0 to 2 mm	☐ 3 to 5 mm	☐ 6 to 10 mm	☐ >10 mm				
Post sag (70° flex)	☐ 0 to 2 mm	☐ 3 to 5 mm	☐ 6 to 10 mm	☐ >10 mm				
Med jt opening (20° flex) (valgus rot)	☐ 0 to 2 mm	☐ 3 to 5 mm	☐ 6 to 10 mm	☐ >10 mm				
Lat jt opening (20° flex) (varus rot)	☐ 0 to 2 mm	☐ 3 to 5 mm	☐ 6 to 10 mm	☐ >10 mm				
Pivot shift	☐ neg	☐ + (glide)	☐ ++ (clunk)	☐ +++ (gross)				
Reversal pivot shift	☐ equal	☐ glide	☐ marked	☐ gross	☐	☐	☐	☐
5. COMPARTMENTAL FINDINGS								
Crepitus patellofemoral	☐ none		☐ moderate	☐ severe				
Crepitus medial compartment	☐ none		☐ moderate	☐ severe				
Crepitus lateral compartment	☐ none		☐ moderate	☐ severe	☐		☐	☐
6. X-RAY FINDINGS								
Med Joint space narrowing	☐ none		☐ <50%	☐ >50%				
Lat Joint space narrowing	☐ none		☐ <50%	☐ >50%				
Patellofemoral joint narrowing	☐ none		☐ <50%	☐ >50%	☐		☐	☐
7. FUNCTIONAL TEST One leg hop (% of opposite side)	☐ 100 ≥ 90%	☐ 89 to 76%	☐ 75 to 50%	☐ <50%	☐	☐	☐	☐
**FINAL EVALUATION					☐	☐	☐	☐

*Group Grade: The lowest grade within a group determines the group grade. **Final Evaluation: The worst group determines the final evaluation.
In a final evaluation, all 7 groups are to be evaluated. For a quick knee profile, the evaluation of groups, 1 to 4 are sufficient.

*The International Knee Documentation Committee is developing a system of knee evaluation that will allow clinicians to compare the results of knee ligament surgery. The crux of this data collection lies in the assessment of seven variables, each assigned one of four grades, that will separate patients and knees into groups that can be compared.

The data evaluation imposes some arbitrary Committee standards that may require amendment. The Committee recommends these three guidelines when using the evaluation form:

1. The postoperative patient will be graded at the highest activity level accomplished—i.e., Level I: jumping, pivoting, hard cutting (football, soccer); Level II: heavy manual work (skiing, tennis); Level III: light manual work (jogging, running); and Level IV: sedentary work (ADL). Thus, symptoms and function will be linked to activity level.
2. Each of the seven variables will be characterized by the lowest score awarded: normal, nearly normal, abnormal, severely abnormal.
3. Short-term results are those followed a minimum of 2 years; 5 years are required for intermediate-term results; and 10 years minimum for long-term results.

TABLE 11–8. Functional Testing of the Knee*

Starting Position	Action	Function Level
Standing	1. Walking backward 2. Running forward 20° (knee flexion)	6–8 m: Functional 3–6 m: Functionally fair 1–3 m: Functionally poor 0 m: Nonfunctional
Standing	1. Squat 20 to 30° 2. Jump, lifting body off floor	5 to 6 Repetitions: Functional 3 to 4 Repetitions: Functionally fair 1 to 2 Repetitions: Functionally poor 0 Repetitions: Nonfunctional

*Modified from Palmar, M. L., and M. Epler: Clinical Assessment Procedures in Physical Therapy. Philadelphia, J. B. Lippincott, 1990, pp. 275–276.

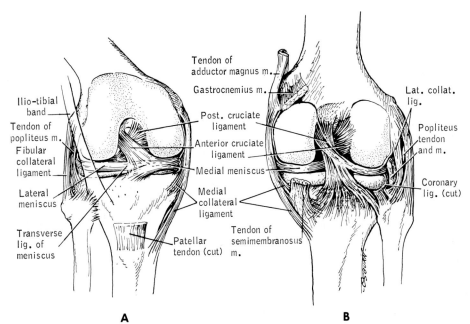

Tendon of adductor magnus m.
Gastrocnemius m.
Ilio-tibial band
Post. cruciate ligament
Anterior cruciate ligament
Tendon of popliteus m.
Fibular collateral ligament
Medial meniscus
Lateral meniscus
Medial collateral ligament
Transverse lig. of meniscus
Patellar tendon (cut)
Tendon of semimembranosus m.

Lat. collat. lig.
Popliteus tendon and m.
Coronary lig. (cut)

A   B

FIGURE 11–22. Anatomic drawings of knee. (A) Anterior view. Patellar tendon is sectioned, the patella is reflected upward, and the knee is flexed. Note that the cruciate ligament rises in front of anterior tibial spine, not from it. Note also that the medial meniscus is firmly attached to the medial collateral ligament. (B) Posterior view with the knee extended. Note that the posterior ligament has been removed. The two layers of the medial collateral ligament are shown, as is the tibial portion of the lateral collateral ligament. The posterior cruciate ligament rises behind the tibia, not on its upper surface. Observe the femoral attachment of the anterior cruciate ligament at the back of the notch. (From O'Donoghue, D. H.: Treatment of Injuries to Athletes, 4th ed. Philadelphia, W. B. Saunders Co., 1984, p. 477.)

stops without using the quadriceps or decelerates in a crouched position (more than 30° flexion of the knee). The effect of the test can be accentuated by having the patient turn away from the affected leg just as the patient is about to stop.[17]

For the "*disco test,*" the patient stands on one leg with the knee flexed 10 to 20°. The patient is asked to rotate or twist left and right while holding the flexed position. Apprehension during the test or refusal to do the test is a positive sign for rotary instability. If pain is felt on the joint line, it may be indicative of meniscus pathology, in which case it is called *Merke's sign.*[18] Pain on medial rotation along the joint line implies medial meniscus pathology, and pain on lateral rotation implies lateral meniscus pathology.

Larson[19] advocated the *leaning hop test.* For this test, the patient hops up and down on one leg while abducting the opposite leg. A positive test is apprehension during the test or refusal to do the test and is a positive sign for rotary instability.

Strobel and Stedtfeld[18] put forward the *one-leg hop test.* The patient stands and does a "long jump" hop on one leg while landing on the same leg. The test is repeated three times alternately with each leg. If rotary instability is evident, the distance for the affected leg will be less than that for the normal leg.

Ligament Stability

Because the knee, more than any other joint in the body, depends on its ligaments to maintain its integrity, it is imperative that the ligaments be tested.

The ligaments of the knee joint act as primary stabilizers and guide the movement of the bones in proper relation to one another. There are several ligaments around the knee, but four deserve special mention (Fig. 11–22).

Collateral and Cruciate Ligaments

Collateral Ligaments. The *medial (tibial) collateral ligament* lies more posteriorly than anteriorly on the medial aspect of the tibiofemoral joint. It is made up of two layers—one superficial and one deep. The deep layer is a thickening of the joint capsule and blends with the *medial meniscus.* (It is sometimes called the *medial capsular ligament.*) The superficial layer is a strong, broad triangular strap. It starts distal to the adductor tubercle and extends to the medial surface of the tibia approximately 6 cm below the joint line. It blends with the posterior capsule and is separated from the capsule and medial meniscus by a bursa.

The entire medial collateral ligament is tight throughout the full range of motion, although there is greater stress placed on different parts of the ligament as it goes through the range of motion because of the shape of the femoral condyles. All of its fibers are taut on full extension. In flexion, the anterior fibers are the most taut; in midrange, the posterior fibers are the most taut.[20]

The *lateral (fibular) collateral ligament* is round, lying under the tendon of the biceps femoris muscle. It also lies more posteriorly than anteriorly when the tibiofemoral joint is in extension. As the knee flexes, it provides protection to the lateral aspect of the knee. It is not attached to the lateral meniscus but rather is separated from it by a small fat pad.[20]

Cruciate Ligaments. The cruciate ligaments cross each other and are the primary rotary stabilizers of the knee.[21] These strong ligaments are named in relation to their attachment to the tibia and are intracapsular but extrasynovial. Each ligament has an anteromedial and a posterolateral portion. The *anterior cruciate ligament* also has an intermediate portion.

The anterior cruciate ligament extends superiorly, posteriorly, and laterally, twisting on itself as it extends from the tibia to the femur. Its main functions are to prevent anterior movement of the tibia on the femur, check external rotation of the tibia in flexion, and to a lesser extent, check extension and hyperextension at the knee. It also helps to control the normal rolling and gliding movement of the knee. The anteromedial bundle is tight in both flexion and extension, whereas the posterolateral bundle is tight on extension. As a whole, the ligament has the least amount of stress on it between 30° and 60° flexion.[20-23]

The *posterior cruciate ligament* extends superiorly, anteriorly, and medially from the tibia to the femur. This strong fan-shaped ligament, the stoutest ligament in the knee, is a primary stabilizer of the knee against posterior movement of the tibia on the femur, and it checks extension and hyperextension. In addition, the ligament helps to maintain rotary stability and functions as the knee's central axis of rotation. Along with the anterior cruciate ligament, it acts as a rotary guide to the "screwing home" mechanism of the knee.[20, 23]

As with the medial and lateral collateral ligaments, both cruciate ligaments are taut throughout the full range of motion, although the amount of tightness will vary. For example, for the posterior cruciate ligament, the bulk of the fibers are tight at 30° flexion, but the posterolateral fibers are loose in early flexion.

With lateral rotation of the tibia, both collateral ligaments become more taut, and the cruciate ligaments become relaxed (Fig. 11–23). With medial rotation of the tibia, the reverse action occurs; the collateral ligaments become more relaxed, and the cruciate ligaments become tighter.[20, 24]

Testing of Ligaments

When testing the ligaments of the knee, the examiner must watch for four one-plane instabilities and four rotational instabilities (Table 11–9). Thus, this section includes tests for the following:

1. One-plane medial instability.
2. One-plane lateral instability.

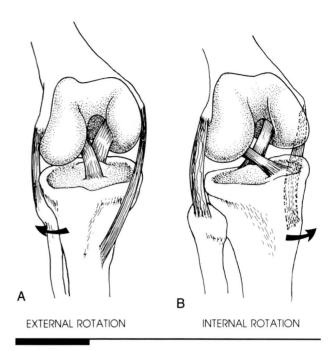

EXTERNAL ROTATION   INTERNAL ROTATION

FIGURE 11–23. *Effect of tibial rotation on cruciate and collateral ligaments. (A) The collateral ligament is taut; the cruciate ligament is lax. (B) The collateral ligament is lax; the cruciate ligament is taut.*

3. One-plane anterior instability.
4. One-plane posterior instability.
5. Anteromedial rotary instability.
6. Anterolateral rotary instability.
7. Posteromedial rotary instability.
8. Posterolateral rotary instability.

There are a number of tests for each type of instability. The examiner may use the one or two tests that obtain the best results. It is not essential to do all of the tests discussed. The techniques chosen must be practiced diligently so the examiner becomes proficient at doing them; only with practice will the examiner be able to determine which structures are injured.

When testing for ligament stability of the knee, the examiner should keep the following in mind:

1. The normal knee is tested first to establish a baseline as well as show the patient what to expect. This action helps to gain the patient's confidence by showing what the test involves.

2. The appropriate stress should be applied gently.

3. The stress is repeated several times and increased to the point of pain to demonstrate maximum laxity without causing muscle spasm.

4. It is not only the degree of opening but also the quality of the opening (i.e., the end feel) that are of concern.

TABLE 11–9. Tests for Ligamentous Instability Around the Knee

Instability	Tests Used to Determine Instability	Structures Injured to Some Degree if Test Positive*	Notes
One-plane medial (straight medial)	1. Abduction (valgus) stress with knee *in full extension*	1. Medial collateral ligament (superficial and deep fibers) 2. Posterior oblique ligament 3. Posteromedial capsule 4. Anterior cruciate ligament 5. Posterior cruciate ligament 6. Medial quadriceps expansion 7. Semimembranosus muscle	If either cruciate ligament torn (third-degree sprain) or stretched, rotary instability will also be evident
	2. Abduction (valgus) stress with knee *slightly flexed* (20 to 30°)	1. Medial collateral ligament (superficial and deep fibers) 2. Posterior oblique ligament 3. Posterior cruciate ligament	1. If posterior cruciate ligament torn (third-degree sprain), rotary instability will also be evident 2. Opening of 12 to 15° signifies injury to posterior cruciate ligament 3. If tibia externally rotated, stress is taken off posterior cruciate ligament 4. If tibia is internally rotated, stress is increased on cruciate ligaments while medial collateral ligament relaxes
One-plane lateral (straight lateral)	1. Adduction (varus) stress with knee *in full extension*	1. Lateral collateral ligament 2. Posterolateral capsule 3. Arcuate-popliteus complex 4. Biceps femoris tendon 5. Posterior cruciate ligament 6. Anterior cruciate ligament 7. Lateral gastrocnemius muscle	If either cruciate ligament is torn (third-degree sprain) or stretched, rotary instability will also be evident
	2. Adduction (varus) stress with knee *slightly flexed* (20 to 30°) and tibia *externally rotated*	1. Lateral collateral ligament 2. Posterolateral capsule 3. Arcuate-popliteus complex 4. Iliotibial band 5. Biceps femoris tendon	1. If tibia not externally rotated, maximum stress will not be placed on lateral collateral ligament 2. External rotation of tibia results in relaxation of both cruciate ligaments 3. With flexion, the iliotibial band lies over the center of the lateral joint line 4. If tibia is internally rotated, stress is increased on both cruciate ligaments while lateral collateral ligament relaxes
One-plane anterior	1. Lachman test (20 to 30° knee flexion)	1. Anterior cruciate ligament 2. Posterior oblique ligament 3. Arcuate-popliteus complex	1. Medial collateral ligament and iliotibial band lax in this position 2. Tests primarily posterolateral bundle of anterior cruciate ligament
	2. Anterior drawer sign (90° knee flexion)	1. Anterior cruciate ligament 2. Posterolateral capsule 3. Posteromedial capsule 4. Medial collateral ligament 5. Iliotibial band 6. Posterior oblique ligament 7. Arcuate-popliteus complex	1. Tests primarily anteromedial bundle of anterior cruciate ligament 2. If anterior cruciate ligament and medial or lateral structures torn (third-degree sprain) or stretched, rotary instability will also be evident

TABLE 11–9. Tests for Ligamentous Instability Around the Knee *Continued*

Instability	Tests Used to Determine Instability	Structures Injured to Some Degree if Test Positive*	Notes
One-plane posterior	1. Posterior drawer sign (90° knee flexion) 2. Posterior sag sign	1. Posterior cruciate ligament 2. Arcuate-popliteus complex 3. Posterior oblique ligament 4. Anterior cruciate ligament	If posterior cruciate ligament and medial or lateral structures torn (third-degree sprain) or stretched, rotary instability will also be evident
Anteromedial rotary	Slocum test (foot laterally rotated 15°)	1. Medial collateral ligament (superficial and deep fibers) 2. Posterior oblique ligament 3. Posteromedial capsule 4. Anterior cruciate ligament	Test must *not* be done in extreme lateral rotation of tibia because passive stabilizing will result from "coiling" to maximum rotation
Anterolateral rotary	1. Slocum test (foot medially rotated 30°) 2. Losee test 3. Jerk test of Hughston	1. Anterior cruciate ligament 2. Posterolateral capsule 3. Arcuate-popliteus complex 4. Lateral collateral ligament 5. Iliotibial band	1. Tests bring about anterior subluxation of tibia on femur, causing patient to experience "giving way" sensation 2. Slocum test must *not* be done in extreme medial rotation of tibia because passive stabilization will result from "coiling" to maximum rotation
	1. Lateral pivot shift test of Macintosh 2. Slocum's "ALRI" test 3. Crossover test 4. Flexion-rotation drawer test	1. Anterior cruciate ligament 2. Posterolateral capsule 3. Arcuate-popliteus complex 4. Lateral collateral ligament 5. Iliotibial band	Tests cause reduction of subluxed tibia on femur
Posteromedial rotary	Hughston's posteromedial drawer sign	1. Posterior cruciate ligament 2. Posterior oblique ligament 3. Medial collateral ligament (superficial and deep fibers) 4. Semimembranosus muscle 5. Posteromedial capsule 6. Anterior cruciate ligament	
Posterolateral rotary	1. Hughston's posterolateral drawer sign 2. Jakob test (reverse pivot shift maneuver) 3. External rotational recurvatum test	1. Posterior cruciate ligament 2. Arcuate-popliteus ligament 3. Lateral collateral ligament 4. Biceps femoris tendon 5. Posterolateral capsule 6. Anterior cruciate ligament	

*The amount of displacement will give an indication of how badly and how many of the structures are injured (i.e., first-, second-, or third-degree sprain).

5. If the ligament is intact, there should be an abrupt stop or end feel when the ligament is stressed. A soft or indistinct end feel usually signifies ligamentous injury.

6. Ligaments of the knee tend to act in concert to maintain stability, and individual ligaments are difficult to isolate in terms of their function. Thus, more than one test may be found to be positive in assessments for the different instabilities. For example, a patient may exhibit a one-plane medial instability as well as an anteromedial and/or anterolateral rotary instability, depending on the severity of the injury to the various ligamentous structures.

7. Tests for ligament instability are more accurate for assessment of a chronic injury than for assessment of an acute injury in the unanesthetized knee because of the presence of muscle spasm and swelling in the acutely injured knee.

8. The muscles must be relaxed if the tests are to be valid. Maximum laxity is demonstrated with the patient under anesthesia.

9. For the tests involving rotary instability in which the tibia is moved in relation to the femur, if the movement is into extension, subluxation of the tibia relative to the femur occurs in a positive test. If the movement is into flexion, reduction of the tibia relative to the femur occurs in a positive test.

10. Positive rotational tests should not be repeated too frequently as they may lead to articular cartilage damage, further meniscal tearing, or further damage to injured ligaments.

11. Because the ligamentous tests are subjective tests, the more experience the examiner has in doing the tests, the more accurate will be the interpretation of the test. Thus, the examiner should select only one or two from each group of tests and learn to do them well rather than learn all of the tests and risk doing them poorly.

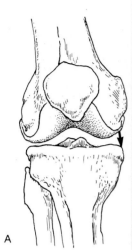

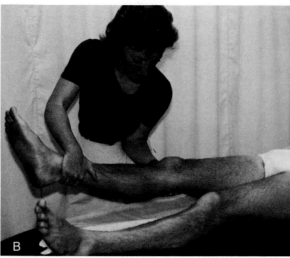

FIGURE 11-24. Abduction (valgus stress) test. (A) "Gapping" on the medial aspect of the knee. (B) Positioning for testing the medial collateral ligament (extended knee).

TESTS FOR ONE-PLANE MEDIAL INSTABILITY

Abduction (Valgus Stress) Test. This test is an assessment for one-plane (straight) medial instability, which means that the tibia moves away from the femur on the medial side (Fig. 11-24). The examiner applies a valgus stress (pushes the knee medially) at the knee while the ankle is stabilized in slight lateral rotation. The knee is first in full extension and then it is slightly flexed so that it is "unlocked" (20 to 30°).

If the test is positive (i.e., if the tibia moves away from the femur an excessive amount when a valgus stress is applied) when the knee is in extension, the following structures may have been injured to some degree:

1. Medial collateral ligament (superficial and deep fibers).
2. Posterior oblique ligament.
3. Posteromedial capsule.
4. Anterior cruciate ligament.
5. Posterior cruciate ligament.
6. Medial quadriceps expansion.
7. Semimembranosus muscle.

The examiner will usually find that one or more of the rotary tests are also positive. A positive finding on full extension is classified as a major disruption of the knee. If the examiner applies lateral rotation to the foot when performing the test in extension and finds excessive lateral rotation on the affected side, it is a sign of possible anteromedial rotary instability.

If the test is positive when the knee is flexed to 20 to 30°, the following structures may have been injured to some degree:

1. Medial collateral ligament.
2. Posterior oblique ligament.

3. Posterior cruciate ligament.
4. Posteromedial capsule.

This part of the valgus stress test would be classified as the true test for one-plane medial instability.

If a stress radiograph is taken when the test is performed in full extension, a 5-mm opening is indicative of a grade 1 injury; up to 10 mm, a grade 2 injury; and more than 10 mm, a grade 3 injury.[20, 25]

TESTS FOR ONE-PLANE LATERAL INSTABILITY

Adduction (Varus Stress) Test. This test is an assessment for one-plane lateral instability (i.e., the tibia moves away from the femur an excessive amount on the lateral aspect of the leg). The examiner applies a varus stress (i.e., pushes the knee laterally) at the knee while the ankle is stabilized (Fig. 11-25). The test is first done in full extension and then in 20 to 30° of flexion. If the tibia is laterally rotated in full extension before the test, the cruciate ligaments will be uncoiled, and maximum stress will be placed on the collateral ligaments.

If the test is positive (i.e., if the tibia moves away from the femur when a varus stress is applied) in extension, the following structures may have been injured to some degree:

1. Fibular or lateral collateral ligament.
2. Posterolateral capsule.
3. Arcuate-popliteus complex.
4. Biceps femoris tendon.
5. Posterior cruciate ligament.
6. Anterior cruciate ligament.
7. Lateral gastrocnemius muscle.
8. Iliotibial band.

The examiner will usually find that one or more rotary instability tests will also be positive. A positive test is indicative of major instability of the knee.

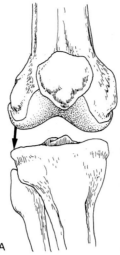

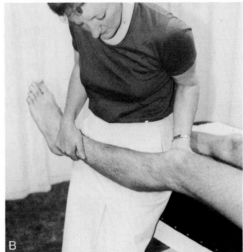

FIGURE 11–25. Adduction (varus stress) test. (A) One-plane lateral instability "gapping" on the lateral aspect. (B) Positioning for testing lateral collateral ligament (slightly flexed knee is illustrated).

A

B

If the test is positive when the knee is flexed 20 to 30° with lateral rotation of the tibia, the following structures may have been injured to some degree:

1. Lateral collateral ligament.
2. Posterolateral capsule.
3. Arcuate-popliteus complex.
4. Iliotibial band.
5. Biceps femoris tendon.

This part of the varus stress test is classified as the true test for one-plane lateral instability.

If a stress radiograph is taken when the test is performed in full extension, a 5-mm opening is indicative of a grade 1 injury; up to 8 mm, a grade 2 injury; and more than 8 mm, a grade 3 injury, to the lateral ligaments of the knee.[20, 25]

Both varus and valgus stress testing (varus-valgus test) can be performed while palpating the joint line. The examiner holds the ankle between the examiner's waist and forearm while the patient lies supine. At the same time, the examiner palpates the medial and lateral joint lines with the fingers. Varus and valgus stresses are applied with the heels of the hands (Fig. 11–26).[18]

TESTS FOR ONE-PLANE ANTERIOR INSTABILITY

Lachman Test. The Lachman test is the best indicator of injury to the anterior cruciate ligament, especially the posterolateral band.[26] It is a test for one-plane anterior instability. The patient lies supine with the involved leg beside the examiner. The examiner holds the patient's knee between full extension and 30° of flexion. This position is close to

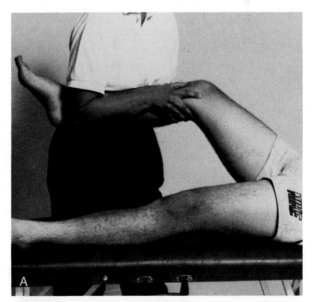

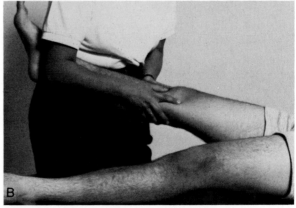

FIGURE 11–26. Varus-valgus test. (A) Knee flexed. (B) Knee extended.

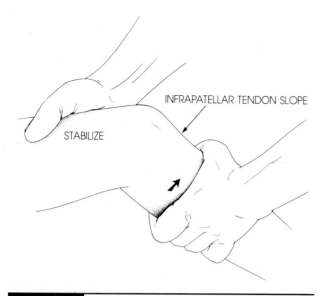

INFRAPATELLAR TENDON SLOPE

STABILIZE

FIGURE 11–27. *Hand position for classic Lachman test.*

the functional position of the knee in which the anterior cruciate ligament plays a major role. The patient's femur is stabilized with one of the examiner's hands while the proximal aspect of the tibia is moved forward with the other hand (Fig. 11–27). A positive sign is indicated by a "mushy" or soft end feel when the tibia is moved forward on the femur and the infrapatellar tendon slope disappears. A positive sign indicates that the following structures may have been injured to some degree:

1. Anterior cruciate ligament (especially the posterolateral bundle).
2. Posterior oblique ligament.
3. Arcuate-popliteus complex.

Other ways of doing the Lachman test have also been advocated. The method that works for the examiner and that the examiner can use competently

should be selected. Another method (modification 1) has the patient sitting with the leg over the edge of the examining table. The examiner sits facing the patient and supports the foot of the test leg on the examiner's thigh so that the patient's knee is flexed 30°. The examiner stabilizes the thigh with one hand and pulls the tibia forward with the other hand (Fig. 11–28). Abnormal forward motion is considered a positive test.[27]

For examiners with small hands, the *stable Lachman test* (modification 2) is recommended. The patient lies supine with the knee resting on the examiner's knee (Fig. 11–29). One of the examiner's hands stabilizes the femur against the examiner's thigh, and the other hand applies an anterior stress.[18]

Modification 3 has the patient lying supine while the examiner stabilizes the foot between the examiner's thorax and arm. Both hands are placed around the tibia, the knee is flexed 20 to 30°, and an "anterior drawer" is performed.[18] This technique allows gravity to control movement of the femur, which may not be sufficient to show a good positive test (Fig. 11–30).

Another way of doing the test (modification 4) is for the patient to lie supine while the examiner stands beside the leg to be tested with the eyes level with the knee. The examiner grasps the femur with one hand and the tibia with the other hand.[18] The tibia is pulled forward, and any abnormal motion is noted (Fig. 11–31). As with the regular Lachman test, the examiner may have difficulty stabilizing the femur if the examiner has small hands.

The Lachman test (modification 5) may also be done with the patient prone.[28, 29] In this method, the examiner stabilizes the foot between the examiner's thorax and arm and places one hand around the tibia. The other hand stabilizes the femur (Fig. 11–32). Gravity will assist anterior movement, but it is

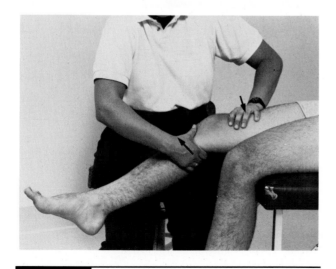

FIGURE 11–28. *Lachman test (modification 1).*

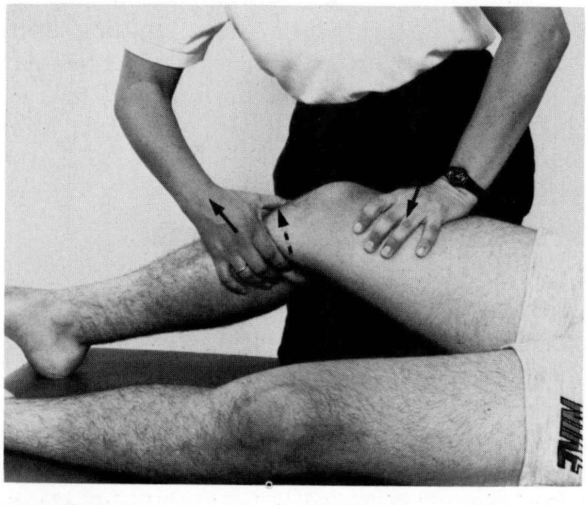

FIGURE 11–29. *Stable Lachman test.*

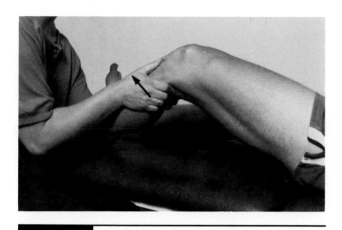

FIGURE 11–30. Lachman test (modification 3).

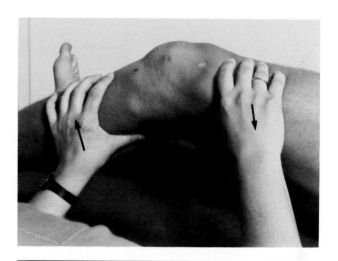

FIGURE 11–31. Lachman test (modification 4).

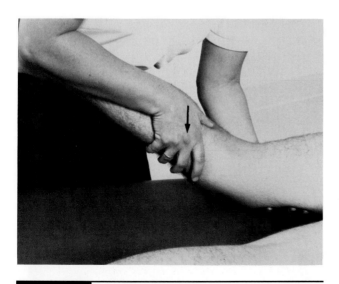

FIGURE 11–32. Prone Lachman test.

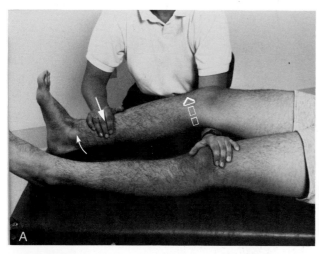 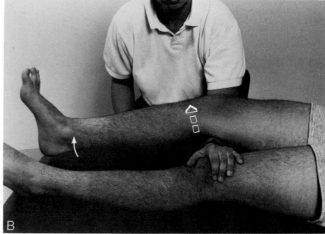

FIGURE 11–33. (A) *Active Lachman (maximum quadriceps) test.* (B) *No-touch Lachman test. Open arrow shows where the examiner watches for shift.*

more difficult to determine the quality of the end feel.

The *active (no touch) Lachman test*[18, 30, 31] is the sixth modification of the original Lachman test. The patient lies supine with the knee flexed over the examiner's forearm so that the knee is flexed approximately 30° (Fig. 11–33). The patient is asked to actively extend the knee, and the examiner watches for anterior displacement of the tibia relative to the unaffected side. The test may also be carried out with the foot held down on the table to increase the pull of the quadriceps. In this case, the test has been called the *maximum quadriceps test.*[18] The examiner must be certain that there is no posterior sag before performing the test.

The Lachman test may be graded with a stress radiograph; a 3- to 6-mm opening is classified as a grade I injury; 6 to 9 mm, grade II; 10 to 16 mm, grade III; and 16 to 20 mm, grade IV.[18]

Drawer Sign or Test. The drawer sign is a test for one-plane anterior and one-plane posterior instabilities.[32] The difficulty with this test is determining the neutral starting position if the ligaments have been injured. The patient's knee is flexed to 90°, and the hip is flexed to 45°. In this position, the anterior cruciate ligament is almost parallel with the tibial plateau. The patient's foot is held on the table by the examiner's body with the examiner sitting on the patient's forefoot and the foot in neutral rotation. The examiner's hands are placed around the tibia to ensure that the hamstring muscles are relaxed (Fig. 11–34). The tibia is then drawn forward on the femur. The normal amount of movement that should be present is approximately 6 mm. This part of the test assesses one-plane anterior instability. If the test is positive (i.e., the tibia moves forward more than 6 mm on the femur), the following structures may have been injured to some degree:

1. Anterior cruciate ligament (especially the anteromedial bundle).
2. Posterolateral capsule.
3. Posteromedial capsule.
4. Medial collateral ligament (deep fibers).
5. Iliotibial band.
6. Posterior oblique ligament.
7. Arcuate-popliteus complex.

If only the anterior cruciate ligament is torn, the test will be negative because other structures (posterior capsule and posterolateral and posteromedial structures) limit movement. In addition, hemarthrosis, a torn medial meniscus (posterior horn) wedged against the medial femoral condyle, and hamstring spasm may result in a false-negative test.

When performing this test, the examiner must ensure that the posterior cruciate ligament is not

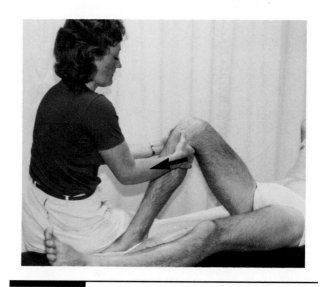

FIGURE 11–34. *Position for drawer sign.*

torn or injured. If it has been torn, it will allow the tibia to drop back on the femur, and when the examiner pulls the tibia forward, a large amount of movement will occur, giving a false-positive sign (see "Posterior Sag Sign"). Thus, the test should be considered positive only if it is shown that the posterior drawer is not present.

Weatherwax[33] described a modified way of testing the anterior drawer. The patient lies supine. The examiner flexes the patient's hip and knee to 90° and supports the lower leg between the examiner's trunk and forearm. The examiner places the hands around the tibia as with the standard test and applies sufficient force to slowly lift the patient's buttock off the table (Fig. 11–35).

If when doing the anterior drawer test there is an audible snap or palpable jerk *(Finochietto's jumping sign)* when the tibia is pulled forward and the tibia moves forward excessively, a meniscus lesion probably accompanies the torn anterior cruciate ligament.[18]

After the anterior movement of the tibia on the femur, the posterior movement of the tibia on the femur should be completed. In this part of the test, the tibia is pushed back on the femur. This phase is a test for one-plane posterior instability. If when the tibia is pushed backward the examiner forcefully rotates the tibia laterally and excessive movement occurs, the test is positive for posterolateral instability. Warren[34] calls this maneuver the *arcuate spin test*. If the test is positive, the following structures may have been injured to some degree:

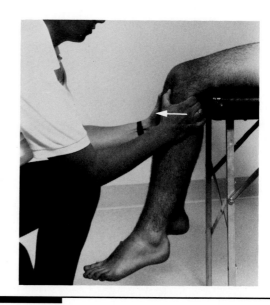

FIGURE 11–36. *Anterior drawer test in sitting. Examiner feels anterior shift with thumbs.*

1. Posterior cruciate ligament.
2. Arcuate-popliteus complex.
3. Posterior oblique ligament.
4. Anterior cruciate ligament.

If the arcuate-popliteus complex remains intact, a positive drawer sign cannot be elicited.

Feagin[28] advocated doing the drawer test with the patient sitting with the leg hanging relaxed over the end of the examining table. The examiner places the hands as with the standardized test and slowly draws the tibia first forward and then backward to test anterior and posterior drawer (Fig. 11–36). The examiner uses the thumbs to palpate the tibia plateau movement relative to the femur. The examiner may also note any rotational deformity, and the posterior sag is eliminated because the effect of gravity is eliminated.

Active Drawer Test. The patient is positioned as for the normal drawer test. The examiner holds the patient's foot down. The patient is asked to try to straighten the leg, and the examiner prevents the patient from doing so (isometric test). If the anterior cruciate ligament is torn, the anterior contour of the knee will change as the tibia is drawn forward, indicating a positive test for a torn anterior cruciate ligament (Fig. 11–37). A second part of the test may be instituted by having the patient contract the hamstrings isometrically so that the tibial plateau moves posteriorly. This part of the test will accentuate the posterior sag for posterior cruciate insufficiency and ensure maximum movement for anterior cruciate insufficiency.[18] If the posterior cruciate ligament is torn, a posterior sag will be evident before the patient contracts the quadriceps. Contraction of the quadriceps will cause the tibia to shift forward

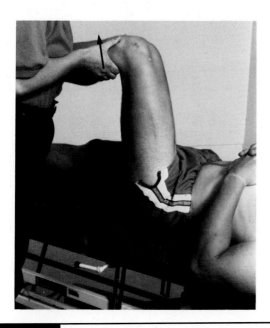

FIGURE 11–35. *Anterior drawer test in 90° flexion with the hip flexed 90°.*

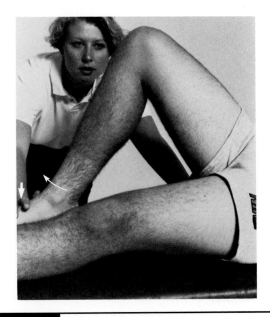

FIGURE 11–37. *Active anterior drawer test. Examiner watches for anterior shift.*

to its normal position, indicating a positive test for a torn posterior cruciate ligament. The active drawer test is a better expression of posterior cruciate insufficiency than of anterior cruciate insufficiency.

With the drawer sign or test, if the anterior and/or posterior cruciate ligaments are torn (third-degree sprain), some rotary instability will be evident when the appropriate ligamentous tests are done (Fig. 11–38).

TESTS FOR ONE-PLANE POSTERIOR INSTABILITY

Posterior "Sag" Sign (Gravity Drawer Test). The patient lies supine with the hip flexed to 45° and the knee flexed to 90°. In this position, the tibia will "drop back," or sag back, on the femur if the posterior cruciate ligament is torn (Fig. 11–39). Posterior tibial displacement is more noticeable when the knee is flexed 90 to 110° than when the knee is only slightly flexed. It is a test for one-plane posterior instability. The examiner must be careful because the position could result in a false-positive anterior drawer test for the anterior cruciate ligament if the sag remains unnoticed. If there is minimal or no swelling, the sag is quite evident because of an obvious concavity distal to the patella. If the posterior sag sign is present, the following structures may have been injured to some degree:

1. Posterior cruciate ligament.
2. Arcuate-popliteus complex.

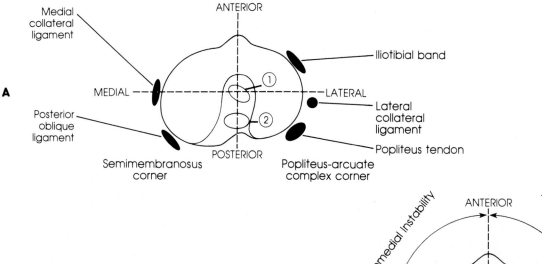

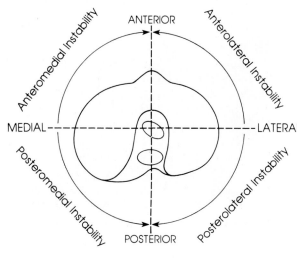

FIGURE 11–38. (A) Axes of the knee. 1 = Anterior cruciate ligament; 2 = Posterior cruciate ligament. (B) Rotary instabilities of the knee.

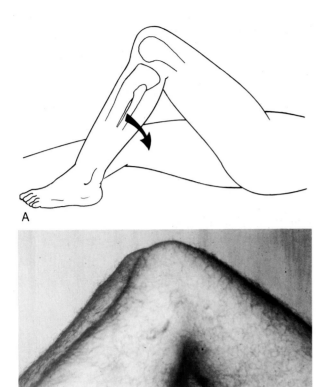

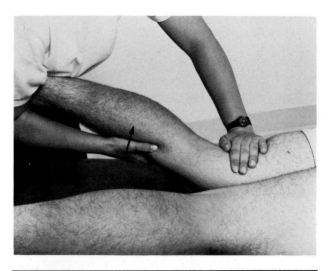

FIGURE 11–40. Reverse Lachman test.

FIGURE 11–39. Sag sign. (A) Illustration of posterior sag sign. (B) Note profile of two knees; the left (nearer) sags backward compared with the normal right knee, indicating posterior cruciate defect. (From O'Donoghue, D. H.: Treatment of Injuries to Athletes, 4th ed. Philadelphia, W. B. Saunders Co., 1984, p. 450.)

posterior drawer test because when the posterior cruciate ligament is torn, the greatest posterior displacement is at 90°.

Drawer Sign or Test (see above).

Active Drawer Test (see above).

Godfrey Test.[18] The patient lies supine and the examiner holds both legs while flexing the patient's hips and knees to 90°. If there is posterior instability, a posterior sag of the tibia will be seen. If manual posterior pressure is applied to the tibia, posterior displacement may increase (Fig. 11–41).

3. Posterior oblique ligament.
4. Anterior cruciate ligament.

If it appears that the patient has a positive posterior sag sign, the patient should carefully extend the knee while the examiner holds the thigh in 90 to 100° of flexion. This action is sometimes called the *voluntary anterior drawer sign*, and the results are similar to those of the active anterior drawer test. As the patient does this slowly, the tibial plateau will move or shift forward to its normal position, indicating that the tibia had previously been posteriorly subluxed on the femur.

Reverse Lachman Test.[18] The patient lies prone with the knee flexed to 30°, and the examiner grasps the tibia with one hand while fixing the femur with the other hand (Fig. 11–40). The examiner ensures that the hamstring muscles are relaxed. The examiner then pulls up the tibia (posteriorly), noting the amount of movement and the quality of the end feel. It is a test for the posterior cruciate ligament. The examiner should be wary of a false-positive test if the anterior cruciate ligament has been torn, because gravity may cause an anterior shift. This test is not as accurate for the posterior cruciate ligament as the

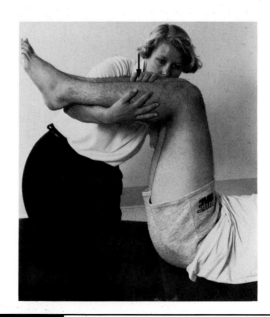

FIGURE 11–41. Godfrey test. Examiner watches for posterior shift.

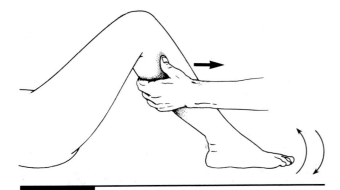

FIGURE 11–42. *Slocum test.*

TESTS FOR ANTEROMEDIAL ROTARY INSTABILITY

Slocum Test. The Slocum test assesses both anterior rotary instabilities.[35] The patient's knee is flexed to 80 or 90°, and the hip is flexed to 45°. The foot is first placed in 30° medial rotation (Fig. 11–42). The examiner then sits on the patient's forefoot to hold the foot in position and draws the tibia forward; if the test is positive, movement will occur primarily on the lateral side of the knee. This movement would be excessive relative to the unaffected side and indicates anterolateral rotary instability. It also indicates that the following structures may have been injured to some degree:

1. Anterior cruciate ligament.
2. Posterolateral capsule.
3. Arcuate-popliteus complex.
4. Lateral collateral ligament.
5. Posterior cruciate ligament.
6. Iliotibial band.

If the examiner finds anterolateral instability during this first position of the Slocum test, the second part of the test, which assesses anteromedial rotary instability in this position, is of less value.[36]

In the second part of the test, the foot is placed in 15° of lateral rotation, and the tibia is drawn forward by the examiner. If the test is positive, the movement will occur primarily on the medial side of the knee. This movement would be excessive relative to the unaffected side and indicates anteromedial rotary instability. It also indicates that the following structures may have been injured to some degree:

1. Medial collateral ligament (especially the superficial fibers, although the deep fibers may also be affected).
2. Posterior oblique ligament.
3. Posteromedial capsule.
4. Anterior cruciate ligament.

For the Slocum test, it is imperative that the examiner medially or laterally rotate the foot to the degrees shown. If the examiner rotates the tibia as

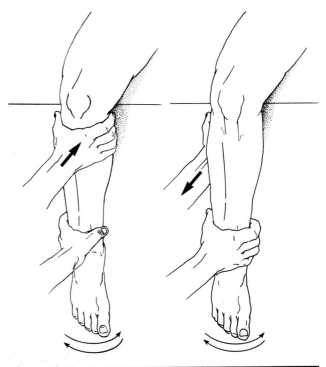

FIGURE 11–43. *Slocum test with the patient in the sitting position.*

far as it will go, the test will be negative because this action tightens all of the remaining structures.

If a stress radiograph is taken during the test, minimal or no movement indicates a negative test; 1 mm or less, a grade 1 injury; 1 to 2 mm, a grade 2 injury; and more than 2 mm, a grade 3 injury.[25]

The test may also be performed with the patient sitting with the knees flexed over the edge of the examining table (Fig. 11–43).[20] The examiner applies an anterior or a posterior force while holding the foot medially or laterally rotated. If this procedure is used, the examiner must remember that use of the anterior force tests for anterior rotary instability, whereas use of the posterior force tests for posterior rotary instability (see "Hughston's Posteromedial and Posterolateral Drawer Sign" in a later section). The examiner should note whether the movement is excessive on the medial or the lateral side of the knee relative to the normal knee. Excessive movement indicates a positive test.

TESTS FOR ANTEROLATERAL ROTARY INSTABILITY

Slocum Test (see above).

Lateral Pivot Shift Maneuver (Test of MacIntosh or Lemaire Test). This is the primary test used to assess anterolateral rotary instability of the knee and is an excellent test for anterior cruciate ligament ruptures (Fig. 11–44).[37–40] During this test, the tibia moves away from the femur on the lateral side and moves anteriorly in relation to the femur.

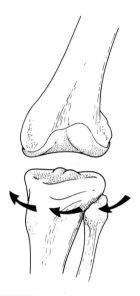

FIGURE 11–44. Anterolateral rotary instability.

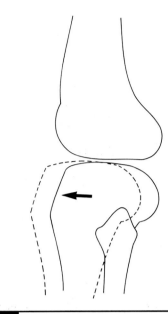

FIGURE 11–45. Anterior shift of the tibia during the lateral pivot shift test.

Normally, the knee's center of rotation changes constantly through its range of motion as a result of the shape of the femoral condyles, ligamentous restraint, and muscle tension. The path of movement of the tibia on the femur is described as a combination of rolling and sliding, with rolling predominating when the instant center is near the joint line and sliding predominating when the instant center shifts distally from the contact area. The MacIntosh test is a duplication of the anterior subluxation-reduction phenomenon that occurs during the normal gait cycle when the anterior cruciate ligament is torn. Thus, it illustrates a dynamic subluxation. This shift occurs between 20 and 40° of flexion (0° being the knee in the extended position). It is this phenomenon that gives the patient the clinical description of feeling the knee "give way" (Fig. 11–45).

The patient lies supine with the hip flexed to 30° and relaxed in slight medial rotation (20°). The examiner holds the patient's foot with one hand while the other hand is placed at the knee. This is done by placing the heel of the hand behind the fibula over the lateral head of the gastrocnemius muscle with the tibia medially rotated, causing the tibia to sublux anteriorly as the knee is taken into extension (Fig. 11–46). In extension, the secondary restraints (i.e., hamstrings, lateral femoral condyle, and lateral meniscus) are less efficient than in flexion. The examiner then applies a valgus stress to the knee while maintaining a medial rotation torque on the tibia at the ankle. The leg is then flexed, and at approximately 30 to 40°, the tibia will reduce or "jog" backward and the patient will say that is what the "giving way" feels like, indicating a positive

test. The reduction of the tibia on the femur is due to the change in position of the iliotibial band when it switches from an extensor function to a flexor function, pulling the tibia back into its normal position. The test involves two phases—first subluxation and then reduction. The iliotibial band must be intact for the test to work. Thus, in cases of

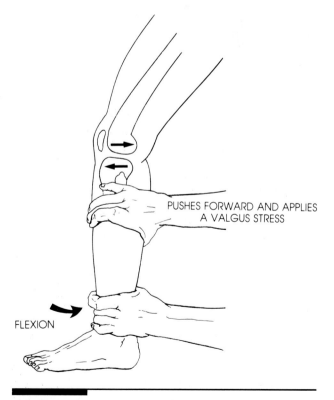

PUSHES FORWARD AND APPLIES A VALGUS STRESS

FLEXION

FIGURE 11–46. Lateral pivot shift test.

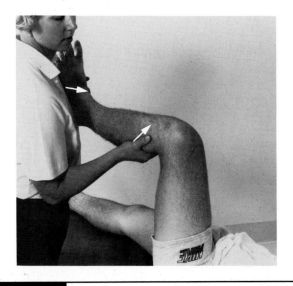

FIGURE 11–47. *Soft pivot shift test. Examiner watches for anterior shift.*

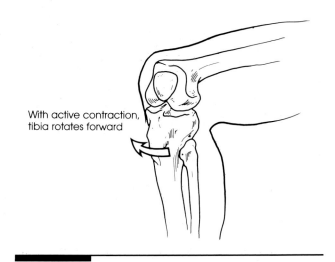

With active contraction, tibia rotates forward

FIGURE 11–48. *Active pivot shift test.*

anterolateral instability in which the iliotibial band has also been torn, the test will not work. In addition, if either meniscus has been torn, it may limit or prevent the subluxation reduction motion seen in the test. If the patient is tense or apprehensive, the test can be modified; this is called the *soft pivot shift test* (Fig. 11–47). The patient lies supine and the examiner supports the test foot with one hand while placing the other hand over the calf muscle 10 to 20 cm distal to the knee joint. The examiner flexes and extends the knee slowly and gently. After three to five cycles, the examiner applies axial compression while the hand over the calf exerts an anterior pressure. In a positive test, the tibia will sublux and reduce but not with the same apprehensive jerky feeling.[18] Kennedy[25] advocated pushing on the fibula with the thumb when performing this maneuver. Because hip abduction/adduction has an effect on the iliotibial band, hip position plays an important role in the test. Subluxation is most obvious when the hip is abducted and least obvious when it is adducted. In addition, lateral rotation of the tibia allows greater subluxation because, like abduction, it decreases the stress on the iliotibial band.[18] If the test is positive, the following structures have probably been injured to some degree:

1. Anterior cruciate ligament.
2. Posterolateral capsule.
3. Arcuate-popliteus complex.
4. Lateral collateral ligament.
5. Iliotibial band.

Active Pivot Shift Test.[41] The patient sits with the foot on the floor in neutral rotation and the knee flexed 80 to 90°. The patient is asked to isometrically contract the quadriceps while the examiner stabilizes the foot. A positive test is indicated by antero-lateral subluxation of the lateral tibial plateau and is indicative of anterolateral instability (Fig. 11–48).

Losee Test. The patient lies supine while relaxed.[42] The examiner holds the patient's ankle and foot so that the leg is laterally rotated and braced against the examiner's abdomen. The knee is then flexed to 30°, and the examiner ensures that the hamstring muscles are relaxed (Fig. 11–49). The lateral rotation ensures that the subluxation of the knee is reduced at the beginning of the test. With the examiner's other hand positioned so that the fingers lie over the patella and the thumb is hooked behind the fibular head, a valgus force is applied to the knee; the examiner uses the abdomen as a fulcrum while extending the patient's knee and applying forward pressure behind the fibular head with the thumb. The valgus stress compresses the structures in the lateral compartment and makes the anterior subluxation, if present, more noticeable. At the same time, the foot and ankle are allowed to drift into medial rotation. If the foot and ankle are not allowed to rotate medially, the anterior subluxation of the lateral tibial plateau may be prevented. Just before full extension of the knee, there will be a "clunk" forward if the test is positive, and the patient must recognize the movement as the instability that was previously experienced. This clunk means that the tibia has subluxed anteriorly and indicates injury to the same structures as indicated by the pivot shift maneuver.

Jerk Test of Hughston.[43] This test is similar to the pivot shift maneuver. The positioning of the patient and the examiner are the same, except that the patient's hip is flexed to 45°. With this test, the knee is first flexed to 90°. The leg is then extended, maintaining medial rotation and a valgus stress. At approximately 20 to 30° of flexion, the tibia will shift forward, causing a subluxation of the lateral tibial plateau with a jerk if the test is positive. If the

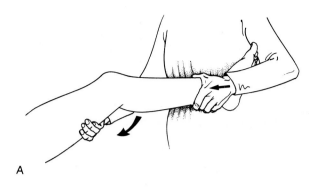

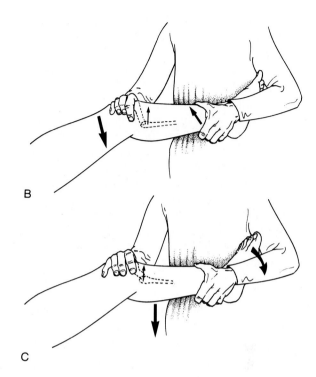

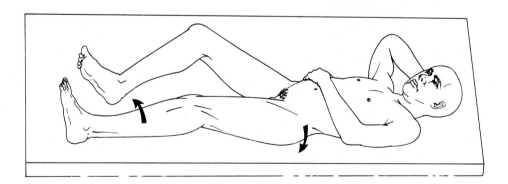

FIGURE 11–49. Losee test. (A) The foot is laterally rotated and cradled in the examiner's hand; the abdomen is against the fibula; and the leg is flexed to relax the hamstrings. (B) The examiner's right thumb pushes the fibula forward while valgus stress is applied with the abdomen. (C) The patient's knee is extended while the foot is allowed to internally rotate; valgus stress is still applied, and the fibula is pushed forward.

leg is carried into further extension, it will spontaneously reduce. A positive jerk test indicates that the same structures are injured as indicated by the pivot shift maneuver and assesses anterolateral rotary instability. According to the literature,[20] this test is not as sensitive as the pivot shift test.

Slocum's "ALRI" Test. The Slocum ALRI test also assesses anterolateral rotary instability.[20, 36] The patient is in the side lying position (approximately 30° from supine). The bottom leg is the uninvolved leg. The knee of the uninvolved leg is flexed to add stability (Fig. 11–50). The foot of the involved leg

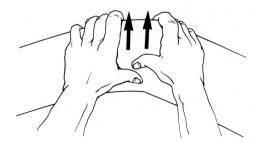

FIGURE 11–50. Slocum's anterolateral rotary instability test.

rests and is stabilized on the examining table with the patient's foot in medial rotation and the knee in extension and valgus. This position helps to eliminate hip rotation during the test. The examiner applies a valgus stress to the knee while flexing the knee. The subluxation of the knee will reduce during this test between 25 and 45° of flexion if the test is positive. A positive test indicates that the same structures are injured as indicated in the pivot shift maneuver. The main advantage of this particular test is that it aids in relaxation of the patient's hamstring muscles and is easier to perform on heavy or tense patients.

Crossover Test of Arnold. The patient is asked to cross the uninvolved leg in front of the involved leg (Fig. 11–51). The examiner then carefully steps on the patient's involved foot to stabilize it and instructs the patient to rotate the upper torso away from the injured leg approximately 90° from the fixed foot. When this position is achieved, the patient contracts the quadriceps muscles, producing the same symptoms and testing the same structures as in the lateral pivot shift test.

Noyes (Flexion-Rotation Drawer) Test. Described by Noyes,[44] this test is a modification of the pivot shift test. The patient lies supine and the examiner holds the patient's ankle between the examiner's trunk and arm with the hands around the tibia (Fig.

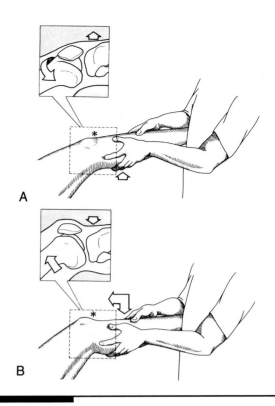

FIGURE 11–52. *Noyes (flexion-rotation drawer) test. (A) Test in subluxated position. With the leg held in neutral rotation, the weight of the thigh causes the femur to drop back posteriorly and, more importantly, to rotate externally, producing anterior subluxation of the lateral tibial plateau. (B) Test in reduced position. Gentle flexion and a downward push on the leg (as in a posterior drawer test) reduce the subluxation. This test assesses the function of the anterior cruciate ligament in the control of both translation and rotation. (From Noyes, F. R., et al.: J. Bone Joint Surg. 62A:687–695, 1980.)*

11–52). The examiner flexes the patient's knee to 20 to 30° while maintaining the tibia in neutral rotation. The tibia is then pushed posteriorly as is done in a posterior drawer test. This posterior movement reduces the subluxation of the tibia, indicating a positive test for anterolateral rotary instability. If the tibia is alternately pushed posteriorly and released and the femur is allowed to rotate freely, the reduction and subluxation will be seen and felt as the femur rotates medially and laterally.

Flexion-Extension-Valgus Test. The patient lies supine and the examiner holds the patient's leg as in the Noyes test above. The examiner palpates the joint line with the thumb and fingers of both hands, and a valgus stress and axial compression are applied while the knee is flexed and extended (Fig. 11–53). If the anterior cruciate ligament is torn, the examiner will feel the reduction and subluxation. The tibia is not rotated, so the subluxation is easily felt.[45]

Nakajima ("N") Test.[18] The patient lies supine and the examiner stands on the side of the test leg.

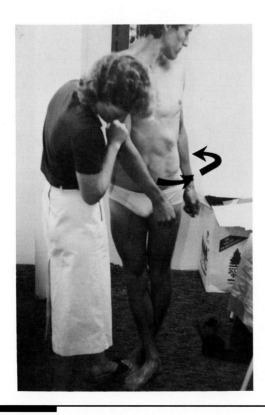

FIGURE 11–51. *Crossover test.*

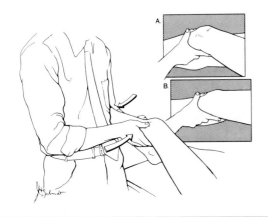

FIGURE 11–53. *Flexion-extension-valgus test. The leg is supported between the examiner's arm and chest. The thumb and fingers palpate the joint margins and/or rest on the tibial metaphysis. Valgus stress and axial compression are applied while flexing the knee (position A) and extending the knee (position B). In position A, when the knee is flexed from 0 to 15 to 20°, a definite "clunk" or external rotation of the lateral tibial plateau is visible or palpable. The phenomenon may also be elicited by reversing the maneuver. (From Hanks, G. A., et al.: Am. J. Sports Med. 9:226, 1981.)*

The patient's foot is held with one hand, which medially rotates the tibia. The knee is flexed to 90°. The examiner's other hand is placed over the lateral femoral condyle with the thumb behind the head of the fibula and pushing it forward. The examiner slowly extends the knee while pushing the head of the fibula forward, noting whether subluxation occurs, which indicates a positive test.

Martens Test.[18] The patient and examiner are positioned as for the Noyes test. The examiner grips the patient's leg distal to the knee joint with one hand and pushes the femur posteriorly with the other hand. A valgus stress is applied to the knee as the knee is flexed until the tibia reduces, indicating a positive test (Fig. 11–54).

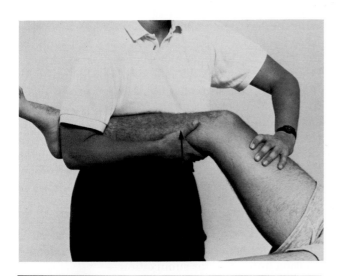

FIGURE 11–54. *Martens test.*

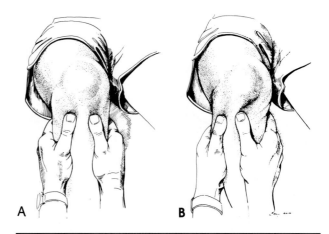

FIGURE 11–55. *Posterolateral drawer test, anterior view. (A) Starting position for posterolateral drawer test. (B) Positive posterolateral drawer test with posterior and lateral rotation of the lateral tibial condyle. (From Hughston, J. C., and L. A. Norwood: Clin. Orthop. Relat. Res. 147:83, 1980.)*

TESTS FOR POSTEROMEDIAL ROTARY INSTABILITY

Hughston's Posteromedial and Posterolateral Drawer Sign. The patient lies supine with the knee flexed to 80 to 90° and the hip flexed to 45° (Fig. 11–55).[46] The examiner medially rotates the patient's foot slightly and sits on the foot to stabilize it. The examiner then pushes the tibia posteriorly. If the tibia moves or rotates posteriorly on the medial aspect an excessive amount relative to the normal knee, the test is positive and indicative of posteromedial rotary instability. A positive test indicates that the following structures have probably been injured to some degree:

1. Posterior cruciate ligament.
2. Posterior oblique ligament.
3. Medial collateral ligament (superficial and deep fibers).
4. Semimembranosus muscle.
5. Posteromedial capsule.
6. Anterior cruciate ligament.

The medial tibial tubercle will rotate posteriorly around the posterior cruciate ligament when the tibia is in mild medial rotation. If the posterior cruciate ligament is also torn, the posteromedial movement will be greater, and the tibia will sublux posteriorly (Fig. 11–56).

The test may also be done with the patient sitting with the knee flexed over the edge of the examining table. The examiner pushes posteriorly while holding the patient's leg in medial rotation, watching for the same excessive movement.

Posterolateral rotary instability may be tested in a similar fashion.[46] The patient and examiner are in

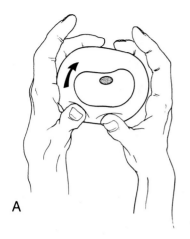
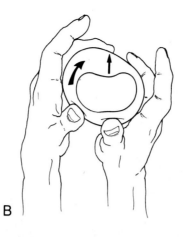

A   B

FIGURE 11–56. *Posterolateral drawer test. (A) If the posterior cruciate ligament is intact, the tibia will rotate posterolaterally. (B) If the posterior cruciate ligament is torn, the tibia will rotate posterolaterally and sublux posteriorly.*

the same position, but the patient's foot is slightly laterally rotated. If the tibia rotates posteriorly on the lateral side an excessive amount relative to the uninvolved leg when the examiner pushes the tibia posteriorly, the test is positive for posterolateral rotary instability. The test will be positive only if the posterior cruciate ligament is torn. The examiner may palpate the fibula while doing the movement to feel for excessive movement. The test indicates that the following structures have probably been injured to some degree:

1. Posterior cruciate ligament.
2. Arcuate-popliteus complex.
3. Lateral collateral ligament.
4. Biceps femoris tendon.

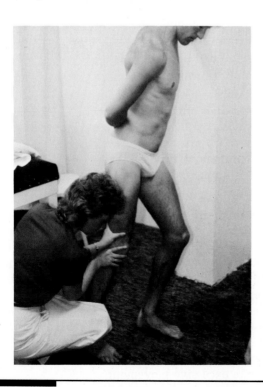

FIGURE 11–57. *Jakob test (method 1 showing valgus stress and flexion).*

5. Posterolateral capsule.
6. Anterior cruciate ligament.

TESTS FOR POSTEROLATERAL ROTARY INSTABILITY

Hughston's Posteromedial and Posterolateral Drawer Sign (see above).

Jakob Test (Reverse Pivot Shift Maneuver). This is a test for posterolateral rotary instability,[20, 47] and it can be performed in two ways (Figs. 11–57 and 11–58).

METHOD 1. The patient stands and leans against a wall with the uninjured side adjacent to the wall and the body weight distributed equally between the two feet. The examiner's hands are placed above and below the involved knee, and a valgus stress is exerted while flexion of the patient's knee is initiated. If there is a jerk in the knee or the tibia shifts posteriorly and the "giving way" phenomenon occurs during this maneuver, it indicates injury to the same structures as indicated by a positive Hughston's posterolateral drawer sign.

METHOD 2. The patient lies in the supine position with the hamstring muscles relaxed. The examiner faces the patient, lifts the patient's leg, and supports the leg against the examiner's pelvis. The examiner's other hand supports the lateral side of the calf with the palm on the proximal fibula. The knee is flexed to 70 to 80° of flexion and the foot is laterally rotated, causing the lateral tibial plateau to sublux posteriorly (Fig. 11–58A). The knee is taken into extension by its own weight while the examiner leans on the foot to impart a valgus stress to the knee through the leg. As the knee approaches 20° of flexion, the lateral tibial tubercle will shift forward or anteriorly into the neutral rotation and reduce the subluxation, indicating a positive test (Fig. 11–58B). The leg is then flexed again, and the foot falls back into lateral rotation and posterior subluxation.

External Rotation Recurvatum Test. There are two methods for performing this test.

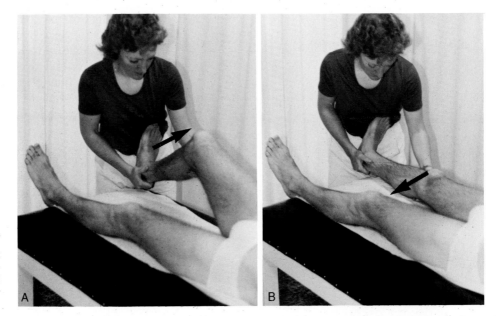

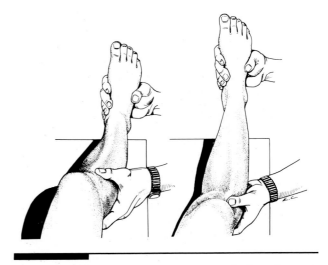

FIGURE 11–58. Reverse pivot shift test. (A) Position causes lateral tibial tubercle to sublux. (B) Position causes lateral tibial tubercle to reduce.

METHOD 1. The patient lies in the supine position with the lower limbs relaxed. The examiner gently grasps the big toe of each foot and lifts both feet off the examining table (Fig. 11–59).[46] The patient is told to keep the quadriceps muscles relaxed. While elevating the legs, the examiner watches the tibial tuberosities. For the test to be positive, the affected knee will go into relative hyperextension on the lateral aspect, with the tibia and tibial tuberosity rotating laterally. The affected knee will have the appearance of a relative genu varum. It is a test for posterolateral rotary instability in extension and assesses the same structures previously mentioned.

METHOD 2. The patient lies supine and the examiner's hand holds the patient's heel or foot and flexes the knee to 30 to 40° (Fig. 11–60).[46] The examiner's other hand holds the posterolateral aspect of the patient's knee and slowly extends it. With the hand on the knee, the examiner will feel the relative hyperextension and lateral rotation occurring in the injured limb compared to the uninjured limb. This is a test for posterolateral rotary instability and assesses the same structures as previously mentioned.

Dynamic Posterior Shift Test.[48] The patient lies supine and the examiner flexes the hip and knee of

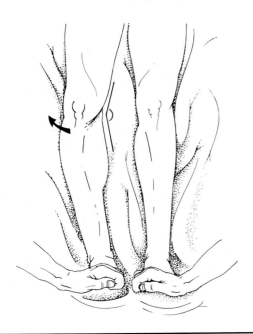

FIGURE 11–59. External rotational recurvatum test.

FIGURE 11–60. External recurvatum test (method 2). The test is begun by holding the knee in flexion (left). As the knee is slowly extended, the hand at the knee will feel the external rotation and recurvatum at the posterolateral aspect of the knee. (From Hughston, J. C., and L. A. Norwood: Clin. Orthop. Relat. Res. 147:86, 1980.)

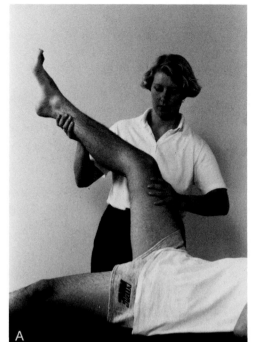

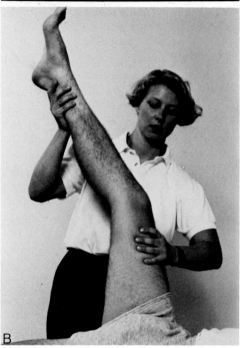

FIGURE 11–61. *Dynamic posterior shift test. (A) Starting position in flexion. (B) Extended position in which posterior shift will occur.*

the test leg to 90° with the femur in neutral rotation. One hand of the examiner stabilizes the anterior thigh while the other hand extends the knee. If the test is positive, the tibia will reduce anteriorly with a clunk as extension is reached. The test is positive for posterior and posterolateral instabilities. If the knee is painful before extension is accomplished,

the hip flexion may be decreased, but the hamstrings must be kept tight (Fig. 11–61).

Active Posterolateral Drawer Sign.[49] The patient sits with the foot on the floor in neutral rotation. The knee is flexed to 90°. The patient is asked to isometrically contract the hamstrings, primarily the lateral one (biceps femoris), while the examiner stabilizes the foot. A positive test for posterolateral instability is posterior subluxation of the lateral tibial plateau (Fig. 11–62).

Loomer's Posterolateral Rotatory Instability Test.[50] The patient lies supine and flexes both hips and both knees to 90°. The examiner then grasps the feet and maximally laterally rotates both tibia. The test is considered positive if the injured tibia laterally rotates excessively and there is a posterior sag of the affected tibial tubercle; both signs must be present for a positive test.

Special Tests

Although special tests in the knee are done only if the examiner suspects certain pathologies and wants to do a confirming test, tests for swelling should always be done.

Tests for Meniscus Injury

Although there are several tests for a meniscus injury, none can be considered definitive without considerable experience on the part of the examiner. Because the menisci are avascular and have no nerve supply on their inner two thirds, an injury to the meniscus can result in no pain or swelling, making diagnosis even more difficult.

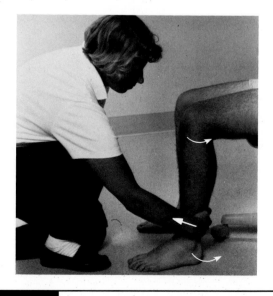

FIGURE 11–62. *Active posterolateral drawer sign or test. Examiner watches for posterolateral shift.*

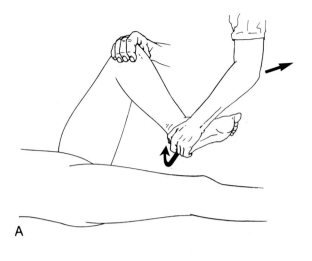

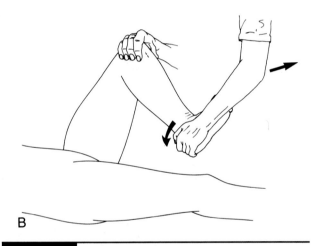

FIGURE 11–63. McMurray test (method 2). (A) Medial meniscus. (B) Lateral meniscus.

McMurray Test. The patient lies in the supine position with the knee completely flexed (the heel to the buttock).[51] The examiner then medially rotates the tibia (Fig. 11–63). If there is a loose fragment of the lateral meniscus, this action will cause a snap or click that is often accompanied by pain. By repeatedly changing the amount of flexion, the examiner can test the entire posterior aspect of the meniscus from the posterior horn to the middle segment. The anterior half of the meniscus is not as easily tested because the pressure on the meniscus is not as great. To test the medial meniscus, the examiner performs the same procedure with the knee laterally rotated.

The test may be modified by medially rotating the tibia, extending the knee, and moving through the full range of motion to test the lateral meniscus. The process is repeated several times. The tibia is then laterally rotated, and the process is repeated to test the medial meniscus. Both methods are described by McMurray.[51]

"Bounce Home" Test. The patient lies in the supine position, and the heel of the patient's foot is cupped in the examiner's hand (Fig. 11–64). The patient's knee is completely flexed, and the knee is passively allowed to extend. If extension is not complete or has a rubbery end feel ("springy block"), there is something blocking full extension. The most likely cause of a block is a torn meniscus.

O'Donoghue's Test. If a patient complains of pain along the joint line, the patient is asked to lie in the supine position. The examiner flexes the knee to 90°, rotates it medially and laterally twice, and then fully flexes and rotates it both ways again. A positive sign is indicated by increased pain on rotation in either or both positions and is indicative of capsular irritation or a meniscus tear.

Apley's Test.[52] The patient lies in the prone position with the knee flexed to 90°. The patient's thigh is then anchored to the examining table with the examiner's knee (Fig. 11–65). The examiner medially and laterally rotates the tibia, combined first with distraction, while noting any restriction, excessive movement, or discomfort. The process is repeated using compression instead of distraction. If rotation plus distraction is more painful, the lesion is probably ligamentous. If the rotation plus compression is more painful, the lesion is probably a meniscus injury.

Modified Helfet Test.[53] In the normal knee, the tibial tuberosity is in line with the midline of the patella when the knee is flexed to 90°. When the knee is extended, however, the tibial tubercle is in line with the lateral border of the patella (Fig. 11–

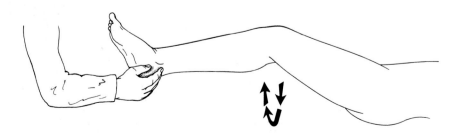

FIGURE 11–64. Bounce home test.

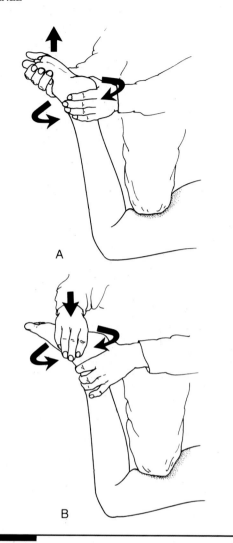

A

B

FIGURE 11–65. *Apley's test. (A) Distraction. (B) Compression.*

66). If this change does not occur with the change in movement, rotation is blocked, indicating injury to the meniscus or a possible cruciate injury.

Test for a Retreating or Retracting Meniscus. The patient sits on the edge of the examining table or lies in the supine position with the knee flexed to 90°.[53] The examiner places one finger over the joint line of the patient's knee anterior to the medial collateral ligament where the curved margin of the medial femoral condyle approaches the tibial tuberosity (Fig. 11–67). The patient's leg and foot are then passively laterally rotated, and the meniscus will normally disappear. The leg is medially and laterally rotated several times. The knee must be flexed and the muscles relaxed to do the test. If the meniscus does not disappear, a torn meniscus is indicated because rotation of the tibia is not occurring. The examiner must palpate carefully because a distinct structure is difficult to palpate. If the examiner medially and laterally rotates the unaffected leg several times first, the meniscus can be felt pushing against the finger on medial rotation and will disappear on lateral rotation.

Steinman's Tenderness Displacement Test. The Steinman sign is indicated by point tenderness and pain on the joint line that appears to move anteriorly when the knee is extended and moves posteriorly when the knee is flexed. It is indicative of a possible meniscus tear. Medial pain is elicited on the lateral rotation, and lateral pain is elicited on medial rotation.

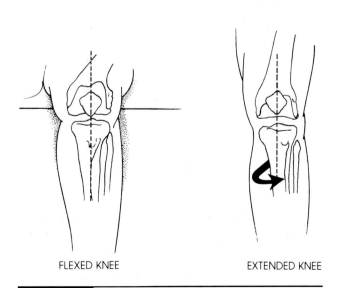

FLEXED KNEE   EXTENDED KNEE

FIGURE 11–66. *Modified Helfet test (negative test shown).*

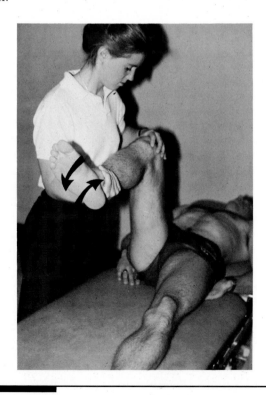

FIGURE 11–67. *Test for a retreating meniscus.*

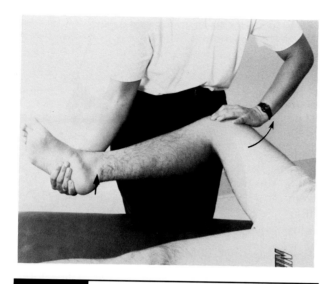

FIGURE 11–68. Payr's sign for a meniscus lesion.

Payr's Test. The patient lies supine with the test leg in the figure-four position (Fig. 11–68). If pain is elicited on the medial joint line, the test is considered positive for a meniscus lesion, primarily in the middle or posterior part of the meniscus.[18]

Bohler's Sign. The patient lies in the supine position, and the examiner applies varus and valgus stresses to the knee. Pain in the opposite joint line (valgus stress for lateral meniscus) on stress testing is a positive sign for meniscus pathology.[18]

Bragard's Sign. The patient lies supine and the examiner flexes the patient's knee. The examiner then laterally rotates the tibia and extends the knee (Fig. 11–69). Pain and tenderness on the medial joint line are indicative of medial meniscus pathology. If the examiner then medially rotates the tibia

and flexes the knee, the pain and tenderness will decrease.[18] Both of these symptoms are indicative of medial meniscus pathology.

Kromer's Sign. This test is similar to Bohler's sign except the knee is flexed and extended while the varus and valgus stresses are applied.[18] A positive test is indicated by the same pain on the opposite joint line.

Childress' Sign. The patient squats and performs a "duck walk."[18] Pain, snapping, or a click is considered positive for a posterior horn lesion.

Anderson Medial-Lateral Grind Test.[54] The patient lies supine. The examiner holds the test leg between the trunk and the arm while the index finger and thumb of the opposite hand are placed over the anterior joint line (Fig. 11–70). A valgus stress is applied to the knee as it is passively flexed to 45°; then, a varus stress is applied to the knee as it is passively extended, producing a circular motion to the knee. The motion is repeated, increasing the varus and valgus stresses with each rotation. A distinct grinding is felt on the joint line if there is meniscus pathology. The test may also show a pivot shift if the anterior cruciate ligament has been torn.

Passler Rotational Grinding Test.[18] The patient sits with the test knee extended and held at the ankle between the examiner's legs proximal to the examiner's knees. The examiner places both thumbs over the medial joint line and moves the knee in a circular fashion, medially and laterally rotating the tibia while the knee is rotated through various flexion angles. Simultaneously, the examiner applies a varus or a valgus stress (Fig. 11–71). Pain elicited on the joint line is indicative of a meniscal lesion.

Cabot's Popliteal Sign.[18] The patient lies supine and the examiner positions the test leg in the figure-four position. The examiner palpates the joint line

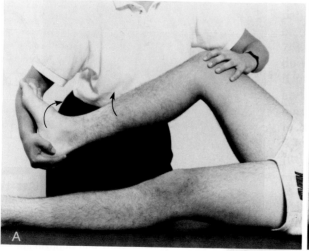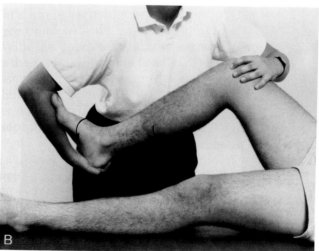

FIGURE 11–69. Bragard's sign for a meniscus lesion. (A) Medial meniscus. (B) Lateral meniscus.

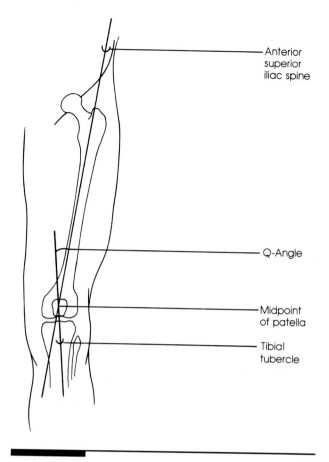

Anterior superior iliac spine

Q-Angle

Midpoint of patella

Tibial tubercle

FIGURE 11-81. *Quadriceps angle (Q-angle).*

Other Special Tests

Q-Angle or the Patellofemoral Angle. The Q-angle (quadriceps angle) is defined as the angle between the quadriceps muscles (primarily the rectus femoris) and the patellar tendon (Fig. 11-81). The angle is obtained by first ensuring the lower limbs are at a right angle to the line joining each ASIS. A line is then drawn from the ASIS to the midpoint of the patella and from the tibial tubercle to the midpoint of the patella. The angle formed by the crossing of these two lines is called the Q-angle. The foot should be placed in a neutral position relative to supination and pronation and the hip in a neutral position relative to medial and lateral rotation as it has been found that different foot and hip positions alter the Q-angle.[58] Normally, the Q-angle is 13 to 18° (13° for males, and 18° for females) when the knee is straight (Fig. 11-82). Any angle less than 13° may be associated with chondromalacia patellae or patella alta. Any angle greater than 18° is often associated with chondromalacia patellae, subluxing patella, increased femoral anteversion, genu valgum, or increased lateral tibial torsion. During the test, which may be done either with radiographs or physically on the patient, the quadriceps should be relaxed. If measured with the patient in the sitting position, the Q-angle should be 0° (Fig. 11-83). While the patient is in a sitting

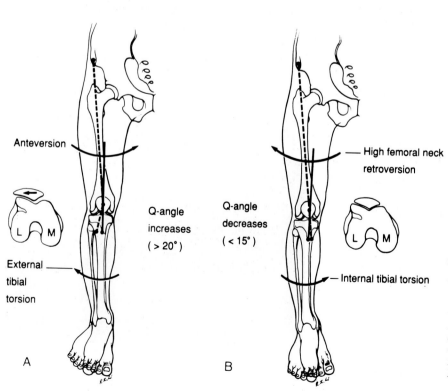

Anteversion

External tibial torsion

Q-angle increases (>20°)

Q-angle decreases (<15°)

A

B

High femoral neck retroversion

Internal tibial torsion

FIGURE 11-82. *(A) Femoral neck anteversion and external tibial torsion increase the Q-angle and lead to lateral tracking of the patella on the femoral sulcus. (B) Femoral neck retroversion and internal tibial torsion decrease the Q-angle and tend to centralize the tracking of the patella. (From Tria, A. J., and R. C. Palumbo: Semin. Orthop. 5:116–117, 1990.)*

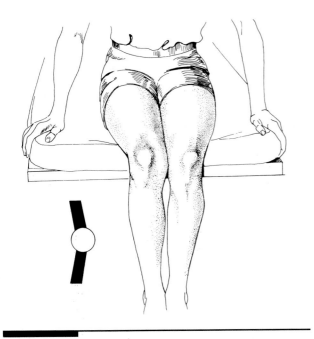

FIGURE 11–83. Q-angle in flexed position. Exaggerated Q-angle in the patient's right knee is seen as residual positive Q-angle with the knee flexed. Normally, the Q-angle in flexion should be 0°. (From Hughston, J. C., et al.: Patellar Subluxation and Dislocation. Philadelphia, W. B. Saunders Co., 1984, p. 24.)

position, the presence of the "bayonet" sign, which indicates an abnormal alignment of the quadriceps musculature, patellar tendon, and tibial shaft, should be noted (Fig. 11–84).

Hughston advocates doing the test with the quadriceps contracted.[43] If performed with the quadriceps contracted and the knee fully extended, the Q-angle should be 8 to 10°. Anything greater than 10° would be considered abnormal.

Daniel's Quadriceps Neutral Angle Test.[59] The patient lies supine and the unaffected leg is tested first. The patient's hip is flexed to 45° and the knee is flexed to 90° with the foot flat on the examining table. The patient is asked to extend the knee isometrically while the examiner holds down the foot. If tibial displacement is noted, knee flexion is decreased (posterior tibial displacement) or increased (anterior tibial displacement). The process is repeated until the angle at which there is no tibial displacement (average, 70°; range, 60 to 90°) is reached. This is the quadriceps neutral angle position. The injured knee is placed in the same neutral angle position, and the patient is asked to contract the quadriceps. Any anterior displacement is indic-

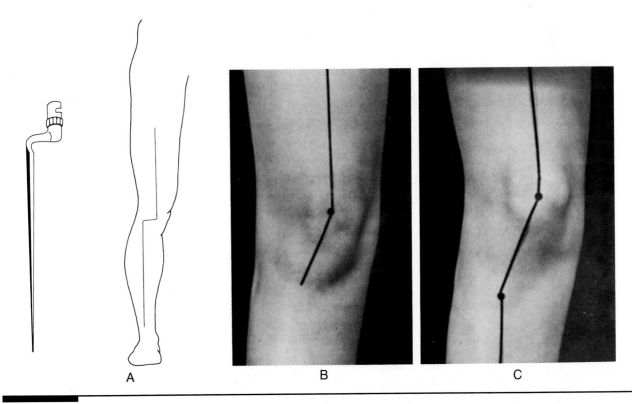

A   B   C

FIGURE 11–84. Increased Q-angle. (A) Bayonet sign. Tibia vara of proximal third causes a markedly increased Q-angle. Alignment of the quadriceps, patellar tendon, and tibial shaft resembles a French bayonet. (From Hughston, J. C., et al.: Patellar Subluxation and Dislocation. Philadelphia, W. B. Saunders Co., 1984, p. 26.) (B) Q-angle with the knee in full extension is only slightly increased over normal. (C) However, with the knee flexed at 30°, there is failure of the tibia to derotate normally and of the patellar tendon to line up with the anterior crest of the tibia. This is not an infrequent finding in patients with patellofemoral arthralgia. (From Ficat, R. P., and D. S. Hungerford: Disorders of the Patello-Femoral Joint. Baltimore, Williams & Wilkins, 1977, p. 117.)

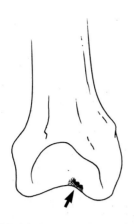

FIGURE 11–85. *Classic site of osteochondritis dissecans.*

ative of posterior cruciate ligament insufficiency. The quadriceps neutral angle is primarily used for machine testing of laxity (e.g., KT1000 arthrometer, Stryker knee laxity tester, CALT testing apparatus).

Wilson Test. This is a test for osteochondritis dissecans. The patient sits with the knee flexed over the examining table. The knee is then actively extended with the tibia medially rotated. At approxi-

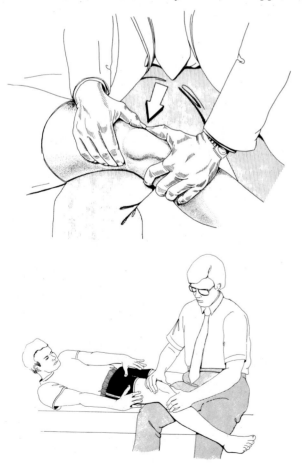

FIGURE 11–86. *Apprehension test. (From Hughston, J. C., et al.: Patellar Subluxation and Dislocation. Philadelphia, W. B. Saunders Co., 1984, p. 31.)*

mately 30° of flexion (0° being straight leg), the pain in the knee increases and the patient is asked to stop the flexion movement. The patient is then asked to rotate the tibia laterally, and the pain disappears. This finding indicates a positive test, which is indicative of osteochondritis dissecans of the femur. The test would be positive only if the lesion is at the classic site for osteochondritis dissecans of the knee, namely, the medial femoral condyle near the intercondylar notch (Fig. 11–85).

Fairbank's Apprehension Test. This is a test for dislocation of the patella.[43, 60] The patient lies in the supine position with the quadriceps muscles relaxed and the knee flexed to 30° while the examiner carefully and slowly pushes the patella laterally (Fig. 11–86). If the patient feels like the patella is going to dislocate, the patient will contract the quadriceps muscles to bring the patella back "into line." This action indicates a positive test. The patient will also have an apprehensive look.

Noble Compression Test. This is a test for iliotibial band friction syndrome.[61] The patient lies in the supine position, and the examiner flexes the patient's knee to 90°, accompanied by hip flexion (Fig. 11–87). Pressure is then applied to the lateral femoral epicondyle or 1 to 2 cm proximal to it with the thumb. While the pressure is maintained, the patient's knee is passively extended. At approximately 30° of flexion (0° being straight leg), the patient will complain of severe pain over the lateral femoral condyle. Pain indicates a positive test. The patient

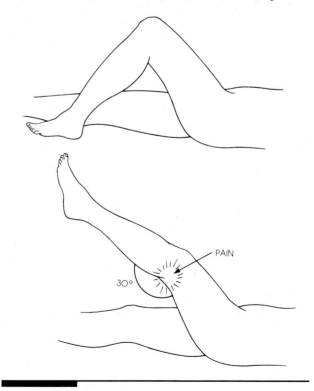

FIGURE 11–87. *Noble compression test.*

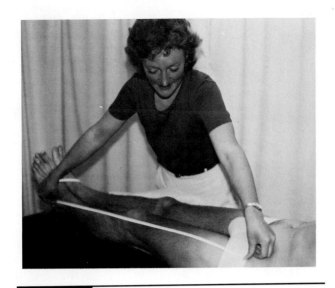

FIGURE 11–88. *Measuring leg length (to the lateral malleolus).*

will state that it is the same pain that occurs with activity.

Functional Test for Quadriceps Contusion. The patient lies in the prone position while the examiner passively flexes the knee as much as possible. If passive knee flexion is 90° or more, it is only a mild contusion. If passive knee flexion is less than 90°, the contusion is moderate to severe, and the patient should not be allowed to bear weight. Normally, the heel-to-buttock distance should not exceed 10 cm in men and 5 cm in women.

Measurement of Leg Length. The patient lies in the supine position with the legs at a right angle to a line joining each ASIS. The patient's feet should face straight up (Fig. 11–88). With a tape measure, the examiner obtains the distance from one ASIS to the lateral malleolus on that side, placing the metal end of the tape measure immediately distal to and pushed up against the ASIS. The tape is stretched so that the other hand pushes the tape against the distal aspect of the lateral malleolus, and the reading on the tape measure is noted. The other side is tested similarly. A difference between the two sides of as much as 1.0 to 1.5 cm is considered normal. However, the examiner must remember that even this difference may result in pathology. If there is a difference, the examiner can determine its site of occurrence by measuring from the high point in the iliac crest to the greater trochanter (for coxa vara), from the greater trochanter to the lateral knee joint line (for femoral length), and from the medial knee joint line to the medial malleolus (for tibial length). The two legs are then compared. The examiner must also remember that torsion deformities to the femur or tibia can alter leg length.

Functional Leg Length. The patient stands in the normal relaxed stance. The examiner palpates the anterior superior iliac spines and then the posterior superior iliac spines and notes any differences. The examiner then positions the patient so that the patient's subtalar joints are in neutral while weight bearing (see Chapter 12). While the patient holds this position with the toes straight ahead and the knees straight, the examiner repalpates the anterior superior iliac spines and the posterior superior iliac spines. If the previously noted differences remain, the pelvis and sacroiliac joints should be further evaluated. If the previously noted differences disappear, the examiner should suspect a functional leg length difference due to hip, knee, or ankle and foot problems—primarily, ankle and foot problems.

Measurement of Muscle Bulk (Anthropometric Measurements for Effusion and Atrophy). The examiner selects areas where muscle bulk or swelling is greatest and measures the circumference of the leg. It is important to note on the patient's chart how far above or below the apex or base of the patella one is measuring and whether the tape measure is placed above or below that mark. The following values are common measurement points:

15 cm below the apex of the patella.
Apex of the patella or joint line.
5 cm above the base of patella.
8 cm above the base of patella.
15 cm above the base of patella.
23 cm above the base of patella.

The examiner must also note, if possible, whether swelling or muscle bulk is being measured and remember that there is no correlation between muscle bulk and strength.

Reflexes and Cutaneous Distribution

Having completed the ligamentous and other tests of the knee, if a scanning examination has not been carried out, the examiner next determines whether the reflexes around the knee joint are normal (Fig. 11–89). The patellar (L3, L4) and medial hamstring (L5, S1) reflexes should be checked for differences between the two sides.

The examiner must keep in mind the dermatomal patterns of the various nerve roots (Fig. 11–90) as well as the cutaneous distribution of the peripheral nerves (Fig. 11–91). To test for altered sensation, the relaxed hands and fingers should cover all aspects of the thigh, knee, and leg. Any differences in sensation should be noted and can be further mapped out using a pinwheel, pin, cotton batten, or brush.

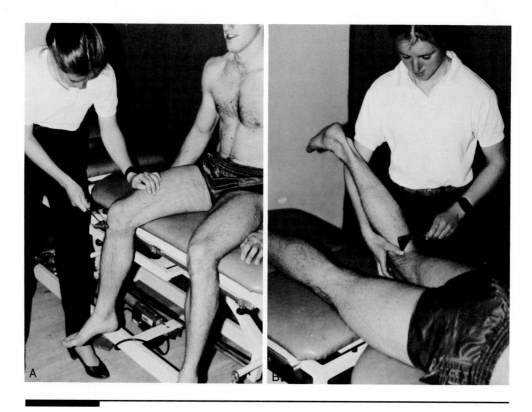

FIGURE 11–89. Reflexes of the knee. (A) Patellar (L3, L4). (B) Medial hamstrings (L5, S1).

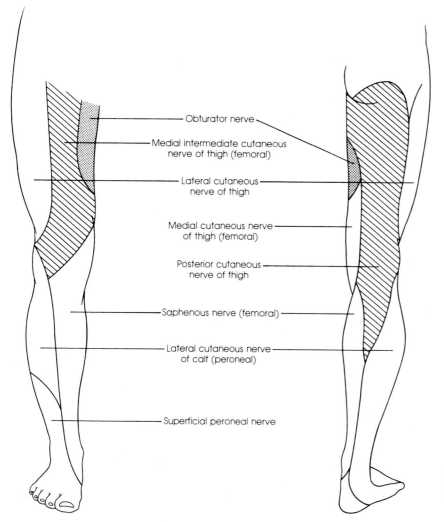

Obturator nerve

Medial intermediate cutaneous nerve of thigh (femoral)

Lateral cutaneous nerve of thigh

Medial cutaneous nerve of thigh (femoral)

Posterior cutaneous nerve of thigh

Saphenous nerve (femoral)

Lateral cutaneous nerve of calf (peroneal)

Superficial peroneal nerve

FIGURE 11–90. Peripheral nerve sensory distribution around the knee.

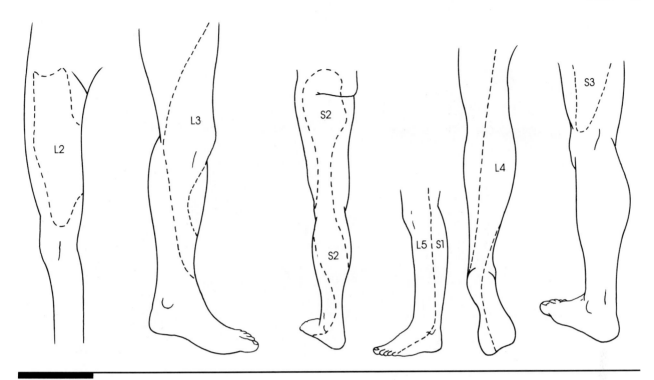

FIGURE 11–91. *Dermatomes about the knee.*

True knee pain tends to be localized to the knee, but it may also be referred to the hip or ankle (Fig. 11–92). In a similar fashion, pain may be referred to the knee from the lumbar spine, hip, and ankle. Sometimes a lesion of the medial meniscus will lead to irritation of the infrapatellar branch of the saphenous nerve. The result is a hyperaesthetic area the size of a quarter on the medial side of the knee. This finding is called *Turner's sign.*[18]

Joint Play Movement

For joint play movements on the knee, the patient is in the supine position. The movement on the affected side is compared with that on the normal side.

The following movements should be carried out at the knee (Fig. 11–93):

1. Backward and forward movements of the tibia on the femur.
2. Medial and lateral translation of the tibia on the femur.
3. Medial and lateral displacements of the patella.
4. Depression (distal movement) of the patella.
5. Anteroposterior movement of the fibula on the tibia.

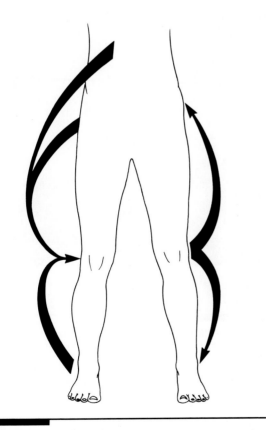

FIGURE 11–92. *Patterns of referred pain to and from the knee.*

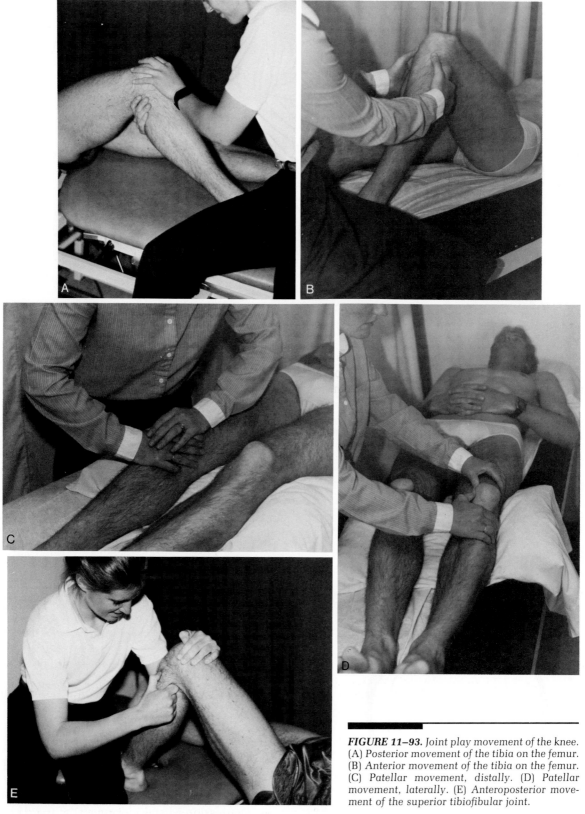

FIGURE 11–93. Joint play movement of the knee.
(A) Posterior movement of the tibia on the femur.
(B) Anterior movement of the tibia on the femur.
(C) Patellar movement, distally. (D) Patellar
movement, laterally. (E) Anteroposterior move-
ment of the superior tibiofibular joint.

Backward and Forward Movements of Tibia on Femur

The patient is asked to lie in the supine position with the test knee flexed to 90° and the hip flexed to 45°. The examiner then places the heel of the hand over the tibial tuberosity while stabilizing the patient's limb with the other hand and pushing backward with the heel of the hand. The end feel of the movement should normally be tissue stretch. To perform the forward movement, the examiner places both hands around the posterior aspect of the tibia. Before performing the joint play movement, the examiner must ensure that the hamstrings and gastrocnemius muscles are relaxed. The tibia is then drawn forward on the femur. The examiner feels the quality of the movement, which normally is tissue stretch.

These joint play movements are similar to the anterior and posterior drawer tests for ligamentous stability.

Medial and Lateral Translation of Tibia on Femur

The patient lies supine and the patient's leg is held between the examiner's trunk and arm. To test medial translation, the examiner puts one hand on the lateral side of the tibia and one hand on the medial side of the femur. The tibia is then pushed medially on the femur. Excessive movement may indicate a torn anterior cruciate ligament (Fig. 11–94). To test lateral translation, the examiner puts one hand on the medial side of the tibia and one hand on the lateral side of the femur. The tibia is then pushed laterally on the femur. Excessive movement may indicate a torn posterior cruciate ligament. The normal end feel of each movement is tissue stretch.[18]

Medial and Lateral Displacements of Patella

The patient is in the supine position with the knee slightly flexed on a pillow or over the examiner's knee (30° flexion). The examiner's thumbs are placed against the medial or lateral edge of the patella, and a force is applied to the side of the patella, with the fingers used to stabilize. The process is then repeated, with pressure applied to the other side of the patella. The other knee is tested as a comparison.

This joint play is similar to the passive movements of the patella; as in the passive test, the patella can be displaced approximately half of its width medially and laterally. The examiner must do the movements slowly and carefully to ensure that the patella is not prone to dislocation.

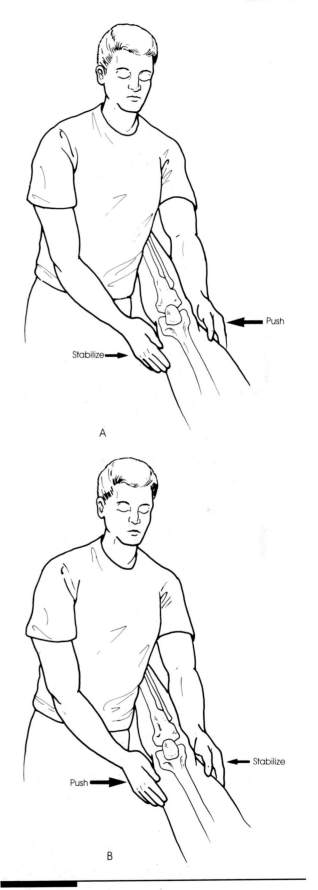

FIGURE 11–94. Medial and lateral shift of tibia on femur. (A) Medial translation for anterior cruciate pathology. (B) Lateral translation for posterior cruciate pathology.

Depression (Distal Movement) of Patella

The patient is in a supine position with the knee slightly flexed. The examiner then places one hand over the patient's patella so that the pisiform bone rests over the base of the patella. The other hand is placed so that the finger and thumb can grasp the medial and lateral edges of the patella to direct the movement of the patella. The examiner then rests the first hand over the second hand and applies a caudal force to the base of the patella and directs the caudal movement with the second hand so that the patella does not grind against the femoral condyles.

Anteroposterior Movement of Fibula on Tibia

The patient is supine with the knee flexed to 90° and the hip flexed to 45°. The examiner then sits on the patient's foot and places one hand around the patient's knee to stabilize the knee and leg. The mobilizing hand is placed around the head of the fibula. The fibula is drawn forward on the tibia, and the movement and end feel are tested. The fibula will then slide back to its resting position of its own accord. The movement is tested several times and compared with that of the other side.

Care must be taken when performing this technique because the common peroneal nerve, which winds around the head of the fibula, may be easily compressed, causing pain. If the superior tibiofibular joint is stiff or hypomobile, the test itself will cause discomfort.

Palpation

The patient lies supine with the knee slightly flexed. In fact, it is wise to put the knee in several positions during palpation. For example, meniscal cysts are best palpated at 45°, whereas the joint line is easiest to palpate at 90°. When palpating, the examiner looks for abnormal tenderness, swelling, nodules, or abnormal temperature. The following structures should be palpated (Fig. 11–95):

Anteriorly With Knee Extended

Patella, Patellar Tendon, Patellar Retinaculum, Associated Bursa, Cartilaginous Surface of the Patella, and Plica (if Present). The *patella* can be easily palpated over the anterior aspect of the knee. The base of the patella lies superiorly, and the apex lies distally. After palpating the apex of the patella (jumper's knee?), the examiner moves distally, palpating the *patellar tendon* (tendinitis?) and overly-

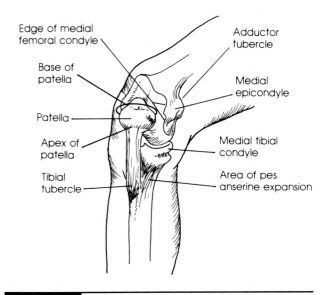

FIGURE 11–95. *Landmarks of the knee. (Adapted from Reilly, B. M.: Practical Strategies in Outpatient Medicine. Philadelphia, W. B. Saunders Co., 1991, p. 1175.)*

ing infrapatellar bursa (Parson's knee?) as well as the fat pad that lies behind the tendon. When the knee is extended, the fat pad will often extend beyond the sides of the tendon. Moving distally, the examiner will come to the tibial tuberosity, which should be palpated for enlargement (Osgood-Schlatter disease?).

Returning to the patella, the examiner can palpate the skin lying over the patella for pathology (is there prepatellar bursitis, or housemaid's knee?) and then extend medially and laterally to palpate the *patellar retinaculum* on either side of the patella. With the examiner pushing down on the lateral aspect of the patella, the medial retinaculum can be brought under tension and then palpated for tender areas. The lateral retinaculum can be palpated in a similar fashion with the examiner pushing down on the medial aspect of the patella. By stressing the retinaculum, the examiner is separating the retinaculum from the underlying tissue.

With the quadriceps muscles relaxed, the articular facets of the patella are palpated for tenderness (chondromalacia patella?) as shown in Figure 11–96. This palpation is often facilitated by carefully pushing of the patella medially to palpate the medial facets and laterally to palpate the lateral facet.

As the medial edge of the patella is palpated, the examiner should carefully feel for the presence of a mediopatellar *plica*. The plica, if pathological, may be palpated as a thickened ridge medial to the patella. To help confirm the presence of the plica, the examiner flexes the patient's knee to 30° and pushes the patella medially. If the plica is present and pathological, this maneuver will often cause pain.

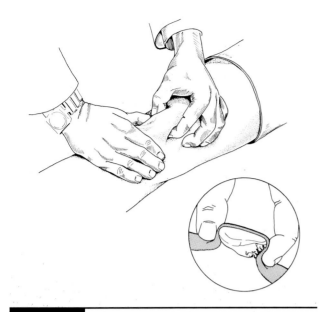

FIGURE 11–96. *Facet tenderness. The medial and lateral facets are checked for tenderness, although tenderness may be related to structures other than patellar surfaces beneath the examining finger. (From Hughston, J. C., et al.: Patellar Subluxation and Dislocation. Philadelphia, W. B. Saunders Co., 1984, p. 28.)*

Suprapatellar Pouch. Returning to the anterior surface of the patella and moving proximally beyond the base of the patella, the examiner's fingers will lie over the suprapatellar pouch. The examiner then lifts the skin and underlying tissue between the thumb and fingers (Fig. 11–97). In this way, the synovial membrane of the suprapatellar pouch, which is continuous with that of the knee joint, can be palpated. The examiner should feel for any thickness, tenderness, or nodules, the presence of which may indicate pathology.

Quadriceps Muscles (Vastus Medialis, Vastus Intermedius, Vastus Lateralis, and Rectus Femoris) and Sartorius. After palpating the suprapatellar pouch, the examiner palpates the quadriceps muscles for tenderness (first- or second-degree strain?), defects (third-degree strain?), or hard masses (myositis ossificans?).

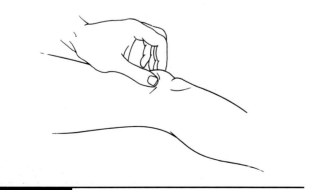

FIGURE 11–97. *Palpation of the synovial membrane.*

Medial Collateral Ligament. If the examiner moves medially from the patella so the fingers lie over the medial aspect of the tibiofemoral joint, the fingers will lie over the medial collateral ligament, which should be palpated along its entire length for tenderness (sprain?) or other pathology (e.g., Pellegrini-Stieda disease).

Pes Anserinus. Medial and slightly distal to the tibial tuberosity, the examiner may palpate the pes anserinus or the common aponeurosis of the tendons of gracilis, semitendinosus, and sartorius muscles for tenderness. Any associated swelling may indicate pes anserine bursitis.

Tensor Fasciae Latae (Iliotibial Band and Head of Fibula). As the examiner moves laterally from the tibial tuberosity, the head of the fibula can be palpated. Medial and slightly superior to the fibula, the examiner palpates the insertion of the iliotibial band into the lateral condyle of the tibia. When the knee is extended, it stands out as a strong, visible ridge anterolateral to the knee joint. As the examiner moves proximally, the iliotibial band is palpated along its entire length.

Anteriorly With Knee Flexed

Flexion at 45°—Tibiofemoral Joint Line and Meniscal Cysts. The examiner palpates the joint line, especially on the lateral aspect, for any evidence of swelling (meniscal cyst?), tenderness, or other pathology.

Flexion at 90°—Tibiofemoral Joint Line, Tibial Plateau, Femoral Condyles, and Adductor Muscles. If the examiner returns to the patella, palpates the apex of the patella, and moves medially or laterally, the fingers will lie on the tibiofemoral joint line, which should be palpated along its entire length. As the joint line is palpated, the examiner should also palpate the tibial plateau (coronary ligament sprain?) medially and laterally and the femoral condyles.

Both condyles should be carefully palpated for any tenderness (e.g., osteochondritis dissecans?). Beginning at the superior aspect of the femoral condyles, the examiner should note that the lateral condyle extends further anteriorly (i.e., higher) than the medial condyle. The trochlear groove between the two condyles can then be palpated. As the medial condyle is palpated, a sharp edge appears on the condyle medially. If the edge is followed posteriorly, the adductor tubercle will be palpated on the posteromedial portion of the medial femoral condyle. After palpating the adductor tubercle, the examiner moves proximally, palpating the adductor muscles of the hip for tenderness or other signs of pathology.

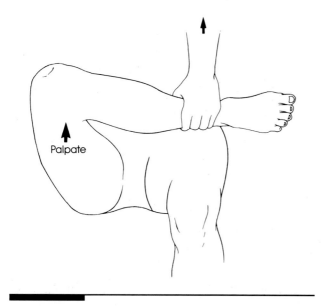

FIGURE 11–98. Palpation of the lateral (fibular) collateral ligament.

Anteriorly With Foot of Test Leg Resting on Opposite Knee—Lateral Collateral Ligament

Kennedy[25] has advocated palpating the lateral collateral ligament by having the patient in the sitting or lying position (Fig. 11–98). The patient's knee is flexed to 90° and the hip is laterally rotated so that the ankle of the test leg rests on the knee of the other leg. The examiner then places the knee into a varus position, and the ropelike ligament stands out if the ligament is intact.

Posteriorly With the Knee Slightly Flexed

Posterior Aspect of Knee Joint. The soft tissue on the posterior aspect of the knee should be palpated for tenderness or swelling (e.g., Baker's cyst?). In some individuals, the popliteal artery may be palpated by running the hand down the center of the posterior knee.

Posterolateral Aspect of Knee Joint. The posterolateral corner of the knee is sometimes called the *popliteus corner.* The examiner should attempt to palpate the arcuate-popliteus complex, lateral gastrocnemius muscle, biceps femoris muscle, and possibly the lateral meniscus in this area. A sesamoid bone is sometimes found inserted in the tendon of the lateral head of the gastrocnemius muscle. This bone, referred to as the *fabella*, may be interpreted as a loose body in the posterolateral aspect of the knee by an unwary examiner.

Posteromedial Aspect of Knee Joint. The posteromedial corner of the knee joint is sometimes referred to as the *semimembranosus corner.* The examiner should attempt to palpate the posterior oblique ligament, the semimembranosus muscle, and possibly the medial meniscus in this area for tenderness or pathology.

Hamstring and Gastrocnemius Muscles. After the various parts of the posterior aspect of the knee have been palpated, the tendons and muscle bellies of the hamstring muscle group (biceps femoris, semitendinosus, and semimembranosus) proximally and gastrocnemius muscle distally should be palpated for tenderness, swelling, or other signs of pathology.

Radiographic Examination

Anteroposterior View. When looking at radiographs of the knee (Fig. 11–99), the examiner should note any possible fractures (e.g., osteochondral), diminished joint space (osteoarthritis—Fig. 11–100), epiphyseal damage, lipping, loose bodies, alterations in bone texture, abnormal calcification or tumors, accessory ossification centers, varus or valgus deformity, patella alta (Figs. 11–101 and 11–102) or baja, and asymmetry of femoral condyles.[62] Stress radiographs of this view will illustrate excessive gapping medially or laterally, indicating ligamentous instability (Fig. 11–103). The examiner should also remember the possible presence of the fabella, which is seen in 20 per cent of the population. Epiphyseal fractures (Fig. 11–104) and osteochondritis dissecans (Fig. 11–105) may also be seen in this view.

Lateral View. With this view,[43, 62] the examiner should note the same structures as seen with the anteroposterior view (Figs. 11–106 and 11–107). In addition, several patellar measurements, if desired, can be made, as shown in Figure 11–100. This view also illustrates Osgood-Schlatter disease (Fig. 11–108) and the presence of the fabella (Fig. 11–109).

Intercondylar Notch (Tunnel View X-ray). With this view (knee flexed to 90°), the tibia and intercondylar attachments of the cruciate ligaments can be examined. Also, any loose bodies or possibility of osteochondritis dissecans, subluxation, patellar tilt (lateral or medial), or dislocation should be noted.

Skyline View. This 30° tangential view is primarily used for suspected patellar problems.[63] It may be taken at different angles, as shown in Figures 11–110 and 11–111, or it may be used to determine the type of patella present, as shown in Figure 11–112. Figure 11–113 illustrates abnormal patellar forms.

Text continued on page 438

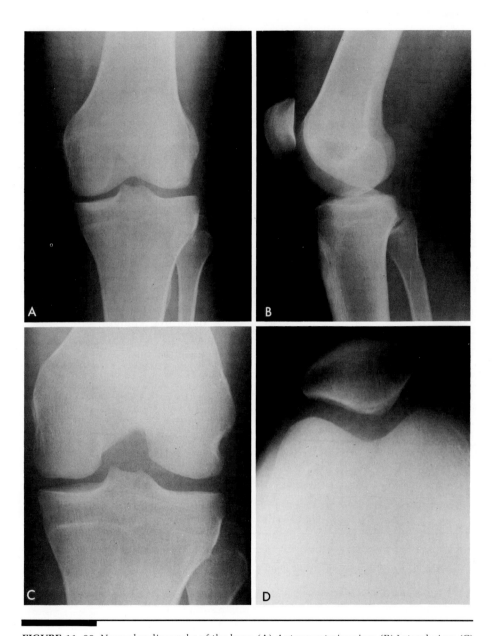

FIGURE 11–99. *Normal radiographs of the knee. (A) Anteroposterior view. (B) Lateral view. (C) "Tunnel" view. (D) "Skyline" view. (From Reilly, B. M.: Practical Strategies in Outpatient Medicine. Philadelphia, W. B. Saunders Co., 1991, p. 1188.)*

VIEW	KNEE FLEXION	PATIENT POSITION	MEASUREMENT		MISCELLANEOUS
AP	0 degrees	Standing, feet straight ahead	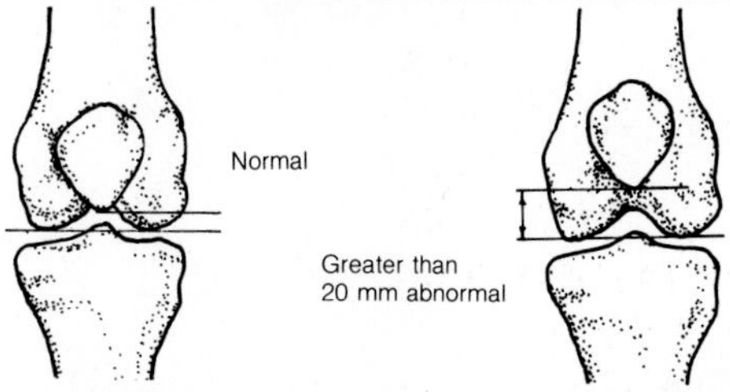 Normal	Greater than 20 mm abnormal	—Hypoplastic patella —Lateral subluxation of patella —Bipartite patella —Asymmetry of femoral condylar (abnormal femoral anteversion or femoral rotation)
Lateral	90 degrees	Supine	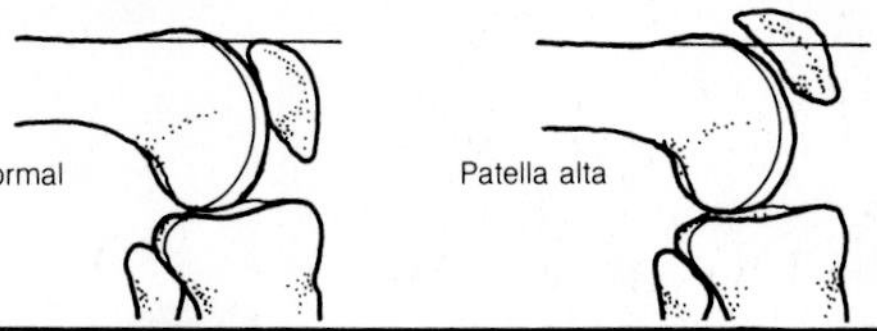 Normal	Patella alta	—Patella infera —Patellar fracture
	Approx. 30 degrees	Supine	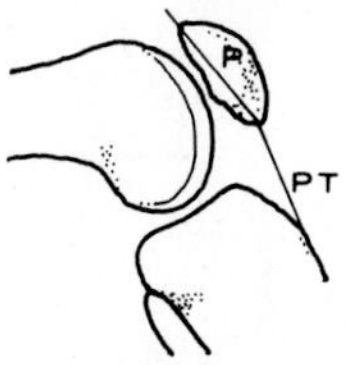 Ratio of P:PT = 1.0 More than 20% variation is abnormal		
	30 degrees	Supine	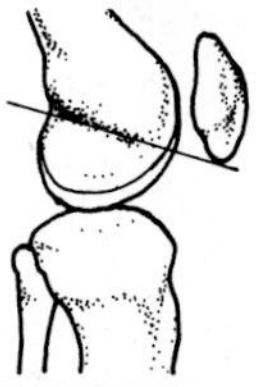 Blumensaat's line (see text)		

FIGURE 11–100. Summary of radiographic findings in patella alta. (From Carson, W. A., et al.: Clin. Orthop. Relat. Res. 185:179, 1984.)

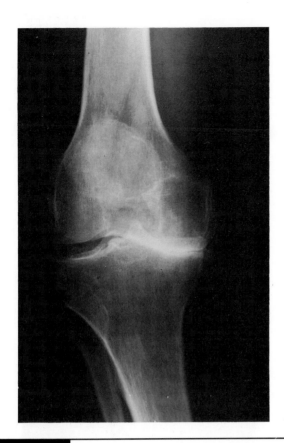

FIGURE 11–101. Degenerative arthritis of the knee in a 63-year-old man. He complained of chronic pain, stiffness, and swelling of both knees. The radiograph demonstrates extensive degenerative arthritis with marked narrowing of the medial joint space and hypertrophic bony changes throughout the joint. There is a valgus deformity of the knee as a result of the osteoarthritis. This patient ultimately required a total knee replacement for amelioration of symptoms. (From Reilly, B. M.: Practical Strategies in Outpatient Medicine. Philadelphia, W. B. Saunders Co., 1991, p. 1207.)

FIGURE 11–102. Anteroposterior view of the knee. (A) Normal patellar position. (B) Patella alta. (C) Patella baja. (From Hughston, J. C., et al.: Patellar Subluxation and Dislocation. Philadelphia, W. B. Saunders Co., 1984, p. 50.)

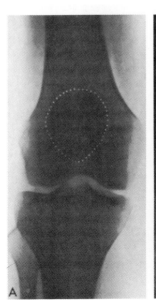
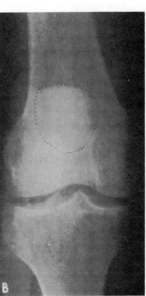
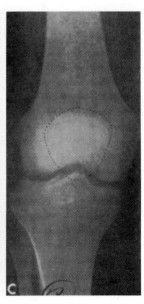

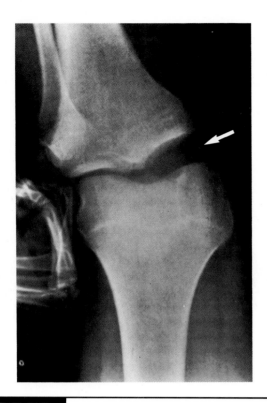

FIGURE 11–103. This valgus stress radiograph shows the patient's knee in full extension. Note the gapping on the medial side (arrow). (Modified from Mital, M. A., and L. I. Karlin: Orthop. Clin. North Am. 11:775, 1980.)

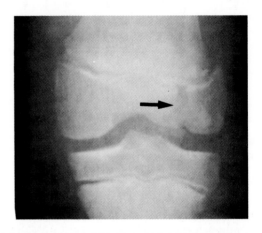

FIGURE 11–104. A Salter-Harris type III injury (arrow) of the growth plate and the epiphysis. Main attention should be directed toward restitution of the joint surface. (From Ehrlich, M. G., and R. E. Strain: Orthop. Clin. North Am. 10:93, 1979.)

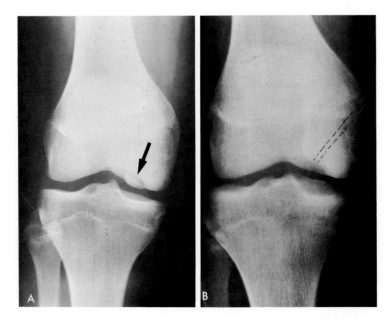

FIGURE 11–105. (A) Osteochondritis dissecans (actually an osteochondral fracture [arrow] of the femoral condyle), with almost the entire femoral attachment of the posterior cruciate ligament remaining attached to the fragment. (B) Three months after repair of posterior cruciate to femur. Excellent function is restored. Complete filling in of this defect is unlikely at this age. (From O'Donoghue, D. H.: Treatment of Injuries to Athletes, 4th ed. Philadelphia, W. B. Saunders Co., 1984, p. 575.)

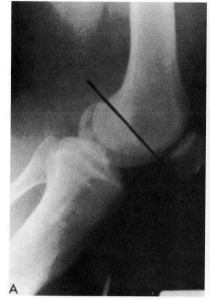
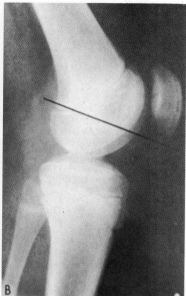

FIGURE 11–106. Lateral view of the patella at 45°. (A) Normal patellar position in relation to the intercondylar notch. (B) Patella alta. (From Hughston, J. C., et al.: Patellar Subluxation and Dislocation. Philadelphia, W. B. Saunders Co., 1984, p. 52.)

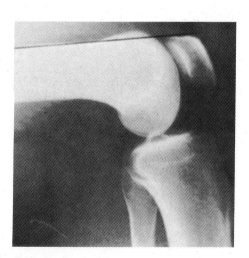

FIGURE 11–107. Lateral view at 90° shows the normal position of the patella. (From Hughston, J. C., et al.: Patellar Subluxation and Dislocation. Philadelphia, W. B. Saunders Co., 1984, p. 52.)

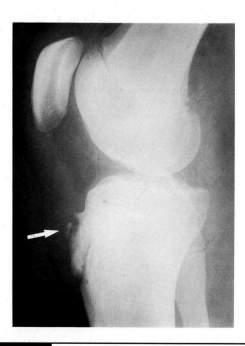

FIGURE 11–108. Osgood-Schlatter disease, showing epiphysitis of the entire epiphysis (arrow), with irregularity of the epiphyseal line. Because this epiphyseal cartilage is continuous with that of the upper tibia, it should not be disturbed. If surgery is used, exposure should be superficial to the epiphyseal cartilage. (Modified from O'Donoghue, D. H.: Treatment of Injuries to Athletes, 4th ed. Philadelphia, W. B. Saunders Co., 1984, p. 574.)

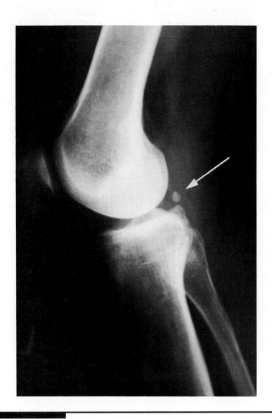

FIGURE 11–109. Sesamoid bone (fabella) in the gastrocnemius muscle.

TANGENTIAL VIEW	KNEE FLEXION	TECHNIQUE AND POSITION	MEASUREMENTS	MISCELLANEOUS

Hughston	55 degrees	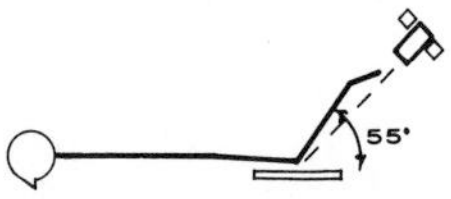 Prone position. Beam directed cephalad and inferior, 45 degrees from vertical.	1) Sulcus angle: 118°
			
			2) Patella index:
			$$\frac{AB}{XB - XA}$$
			NL: Male 15
			Female 17 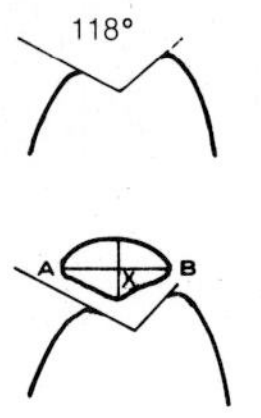
				—Patellar dislocation
				—Osteochondral fracture
				—Soft tissue calcification (old dislocated patella or fracture)
				—Patellar subluxation
				  Patellar tilt
				  Increased medial joint space
				  Apex of patella lateral to apex of femoral sulcus
				  Lateral patella edge lateral to femoral condyle
				  Hypoplastic lateral femoral condyle (usually proximal)
				—Patellofemoral osteophytes
				—Subchondral trabeculae orientation (increase or decrease)
				—Patellar configuration (Wiberg-Baugartl) 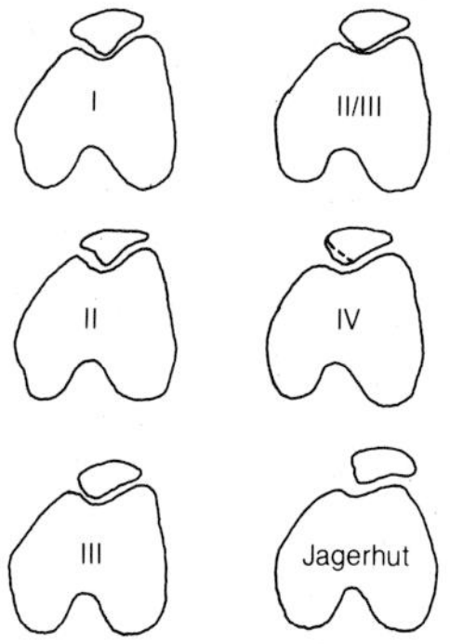

Merchant	45 degrees	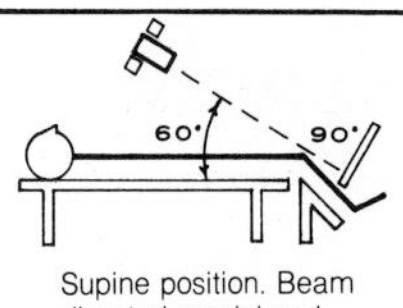 Supine position. Beam directed caudal and inferior, 30 degrees from vertical.	1) Sulcus angle: 138° 2) Congruence angle: Med. −6° Lat. 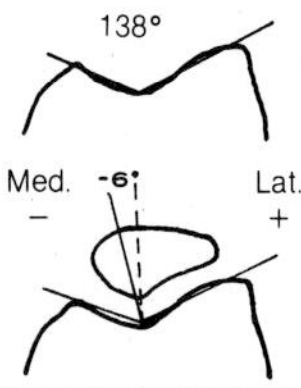 − +	I II/III II IV III Jagerhut
Laurin	20 degrees	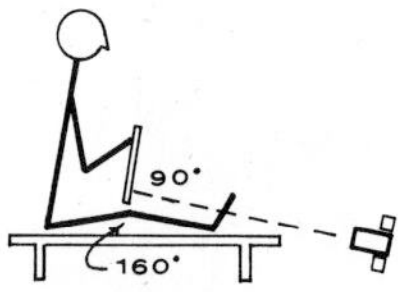 Sitting position. Beam directed cephaled and superior, 160 degrees from vertical.	1) Lateral patellofemoral angle: LAT. NL: ABNL: ABNL: 2) Patellofemoral index: Ratio A/B Med. Lat. Normal = 1.6 or less 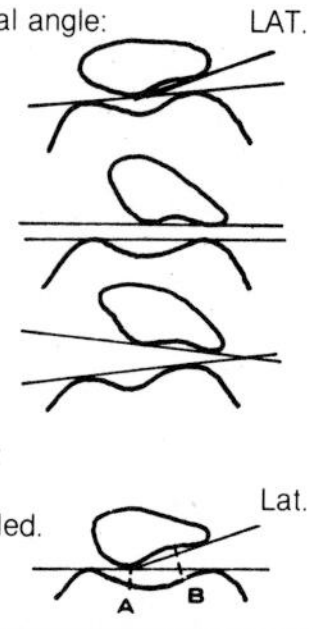	

FIGURE 11–110. Summary of radiographic findings, tangential view. (From Carson, W. A., et al.: Clin. Orthop. Relat. Res. 185:182, 1984.)

436

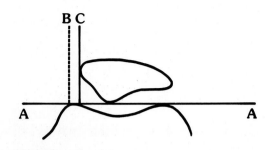

FIGURE 11–111. Lateral patellar displacement. A line is drawn through the highest points of the medial and lateral femoral condyles (line AA). A perpendicular to that line, at the medial edge of the medial femoral condyle (line B), normally lies 1 mm or less medial to the patella (line C). (From Laurin, C. A., R. Dussault, and H. P. Levesque. Clin Orthop. 144:16, 1979.)

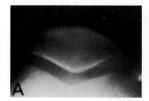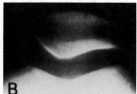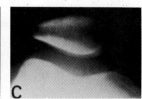

FIGURE 11–112. Examples of patellar variations. (A) Wiberg type I. (B) Wiberg type II. (C) Wiberg type III. (From Ficat, R. P., and D. S. Hungerford: Disorders of the Patello-Femoral Joint. Baltimore, Williams & Wilkins, 1977, p. 53.)

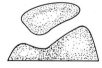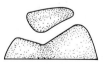

Baumgartl Wiberg III Alpine hunter's cap

FIGURE 11–113. Variations in patellar form that are considered dysplastic. (Modified from Ficat, R. P., and D. S. Hungerford: Disorders of the Patello-Femoral Joint. Baltimore, Williams & Wilkins, 1977, p. 55.)

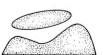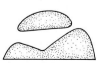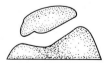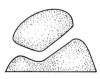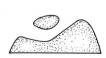

Pebble Half-moon Patella magna Patella parva

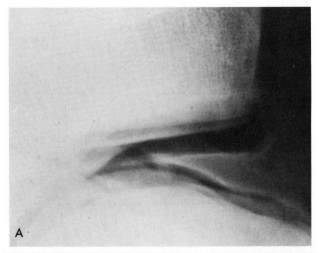
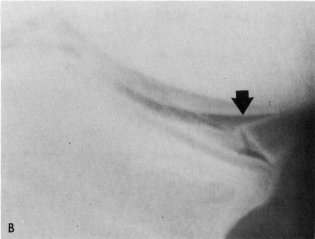

FIGURE 11–114. Arthrogram demonstrating a torn meniscus. The normal meniscus on the lateral side (A) is compared here with the easily demonstrated tear in the medial meniscus (arrow) in the same patient (B). (From Reilly, B. M.: Practical Strategies in Outpatient Medicine. Philadelphia, W. B. Saunders Co., 1991, p. 1198.)

Arthrogram. Arthrograms of the knee are used primarily to diagnose tears in the menisci (Fig. 11–114) and plica (Fig. 11–115). Double-contrast arthrograms are also used (Fig. 11–116).

Arthroscope. The arthroscope is being used increasingly more frequently to diagnose lesions of the knee as well as to repair many of them surgically.[64–66] By using various approaches to the knee, the surgeon is able to view all of the structures to determine if they have been injured (Fig. 11–117).

CT Scans. CT scans are often used to view soft tissue as well as bone (Fig. 11–118).

MRI. MRI is advantageous because of its ability to show soft tissue as well as bone tissue while providing no exposure to ionizing radiation. MRI has been found to be useful in diagnosing lesions of the menisci and cruciate ligaments (Figs. 11–119, 11–120, 11–121, and 11–122).[17]

Xerography. Xerography may be used to delineate the edge of bone (Fig. 11–123).

Text continued on page 444

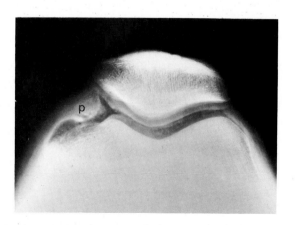

FIGURE 11–115. Tangential patellar view after arthrography shows thinning and slight roughening of the patellar cartilage, especially medially. The mediopatellar plica (p) is noted to be markedly thickened. (From Weissman, B. N. W., and C. B. Sledge: Orthopedic Radiology. Philadelphia, W. B. Saunders Co., 1986, p. 536.)

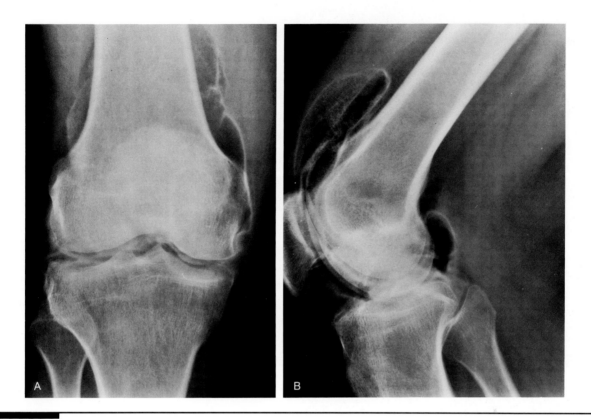

FIGURE 11–116. Double-contrast arthrogram. (A) The anteroposterior view demonstrates the menisci and articular cartilage. (B) The lateral projection illustrates the extent of the joint space. (From Forrester, D. M., and J. C. Brown: The Radiology of Joint Disease. Philadelphia, W. B. Saunders Co., 1987, p. 200.)

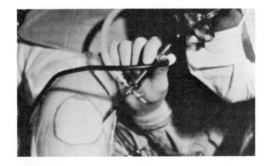

FIGURE 11–117. Arthroscopy of the knee. (From Patel, D.: Orthop. Clin. North Am. 13:301, 1982.)

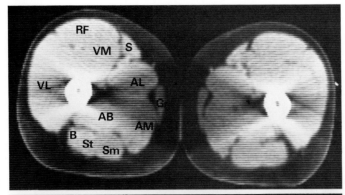

A

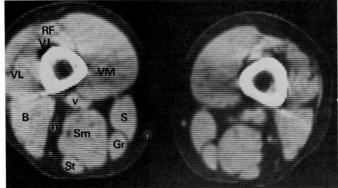

B

FIGURE 11–118. Muscular anatomy as shown on scan. CT images through the upper femur (A) and lower third of femur (B). Ab = adductor brevis, AL = adductor longus, AM = adductor magnus, B = biceps femoris, g = ■, Gr = gracilis, n = tibial and common peroneal nerves, RF = rectus femoris, S = sartorius, Sm = semimembranosus, St = semitendinosus, V = deep femoral vein and artery, VI = vastus intermedius, VL = vastus lateralis, VM = vastus medialis. (From Weissman, B. N. W., and C. B. Sledge: Orthopedic Radiology. Philadelphia, W. B. Saunders Co., 1986, p. 504.)

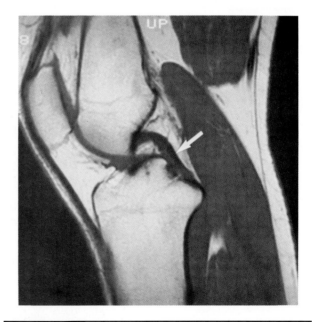

FIGURE 11–119. MRI showing intact posterior cruciate ligament (arrow). (From Strobel, M., and H. W. Stedtfeld: Diagnostic Evaluation of the Knee. Berlin, Springer-Verlag, 1990, p. 243.)

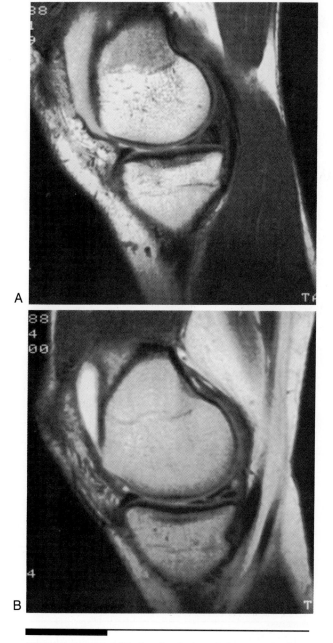

FIGURE 11–120. MRI showing lesion of the posterior horn of the medial meniscus (A). In some cases contrast can be enhanced by the intra-articular injection of gadolinium diethylenetriamene penta-acetic acid (DTPA). (B) Inferior longitudinal tear with an associated horizontal tear. (From Strobel, M., and H. W. Stedtfeld: Diagnostic Evaluation of the Knee. Berlin, Springer-Verlag, 1990, p. 240.)

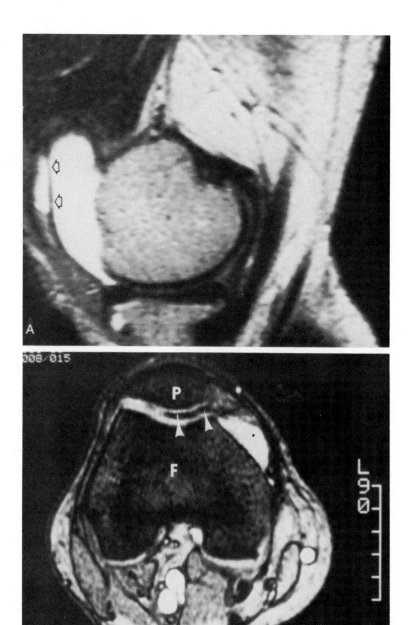

FIGURE 11–121. MRI of medial patellar plica. (A) Sagittal, T2-weighted image medial to the patella shows a white-appearing effusion within the knee joint. A vertical linear band within the joint (open arrows) represents the medial plica. (B) Transaxial STIR image through the patellofemoral joint shows the effusion (arrowheads), which appears bright and surrounds a tonguelike extension of tissue arising from the medial joint line and located between the patella (P) and femur (F). This tissue represents a medial plica. In this location, plicae can become hypertrophied and lead to symptoms and signs of internal derangement. (From Kursunoglu-Brahme, S., and D. Resnick: Orthop. Clin. North Am. 21:571, 1990.)

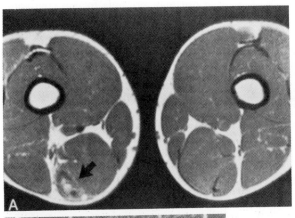

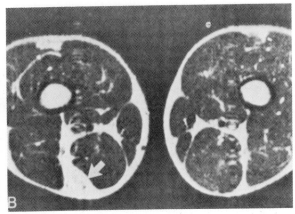

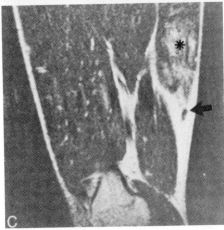

FIGURE 11–122. MRI showing tendon rupture in a 22-year-old athlete who pulled his hamstring on two occasions and was unable to run. Seven centimeters above the patella, (A) axial T1-weighted (TR, 600 msec; TE, 20 msec) and (B) T2-weighted (TR, 2,000 msec; TE, 85 msec) MRIs show abnormally high signal intensity of the right semitendinosus muscle (arrows) compared with the normal left side. (C) A sagittal T2-weighted MRI (TR, 2,000 msec; TE, 85 msec) shows that the retracted semitendinosus muscle (asterisk) has an abnormally high signal intensity. The arrow indicates a torn musculotendinous junction. (From Bassett, L. W., and R. H. Gold.: Clin. Orthop. Relat. Res. 244:20, 1989.)

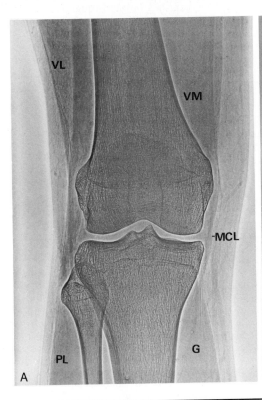

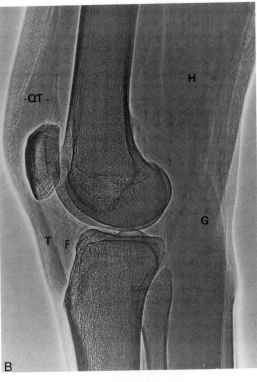

FIGURE 11–123. Xerography of the knee. F = infrapatellar fat pad, G = gastrocnemius, H = hamstrings, MCL = medial collateral ligament, PL = peroneus longus, QT = quadriceps tendon, T = patellar tendon, VL = vastus lateralis, VM = vastus medialis. (From Weissman, B. N. W., and C. B. Sledge: Orthopedic Radiology. Philadelphia, W. B. Saunders Co., 1986, p. 504.)

PRÉCIS OF THE KNEE ASSESSMENT*

History
Observation
Examination
  Active movements
    Knee flexion
    Knee extension
    Medial rotation of the tibia on the femur
    Lateral rotation of the tibia on the femur
  Functional assessment
  Passive movements (as in active movements)
  Resisted isometric movements
    Knee flexion
    Knee extension
    Ankle plantar flexion
    Ankle dorsiflexion
  Tests for ligament stability
    Test for one-plane medial instability
    Test for one-plane lateral instability
    Tests for one-plane anterior and posterior instabilities
    Tests for anteromedial and anterolateral rotary instabilities
    Tests for posteromedial and posterolateral rotary instabilities
  Special tests
    Tests for meniscus injury
    Plica tests
    Tests for swelling
    Other special tests
  Reflexes and cutaneous distribution
  Joint play movements
    Backward and forward movements of the tibia on the femur
    Medial and lateral displacements of the patella
    Depression of the patella
    Anteroposterior movement of the fibula on the tibia
  Palpation
  Radiographic examination

After any examination, the patient should always be warned of the possibility of exacerbation of symptoms as a result of the assessment.

*Although examination of the knee may be carried out with the patient in the supine position, some of the tests may require the patient to move to other positions (e.g., standing, lying, prone, sitting, and so on). When these tests are used, the examination should be planned in such a way that the movement and, therefore, discomfort of the patient are kept to a minimum. Thus, the sequence should be from standing to sitting, to supine lying, to side lying, and, finally, to prone lying.

CASE STUDIES

When doing these case studies, the examiner should list the appropriate questions to be asked and why they are being asked, what to look for and why, and what things should be tested and why. Depending on the answers of the patient (and the examiner should consider different responses), several possible causes of the patient's problem may become evident (examples are given in parentheses). If so, a differential diagnosis chart should be made. The examiner can then decide how different diagnoses may affect the treatment plan.

1. A 59-year-old man presents to you complaining of moderate pain and swelling of 4 months' duration in his right knee. There is no history of trauma. The pain and swelling have become worse during the past month. Describe your assessment plan for this patient (osteoarthritis versus meniscus pathology).

2. A 24-year-old male football player is referred to you for treatment after a surgical repair to his anterior cruciate and medial collateral ligaments of the right knee. He is still in a splint, but the surgeon says the splint can be removed for treatment. Describe your assessment plan for this patient.

3. A 54-year-old man comes to you for treatment. He complains of difficulty when walking and pain in the left hamstrings that is referred into the area of the gluteal fold. There is ecchymosis evident in the posterior knee and a small amount in the superior calf area. Describe your assessment plan for this patient (hamstring strain versus sciatica).

4. An 18-year-old woman presents to your clinic complaining of anterior knee pain. Design your assessment plan for this patient (chondromalacia patella versus plica syndrome).

5. A 16-year-old female volleyball player comes to you complaining of knee pain. Her knee is painful when she plays, and she sometimes feels a clicking when going up and down stairs. Describe your assessment plan for this patient (meniscus pathology versus plica syndrome).

6. A 17-year-old male soccer player comes to you complaining that his knee feels unstable. He says he was playing soccer, twisted to challenge a player, and felt a pop in his knee. Describe your assessment plan for this patient (osteochondral fracture versus anterior cruciate sprain).

7. A 10-year-old boy is brought to you by his parents. He is complaining of anterior knee pain. Describe your assessment plan for this patient (Osgood-Schlatter's disease versus chondromalacia patellae).

8. A 20-year-old female rugby player comes to you complaining of lateral knee pain that is sometimes referred down the leg. The knee hurts when she walks. She vaguely remembers being kicked in the knee while playing rugby 10 days earlier. Describe your assessment plan for this patient (superior tibiofibular joint subluxation versus common peroneal nerve neuropraxia).

9. An 18-year-old female swimmer presents to you complaining of medial knee pain. She has just increased her training to 10,000 m per day. Describe your assessment plan for this patient (medial collateral ligament sprain versus chondromalacia patella).

REFERENCES

CITED REFERENCES

1. Kaltenborn, F. M.: Mobilization of the Extremity Joints. Oslo, Olaf Norles Bokhandel, 1980.
2. Arnoczsky, S. P.: The blood supply of the meniscus and its role in healing and repair. American Association of Orthopedic Surgeons, Symposium on Sports Medicine: The Knee. St. Louis, C. V. Mosby, 1985.
3. Radin, E. L., F. de Lamotte, and P. Maquet: Role of the menisci in the distribution of stress in the knee. Clin. Orthop. Relat. Res. 185:290, 1984.
4. Seedhom, B. B.: Loadbearing function of the menisci. Physiotherapy 62:223, 1976.
5. Ficat, R. P., and D. S. Hungerford: The Patello-Femoral Joint. Baltimore, Williams & Wilkins, 1977.

6. Goodfellow, J., D. S. Hungerford, and M. Zindel: Patellofemoral joint mechanics and pathology: Functional anatomy of the patellofemoral joint. J. Bone Joint Surg. 58B:287, 1976.

7. Staheli, L. T., and G. M. Engel: Tibial torsion. Clin. Orthop. Relat. Res. 86:183, 1972.

8. Waldron, V. D.: A test for chondromalacia patellae. Orthop. Rev. 12:103, 1983.

9. Jacobson, K. E., and F. C. Flandry: Diagnosis of anterior knee pain. Clin. Sports Med. 8:179, 1989.

10. Segal, P., and M. Jacob: The Knee. Chicago, Year Book Medical Pub., 1983.

11. Kannus, P., M. Jarvinea, and K. Latvala. Knee strength evaluation. Scand. J. Sport Sci. 9:9, 1987.

12. Goslin, B. R., and J. Charteris: Isokinetic dynamometry: Normative data for clinical use in lower extremity (knee) cases. Scand. J. Rehab. Med. 11:105, 1979.

13. Noyes, F. R., G. H. McGinniss, and L. A. Mooar: Functional disability in the anterior cruciate insufficient knee syndrome—Review of knee rating systems and projected risk factors in determining treatment. Sports Med. 1:278, 1984.

14. Insall, J. N., L. D. Dorr, R. D. Scott, and W. N. Scott: Rationale of the Knee Society clinical rating system. Clin. Orthop. Relat. Res. 248:13, 1989.

15. Kettelkamp, D. B., and C. Thompson: Development of a knee scoring scale. Clin. Orthop. Relat. Res. 107:93, 1975.

16. Losee, R. E.: Diagnosis of chronic injury to the anterior cruciate ligament. Orthop. Clin. North Am. 16:83, 1985.

17. Jackson, D. W., L. D. Jennings, R. M. Maywoods, and P. E. Berger: Magnetic resonance imaging of the knee. Am. J. Sports Med. 16:29, 1988.

18. Strobel, M., and H. W. Stedtfeld: Diagnostic Evaluation of the Knee. Berlin, Springer-Verlag, 1990.

19. Larson, R. L.: Physical examination in the diagnosis of rotary instability. Clin. Orthop. Relat. Res. 172:38, 1983.

20. Muller, W.: The Knee: Form, Function and Ligament Reconstruction. New York, Springer-Verlag, 1983.

21. Detenbeck, L. C.: Function of the cruciate ligaments in knee stability. Am. J. Sports Med. 2:217, 1974.

22. Furman, W., J. L. Marshall, and F. G. Girgis: The anterior cruciate ligament: A functional analysis based on postmortem studies. J. Bone Joint Surg. 58A:179, 1976.

23. Girgis, F. G., J. L. Marshall, and A. R. S. Al Monajem: The cruciate ligaments of the knee joint: Anatomical, functional and experimental analysis. Clin. Orthop. Relat. Res. 106:216, 1975.

24. Baker, C. L., L. A. Norwood, and J. C. Hughston: Acute combined posterior and posterolateral instability of the knee. Am. J. Sports Med. 12:204, 1984.

25. Kennedy, J. C.: The Injured Adolescent Knee. Baltimore, Williams & Wilkins, 1979.

26. Jonsson, T., B. Althoff, L. Peterson, and P. Renstrom: Clinical diagnosis of ruptures of the anterior cruciate ligament: A comparative study of the Lachman test and the anterior drawer sign. Am. J. Sports Med. 10:100, 1982.

27. Bechtel, S. L., B. R. Ellman, and J. L. Jordon: Skier's knee: The cruciate connection. Phys. Sports Med. 12:51, 1984.

28. Feagin, J. A.: The Crucial Ligaments. Edinburgh, Churchill Livingstone, 1988.

29. Rebman, L. W.: Lachman's test: An alternative method. J. Orthop. Sports Phys. Ther. 9:381, 1988.

30. Cross, M. J., and K. J. Crichton: Clinical Examination of the Injured Knee. Baltimore, Williams & Wilkins, 1987.

31. Cross, M. J., D. R. Schmidt, and I. G. Mackie: A no-touch test for the anterior cruciate ligament. J. Bone Joint Surg. 69B:300, 1987.

32. Butler, D. L., F. R. Noyes, and E. S. Grood: Ligamentous restraints to anterior-posterior drawer in the human knee. J. Bone Joint Surg. 622A:259, 1980.

33. Weatherwax, R. J.: Anterior drawer sign. Clin. Ortho. Rel. Res. 154:318, 1981.

34. Warren, R. F.: Physical diagnosis of the knee. In Post, M. (ed.): Physical Examination of the Musculoskeletal System. Chicago, Year Book Medical Pub., 1987.

35. Slocum, D. B., and R. L. Larson: Rotary instability of the knee. J. Bone Joint Surg., 50A:211, 1968.

36. Slocum, D. B., S. L. James, R. L. Larson, and K. M. Singer: A clinical test for anterolateral rotary instability of the knee. Clin. Orthop. Relat. Res. 118:63, 1976.

37. Fetto, J. F., and J. L. Marshall: Injury to the anterior cruciate ligament producing the pivot shift sign: An experimental study on cadaver specimens. J. Bone Joint Surg. 61A:710, 1979.

38. Galway, H. R., and D. L. MacIntosh: The lateral pivot shift: A symptom and sign of anterior cruciate ligament insufficiency. Clin. Orthop. Relat. Res. 147:45, 1980.

39. Tamea, C. D., and C. E. Henning: Pathomechanics of the pivot shift maneuver. Am. J. Sports Med. 9:31, 1981.

40. Katz, J. W., and R. F. Fingeroth: The diagnostic accuracy of ruptures of the anterior cruciate ligament comparing the Lachman test, the anterior drawer sign and the pivot shift test in acute and chronic knee injuries. Am. J. Sports Med. 14:88, 1986.

41. Peterson, L., M. I. Pitman, and J. Gold: The active pivot shift: The role of the popliteus muscle. Am. J. Sports Med. 12:313, 1984.

42. Losee, R. E., T. R. J. Ennis, and W. O. Southwick: Anterior subluxation of the lateral tibial plateau: A diagnostic test and operative review. J. Bone Joint Surg. 60A:1015, 1978.

43. Hughston, J. C., W. M. Walsh, and G. Puddu: Patellar Subluxation and Dislocation. Philadelphia, W. B. Saunders Co., 1984.

44. Noyes, F. R., D. L. Butler, E. S. Grood, et al.: Clinical paradoxes of anterior cruciate instability and a new test to detect its instability. Orthop. Trans. 2:36, 1978.

45. Hanks, G. A., D. M. Joyner, and A. Kalenak: Anterolateral instability of the knee. Am. J. Sports Med. 9:225, 1981.

46. Hughston, J. C., and L. A. Norwood: The posterolateral drawer test and external rotational recurvatum test for posterolateral rotary instability of the knee. Clin. Orthop. Relat. Res. 147:82, 1980.

47. Jakob, R. P., H. Hassler, and H. U. Staeubli: Observations on rotary instability of the lateral compartment of the knee. Acta Orthop. Scand. (Suppl. 191) 52:1, 1981.

48. Shelbourne, K. D., F. Benedict, J. R. McCarroll, and A. C. Rettig: Dynamic posterior shift test—An adjunct in evaluation of posterior tibial subluxation. Am. J. Sports Med. 17:275, 1989.

49. Shino, K., S. Horibe, and K. Ono: The voluntary evoked posterolateral drawer sign in the knee with posterolateral instability. Clin. Orthop. Relat. Res. 215:179, 1987.

50. Loomer, R. L.: A test for knee posterolateral rotary instability. Clin. Orthop. Relat. Res. 264:235, 1991.

51. McMurray, T. P.: The semilunar cartilages. Br. J. Surg. 29:407, 1942.

52. Apley, A. G.: The diagnosis of meniscus injuries—Some new clinical methods. J. Bone Joint Surg. 29B:78, 1947.

53. Helfet, A.: Disorders of the Knee. Philadelphia, J. B. Lippincott Co., 1974.

54. Anderson, A. F., and A. B. Lipscomb: Clinical diagnosis of meniscal tears—Description of a new manipulative test. Am. J. Sports Med. 14:291, 1988.

55. Mital, M. A., and J. Hayden: Pain in the knee in children: The medial plica shelf syndrome. Orthop. Clin. North Am. 10:713, 1979.

56. McConnell, J.: The management of chondromalacia patellae: A long term solution. Aust. J. Physiother. 32:215, 1986.

57. Kolowich, P. A., L. E. Paulos, T. D. Rosenberg, and S. Farnsworth: Lateral release of the patella: Indications and contraindications. Am. J. Sports Med. 18:359, 1990.

58. Olerud, C., and P. Berg: The variation of the Q angle with different positions of the foot. Clin. Orthop. Relat. Res. 191:162, 1984.

59. Daniel, D. M., M. L. Stone, P. Barnett, and R. Sachs: Use of the quadriceps active test to diagnose posterior cruciate ligament disruption and measure posterior laxity of the knee. J. Bone Joint Surg. 70A:386, 1988.

60. Fairbank, H. A. T.: Internal derangement of the knee in children and adolescents. Proc. Roy. Soc. Med. 30:427, 1937.

61. Noble, H. B., M. R. Hajek, and M. Porter: Diagnosis and treatment of iliotibial band tightness in runners. Phys. Sportsmed. 10:67, 1984.

62. Carson, W. G., Jr., S. L. James, R. L. Larson, et al: Patellofem-

oral disorders: Physical and radiographic evaluation: I. Physical examination. Clin. Orthop. Relat. Res. 185:165, 1984.

63. Speakman, H. B., and J. Weisberg: The vastus medialis controversy. Physiotherapy 63:249, 1977.

64. Mital, M. A., and L. I. Karlin: Diagnostic arthroscopy in sports injuries. Orthop. Clin. North Am. 11:771, 1980.

65. McClelland, C. J.: Arthroscopy and arthroscopic surgery of the knee. Physiotherapy 70:154, 1984.

66. Noyes, F. R., R. W. Bassett, E. S. Grood, and D. L. Butler: Arthroscopy in acute traumatic hemarthrosis of the knee. J. Bone Joint Surg. 62A:687, 1980.

GENERAL REFERENCES

Adams, J. C.: Outline of Orthopedics. London, E & S Livingstone, Ltd., 1968.

Ahstrom, J. P.: Reliability of history and physical examination in diagnosis of meniscus pathology. Curr. Pract. Orthop. Surg., Vol. 7, St. Louis, C. V. Mosby, 1977.

Aichroth, P., M. A. R. Freeman, I. S. Smillie, and W. A. Souter: A knee function assessment chart. J. Bone Joint Surg. 60B:308, 1978.

Arnold, J. A., T. P. Coker, L. M. Heaton, et al.: Natural history of anterior cruciate tears. Am. J. Sports Med. 7:305, 1979.

Bassett, L. W., and R. H. Gold: Magnetic resonance imaging of the musculoskeletal system—An overview. Clin. Orthop. Relat. Res. 244:17, 1989.

Bassett, L. W., R. H. Gold, and L. L. Seeger: MRI Atlas of the Musculoskeletal System. London, Martin Dunitz, 1989.

Beetham, W. P., H. P. Polley, C. H. Slocumb, and W. F. Weaver: Physical Extremities of the Joints. Philadelphia, W. B. Saunders Co., 1965.

Booker, J. M., and G. A. Thibodeau: Athletic Injury Assessment. St. Louis, C. V. Mosby Co., 1989.

Brantigan, O. C., and A. F. Voshell: The mechanics of the ligaments and menisci of the knee joint. J. Bone Joint Surg. 23:44, 1941.

Bryant, J. T., and T. D. Cooke: A biomechanical function of the ACL: Prevention of medial translation of the tibia. In Feagin, J. A. (ed.): The Crucial Ligaments. Edinburgh, Churchill Livingstone, 1988.

Burk, D. L., M. K. Dalinka, E. Kinal, M. L. Schiebler, E. K. Cohen, R. J. Prorok, W. B. Gefter, and H. Y. Kressel: Meniscal and ganglion cysts of the knee: MR evaluation. Am. J. Radiol. 150:331, 1988.

Cabaud, H. E., and D. B. Slocum: The diagnosis of chronic anterolateral rotary instability of the knee. Am. J. Sports Med. 5:99, 1977.

Cailliet, R.: Knee Pain and Disability. Philadelphia, F. A. Davis Co., 1973.

Clancy, W. G.: Evaluation of acute knee injuries. American Association of Orthopedic Surgeons, Symposium on Sports Medicine: The Knee. St. Louis: C. V. Mosby, 1985.

Clarkson, H. M., and G. B. Gilewich: Musculoskeletal Assessment—Joint Range of Motion and Manual Muscle Strength. Baltimore, Williams & Wilkins, 1989.

Collins, H. R.: Anterolateral rotary instability. American Association of Orthopedic Surgeons, Symposium on the Athlete's Knee. St. Louis: C. V. Mosby, 1980.

Cooper, D. E.: Tests for posterolateral instability of the knee in normal subjects—Results of examination under anaesthesia. J. Bone Joint Surg. 73A:30, 1991.

Crues, J. V., R. Ryu, and F. W. Morgan: Meniscal pathology—The expanding role of magnetic resonance imaging. Clin. Orthop. Relat. Res. 252:80, 1990.

Cyriax, J.: Textbook of Orthopaedic Medicine, vol. 1. Diagnosis of Soft Tissue Lesions. London, Bailliere Tindall, 1975.

Daniel, D. M., and M. L. Stone: Diagnosis of knee ligament injury: Tests and measurements of joint laxity. In Feagin, J. A. (ed.): The Crucial Ligaments. Edinburgh, Churchill Livingstone, 1988.

Davies, G. J., and R. Larson: Examining the knee. Phys. Sportsmed. 6:49, 1978.

De Haven, K. E., and H. R. Collins: Diagnosis of internal derangement of the knee—The role of arthroscopy. J. Bone Joint Surg. 57A:802, 1975.

Donaldson, W. F., R. F. Warren, and T. Wickiewicz: A comparison of acute anterior cruciate ligament examinations—Initial vs examination under anesthesia. Am. J. Sports Med. 13:5, 1985.

Dontigny, R. L.: Terminal extension exercises for the knee. Phys. Ther. 52:45, 1972.

Doppman, J. L.: Baker's cyst and the normal gastrocnemiosemimembranosus bursa. Am. J. Roentgenol. 94:646, 1965.

Ehrlich, M. G., and R. E. Strain: Epiphyseal injuries about the knee. Orthop. Clin. North Am. 10:91, 1979.

Ellison, A. E.: The pathogenesis and treatment of anterolateral rotary instability. Clin. Orthop. Relat. Res. 147:29, 1980.

Fetto, J. F., and J. L. Marshall: The natural history and diagnosis of anterior cruciate ligament insufficiency. Clin. Orthop. Relat. Res. 147:29, 1980.

Fowler, P. J.: The classification and early diagnosis of knee joint instability. Clin. Orthop. Relat. Res. 147:15, 1980.

Francis, R. S., and D. E. Scott: Hypertrophy of the vastus medialis in knee extension. Phys. Ther. 54:1066, 1974.

Frankel, V. H., A. H. Burstein, and D. B. Brooks: Biomechanics of internal derangement of the knee. J. Bone Joint Surg. 53:945, 1971.

Fulherson, J. P.: Evaluation of the peripatellar soft tissues and retinaculum in patients with patellofemoral pain. Clin. Sports Med. 8:197, 1989.

Fulkerson, J. P.: Awareness of the retinaculum in evaluating patellofemoral pain. Am. J. Sports Med. 10:147, 1982.

Gartland, J. J.: Fundamentals of Orthopedics. Philadelphia, W. B. Saunders Co., 1979.

Gersoff, W. K., and W. G. Clancy: Diagnosis of acute and chronic anterior cruciate ligament tears. Clin. Sports Med. 7:727, 1988.

Gillquist, J.: Diagnosis and classification of the instability of the knee joint. Semin. Ortho. 2:18, 1987.

Goodfellow, J., D. S. Hungerford, and M. Zindel: Patellofemoral joint mechanics and pathology: Chondromalacia patellae. J. Bone Joint Surg., 58B:291, 1976.

Gough, J. V., and G. Ladley: An investigation into the effectiveness of various forms of quadriceps exercises. Physiother. 57:356, 1971.

Greenmill, B. J.: The importance of the medial quadriceps expansion in medial ligament injury. Can. J. Surg. 10:312, 1967.

Grood, E. S., S. F. Stowers, and F. R. Noyes: Limits of movement in the human knee—Effect of sectioning the posterior cruciate ligament and posterolateral structures. J. Bone Joint Surg. 70A:88, 1988.

Hardaker, W. G., T. L. Shipple, and F. H. Bassett: Diagnosis and treatment of the plica syndrome of the knee. J. Bone Joint Surg. 62A:221, 1980.

Hollinshead, W. H., and D. B. Jenkins: Functional Anatomy of the Limbs and Back. Philadelphia, W. B. Saunders Co., 1981.

Hoppenfeld, S.: Physical Examination of the Spine and Extremities. New York, Appleton-Century-Crofts, 1976.

Hoppenfeld, S.: Physical examination of the knee joint by complaint. Orthop. Clin. North Am. 10:3, 1979.

Hughston, J. C.: The absent posterior drawer test in some acute posterior cruciate ligament tears of the knee. Am. J. Sports Med. 16:39, 1988.

Hughston, J. C., J. R. Andrews, M. J. Cross, and A. Moschi: Classification of knee ligament instabilities: Part I. The medial compartment and cruciate ligaments. J. Bone Joint Surg. 58A:173, 1976.

Hughston, J. C., J. A. Bowden, J. R. Andrews, and L. A. Norwood: Acute tears of the posterior cruciate ligament. J. Bone Joint Surg. 62A:438, 1980.

Insall, J., K. A. Falvo, and D. W. Wise: Chondromalacia patellae: A prospective study. J. Bone Joint Surg. 58A:1, 1976.

Jackson, J. P.: Internal derangement of the knee-joint. Physiother. 52:229, 1966.

Jakob, R. P.: Pathomechanical and clinical components of the pivot shift sign. Semin. Orthop. 2:9, 1987.

Jakob, R. P., H. U. Staubli, and J. T. Deland: Grading the pivot shift—Objective tests with implications for treatment. J. Bone Joint Surg. 69B:294, 1987.

Jensen, K.: Manual laxity tests for anterior cruciate ligament injuries. J. Orthop. Sports Phys. Ther. 11:474, 1990.

Kapandji, L. A.: The Physiology of the Joints, vol. 2: Lower Limb. New York, Churchill Livingstone, 1970.

Kennedy, J. C., R. Stewart, and D. M. Walker: Anterolateral rotary instability of the knee joint: An early analysis of the Ellison repair. J. Bone Joint Surg. 60A:1031, 1974.

Kursunoglu-Brahme, S., and D. Resnick: Magnetic resonance imaging of the knee. Orthop. Clin. North Am. 21:561, 1990.

Leib, F. J., and J. Perry: Quadriceps function. J. Bone Joint Surg. 50A:1535, 1968.

Losee, R. E.: The pivot shift. In Feagin, J. A. (ed.): The Crucial Ligaments. Edinburgh, Churchill Livingstone, 1988.

Losee, R. E.: Concepts of the pivot shift. Clin. Orthop. Relat. Res. 172:45, 1983.

Lucie, R. S., J. D. Wiedel, and D. G. Messner: The acute pivot shift: Clinical correlation. Am. J. Sports Med. 12:189, 1984.

Macnicol, M. F.: The Problem Knee—Diagnosis and Management in the Younger Patient. London, Wm. Heinemann Med. Books, 1986.

Major, D.: Anatomical and functional aspects of the knee joint. Physiother. 52:224, 1966.

Malek, M. M., and R. E. Manjini: Patellofemoral pain syndrome: A comprehensive and conservative approach. J. Orthop. Sports Phys. Ther. 2:108, 1981.

Malone, T., and S. T. Kegerreis: Evaluation process. In Mangine, R. E. (ed.): Physical Therapy of the Knee. Edinburgh, Churchill Livingstone, 1988.

Mandelbaum, B. R., G. A. Finerman, M. A. Reicher, S. Hartzman, L. W. Bassett, R. H. Gold, W. Rauschning, and F. Dorey: Magnetic resonance imaging as a tool for evaluation of traumatic knee injuries. Am. J. Sports Med. 14:361, 1986.

McRae, R.: Clinical Orthopaedic Examination. New York, Churchill Livingstone, 1976.

Moran, D. J., and R. T. Floyd: The Lachman test: Alternative techniques and applications for anterior cruciate ligament evaluation. Sports Med. Update 5:3, 1990.

Norwood, L. A., and J. C. Hughston: Combined anterolateral-anteromedial instability of the knee. Clin. Orthop. Relat. Res. 147:62, 1980.

Noyes, F. R., and E. S. Grood: Diagnosis of knee ligament injuries: Clinical concepts. In Feagin, J.A. (ed.): The Crucial Ligaments. Edinburgh, Churchill Livingstone, 1988.

Nunn, K. D., and J. L. Mayhew: Comparison of three methods of assessing strength imbalances at the knee. J. Orthop. Sports Phys. Ther. 10:134, 1988.

O'Donoghue, D. H.: Treatment of Injuries to Athletes, 4th ed. Philadelphia, W. B. Saunders Co., 1984.

Palmer, M. L., and M. Epler: Clinical Assessment Procedures in Physical Therapy. Philadelphia, J. B. Lippincott Co., 1990.

Patel, D.: Superior lateral-medial approach to arthroscopic meniscectomy. Orthop. Clin. North Am. 13:299, 1982.

Percy, E. C., and R. T. Strother: Patellalgia. Phys. Sports Med. 13:43, 1985.

Perry, J.: Function of quadriceps. J. Can. Physiother. Assoc. 24:130, 1972.

Pickett, J. C., and E. L. Radin: Chondromalacia of the Patella. Baltimore, Williams & Wilkins, 1983.

Pipkin, G.: Knee injuries: The role of the suprapatellar plica and suprapatellar bursa in simulating internal derangements. Clin. Orthop. Relat. Res. 74:161, 1971.

Reid, D. C.: Functional Anatomy and Joint Mobilization. Edmonton: University of Alberta Bookstore, 1980.

Reider, B., J. L. Marshall, B. Koslin, B. Ring, and F. G. Girgis: The anterior aspect of the knee joint. J. Bone Joint Surg. 63A:351, 1981.

Reilly, B. M.: Practical Strategies in Outpatient Medicine. Philadelphia, W. B. Saunders Co., 1984.

Renstrom, P., and R. J. Johnson: Anatomy and biomechanics of the menisci. Clin. Sports Med. 9:523, 1990.

Rovere, G. D., and D. M. Adair: Anterior cruciate-deficient knees: A review of the literature. Am. J. Sports Med. 11:412, 1983.

Rusche, K., and R. E. Mangine: Pathomechanics of injury to the patellofemoral and tibiofemoral joint. In Mangine, R. E. (ed.): Physical Therapy of the Knee. Edinburgh, Churchill Livingstone, 1988.

Segal, P., and M. Jacob: The Knee. Chicago, Year Book Medical Pub., 1983.

Smillie, I. S.: Diseases of the knee joint. Physiother. 70:144, 1984.

Tachdjian, M. O.: Pediatric Orthopedics. Philadelphia, W. B. Saunders Co., 1972.

Torg, J. S., W. Conrad, and V. Allen: Clinical diagnosis of anterior cruciate ligament instability in the athlete. Am. J. Sports Med. 4:84, 1976.

Tria, A. J., and R. C. Palumbo: Conservative treatment of patellofemoral pain. Semin. Orthop. 5:115, 1990.

Trickey, E. L.: Injuries to the posterior cruciate ligament: Diagnosis and treatment of early injuries and reconstruction of late instability. Clin. Orthop. Relat. Res. 147:76, 1980.

Turner, J. S., and I. S. Smillie: The effect of tibial torsion on the pathology of the knee. J. Bone Joint Surg. 63B:396, 1981.

Wallace, L. A., R. E. Mangine, and T. R. Malone: The knee. In Gould, J. A. (ed.): Orthopedic and Sports Physical Therapy. St. Louis, C. V. Mosby Co., 1990.

Warren, L. F., J. Marshall, and F. Girgis: The prime static stabilizer of the medial side of the knee. J. Bone Joint Surg. 56A:665, 1974.

Warren, L. F., and J. Marshall: The supporting structures and layers on the medial side of the knee. J. Bone Joint Surg. 61A:56, 1979.

Weiss, J. R., J. J. Irrganj, R. Sawhney, S. Dearwater, and F. H. Fu: A functional assessment of anterior cruciate ligament deficiency in an acute and clinical setting. J. Orthop. Sports Phys. Ther. 11:372, 1990.

Weissman, B. N. W., and C. B. Sledge: Orthopedic Radiology. Philadelphia, W. B. Saunders Co., 1986.

Welsh, R. P.: Knee joint structure and function. Clin. Orthop. Relat. Res. 147:7, 1980.

Wiles, P., and R. Sweetnam: Essentials of Orthopedics. London, J & A Churchill, Ltd., 1965.

Lower Leg, Ankle, and Foot

At least 80 per cent of the general population has foot problems that can often be corrected by proper assessment, treatment, and, above all, care of the feet. Lesions of the ankle and foot can alter the mechanics of gait and, as a result, cause stress on other lower limb joints; this in turn may lead to pathology in these joints.

The foot and ankle combine flexibility with stability because of the many bones they comprise and because of their shapes. The lower leg, ankle, and foot have two principal functions—propulsion and support. For propulsion, they act like a flexible lever; for support, they act like a rigid structure that holds up the entire body. The functions of the foot include the following:

1. Acting as a support base that provides the necessary stability for upright posture with minimal muscle effort.
2. Providing a mechanism for rotation of the tibia and fibula during the stance phase of gait.
3. Providing flexibility to adapt to uneven terrain.
4. Providing flexibility for absorption of shock by becoming a rigid structure in the pronated position.
5. Acting as a lever during "push-off."

Although the joints of the lower leg, ankle, and foot are discussed separately, they act as functional groups, not as isolated joints. The movement occurring at each individual joint is minimal. However, when combined, there normally is sufficient range of motion in all of the joints to allow functional mobility as well as functional stability. For ease of understanding, the joints of the foot are divided into three sections—hindfoot, midfoot, and forefoot.

APPLIED ANATOMY

Hindfoot

Tibiofibular Joints. The inferior (distal) tibiofibular joint is a fibrous or syndesmosis type of joint. It is supported by the anterior tibiofibular, posterior tibiofibular, and inferior transverse ligaments as well as the interosseous ligament. The movements at this joint are minimal but allow a small amount of "spread" (1 to 2 mm) at the ankle joint during dorsiflexion. The joint is supplied by the deep peroneal and tibial nerves.

Talocrural Joint. The talocrural joint (ankle joint) is a uniaxial, modified hinge synovial joint located between the *talus*, the *medial malleolus* of the tibia, and the *lateral malleolus* of the fibula. The talus is shaped so that in dorsiflexion it is wedged between the malleoli, allowing little or no inversion or eversion at the ankle joint. The talus is approximately 2.4 mm wider anteriorly than posteriorly. The medial malleolus is shorter, extending halfway down the talus, whereas the lateral malleolus extends almost to the level of the talocalcanean joint.

The talocrural joint is designed for stability, not mobility. Its close packed position is maximum dorsiflexion, and its capsular pattern is more limitation of plantar flexion than dorsiflexion. This joint is strongest in the dorsiflexed position. The resting position is 10° of plantar flexion midway between maximum inversion and eversion.

On the medial side of the joint, the major ligament is the *deltoid*, or *medial collateral ligament*, which consists of four separate ligaments: (1) the *tibio-*

navicular, (2) *tibiocalcanean*, and (3) *posterior tibiotalar ligaments* superficially, which resist talar abduction, and (4) the *anterior tibiotalar ligament* deep, which resists lateral translation and lateral rotation of the talus.

On the lateral aspect, the talocrural joint is supported by (1) the *anterior talofibular ligament*, which provides stability against excessive inversion of the talus; (2) the *posterior talofibular ligament*, which resists ankle dorsiflexion, adduction ("tilt"), medial rotation, and medial translation of the talus; and (3) the *calcaneofibular ligament*, which provides stability against maximum inversion at the ankle and subtalar joints. The talocrural joint has one degree of freedom, and the movements possible at this joint are dorsiflexion and plantar flexion.

Subtalar (Talocalcanean) Joint. The subtalar joint is a synovial joint having three degrees of freedom and a close packed position of supination. Supporting the subtalar joint are the lateral talocalcanean and medial talocalcanean ligaments. In addition, the interosseous talocalcanean and cervical ligaments limit eversion.

The movements possible at the subtalar joint are gliding and rotation. In addition, medial rotation of the leg causes a valgus (outward) movement of the calcaneus, whereas lateral rotation of the leg produces a varus (inward) movement of the calcaneus. The axis of the joint is at an angle of 40 to 45° inclined vertically and 15 to 18° to the sagittal plane.

Midfoot (Midtarsal Joints)

Talocalcaneonavicular Joint. The talocalcaneonavicular joint is a "ball-and-socket" synovial joint with three degrees of freedom. Its close packed position is supination, and the dorsal talonavicular ligament, bifurcated ligament, and plantar calcaneonavicular (spring) ligament support the joint. Movements possible at this joint are gliding and rotation.

Cuneonavicular Joint. The cuneonavicular joint is a plane synovial joint with a close packed position of supination. The movements possible at this joint are slight gliding and rotation.

Cuboideonavicular Joint. The cuboideonavicular joint is fibrous, its close packed position being supination. The movements possible at this joint are slight gliding and rotation.

Intercuneiform Joints. The intercuneiform joints are plane synovial joints with a close packed position of supination. The movements possible at these joints are slight gliding and rotation.

Cuneocuboid Joint. The cuneocuboid joint is a plane synovial joint with a close packed position of supination. The movements of slight gliding and rotation are possible at this joint.

Calcaneocuboid Joint. The calcaneocuboid joint is saddle shaped with a close packed position of supination. Supporting this joint are the bifurcated ligament, the calcaneocuboid ligament, and the long plantar ligaments. The movement possible at this joint is gliding with conjunct rotation.

Forefoot

Tarsometatarsal Joints. The tarsometatarsal joints are plane synovial joints with a close packed position of supination. The movement possible at these joints is gliding.

Intermetatarsal Joints. The four intermetatarsal joints are plane synovial joints with a close packed position of supination. The movement possible at these joints is gliding.

Metatarsophalangeal Joints. The five metatarsophalangeal joints are condyloid synovial joints with two degrees of freedom. Their close packed position is full extension. Their capsular pattern is variable for the lateral four joints and more limitation of extension than flexion for the medial joint, and their resting position is 10° of extension. The movements possible at these joints are flexion, extension, abduction, and adduction.

Interphalangeal Joints. The interphalangeal joints are synovial hinge joints with one degree of freedom. The close packed position is full extension, and the capsular pattern is more limitation of extension than flexion. The resting position of the distal and proximal interphalangeal joints is slight flexion. The movements possible at these joints are flexion and extension.

PATIENT HISTORY

It is important to take a detailed and complete history when assessing the lower leg, ankle, and foot. The examiner should determine the following information:

1. What is the patient's usual activity or pastime? Answers to this question should give some idea of the stresses placed on the lower leg, ankle, and foot.

2. What is the patient's occupation? Whether the patient stands a great deal and the type of surfaces on which the patient usually stands may have bearings on what is causing the problem.

3. Is there any history of previous injury or affliction? For example, poliomyelitis may lead to a pes cavus. Systemic conditions such as diabetes, gout, psoriasis, and collagen diseases may manifest themselves first in the foot.

4. What types of shoes does the patient wear? What type of heel do the shoes have? Are the shoes in good condition? Does the patient make use of orthotics? If so, are they still functional? When an appointment is being made for an assessment, the patient should be told not to wear new shoes so the examiner can use the shoes to determine the individual's usual wear pattern. The examiner should also note whether the shoe offers proper support. Any orthotics should also be brought to the assessment.

5. Does walking on various terrains make a difference in regard to the foot problem? If so, which terrains cause the most obvious problem? For example, walking on grass (an uneven surface) may bother a person more than walking on a sidewalk (a relatively even surface).

6. Does activity make a difference? Pain after activity suggests overuse. Pain during the activity suggests stress on the injured structure.

7. What was the mechanism of injury? Ankle sprains occur most often when the foot is inverted, with injury to the anterior talofibular ligament.[1] Achilles tendinitis often arises as the result of overuse, increased activity, or change in a high-stress training program.

8. Are symptoms improving, becoming worse, or staying the same? It is important to know the type of onset and the duration and intensity of symptoms.

9. What are the sites and boundaries of pain or abnormal sensation? The examiner should note whether the pattern is one of a dermatome, a peripheral nerve, or another painful structure.

10. Did the patient notice a transient or fixed deformity of the foot or ankle at the time of injury? Was there any transitory locking (e.g., a loose body)?

11. Was the patient able to continue the activity after the injury? If so, the injury is probably not too severe, provided there is no loss of stability.

12. Was there any swelling or bruising (ecchymosis)? How quickly and where did it develop? This question can elicit some idea of the type of swelling (e.g., blood, synovial, or purulent) and whether it is intracapsular or extracapsular.

13. For active people, especially runners or joggers, the following questions should also be considered[2]:

a. How long has the patient been running or jogging?

b. On what type of terrain and surface does the patient train?

c. In what type of workouts does the patient participate? Have the workouts changed lately? How many workouts are done per week? How far does the patient run per week? (Joggers run approximately 2 to 30 km per week at a pace of 5 to 10 min/km, and sports runners run 30 to 65 km per week at a pace of 5 to 6 min/km. Long-distance runners run 60 to 180 km per week at a pace of 4 to 5 min/km. Elite runners run 100 to 270 km per week at a pace of 3.3 to 4 min/km.

d. What types of warm-up, stretching, and "warm-down" does the patient do? The answers will give the examiner some idea of whether the warm-up and stretching activities are static or ballistic and whether these activities might be detrimental.

e. What type and style of athletic shoes does the patient wear? (The patient should have the shoes at the examination.) Are they "control" or "cushioning" shoes? The examiner should be able to tell if the shoes fit properly.

f. Does the patient wear socks while training? If so, what kind (e.g., cotton, wool, nylon), and how many pairs?

g. When was the patient's last race? How long was it? When is the patient's next race? The answers will give the examiner some idea of how long the problem has been present and how long it will be until maximum stress is again placed on the joints.

OBSERVATION

When performing the observation, one should remember to compare the weight-bearing (closed-chain) with the non–weight-bearing (open-chain) posture of the foot. During open-chain motion, the talus is considered fixed; during closed-chain motion, the talus moves. Even though the calcaneus is touching a surface in closed-chain movement, for descriptive purposes, it is still considered to be moving. The weight-bearing stance of the foot shows how the body compensates for structural abnormalities (Fig. 12–1). The non–weight-bearing posture shows functional and structural abilities without compensation (Fig. 12–2). Thus, the observation includes looking at the patient from the front, from the side, and from behind in weight-bearing position and from the front, from the side, and from behind in the sitting position with the legs and feet not bearing weight. The examiner should note the patient's willingness and ability to use the feet. The bony and soft-tissue contours of the foot should be normal, and any deviation should be noted. Often, painful callosities may be found over abnormal bony prominences. Any scars or sinuses should also be noted.

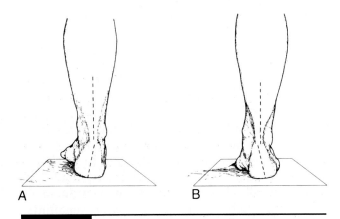

FIGURE 12–1. (A) Closed-chain (weight-bearing) supination of the subtalar joint. Supination of the subtalar joint in the weight-bearing foot results in motion of both the calcaneus and the talus. The calcaneus moves in the frontal plane, and the talus moves in the transverse and sagittal planes. The calcaneus inverts, whereas the talus simultaneously abducts and dorsiflexes relative to the calcaneus. The leg follows the motion of the talus in the transverse plane and externally rotates. The leg also follows the sagittal plane motion of the talus, to some degree. Therefore, the dorsiflexion motion of the talus on the calcaneus tends to impart a slight extension motion to the knee. (B) Closed-chain (weight-bearing) pronation of the subtalar joint. Pronation of the subtalar joint in the weight-bearing foot results in eversion of the calcaneus, and the talus adducts and plantar flexes relative to the calcaneus. The leg follows the talus in a transverse plane and internally rotates. In a sagittal plane, the leg also moves with the talus, to some extent. As the talus plantarflexes, the proximal aspect of the tibia moves forward to slightly flex the knee. (From Root, M. L., et al.: Normal and Abnormal Function of the Foot. Los Angeles, Clinical Biomechanics Corp., 1977, p. 30.)

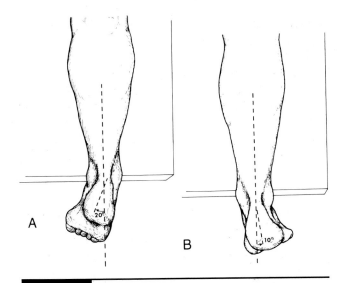

FIGURE 12–2. (A) Open-chain (non–weight-bearing) supination of the subtalar joint. When the non–weight-bearing foot is moved at the subtalar joint in the direction of supination, the talus is stable, and the calcaneus and foot move around the talus. The calcaneus and foot invert, plantarflex, and adduct. These positional changes, associated with subtalar joint supination, are readily visible compared with the pronated position of the subtalar joint. (B) Open-chain (non–weight-bearing) pronation of the subtalar joint. When the subtalar joint is moved into a pronated position in the non–weight-bearing foot, the foot abducts, everts, and dorsiflexes around the stable talus. The positional variances can best be appreciated by comparing this illustration with the supinated position of the subtalar joint. (From Root, M. L., et al.: Normal and Abnormal Function of the Foot. Los Angeles, Clinical Biomechanics Corp., 1977, p. 29.)

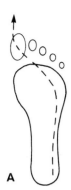 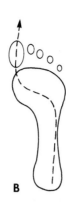

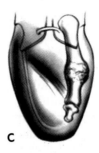

FIGURE 12–7. Weight-bearing patterns in hallux rigidus. (A) Hallux rigidus gait pattern. (B) Normal gait pattern. (C) Shoe develops oblique creases with hallux rigidus. (C is from Jahss, M. H.: Disorders of the Foot. Philadelphia, W. B. Saunders Co., 1991, p. 60.)

weight distribution pattern in gait is shown in Figure 12–7.

The second (chronic) type of hallux rigidus is much more common and is seen primarily in adults—again, in men more frequently than in women. It is frequently bilateral and is usually the result of repeated minor trauma resulting in osteoarthritic changes to the metatarsophalangeal joint of the big toe. The toe stiffens gradually, and the pain, once established, persists. The patient primarily complains of pain at the base of the big toe on walking.

Hallux rigidus may also be due to an anatomic abnormality of the foot, an abnormally long first metatarsal bone (index plus type forefoot), pronation of the forefoot, or trauma.

Hammer Toes

A hammer-toe deformity consists of an extension contracture at the metatarsophalangeal joint and flexion contracture at the proximal interphalangeal joint; the distal interphalangeal joint may be flexed, straight, or hyperextended (see Fig. 12–5A). The interosseus muscles are unable to hold the proximal phalanx in the neutral position, thus losing their flexion effect; this results in the long flexors and extensors clawing the toe, leading to and accentuating the deformity. The causes of hammer toe include an imbalance of the synergic muscles, hereditary factors, or mechanical factors such as poorly fitting shoes or hallux valgus. It is usually seen only in one toe—the second toe. Often, there is a callus or corn over the dorsum of the flexed joint. The condition is often asymptomatic, especially if the hammer toe is flexible or semiflexible. The rigid type of hammer toe is likely to cause the greatest problems.

Mallet Toe

Mallet toe is associated with a flexion deformity of the distal interphalangeal joint (see Fig. 12–5B). It can occur on any of the four lateral toes. Often, a corn or callus is present over the dorsum of the affected joint. The condition is usually asymptomatic.

Hallux Valgus

Medial deviation of the head of the first metatarsal bone occurs in relation to the center of the body, and lateral deviation of the head occurs in relation to the center of the foot (Fig. 12–8). As the metatarsal bone moves medially, the base of the proximal phalanx is carried with it, and the phalanx pivots around the adductor hallucis muscle that inserts into it, causing the distal end as well as the distal phalanx to deviate laterally. The long flexor and extensor muscles then have a "bowstring" effect as they are displaced to the lateral side of the joint.

A callus develops over the medial side of the head of the metatarsal bone, and the bursa becomes thickened and inflamed; excessive bone (exostosis) forms, resulting in a *bunion* (Fig. 12–9). These three changes—callus, thickened bursa, and exostosis—make up the bunion, a condition separate from hallux valgus, although it is the result of hallux valgus.

In normal individuals, the metatarsophalangeal angle (angle between the longitudinal axis of the metatarsal bone and the proximal phalanx) is 8 to 20° (Fig. 12–10). This angle is increased in hallux valgus, depending on the type of hallux valgus present.

The first type (*congruous*) is a simple exaggeration of the normal foot. The deformity does not progress, and the valgus deformity is between 20 and 30°. The opposing joint surfaces are congruent.

The second type (*pathological*) is a potentially progressive deformity, increasing from 20 to 60°. The joint surfaces are no longer congruent, and some may even go to subluxation. This type may occur in *deviated* (early) and *subluxed* (later) stages.

When looking at the foot, the examiner may find that there is a widening gap between the first and second metatarsal bones (increased intermetatarsal

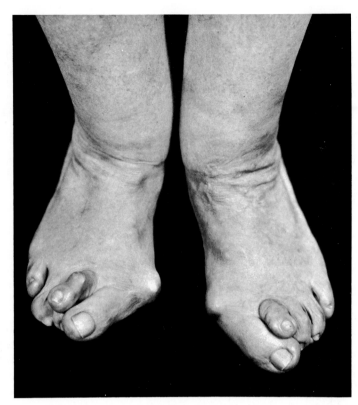

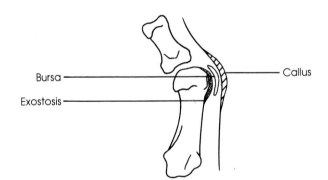

FIGURE 12–8. Hallux valgus with bilateral bunions and overlapped toes. Note how the deviating big toe (hallux) rotates and pushes under the second toe. (From Gartland, J. J.: Fundamentals of Orthopedics. Philadelphia, W. B. Saunders Co., 1987, p. 401.)

Bursa

Exostosis

Callus

FIGURE 12–9. Bunion.

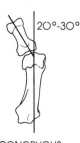
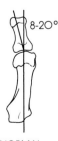
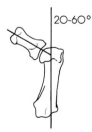

NORMAL

CONGRUOUS

PATHOLOGIC

FIGURE 12–10. Metatarsophalangeal angle.

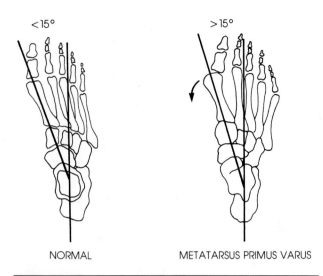

FIGURE 12–11. *Normal foot and metatarsus primus varus. (Note increased intermetatarsal angle.)*

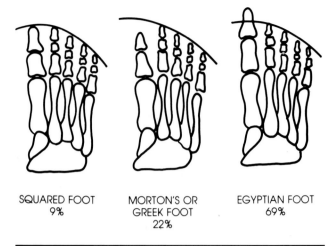

FIGURE 12–12. *Types of feet seen in the general population. (Modified from Viladot: Patologia del Antepié. Barcelona, Ediciones Toray, S. A., 1975.)*

angle) and a lateral deflection of the phalanx at the metatarsophalangeal joint. The joint capsule lengthens on the medial aspect and is contracted on the lateral aspect. The toes rotate on a long axis so that the toenail faces medially because of the pull of the adductor hallucis muscle. Sometimes, the big toe will deviate so far that it lies over or under the second toe.

The etiology of hallux valgus is varied. It may be due to a hereditary factor and is often familial. Women tend to be affected more than men. Trying to keep up with fashion may be a contributing factor if the person wears tight or pointed shoes or tight stockings. Of all hallux valgus cases, 80 per cent are caused by *metatarsus primus varus*, in which the intermetatarsal or metatarsal angle is increased to more than 15° (Fig. 12–11).[7, 8] Metatarsus primus varus is an abduction deformity of the first metatarsal bone in relation to the other metatarsal bones so that the medial border of the forefoot is curved. Normally, this angle is between 0° and 15°.

Morton's (Atavistic or Grecian) Foot

In Morton's foot, the second toe is longer than the first. Increased stress is put on this longer toe, and the big toe tends to be hypomobile. There is often hypertrophy of the second metatarsal bone because there is more stress put through the second toe. The different types of feet and their proportional representations in the population are shown in Figure 12–12.

Morton's Metatarsalgia (Interdigital Neuroma)

In Morton's neuroma, a digital nerve is affected, usually the one between the third and fourth toes

(Fig. 12–13). While walking, the patient is suddenly seized with an agonizing pain on the outer border of the forefoot. The pain is often intermittent, like a cramp, shooting up the side of and to the tip of the toe or the adjacent two toes. If the metatarsal bones are squeezed together, pain will be elicited because

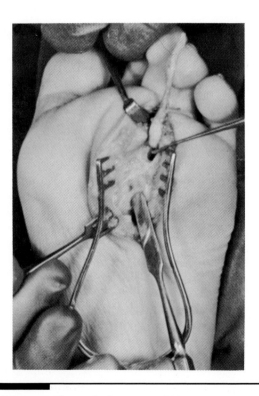

FIGURE 12–13. *The applied anatomy of Morton's metatarsalgia. The interdigital nerve to the 3–4 space has been divided 2 cm above the "neuroma" and is reflected downward. The plantar digital vessels are seen entering the neuroma. The end of the flat dissector is on the upper margin of the transverse ligament. The end of the probe points to the intermetatarsophalangeal bursa. (From Klenerman, L.: The Foot and Its Disorders. Boston, Blackwell Scientific Publications, 1982, p. 143.)*

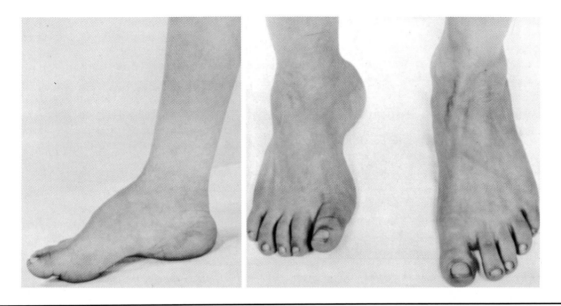

FIGURE 12-14. Pes cavus ("hollow foot"). Note the high medial longitudinal arch, early clawing of the big toe, and the heel in varus. (From Klenerman, L.: The Foot and Its Disorders. Boston, Blackwell Scientific Publications, 1982, p. 72.)

of the pressure on the digital nerve. The condition tends to be more frequent in women than in men.

Pes Cavus ("Hollow Foot" or Rigid Foot)

A pes cavus may be due to a congenital problem; a neurogenic problem such as spina bifida, poliomyelitis, or Charcot-Marie-Tooth disease; talipes equinovarus; or muscle imbalance. There may also be a genetic factor, because it tends to run in families.

The longitudinal arches are accentuated (Fig. 12-14), and the metatarsal heads are lower in relation to the hindfoot so there is a "dropping" of the forefoot. The soft tissues of the sole are abnormally short, which gives the foot a shortened appearance. If the deformity persists, the bones will eventually alter their shape, perpetuating the deformity. The heel is normal, at least initially. Claw toes are often associated with the condition. The examiner will often find painful callosities beneath the metatarsal heads and tenderness along the deformed toes. There is pain in the tarsal region after a period of time because of osteoarthritic changes in these joints.

The longitudinal arches are high, both on the medial and lateral aspects, and the forefoot is thickened and splayed (spread out) (Table 12-1). The metatarsal heads are prominent on the sole of the foot, and the toes do not touch the ground, even on active or passive movement. Individuals with pes cavus have difficulty tolerating prolonged activities, such as long-distance running and ballet.

Pes Planus (Flatfoot or Mobile Foot)

Flatfoot may be congenital or the result of muscle weakness, ligament laxity or "dropping" of the talar head, paralysis, or a pronated foot. Pes planus may also be due to trauma. For example, a traumatic case of flatfoot may follow the fracture of the calcaneus. It may also result from a postural deformity, such as medial rotation of the hips or medial tibial torsion.

TABLE 12-1. Pes Cavus Classification

Classification	Features
1. Mild	Longitudinal arch appears high N.W.B. Longitudinal arch almost normal W.B. Toes clawed N.W.B. Toes may be normal W.B. May have hindfoot varus
2. Moderate	Longitudinal arch high N.W.B. and W.B. Claw toes evident N.W.B. and W.B. Calluses under prominent metatarsal heads Dorsiflexion may be limited Forefoot plantar flexed on hindfoot
3. Severe	Calcaneus cannot pronate past 5° varus Heel in varus, foot in valgus Decreased R.O.M. in foot

N.W.B. = non–weight bearing; W.B. = weight bearing; R.O.M. = range of motion.

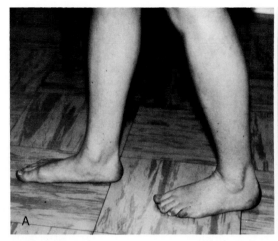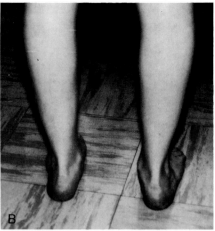

FIGURE 12–15. *Pes planus (flatfoot).* (A) *Side view.* (B) *Posterior view. Note how the foot is pronated.*

It must be remembered that all infants have flat feet initially up to approximately 2 years of age. This appearance is in part due to the fat pad in the longitudinal arch and in part due to the incomplete formation of the arches.

The medial longitudinal arch is reduced so that on standing its borders are close to or in contact with the ground. If the condition persists into adulthood, it becomes a permanent structural deformity, leading to a defect or alteration of the tarsal bones as well as of the talonavicular joints.

There are two types of flatfoot. The first type (*rigid* or *congenital*) is relatively rare. The calcaneus is found in a valgus position, whereas the midtarsal region is in pronation. The talus faces medially and downward, and the navicula is displaced dorsally and laterally on the talus. There are accompanying soft-tissue contractures. The second type is *acquired* or *flexible* (Fig. 12–15). In this case, the deformity is similar to the rigid flatfoot, but the foot is mobile (Table 12–2). It is usually due to hereditary factors and is sometimes called a *hypermobile flatfoot.* Flexible flatfoot may be due to tibial or femoral torsion, coxa vara, or a defect in the subtalar joint. If the patient is asked to stand on tiptoes and the arch appears, it is an indication that the patient has a mobile flatfoot.

TABLE 12–2. Pes Planus Classification

Classification	Features
1. Mild	4 to 6° hindfoot valgus 4 to 6° forefoot varus
2. Moderate	6 to 10° hindfoot valgus 6 to 10° forefoot varus Poor shock absorption at heel strike
3. Severe	10 to 15° hindfoot valgus 8 to 10° forefoot varus Equinus deformity may be present

"Rocker Bottom" Foot

In the rocker bottom foot deformity, the forefoot is dorsiflexed on the hindfoot; this results in a "broken midfoot," so the medial and longitudinal arches are absent.

Standing—Weight Bearing (Anterior View)

Figure 12–16 shows the anterosuperior view of the feet in the weight-bearing stance. Is there any supination or pronation of the foot? *Supination* of the foot involves inversion of the heel, adduction of the forefoot, and plantar flexion at the subtalar joint and midtarsal joints (Fig. 12–17A). In addition, there is lateral rotation of the leg relative to the foot. Supi-

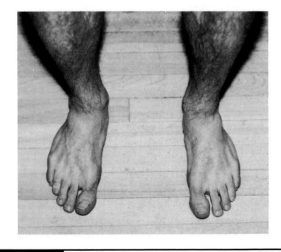

FIGURE 12–16. *Anterosuperior view of the feet (weight-bearing position).*

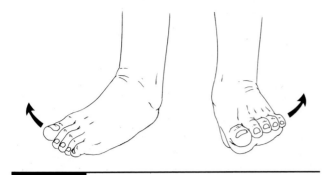

FIGURE 12–17. *Supination (A) and pronation (B) of the foot.*

nation of the foot causes the proximal aspect of the tibia to move posteriorly. Supination is required during propulsion to give rigidity to the foot and requires less muscle work than pronation.

Pronation of the foot involves eversion of the heel, abduction of the forefoot, medial rotation of the leg relative to the foot, and dorsiflexion of the subtalar and midtarsal joints (Fig. 12–17B). This movement causes the proximal aspect of the tibia to move anteriorly. The pronated foot has greater subtalar motion than the supinated foot and requires more muscle work to maintain stance stability than the supinated foot. The foot is much more mobile in this position.

The definitions used in this chapter are the ones preferred by orthopedists and podiatrists. For example, anatomists and kinesiologists such as Kapandji[9] refer to *inversion* as a combination of adduction and supination and to *eversion* as a combination of abduction and pronation. Lipscomb and Ibrahim[10] as well as Williams and Warwick[11] define *supination* and *pronation* as opposite the terms just mentioned. Because of the confusion in terminology concerning the terms supination and pronation, readers of books and articles on the foot must be careful to discern exactly what each author means.

In the infant, the foot is pronated. As the child matures, the foot begins to supinate, accompanied by development of the medial longitudinal arch. The foot also appears more pronated in the infant because of the fat pad in the medial longitudinal arch.

How does the patient stand or walk? Normally, in standing, 50 to 60 per cent of the weight is taken on the heel and 40 to 50 per cent is taken by the metatarsal heads. The foot forms an angle (the Fick angle), which is approximately 12 to 18° from the sagittal axis of the body, developing from 5° in children (Fig. 12–18).[12] During movement, the foot is subjected to high loading, and pathology may cause the gait to be altered. The accumulative force to which each foot is subjected during the day is the equivalent of 639 metric tons in a person who weighs approximately 90 kg and is estimated as

walking 13 km per day. In walking, the foot is subjected to weight that is 1.2 times that of the body; in running, the weight is 2 times body weight; and in jumping from a height of 60 cm, the weight is 5 times body weight.

In normal weight bearing, if the relation of the foot to the ankle is normal, all of the metatarsal bones bear weight, and all of the metatarsal heads lie in the same transverse plane. The forefoot and hindfoot should be parallel to each other and the floor. The midtarsal joints are in maximum pronation, and the subtalar joint is in neutral position. The subtalar and talocrural joints should be parallel to the floor. Finally, the posterior bisection of the calcaneus and distal one third of the leg should form two vertical, parallel lines.[13]

The patient should be asked to walk on the toes, heels, and outer and inner borders of the feet. This action gives an indication of the patient's muscle power and functional range of motion. With a third-degree strain of the Achilles tendon, the patient will not be able to walk on the toes. Lack of dorsiflexion, or at least the anatomic position, will make it difficult for the individual to walk on the heels. When the patient walks on the inner or outer border of the

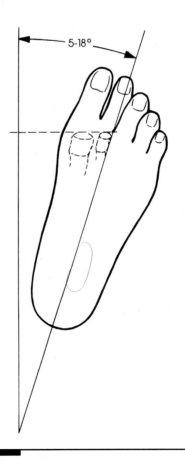

FIGURE 12–18. *Fick angle. (From Viladot: Patologia del Antepié. Barcelona, Ediciones Toray, S. A., 1975.)*

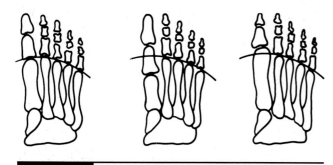

FIGURE 12–19. Metatarsal classifications. (From Viladot: Patologia del Antepié. Barcelona, Ediciones Toray, S. A., 1975.)

appear in three ways,[14] based on the length of the metatarsal bones (Fig. 12–19):

1. *Index plus type.* The first metatarsal (1) is longer than the second (2), with the others (3, 4, and 5) of progressively decreasing lengths so that 1 > 2 > 3 > 4 > 5.

2. *Index plus-minus type.* The first metatarsal is equal in length to the second metatarsal, with the others progressively diminishing in length so that 1 = 2 > 3 > 4 > 5.

3. *Index minus type.* The second metatarsal is longer than the first and third metatarsals. The fourth and fifth metatarsals are progressively shorter than the third so that 1 < 2 > 3 > 4 > 5. Figure 12–19 illustrates this concept and shows the proportional representation of each in the population.

Do the toenails appear normal? The examiner should look for warts, calluses, and corns. Warts are especially tender to the pinch (but not to direct pressure), but calluses are not. Plantar warts also tend to separate from the surrounding tissues, but calluses do not.

Is there any swelling or pitting edema within the ankle (Fig. 12–20)? If there is any swelling, is it intracapsular or extracapsular? The examiner should also check the patient's gait for the position of the foot at heel strike, at foot flat, and at "toe-off" positions. The gait cycle is described in greater detail in Chapter 14.

One should also look at the tibia to note any local or general bone swelling (Fig. 12–21). Does the tibia have a normal shape, or is it bowed? Is there any torsional deformity? The medial malleolus usually lies anterior to the lateral malleolus. "Pigeon toes" are the result of a medial tibial torsion deformity;

feet, pain and difficulty will be experienced in the presence of a subtalar lesion.

Does the patient use a cane or other walking aid? Using a cane in the opposite hand diminishes the stress on the ankle joint and foot by approximately one third.

One should also check the efficiency of the toes. Are the toes straight and parallel? Is the patient able to flex, extend, adduct, and abduct the toes? The toes have a primarily ambulatory function, although with training, they can develop a prehensile function. The toes extend the weight-bearing area forward and, by so doing, reduce the load on the metatarsal heads. The great toe also has a primary function of "pushing off" during gait.

Are there any prominent bumps or exostoses? Is there any splaying (widening) of the forefoot? Splaying of the forefoot and metatarsus primus varus are more evident in weight bearing. The forefoot can

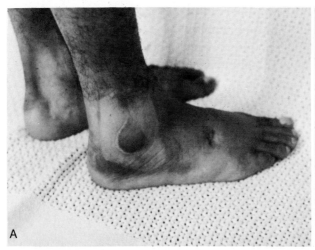
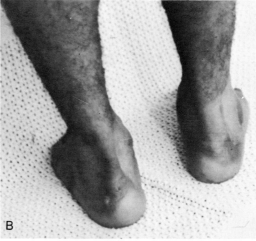

FIGURE 12–20. Ankle sprain. (A) Note pattern of pitting edema on top of the right foot. (B) The swelling is intracapsular, as indicated by swelling on both sides of the right Achilles tendon.

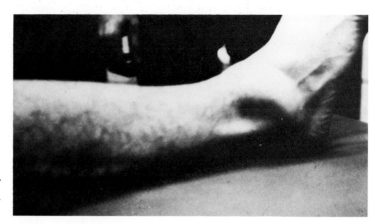

FIGURE 12-21. Swelling within the talocrural and subtalar joint capsule.

they do not constitute a foot deformity (Table 12–3).

With the patient in a standing position, the examiner should observe whether the patient's hips and trunk are in normal position. Excessive lateral rotation of the hip or rotation of the trunk away from the opposite hip elevates the medial longitudinal arch of the foot, whereas medial rotation of the hip or trunk rotation toward the opposite hip tends to flatten the arch (Fig. 12–22). Medial rotation of the hip can also cause pigeon toes. If the iliotibial band is tight, the tightness may cause eversion and lateral rotation of the foot.

Any vasomotor changes should be recorded, including loss of hair on the foot, toenail changes, osteoporosis as seen on radiographs, and possible differences in temperature between the limbs. Sys-

temic diseases such as diabetes can also lead to foot problems as a result of altered sensation, thus facilitating easier injury.

The examiner should look for any circulatory impairment or presence of varicose veins. Brick-red color or cyanosis when the limb is dependent is an indication of impairment. Does this condition change to rapid blanching, or does it stay normal on elevation of the limbs?

Standing—Weight Bearing (Posterior View)

From behind, the examiner compares the bulk of the calf muscles and notes any differences. Variation may be due to peripheral nerve lesions, nerve root problems, or atrophy caused by disuse after injury. The Achilles tendons on each side should be compared. If a tendon appears to curve out (Fig. 12–23), it may be caused by a fallen medial longitudinal arch, resulting in a pes planus (flatfoot condition).

The examiner notes the calcaneus for normality of shape and position. Runners often build up bone and a callus on the heel, resulting in a pump bump as a result of pressure on the heel (Fig. 12–24).

The malleoli are compared for positioning. Normally, the lateral malleolus extends further distally than the medial malleolus; however, the medial malleolus extends further anteriorly.

Standing—Weight Bearing (Lateral View)

With the side view, the examiner is primarily observing the longitudinal arches of the foot (Fig. 12–25). The examiner should note whether the medial arch is higher than the lateral arch (as would be expected). One can often determine any differences in the arches by looking at the footprint patterns (Fig. 12–26). The footprint pattern can be estab-

TABLE 12–3. Etiology of Toeing-In and Toeing-Out in Children*

Level of Affection	Toe-In	Toe-Out
Feet-ankles	Pronated feet (protective toeing-in) Metatarsus varus Talipes varus and equinovarus	Pes valgus due to contracture of triceps surae muscle Talipes calcaneovalgus Congenital convex pes planovalgus
Leg-knee	Tibia vara (Blount's disease) and developmental genu varum Abnormal internal tibial torsion Genu valgum—developmental (protective toeing-in to shift body center of gravity medially)	External tibial torsion Congenital absence of hypoplasia of the fibula
Femur-hip	Abnormal femoral antetorsion Spasticity of internal rotators of hip (cerebral palsy)	Abnormal femoral retroversion Flaccid paralysis of internal rotators of hip
Acetabulum	Maldirected—facing anteriorly	Maldirected—facing posteriorly

*From Tachdjian, M. O.: Pediatric Orthopedics. Philadelphia, W. B. Saunders Co., 1990, p. 2817.

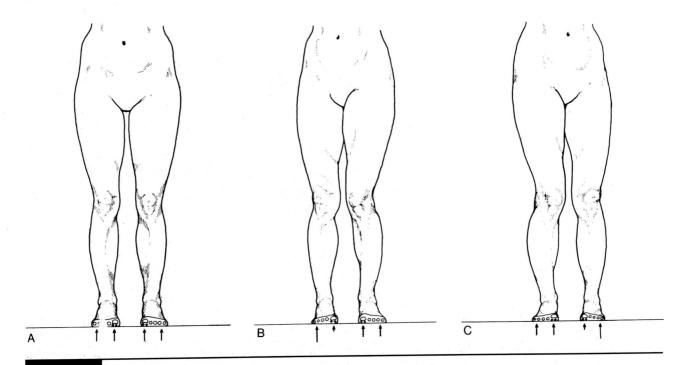

FIGURE 12–22. (A) During static stance, ground reaction forces (arrows) directed upward against the plantar aspect of both feet maintain the transverse plane equilibrium and stability of the lower extremities and pelvis. Equal ground reaction forces are exerted on the lateral and medial plantar surfaces of both feet. (B) When the trunk is rotated to the right, the right foot supinates and the left pronates. The right forefoot inverts from the ground, and vertical ground reaction forces are greater against the lateral side of the forefoot (large arrow) and less against the medial side of the forefoot (small arrow). The left forefoot remains flat on the ground, and vertical ground reaction forces are distributed evenly against the forefoot (equal arrows). (C) When the trunk is rotated to the left, ground reaction exerts unequal forces against the left forefoot and even forces against the right forefoot. (From Root, M. L., et al.: Normal and Abnormal Function of the Foot. Los Angeles, Clinical Biomechanics Corp., 1977, p. 102.)

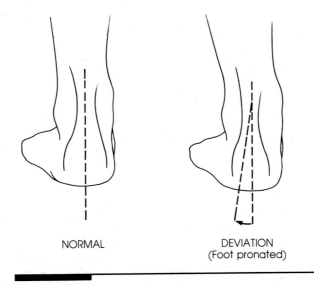

NORMAL   DEVIATION
                        (Foot pronated)

FIGURE 12–23. Normal and deviated Achilles tendons. The deviation is often seen with pes planus (flatfoot) and when the medial longitudinal arch is lower or has "dropped."

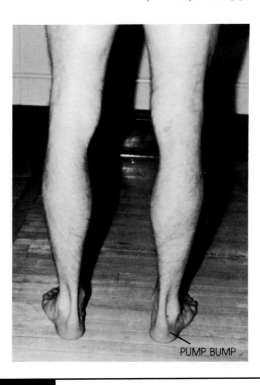

FIGURE 12–24. *Posterior view of the leg and foot. Note "pump bumps."*

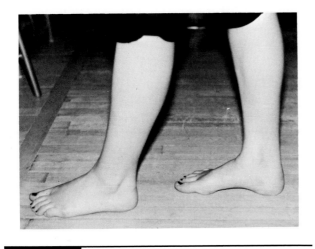

FIGURE 12–25. *Lateral and medial views of the feet showing longitudinal arches.*

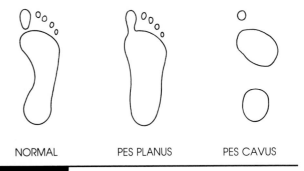

FIGURE 12–26. *Footprint patterns.*

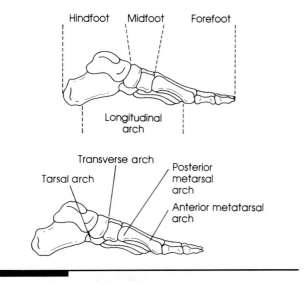

FIGURE 12–27. *Divisions and arches of the foot (medial view).*

lished by putting a light film of baby oil and then powder on the patient's foot and asking the patient to step down on a piece of colored paper. The footprint pattern will then become evident.

The arches of the feet (Fig. 12–27) are maintained by three mechanisms[15]: (1) wedging of the interlocking tarsal and metatarsal bones takes place; (2) the ligaments on the plantar aspect of the foot play a significant role; and (3) the intrinsic and extrinsic muscles of the foot and their tendons help to support the arches. The longitudinal arches form a cone as a result of the angle formed by the metatarsal bones with the floor. With the medial longitudinal arch being more evident, this angle is greater on the medial side. The angle formed by each of the metatarsals with the floor is shown in Figure 12–28.

The *medial longitudinal arch* consists of the calcaneal tuberosity, the talus, the navicular bone, three cuneiforms, and the first, second, and third metatarsal bones (Fig. 12–29). This arch is maintained by the tibialis anterior, tibialis posterior, flexor digitorum longus, flexor hallucis longus, abductor hallucis, and flexor digitorum brevis muscles; the plantar fascia; and the plantar calcaneonavicular ligament (Fig. 12–30).

The calcaneus, cuboid, and fourth and fifth metatarsal bones make up the *lateral longitudinal arch* (Fig. 12–31). This arch is more stable and less adjustable than the medial longitudinal arch. The arch is maintained by the peroneus longus, peroneus brevis, peroneus tertius, abductor digiti minimi, and flexor digitorum brevis muscles; the plantar fascia; the long plantar ligament; and the short plantar ligament.[15]

The *transverse arch* is maintained by the tibialis posterior, tibialis anterior, and peroneus longus muscles and the plantar fascia (Fig. 12–32). This arch consists of the navicular bone, cuneiforms, and cuboid and metatarsal bones. The arch is sometimes divided into three parts: tarsal, posterior metatarsal, and anterior metatarsal. A loss of the anterior metatarsal arch results in callus formation under the heads of the metatarsal bones. The examiner will also note that the metatarsophalangeal joints are slightly extended when the patient is in the normal standing position because the longitudinal arches of the foot curve down toward the toes.[15]

Non–Weight Bearing

With the patient not weight bearing and in a supine position, the examiner should look for abnormal callosities, plantar warts, scars, sinuses, and so forth on the sole of the foot. In addition, by looking at the foot from above (i.e., toes to heel as shown in Fig.

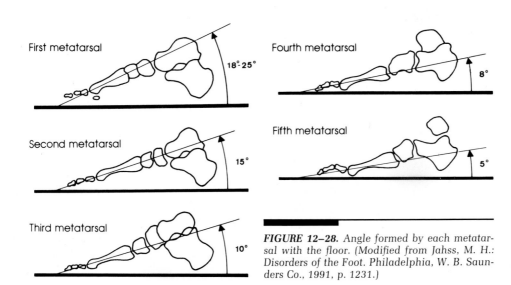

FIGURE 12–28. *Angle formed by each metatarsal with the floor. (Modified from Jahss, M. H.: Disorders of the Foot. Philadelphia, W. B. Saunders Co., 1991, p. 1231.)*

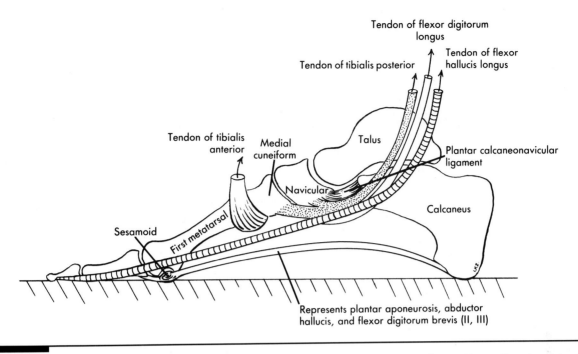

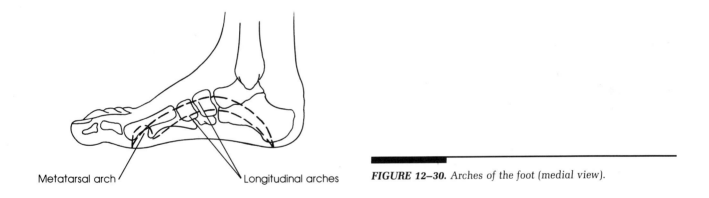

FIGURE 12–29. Supports of the medial longitudinal arch of the foot. (From Hamilton, J. J., and L. K. Ziemer: Functional Anatomy of the Human Ankle and Foot. AAOS Symposium on the Foot and Ankle. St. Louis, C. V. Mosby, 1983, p. 12.)

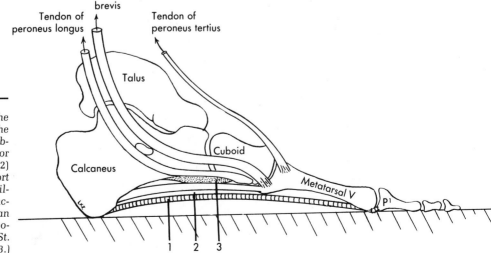

FIGURE 12–30. Arches of the foot (medial view).

FIGURE 12–31. Supports of the lateral longitudinal arch of the foot. (1) Plantar aponeurosis, abductor digiti minimi, and flexor digitorum brevis IV and V. (2) Long plantar ligament. (3) Short plantar ligament. (From Hamilton, J. J., and L. K. Ziemer: Functional Anatomy of the Human Ankle and Foot. AAOS Symposium on the Foot and Ankle. St. Louis, C. V. Mosby, 1983, p. 13.)

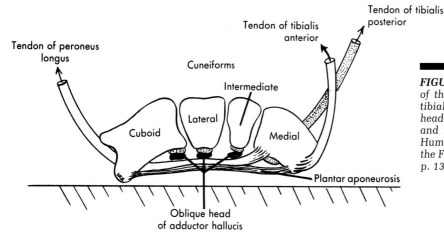

FIGURE 12–32. Supports of the transverse arch of the foot. Stippled tube represents tendon of tibialis posterior; black areas represent oblique head of adductor hallucis. (From Hamilton, J. J., and L. K. Ziemer: Functional Anatomy of the Human Ankle and Foot. AAOS Symposium on the Foot and Ankle. St. Louis, C. V. Mosby, 1983, p. 13.)

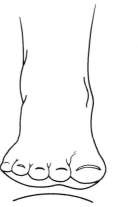

NORMAL   FALLEN ARCH

FIGURE 12–33. Fallen metatarsal arch.

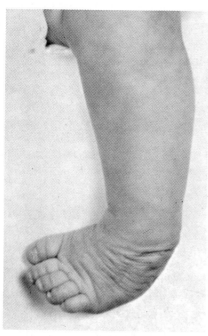
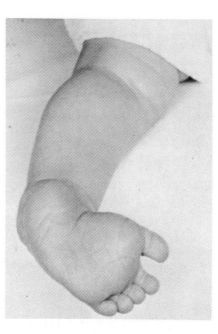

A   B

FIGURE 12–34. Talipes equinovarus (clubfoot) in a child aged 4 months. (A) Anterior view. (B) Posterior view. (From Klenerman, L.: The Foot and Its Disorders. Boston, Blackwell Scientific Publications, 1982, p. 64.)

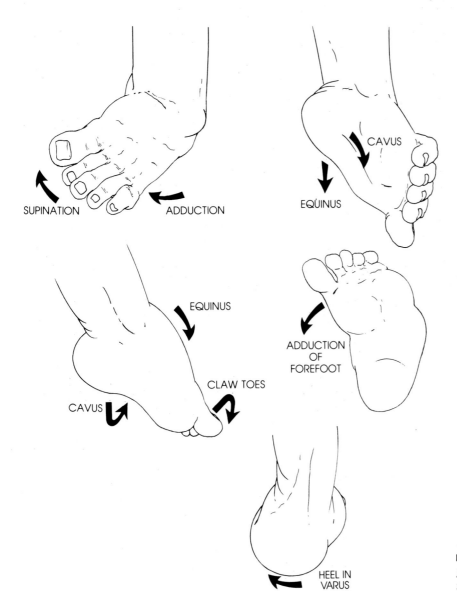

FIGURE 12–35. Components of talipes equinovarus.

12–33), the examiner can note whether the patient has a "fallen" metatarsal arch. Normally, in the non–weight-bearing position, the arch can be seen. If it falls, callosities will often be found over the metatarsal heads. The arch may be reversed or it may fall because of an equinus forefoot, pes cavus, rheumatoid arthritis, short heel cord, or hammer toes.

Young children should be assessed for clubfoot deformities, the most common of which is *talipes equinovarus* (Figs. 12–34 and 12–35). These types

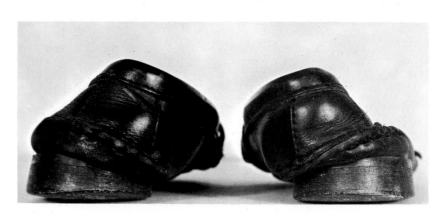

FIGURE 12–36. *Misshapen shoes caused by severely pronated feet. (From Gartland, J. J.: Fundamentals of Orthopedics. Philadelphia, W. B. Saunders Co., 1987, p. 398.)*

of deformities are often associated with other anomalies, such as spina bifida.

Shoes

The examiner looks at the patient's shoes from the inside and the outside for weight-bearing and wear patterns (Figs. 12–36 and 12–37). With the normal foot, the greatest wear on the shoe is beneath the ball of the foot and slightly to the lateral side. If shoes are too small or too narrow, they may pinch the feet, causing deformities and affecting normal growth. If shoes are worn out, they offer little support. If shoes are stiff, they limit proper movement of the foot.

Platform-type shoes often cause painful knees because when wearing these shoes, the patient usually walks with the knees flexed, which may increase the stress on the patella. In addition, these shoes increase the potential for ankle sprains and fractures because a raised center of gravity puts one off balance.

High heels and pointed shoes often contribute to hallux valgus, bunions, march fractures, and Morton's metatarsalgia as a result of the toes' being pushed together. Continuous wearing of high-heeled shoes may also lead to contracture of the calf muscles as well as sore knees and a painful back because the lumbar spine goes into increased lordotic posture to maintain the center of gravity in its normal position.

Shoes with a negative heel (i.e., "earth" shoes) may lead to hyperextension of the knees and chondromalacia patellae. High-cut shoes that cover the medial and lateral malleoli offer more support than low-cut shoes or those that do not cover the malleoli.

Excessive bulging on the medial side of the shoe suggests a valgus or everted foot, whereas excessive bulging on the lateral side suggests an inverted foot. Drop foot resulting from musculature weakness

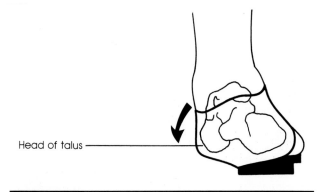

Head of talus ⸻

FIGURE 12–37. *Pes planus (flatfoot) or calcaneus in valgus can lead to misshapen shoes. Note the prominence of the talar head.*

scuffs the toe of the shoe. Oblique forefoot creases in the shoe indicate possible hallux rigidus; absence of forefoot creases indicates no toe-off action during gait.

EXAMINATION

As with any assessment, the examiner must compare one side with the other and note any differences. This comparison is necessary because of the individual differences among normal people.

Active Movements

The first movements are active; painful movements should be done last. In addition, the movements should be done in both non–weight-bearing (long leg sitting or supine lying) and weight-bearing positions, and any differences should be noted. The movements that should be carried out actively in the lower leg, ankle, and foot region are as follows:

Weight Bearing. (Figs. 12–38 and 12–39)

1. Plantar flexion (flexion) (standing on the toes).
2. Dorsiflexion (extension) (standing on the heels).
3. Supination (standing on the lateral edge of the foot).
4. Pronation (standing on the medial edge of the foot).
5. Toe extension.
6. Toe flexion.

Non–Weight Bearing. (Fig. 12–40)

1. Plantar flexion (flexion) (50°).
2. Dorsiflexion (extension) (20°).
3. Supination (45 to 60°).
4. Pronation (15 to 30°).
5. Toe extension (lateral four toes: MTP:40°; PIP: 0°; DIP: 30°/great toe; MTP: 70°; IP: 0°).
6. Toe flexion (lateral four toes. MTP: 40°; PIP: 35°; DIP: 60°/great toe: MTP: 45°; IP: 90°).
7. Toe abduction.
8. Toe adduction.

Plantar Flexion

Plantar flexion of the ankle is approximately 50° (see Fig. 12–40A), and it should be noted that the patient's heel will normally invert when the movement is performed when in weight-bearing position (Fig. 12–41). If heel inversion does not occur, the foot will be unstable.

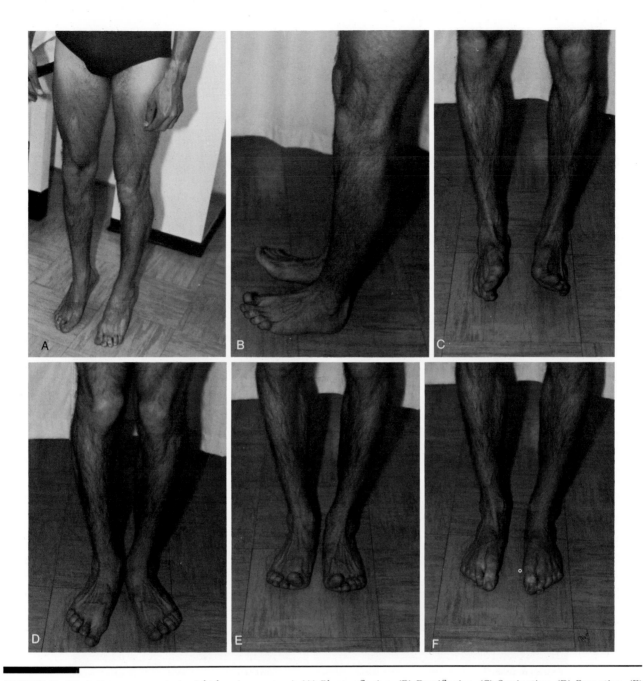

FIGURE 12–38. *Active movements (weight-bearing posture). (A) Plantar flexion. (B) Dorsiflexion. (C) Supination. (D) Pronation. (E) Toe extension. (F) Toe flexion.*

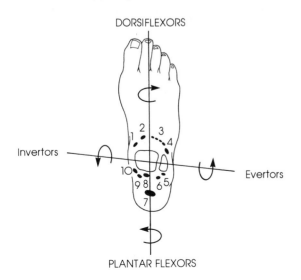

FIGURE 12–39. *Motion diagram of the ankle. (1) Tibialis anterior. (2) Extensor hallucis longus. (3) Extensor digitorum longus. (4) Peroneus tertius. (5) Peroneus brevis. (6) Peroneus longus. (7) Achilles tendon (soleus and gastrocnemius). (8) Flexor hallucis longus. (9) Flexor digitorum longus. (10) Tibialis posterior.*

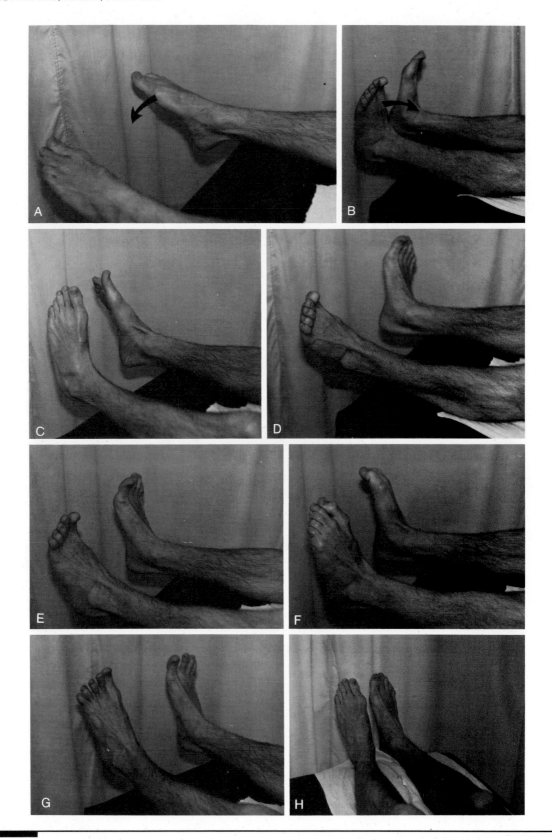

FIGURE 12–40. *Active movements (non–weight-bearing posture).* (A) *Plantar flexion.* (B) *Dorsiflexion.* (C) *Supination.* (D) *Pronation.* (E) *Toe extension.* (F) *Toe flexion.* (G) *Toe abduction.* (H) *Toe adduction.*

Dorsiflexion

Dorsiflexion of the ankle is usually 20° past the anatomic position (foot at 90° to bones of the leg) (see Fig. 12–40*B*). For normal locomotion, 10° of dorsiflexion and 20 to 25° of plantar flexion at the ankle are required. In a baby or young child, there will be greater mobility and flexibility than in an adult. For example, in the newborn, the foot can be readily dorsiflexed so that the toes and dorsum of the foot touch the skin over the tibia.

Supination and Pronation

Supination is 45 to 60° and pronation is 15 to 30°, although there is variability among individuals (see Fig. 12–40*C* and *D*). It is more important to compare the movement with that of the patient's normal side (Figs. 12–42 and 12–43). Supination combines the movements of inversion, adduction, and plantar flexion; pronation combines the movements of eversion, abduction, and dorsiflexion of the foot and ankle. As the patient does the movement, the examiner should watch for the possibility of subluxation of various tendons. The peroneal tendons are especially prone to subluxation, and their subluxation will be evident on eversion (Fig. 12–44).

Toe Extension and Flexion

Movement of the toes occurs at the metatarsophalangeal and proximal and distal interphalangeal joints (see Fig. 12–40*E* and *F*). Extension of the great toe occurs primarily at the metatarsophalangeal joint

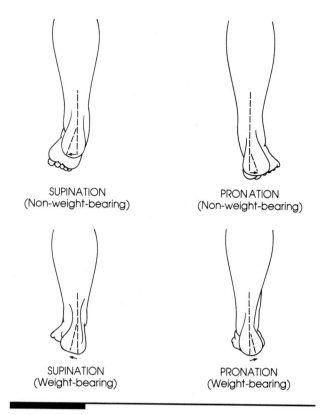

SUPINATION
(Non-weight-bearing)

PRONATION
(Non-weight-bearing)

SUPINATION
(Weight-bearing)

PRONATION
(Weight-bearing)

FIGURE 12–42. *Supination and pronation of the foot in weight-bearing and non–weight-bearing postures (posterior view of the right limb).*

(70°) with minimal or no extension at the interphalangeal joint. For the great toe, 45° flexion occurs at the metatarsophalangeal joint, and 90° occurs at the interphalangeal joint.

For the lateral four toes, extension occurs primarily at the metatarsophalangeal (40°) and distal inter-

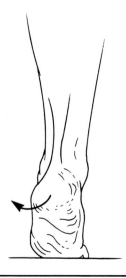

FIGURE 12–41. *Inversion of heel while standing on toes (plantar flexion of ankle).*

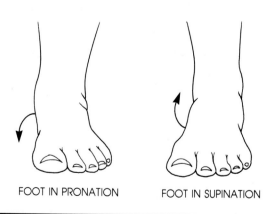

FOOT IN PRONATION

FOOT IN SUPINATION

FIGURE 12–43. *Anterior view of the foot in pronation and supination (weight-bearing stance).*

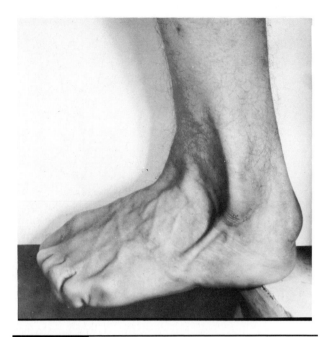

FIGURE 12–44. *Habitual subluxation of the peroneal tendons. The peroneal tendons pass anteriorly to the retrofibular sulcus but not anteriorly to the distal fibula, which is in contradistinction to traumatic subluxation. (From Kelikian, H., and A. S. Kelikian: Disorders of the Ankle. Philadelphia, W. B. Saunders Co., 1985, p. 765.)*

phalangeal joints (30°). Extension at the proximal interphalangeal joints is negligible. For the lateral four toes, 40° flexion occurs at the metatarsophalangeal joints, 35° occurs at the proximal interphalangeal joints, and 60° occurs at the distal interphalangeal joints.

Toe Abduction and Adduction

Abduction and adduction of the toes are measured with the second toe as midline. Although the range of motion of abduction can be measured, it is not usually done. The common practice is to ask the patient to spread the toes and then bring them back together (see Fig. 12–40G and H). The amount and quality of movement are compared with those of the unaffected side.

Nerve Injury

When assessing the active movements, the examiner must remember that peripheral nerve injuries may alter the pattern of movement. For example, the superficial peroneal nerve may be injured as it winds around the head of the fibula, resulting in altered nerve conduction to the peroneus longus and brevis muscles.[16] Thus, the movements controlled by these muscles will be altered. In addition, there will be sensory alterations. Similarly, the tibial nerve may be compressed as it passes through the tarsal tunnel on the medial aspect of the ankle (Fig. 12–45).[17] The tunnel is bordered by the tibiocalcaneal portion of the medial collateral ligament, the medial malleolus, and the calcaneus and talus. All of the intrinsic foot muscles supplied by the tibial nerve and its branches will be affected, as will the sensory distribution.

Passive Movements

The passive movements of the lower leg, ankle, and foot are performed with the patient in the non–weight-bearing posture (Fig. 12–46). As with other joints, if the active range of motion was complete, overpressure could be applied during the active non–weight-bearing movements. The end feel of plantar flexion, dorsiflexion, supination, pronation, toe flexion, and extension is tissue stretch. If the active movements were not full, the following passive movements should be performed:

1. Plantar flexion at the talocrural joint.
2. Dorsiflexion at the talocrural joint
3. Inversion at the subtalar joint.
4. Eversion of the subtalar joint.
5. Adduction at the midtarsal joints.
6. Abduction at the midtarsal joints.
7. Flexion of the toes.
8. Extension of the toes.
9. Adduction of the toes.
10. Abduction of the toes.

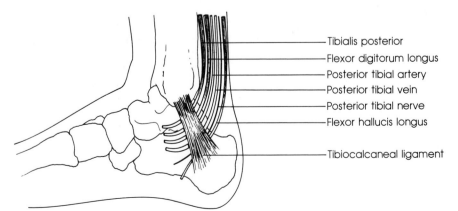

- Tibialis posterior
- Flexor digitorum longus
- Posterior tibial artery
- Posterior tibial vein
- Posterior tibial nerve
- Flexor hallucis longus
- Tibiocalcaneal ligament

FIGURE 12–45. *Tarsal tunnel syndrome.*

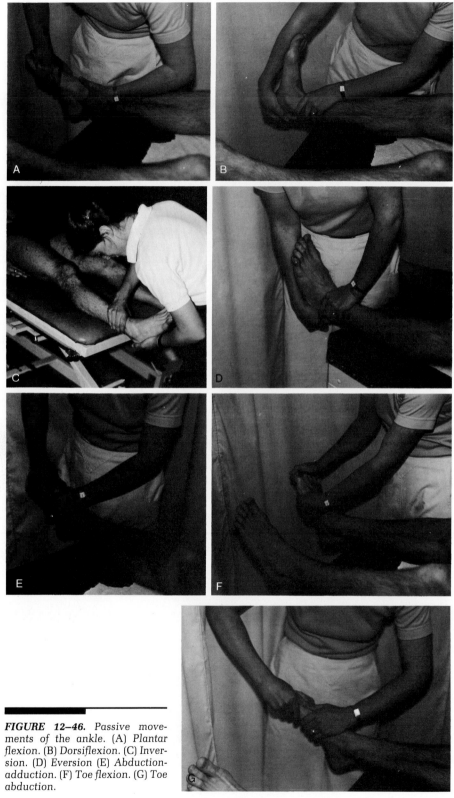

FIGURE 12–46. *Passive movements of the ankle. (A) Plantar flexion. (B) Dorsiflexion. (C) Inversion. (D) Eversion (E) Abduction-adduction. (F) Toe flexion. (G) Toe abduction.*

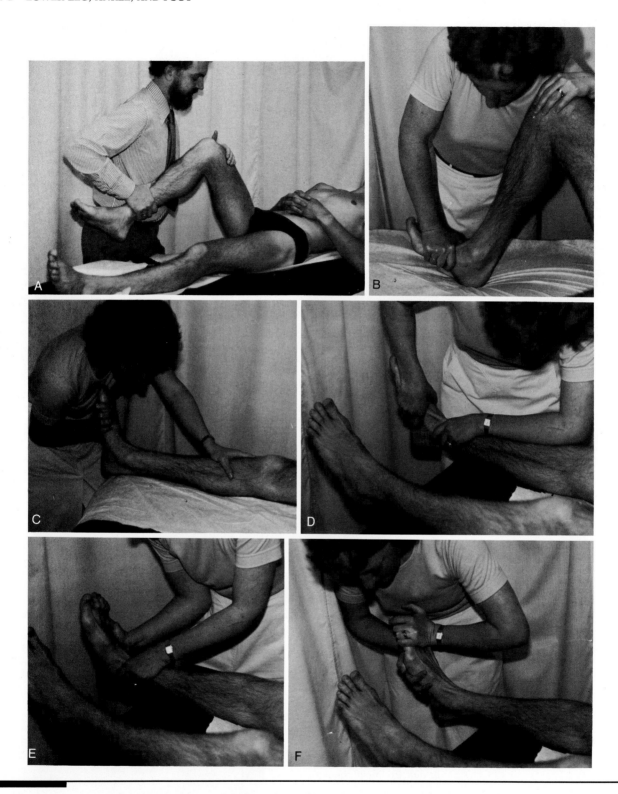

FIGURE 12–47. *Resisted isometric movements of the lower leg, ankle, and foot. (A) Knee flexion. (B) Dorsiflexion. (C) Plantar flexion. (D) Supination. (E) Pronation. (F) Toe extension.*

During the passive movements of the ankle and foot, any capsular patterns should be noted. The capsular pattern of the talocrural joint is more limitation of plantar flexion than of dorsiflexion; the subtalar joint capsular pattern shows more limitation of varus range than of valgus range of motion. The midtarsal joint capsular pattern is dorsiflexion most limited, followed by plantar flexion, adduction, and medial rotation. The first metatarsophalangeal joint has a capsular pattern of extension most limited, followed by flexion. The pattern for the second through fifth metatarsophalangeal joints is variable. The capsular pattern of the interphalangeal joints is extension most limited, followed by flexion.

Resisted Isometric Movements

The resisted isometric movements are done with the patient in the sitting or supine lying position (Fig. 12–47). They are performed to test the contractile tissue around the foot. The patient's foot is placed in the anatomic position. Refer to Table 12–4 for the muscles acting over the foot and ankle. The movements tested isometrically are as follows:

1. Knee flexion.
2. Plantar flexion.
3. Dorsiflexion.
4. Supination.

TABLE 12–4. Muscles of the Lower Limb, Ankle, and Foot: Their Action, and Innervation, and Nerve Root Derivation of the Peripheral Nerves

Action	Muscles Involved	Innervation	Nerve Root Deviation
Plantar flexion (flexion) of ankle	1. Gastrocnemius*	Tibial	S1–S2
	2. Soleus*	Tibial	S1–S2
	3. Plantaris	Tibial	S1–S2
	4. Flexor digitorum longus	Tibial	S2–S3
	5. Peroneus longus	Superficial peroneal	L5, S1–S2
	6. Peroneus brevis	Superficial peroneal	L5, S1–S2
	7. Flexor hallucis longus	Tibial	S2–S3
	8. Tibialis posterior	Tibial	L4–L5
Dorsiflexion (extension) of ankle	1. Tibialis anterior	Deep peroneal	L4–L5
	2. Extensor digitorum longus	Deep peroneal	L5, S1
	3. Extensor hallucis longus	Deep peroneal	L5, S1
	4. Peroneus tertius	Deep peroneal	L5, S1
Inversion	1. Tibialis posterior	Tibial	L4–L5
	2. Flexor digitorum longus	Tibial	S2–S3
	3. Flexor hallucis longus	Tibial	S2–S3
	4. Tibialis anterior	Deep peroneal	L4–L5
	5. Extensor hallucis longus	Deep peroneal	L5, S1
Eversion	1. Peroneus longus	Superficial peroneal	L5, S1–S2
	2. Peroneus brevis	Superficial peroneal	L5, S1–S2
	3. Peroneus tertius	Deep peroneal	L5, S1
	4. Extensor digitorum longus	Deep peroneal	L5, S1
Flexion of toes	1. Flexor digitorum longus	Tibial	S2–S3
	2. Flexor hallucis longus	Tibial	S2–S3
	3. Flexor digitorum brevis	Tibial (medial plantar branch)	S2–S3
	4. Flexor hallucis brevis	Tibial (medial plantar branch)	S2–S3
	5. Flexor accessorius	Tibial (lateral plantar branch)	S2–S3
	6. Interossei	Tibial (lateral plantar branch)	S2–S3
	7. Flexor digiti minimi brevis	Tibial (lateral plantar branch)	S2–S3
	8. Lumbricals (metatarsophalangeal joints)	Tibial (1st by medial plantar branch; 2nd through 4th by lateral plantar branch)	S2–S3
Extension of toes	1. Extensor digitorum longus	Deep peroneal	L5, S1
	2. Extensor hallucis longus	Deep peroneal	L5, S1
	3. Extensor digitorum brevis	Deep peroneal (lateral terminal branch)	S1–S2
	4. Lumbricals (interphalangeal joints)	Tibial (1st by medial plantar branch; 2nd through 4th by lateral plantar branch)	S2–S3
Abduction of toes	1. Abductor hallucis	Tibial (medial plantar branch)	S2–S3
	2. Abductor digiti minimi	Tibial (lateral plantar branch)	S2–S3
	3. Dorsal interossei	Tibial (lateral plantar branch)	S2–S3
Adduction of toes	1. Adductor hallucis	Tibial (lateral plantar branch)	S2–S3
	2. Plantar interossei	Tibial (lateral plantar branch)	S2–S3

*The gastrocnemius and soleus muscles are sometimes grouped together as the triceps surae muscles.

TABLE 12–5. Functional Strength Testing of the Foot and Ankle*

Starting Position	Action	Functional Test
Standing on one leg†	Lift toes and forefeet off ground (dorsiflexion)	10 to 15 Repetitions: Functional 5 to 9 Repetitions: Functionally fair 1 to 4 Repetitions: Functionally poor 0 Repetitions: Nonfunctional
Standing on one leg†	Lift heels off ground (plantar flexion)	10 to 15 Repetitions: Functional 5 to 9 Repetitions: Functionally fair 1 to 4 Repetitions: Functionally poor 0 Repetitions: Nonfunctional
Standing on one leg†	Lift lateral aspect of foot off ground (ankle eversion)	5 to 6 Repetitions: Functional 3 to 4 Repetitions: Functionally fair 1 to 2 Repetitions: Functionally poor 0 Repetitions: Nonfunctional
Standing on one leg†	Lift medial aspect of foot off ground (ankle inversion)	5 to 6 Repetitions: Functional 3 to 4 Repetitions: Functionally fair 1 to 2 Repetitions: Functionally poor 0 Repetitions: Nonfunctional
Seated	Pull small towel up under toes or pick up and release small object (i.e., pencil, marble, cottonball) (toe flexion)	10 to 15 Repetitions: Functional 5 to 9 Repetitions: Functionally fair 1 to 4 Repetitions: Functionally poor 0 Repetitions: Nonfunctional
Seated	Lift toes off ground (toe extension)	10 to 15 Repetitions: Functional 5 to 9 Repetitions: Functionally fair 1 to 4 Repetitions: Functionally poor 0 Repetitions: Nonfunctional

*Modified from Palmer, M. L., and M. Epler: Clinical Assessment Procedures in Physical Therapy. Philadelphia, J. B. Lippincott Co., 1990, pp. 308–310.

†Hand may hold something for balance only.

5. Pronation.
6. Toe extension.
7. Toe flexion.

Dorsiflexion is often tested with the patient's hip flexed to 45° and the knee flexed to 90°, as illustrated in Figure 12–47B. Testing with the patient in this position enables the examiner to exert a greater isometric force. Resisted isometric knee flexion must be performed because the triceps surae (gastrocnemius and soleus muscles together) act on the knee as well as on the ankle and foot.

Functional Assessment

If the patient is able to do the preceding activities with little difficulty, functional tests may be performed to see whether these sequential activities produce pain or other symptoms. The functional activities in order of sequence are as follows:

1. Squatting (both ankles should dorsiflex symmetrically).
2. Standing on toes (both ankles should plantar flex symmetrically).
3. Squatting and bouncing at the end of a squat.
4. Standing on one foot at a time.
5. Standing on the toes, one foot at a time.
6. Going up and down stairs.
7. Walking on the toes.
8. Running straight ahead.
9. Running and twisting.
10. Jumping.
11. Jumping and going into a full squat.

These activities, which are examples only, must be geared to the individual patient. Older patients should not be expected to do some of the activities unless they have, in the recent past, been doing these or similar ones (Table 12–5). Because the functional tests place a stress on the other lower limb joints, the examiner must ensure that these joints exhibit no pathology before all of the tests are completed. As the patient completes the activities, the examiner must assess whether any symptoms occur within a specific time frame (e.g., intermittent claudication or anterior compartment syndrome).[18, 19]

Table 12–6 lists the ranges of motion necessary at the ankle for locomotion.

TABLE 12–6. Range of Motion Necessary at the Foot and Ankle for Selected Locomotion Activities

Activity	Average Range of Motion Necessary
1. Descending stairs	Full dorsiflexion (20°)
2. Walking	Dorsiflexion—10° Plantar flexion—20 to 25°

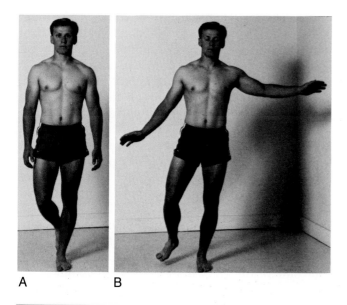

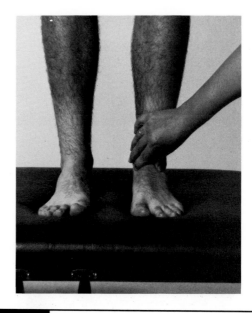

FIGURE 12–48. *Balance and proprioception. (A) One leg, with eyes open. (B) One leg, with eyes closed.*

FIGURE 12–49. *Positioning for determining the neutral position of the subtalar joint in standing position (weight bearing).*

Balance and proprioception are tested by asking the patient to stand on the unaffected leg and then on the affected leg—first with the eyes open, and then with the eyes closed. Any differences in balance time or difficulty in balancing give an idea of proprioceptive ability, especially differences that occurred when the patient's eyes were closed (Fig. 12–48).[20]

Special Tests

When assessing the lower leg, ankle, and foot, it is important to always assess the neutral position of the talus in both weight-bearing and non–weight-bearing situations. Other tests that should be carried out include alignment, functional leg length, and tibial torsion tests. Of the other tests, only those that the examiner wishes to use as confirming tests need be performed.

Tests for Neutral Position of the Talus

Neutral Position of the Talus (Weight Bearing). The patient stands with the feet in a relaxed standing position so that the base width and Fick angle are normal for the patient. The examiner palpates the head of the talus on the dorsal aspect of the foot with the thumb and forefinger of one hand (Fig. 12–49). The patient is asked to slowly rotate the trunk to the right and then to the left, which causes the tibia to medially and laterally rotate so that the talus supinates and pronates. If the foot is positioned so that the talar head does not appear to bulge to either

side, then the subtalar joint will be in its neutral position in weight bearing.[4]

Neutral Position of the Talus (Supine). The patient lies supine with the feet extending over the end of the examining table. The examiner grasps the patient's foot over the fourth and fifth metatarsal heads using the thumb and index finger of one hand. The examiner palpates both sides of the head of the talus with the thumb and index finger of the other hand on the dorsum of the foot (Fig. 12–50). The examiner then gently, passively dorsiflexes the foot until resistance is felt. While the examiner maintains

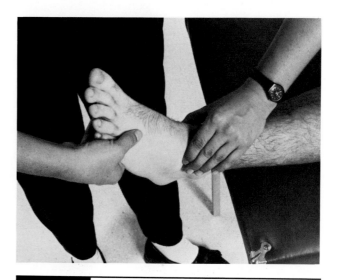

FIGURE 12–50. *Determining the neutral position of the subtalar joint in supine position.*

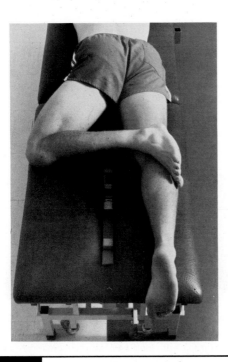

FIGURE 12–51. *Prone lying with legs in figure-4 position to assess neutral position of the subtalar joint in the prone position.*

Neutral Position of the Talus (Prone). The patient lies prone with the feet extended over the end of the examining table. The examiner grasps the patient's foot over the fourth and fifth metatarsal heads with the index finger and thumb of one hand. The examiner palpates both sides of the talus on the dorsum of the foot using the thumb and index finger of the other hand. The examiner then passively and gently dorsiflexes the foot until resistance is felt (Figs. 12–51 and 12–52). While maintaining the dorsiflexed position, the examiner moves the foot back and forth through an arc of supination (talar head bulges laterally) and pronation (talar head bulges medially). As the arc of movement is performed, the examiner will notice that there is a point in the arc at which the foot appears to "fall off" to one side or the other more easily. This point is the neutral position of the subtalar joint, and it is this point that is assumed when looking at forefoot and hindfoot deformities.[4, 5, 13, 21]

Tests for Alignment

Leg-Heel Alignment. The patient lies in the prone position with the feet extending over the end of the examining table. The examiner then places a mark over the midline of the calcaneus at the insertion of the Achilles tendon. The examiner makes a second mark approximately 1 cm distal to the first mark as close to the midline of the calcaneus as possible. A *calcaneal line* is then made to join the two marks.

this position, the foot is passively moved through an arc of supination (talar head bulges laterally) and pronation (talar head bulges medially). If the foot is positioned so that the talar head does not appear to bulge to either side, the subtalar joint will be in its neutral position.[4, 5, 13, 21]

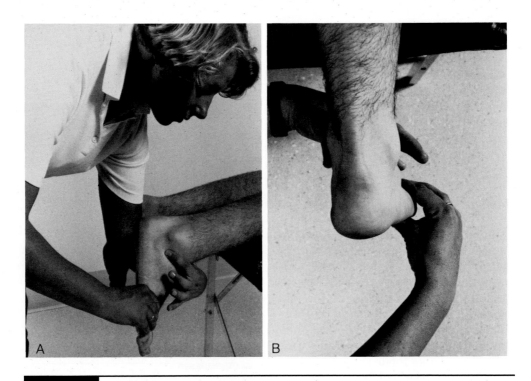

FIGURE 12–52. *Determining the neutral position of the subtalar joints in the prone position. (A) Side View. (B) Superior view.*

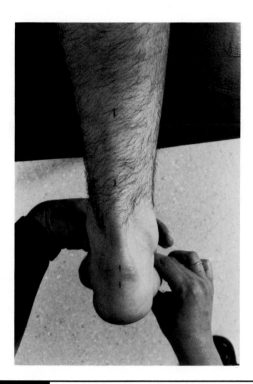

FIGURE 12–53. *Alignment of leg and heel.*

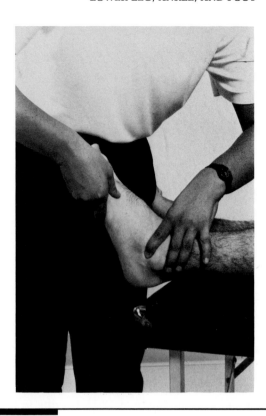

FIGURE 12–54. *Alignment of forefoot and heel.*

Next, the examiner makes two marks on the lower third of the leg in the midline. These two marks are joined, forming the *tibial line*, which represents the longitudinal axis of the tibia. The examiner then places the subtalar joint in neutral position. While the subtalar joint is held in neutral, the examiner looks at the two lines. If the lines are parallel or in slight varus (2 to 8°), the leg-to-heel alignment is considered normal.[21] If the heel is inverted, the patient has hindfoot varus. If the heel is everted, the patient has hindfoot valgus (Fig. 12–53).

Forefoot-Heel Alignment. The patient lies supine with the feet extending over the end of the examining table. The examiner positions the subtalar joint in neutral position. While maintaining this position, the examiner pronates the midtarsal joints maximally. Maintaining this position, the examiner observes the relation between the vertical axis of the heel and the plane of the second through fourth metatarsal heads (Fig. 12–54). Normally, the plane is perpendicular to the vertical axis. If the medial side of the foot is raised, the patient has a forefoot varus. If the lateral side of the foot is raised, the patient has a forefoot valgus.[13, 21]

Tests for Tibial Torsion

Tibial Torsion (Sitting). Tibial torsion is measured by having the patient sit with the knees over the edge of the examining table (Fig. 12–55). The examiner then places the thumb of one hand over

the apex of one malleolus and the index finger of the same hand over the apex of the other malleolus. Next, the examiner visualizes the axes of the knee and of the ankle. The lines are not normally parallel

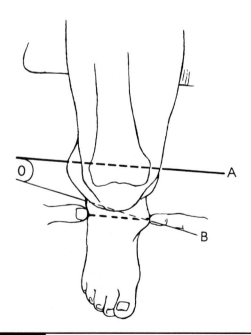

FIGURE 12–55. *Determination of tibial torsion in sitting position. (A) Knee axis. (B) Ankle axis. (Angle) Tibial torsion. (Modified from Fromherz, W. A.: Examination. In Hunt, G. C. (ed.): Physical Therapy of the Foot and Ankle. Clinics in Physical Therapy. New York, Churchill Livingstone, 1988, p. 80.)*

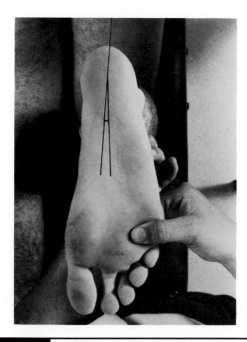

FIGURE 12–56. *Measurement of tibial torsion in the prone position.*

but instead form an angle of 12 to 18° due to lateral rotation of the tibia.[2]

Tibial Torsion (Supine). The patient lies supine. The examiner ensures that the femoral condyle lies in the frontal plane (patella facing straight up). The examiner palpates the apex of both malleoli with one hand and draws a line on the heel representing a line joining the two apices. A second line is drawn on the heel parallel to the floor. The angle formed by the intersection of the two lines indicates the amount of lateral tibial torsion (normal, 13 to 18° in adults, less in children). More than 18° tibial torsion is referred to as a *toe-out position*, whereas less than 13° is referred to as a *toe-in position*.

Tibial Torsion (Prone). The patient lies prone with the knees flexed to 90°. The examiner views from above the angle formed by the foot and thigh (Fig. 12–56) after the subtalar joint has been placed in the neutral position, noting the angle the foot makes with the tibia.[22] This method is most often used in children because it is easier to observe the feet from above.

Tests for Ligamentous Instability

Anterior Drawer Sign of the Ankle. The patient lies supine with the foot relaxed. The examiner stabilizes the tibia and fibula, holds the patient's foot in 20° of plantar flexion, and draws the talus forward in the ankle mortise (Fig. 12–57). In the plantar flexed position, the anterior talofibular ligament is perpendicular to the long axis of the tibia. By adding inversion, which gives an anterolateral stress, the examiner can increase the stress on the anterior talofibular ligament. If straight anterior movement or translation occurs (Fig. 12–58B), the test indicates both medial and lateral ligament insufficiencies. This bilateral finding, which is often more evident in dorsiflexion, means that the superficial and deep deltoid ligaments as well as the anterior talofibular ligament and anterolateral capsule have been torn. If the tear is only on one side (e.g., the lateral side), only that side (lateral in this case) would translate forward, causing medial rotation of the talus; the result would be anterolateral rotary instability (Fig. 12–58C), which is increasingly evident with increasing plantar flexion of the foot.[12, 14, 23–25]

Ideally, the knee should be placed in 90° of flexion to alleviate tension on the Achilles tendon. The test should be performed in plantar flexion and dorsiflexion to test for straight and rotational instabilities.

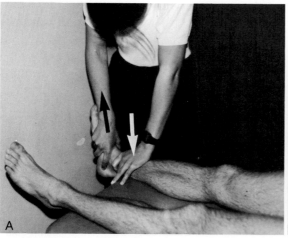
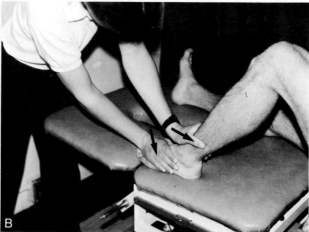

FIGURE 12–57. *Anterior drawer test. (A) Method 1—drawing the foot forward. (B) Method 2—pushing the leg back.*

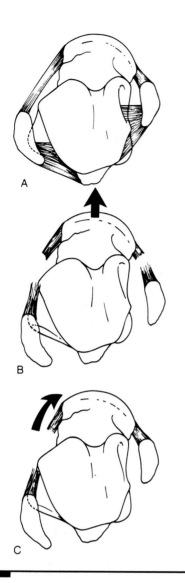

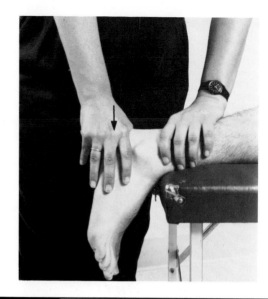

FIGURE 12–59. Prone anterior drawer test.

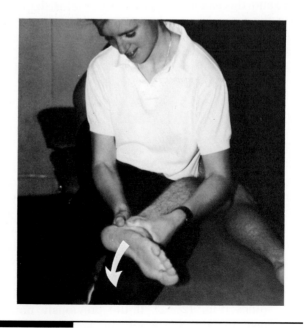

FIGURE 12–58. Anterior drawer test. (A) Normal talar-malleolar relation. (B) Straight anterior translation (one plane anterior instability). (C) Lateral rotary translation (anterolateral rotary instability).

The test may also be performed by stabilizing the foot and talus and pushing the tibia and fibula posteriorly on the talus (see Fig. 12–57B). In this case, excessive posterior movement of the tibia and fibula indicates a positive test.

Prone Anterior Drawer Test.[26] The patient lies prone with the feet extending over the end of the examining table. With one hand, the examiner pushes the heel steadily forward (Fig. 12–59). A positive sign is indicated by excessive anterior movement and a "sucking in" of the skin on both sides of the Achilles tendon. The test is indicative of ligamentous instability, as indicated in the previous test.

Talar Tilt. The patient lies in the supine or side lying position with the foot relaxed (Fig. 12–60).[12, 27] The patient's gastrocnemius muscle may

be relaxed by flexion of the knee to 90°. This test is used to determine whether the calcaneofibular ligament is torn. The foot is held in the anatomic position, which brings the calcaneofibular ligament perpendicular to the long axis of the talus. The talus is then tilted from side to side into adduction and abduction. Adduction tests the calcaneofibular ligament by increasing the stress on the ligament. On a radiograph, this angle may be measured by obtaining the angle between the distal aspect of the tibia and the proximal surface of the talus (see Fig. 12–93). The normal side is tested first for comparison.

Kleiger Test. The patient sits with the knee flexed to 90° and the foot relaxed and non–weight bearing.

FIGURE 12–60. Talar tilt test.

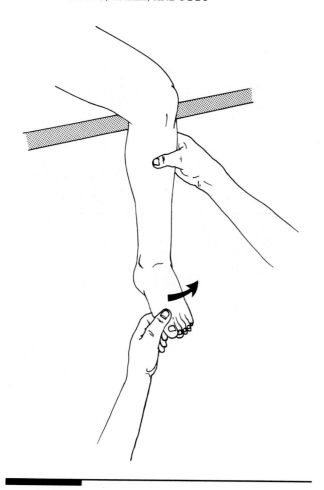

FIGURE 12–61. Kleiger test.

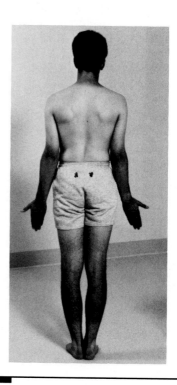

FIGURE 12–62. Functional leg length in the standing position (subtalar joint in neutral).

The examiner gently grasps the foot and rotates it laterally (Fig. 12–61).[1, 14] If the Kleiger test is positive, the patient will have pain medially and laterally, and the examiner may feel the talus displace from the medial malleolus, indicating a tear of the deltoid ligament. On a radiograph, the medial clear space will be increased, suggesting rupture of the ligament (see Fig. 12–93).

Other Special Tests

Functional Leg Length.[28] The patient stands in the normal relaxed stance. The examiner palpates the anterior superior iliac spines and then the posterior superior iliac spines and notes any differences. The examiner then positions the patient so that the patient's subtalar joints are in neutral position while weight bearing. While the patient maintains this position with the toes straight ahead and the knees straight, the examiner repalpates the anterior superior iliac spines and the posterior superior iliac spines (Fig. 12–62). If the previously noted differences remain, the pelvis and sacroiliac joints should be further evaluated. If the previously noted differences disappear, the examiner should suspect

a functional leg length difference resulting from hip, knee, or ankle and foot problems—primarily, ankle and foot problems. (Tables 12–7 and 12–8 show some of the causes and signs of functional leg length differences.) The examiner must then determine what is causing the difference. For example, foot pronation is often seen with forefoot or hindfoot varus, tibial varus, tight muscles (e.g., calf, hamstrings, and hip flexors), and weak muscles (e.g., ankle invertors, piriformis).

Thompson (Simmonds') Test (Sign for Achilles Tendon Rupture). The patient lies prone or kneels on a chair with the feet over the edge of the table or chair (Fig. 12–63). While the patient is relaxed, the examiner squeezes the calf muscles. A positive test is indicated by the absence of plantar flexion when the muscle is squeezed and is indicative of a ruptured Achilles tendon.[29]

One should be careful not to assume that the Achilles tendon is not ruptured if the patient is able to plantar flex the foot while not bearing weight. The long extensor muscles can perform this function in the non–weight-bearing stance even with a rupture (third-degree strain) of the Achilles tendon.

Swing Test for Posterior Tibiotalar Subluxation.[30] The patient sits with feet dangling over the edge of the examining table (Fig. 12–64). The examiner holds the plantar aspect of the patient's feet and uses the fingers to keep the feet parallel to the floor. With the thumbs, the examiner palpates the anterior portion of the talus. The examiner then passively plantar flexes and dorsiflexes the foot and

TABLE 12–7. Functional Limb Length Difference*

Joint	Functional Lengthening	Functional Shortening
Foot	Supination	Pronation
Knee	Extension	Flexion
Hip	Lowering	Lifting
	Extension	Flexion
	External rotation	Internal rotation
Sacroiliac	Anterior rotation	Posterior rotation

*Modified from Wallace, L. A.: Lower Quarter Pain: Mechanical Evaluation and Treatment. *In* Grieve, G. P. (ed.): Modern Manual Therapy of the Vertebral Column. Edinburgh, Churchill Livingstone, 1986, p. 467.

TABLE 12–8. Dynamic Limb Length Evaluation*

Shoe Wear (Asymmetric Wear)	Asymmetric Callus	Asymmetric Posture	Asymmetric
Shoe upper	Medial first DIP	Foot	Toe out
Heel counter	Medial first MP	Ankle	Toe grasp
Varus or valgus	Second and third metatarsal heads	Knee	Patellar alignment over foot
		Hip	Knee flexion
Shoe sole	Fourth and fifth metatarsal heads	Pelvis	Hip drop
Posterior lateral heel			Propulsion
Posterior central heel	Calcaneus		
Posterior medial heel	Lateral		
	Central		
	Medial		

*Modified from Wallace, L. A.: Limb length difference and back pain. *In* Grieve, G. P. (ed.): Modern Manual Therapy of the Vertebral Column. Edinburgh, Churchill Livingstone, 1986, p. 469.

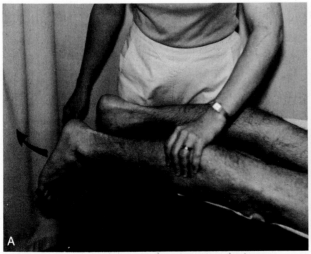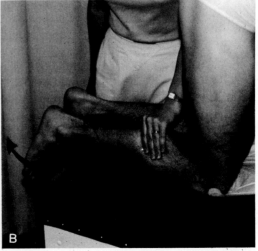

FIGURE 12–63. Thompson test for Achilles tendon rupture. (A) Prone lying position. (B) Kneeling position. Foot will plantar flex (arrow) if test result is negative.

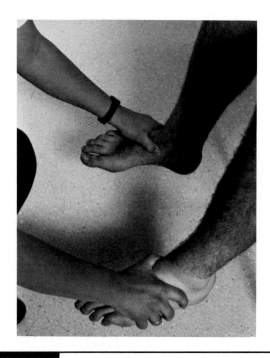

FIGURE 12–64. *Swing test for posterior tibiotalar subluxation.*

compares the quality and degree of movement between feet, especially into dorsiflexion. If resistance to normal dorsiflexion is felt in the injured ankle, it is indicative of a positive test for posterior tibiotalar subluxation.

Feiss Line.[13] The examiner marks the apex of the medial malleolus and the plantar aspect of the first metatarsophalangeal joint while the patient is not weight bearing. The examiner then palpates the lateral aspect of the navicula (navicular tuberosity), noting where it lies relative to a line joining the two

previously made points. The patient then stands with the feet 8 to 15 cm apart. The two points are checked to ensure that they still represent the apex of the medial malleolus and the plantar aspect of the metatarsophalangeal joint. The navicula is again palpated (Fig. 12–65). The navicular tuberosity normally lies on or very close to the line joining the two points. If the navicula falls one third of the distance to the floor, it represents a first-degree flatfoot; if it falls two thirds of the distance, it represents a second-degree flatfoot; and if it rests on the floor, it represents a third-degree flatfoot.

Tinel's Sign at the Ankle. The Tinel sign may be elicited in two places around the ankle. The anterior tibial branch of the deep peroneal nerve may be percussed in front of the ankle (Fig. 12–66). The posterior tibial nerve may be percussed as it passes behind the medial malleolus (see Figs. 12–45 and

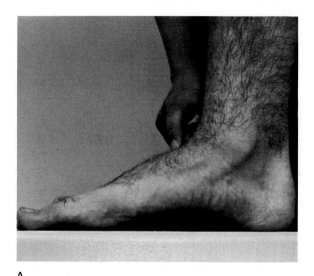

A

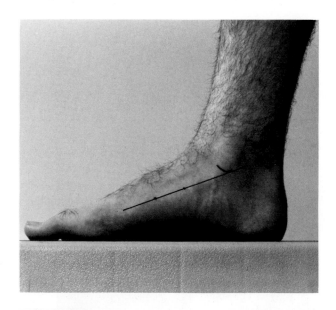

FIGURE 12–65. *Feiss line in weight bearing. Navicular tuberosity is in normal position.*

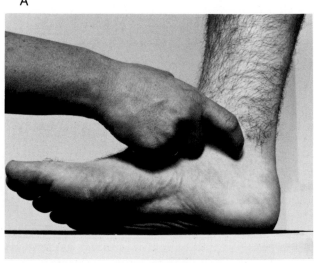

B

FIGURE 12–66. *Tinel's sign. (A) Anterior tibial branch of deep peroneal nerve. (B) Posterior tibial nerve.*

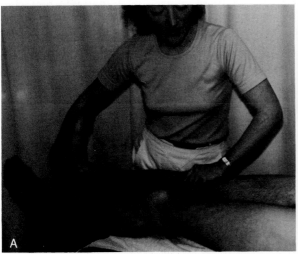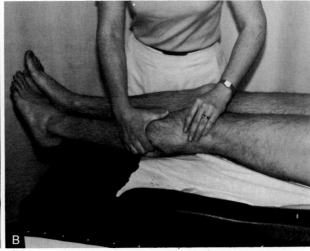

FIGURE 12–67. Homans' sign for thrombophlebitis. (A) Test. (B) Palpation for tenderness in thrombophlebitis.

12–71). In both cases, tingling or paresthesia felt distally is a positive sign.

Homans' Sign. The patient's foot is passively dorsiflexed with the knee extended. Pain in the calf indicates a positive Homans' sign for deep vein thrombophlebitis (Fig. 12–67). Tenderness will also be elicited on palpation of the calf. In addition to these findings, the examiner may find pallor and swelling in the leg as well as a loss of the dorsalis pedis pulse.

Reflexes and Cutaneous Distribution

One must be aware of the sensory distribution of the various peripheral nerves in the foot (especially the superficial peroneal, deep peroneal, and saphenous) and the branches of the tibial nerve (sural, medial plantar, medial calcaneal, and lateral plantar) (Fig. 12–68).

The examiner must also differentiate between the peripheral nerve sensory distribution and the sensory nerve root distribution or dermatomes (Fig. 12–69). Although dermatomes vary among individuals, their pattern will never be identical to the peripheral nerve distribution, which tends to be more consistent among patients.

The patient's sensation should be tested by the examiner running the hands over the anterior, lateral, medial, and posterior surfaces of the patient's leg below the knee, foot, and toes. Any difference in sensation should be noted and can be mapped out more exactly with a pinwheel, pin, cotton batten, and/or brush.

The examiner must test the patient's reflexes. Commonly checked in this region is the Achilles reflex, which is derived from the S1 and S2 nerve roots (Fig. 12–70) and the posterior tibial reflex which is derived from the L5 nerve root (Fig. 12–71). In addition to the S1–S2 nerve root reflex, the examiner should test for pyramidal tract (upper motor neuron) disease. There are various methods for testing the reflexes, including Babinski, Chaddock, Oppenheim, and Gordon reflexes (Fig. 12–72). A positive sign in all of these tests is extension of the big toe. The Babinski reflex also causes fanning of the second through fifth toes. The most common and reliable test is the Babinski test.

One must always remember that pain may be referred to the lower leg, ankle, or foot from the lumbar spine, sacrum, hip, or knee (Fig. 12–73). Conversely, the pain from a lesion in the lower leg, ankle, or foot may be transmitted to the hip or knee.

Joint Play Movements

The joint play movements are done with the patient in the supine or side lying position, depending on which movement is being performed. A comparison of movement between the normal or unaffected side and the injured side should be made.

The following movements should be performed (Figs. 12–74 through 12–77):

1. At the talocrural (ankle) joint.
   a. Long-axis extension (traction).
   b. Anteroposterior glide.
2. At the subtalar joint.
   a. Talar rock.
   b. Side tilt medially and laterally.
3. At the midtarsal joints.
   a. Anteroposterior glide.
   b. Rotation.

Text continued on page 490

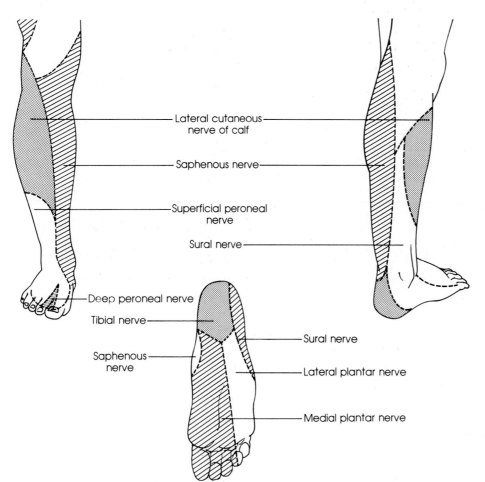

Lateral cutaneous nerve of calf

Saphenous nerve

Superficial peroneal nerve

Sural nerve

Deep peroneal nerve

Tibial nerve

Saphenous nerve

Sural nerve

Lateral plantar nerve

Medial plantar nerve

FIGURE 12–68. Peripheral nerve distribution in the lower leg, ankle, and foot.

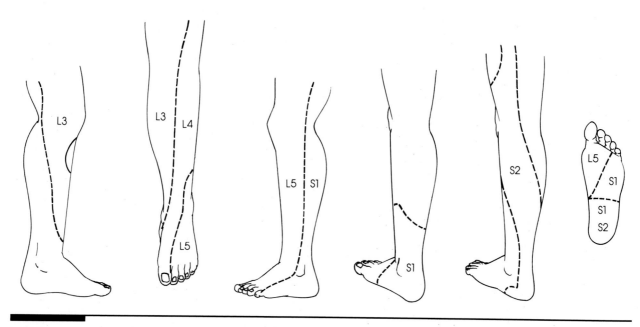

FIGURE 12–69. Dermatomes of the lower leg, ankle, and foot.

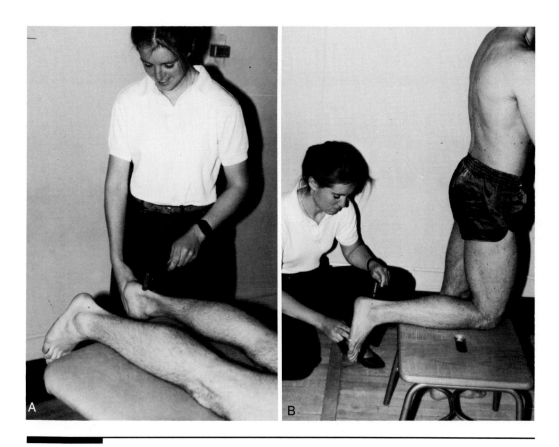

FIGURE 12–70. *Test of the Achilles reflex (S1). (A) Method 1. (B) Method 2.*

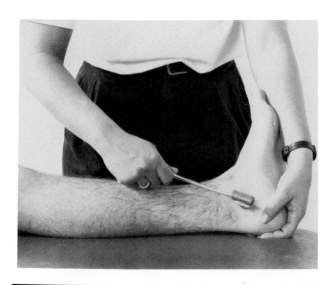

FIGURE 12–71. *Posterior tibial reflex.*

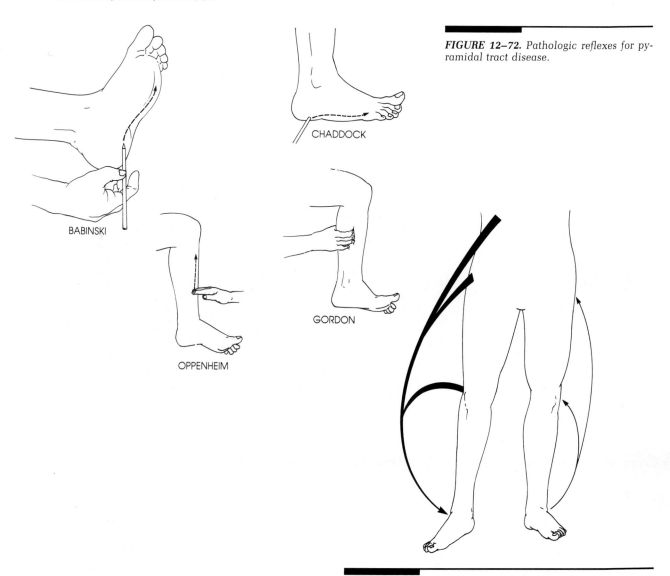

FIGURE **12–72.** *Pathologic reflexes for py-ramidal tract disease.*

BABINSKI

CHADDOCK

OPPENHEIM

GORDON

FIGURE **12–73.** *Pattern of referred pain to and from the ankle.*

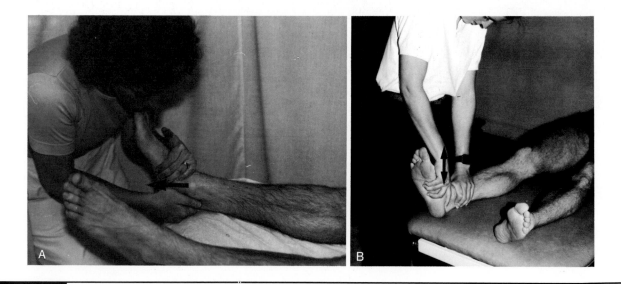

FIGURE **12–74.** *Joint play movements at the talocrural joint. (A) Long-axis extension. (B) Anteroposterior glide at the talocrural joint.*

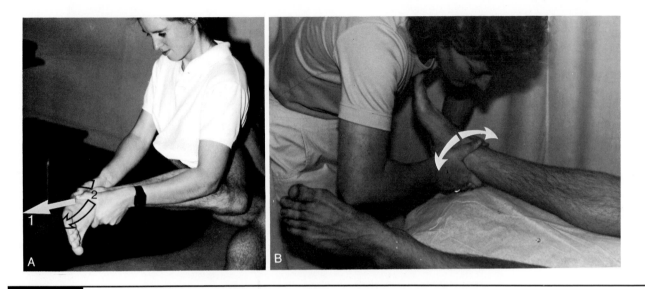

FIGURE 12–75. Joint play movements at the subtalar joint. (A) Talar rock. (1) Slight traction applied. (2) Talus rocked anteriorly and posteriorly. (B) Side tilt.

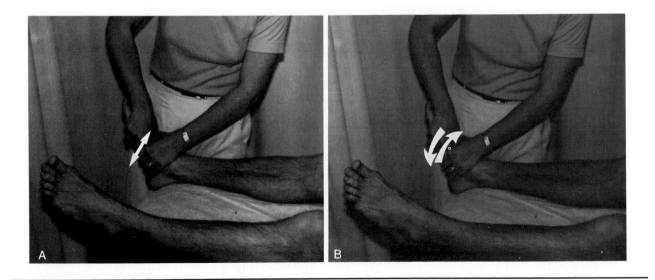

FIGURE 12–76. Joint play movements in the midtarsal and tarsometatarsal joints. (A) Anteroposterior glide. (B) Rotation.

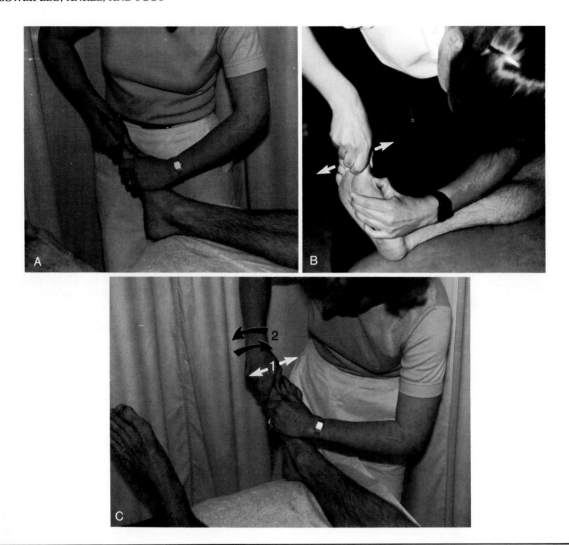

FIGURE 12–77. *Joint play movements at the metatarsophalangeal and interphalangeal joints. (A) Long-axis extension. (B) Anteroposterior glide. (C) Side glide (1) and/or rotation (2).*

4. At the tarsometatarsal joints.
   a. Anteroposterior glide.
   b. Rotation.
5. At the metatarsophalangeal and interphalangeal joints.
   a. Long-axis extension (traction).
   b. Anteroposterior glide.
   c. Lateral or side glide.
   d. Rotation.

Long-Axis Extension

Long-axis extension is performed by stabilizing the proximal segment and applying traction to the distal segment. For example, at the ankle, the examiner stabilizes the tibia and fibula by using a strap or just allows the leg to relax. Both hands are then placed around the ankle, distal to the malleoli, and a distractive force is applied. At the metatarsophalan-

geal and interphalangeal joints, the examiner stabilizes the metatarsal bone or proximal phalanx and applies a distractive force to the proximal or distal phalanx, respectively.

Anteroposterior Glide

Anteroposterior glide at the *ankle joint* is performed by stabilizing the tibia and fibula and drawing the talus and foot forward. To test the posterior movement, the examiner pushes the talus and foot back on the tibia and fibula. There is a difference in the arc of movement between the two actions in tests of joint play. During the anterior movement, the foot should move in an arc into plantar flexion; during the posterior movement, the foot should move in an arc into dorsiflexion.

Anteroposterior glide at the *midtarsal* and *tarsometatarsal joints* is performed in a fashion similar to that of the carpal bones at the wrist. For the midtarsal joints, one stabilizes the navicular, talus, and calcaneus with one hand. The other hand is placed around the distal row of tarsal bones (cuneiforms and cuboid). If the hands are positioned properly, they should touch each other, as in Figure 12–76. An anteroposterior gliding movement of the distal row of *tarsal bones* is applied while the proximal row of tarsal bones is stabilized. The examiner's hands are then moved distally so that the stabilizing hand rests over the distal row of tarsal bones, and the mobilizing hand rests over the proximal aspect of the metatarsal bones. Again, the hands should be positioned so that they touch each other. An anteroposterior gliding movement of the metatarsal bones is applied while stabilizing the distal row of tarsal bones.

Anteroposterior glide at the *metatarsophalangeal* and *interphalangeal joints* is performed by stabilizing the proximal bone (metatarsal or phalanx) and moving the distal bone (phalanx) in an anteroposterior gliding motion in relation to the stabilized bone.

Talar Rock

Talar rock is the only joint play movement performed in the side lying position.[27] Both hips and knees are flexed. The examiner sits with the back to the patient as illustrated (see Fig. 12–75) and places both hands around the ankle just distal to the malleoli. A slight distractive force is applied to the ankle (see Fig. 12–75A, 1), and a rocking movement forward and backward is applied to the foot (see Fig. 12–75A, 2). Normally, the examiner should feel a "clunk" at the extreme of each movement. As with all joint play movements, the movement is compared with that of the unaffected side.

Side Tilt

Side tilt at the *subtalar joint* is performed by placing both hands around the calcaneus (see Fig. 12–75B). The wrists are flexed and extended, side tilting the calcaneus medially and laterally on the talus. The examiner keeps the patient's foot in the anatomic position while performing the movement. The movement is identical to that used to test the calcaneofibular ligament in the talar tilt test.

Rotation

Rotation at the *midtarsal joints* is performed in a similar fashion to the anteroposterior glide at these joints. The proximal row of tarsal bones (navicular, calcaneus, and talus) is stabilized, and the mobilizing hand is placed around the distal tarsal bones (cuneiforms and cuboid). The distal row of bones is then rotated on the proximal row of bones. Rotation at the *tarsometatarsal joints* is performed in a similar fashion.

Rotation at the *metatarsophalangeal* and *interphalangeal joints* is performed by stabilizing the proximal bone with one hand and applying slight traction and rotating the distal bone with the other hand.

Side Glide

Side glide at the *metatarsophalangeal* and *interphalangeal joints* is performed by the examiner's stabilizing the proximal bone with one hand. The examiner then uses the other hand to apply slight traction to the distal bone and moves the distal bone sideways to the right and left in relation to the stabilized bone without causing torsion motion at the joint.

Tests for Tarsal Bone Mobility

Kaltenborn advocates "10 tests" to determine the mobility of the tarsal bones.[31] The sequential movement of the tarsal bones is as follows:

1. Fixate the second and third cuneiforms and mobilize the second metatarsal bone.
2. Fixate the second and third cuneiform bones and mobilize the third metatarsal bone.
3. Fixate the first cuneiform bone and mobilize the first metatarsal bone.
4. Fixate the navicular bone and mobilize the first, second, and third cuneiform bones.
5. Fixate the talus and mobilize the navicular bone.
6. Fixate the cuboid bone and mobilize the fourth and fifth metatarsal bones.
7. Fixate the navicular and third cuneiform bones and mobilize the cuboid bone.
8. Fixate the calcaneus and mobilize the cuboid bone.
9. Fixate the talus and mobilize the calcaneus.
10. Fixate the talus and mobilize the tibia and fibula.

Palpation

The examiner palpates for any swelling, noting whether it is intracapsular or extracapsular. For example, extracapsular swelling around the ankle is indicated by swelling on only one side of the Achilles tendon, whereas intracapsular swelling is indicated by swelling on both sides (see Fig. 12–20). Pitting edema may be present and should be noted. If swelling is present at the end of the day and absent after a night of recumbency, venous insufficiency may be implied owing to a weakening or insufficiency of the action of the muscle pump of the lower leg muscle. Swelling in the ankle may persist for many weeks after the injury as a result of this insufficiency.

One should also notice the texture of the skin and nails. It must be remembered that the skin of an ischemic foot shows a loss of hair and becomes thin and very inelastic. In addition, the nails become coarse, thickened, and irregular. Many of the nail changes seen in the hand in the presence of systemic disease will also be seen in the foot (see Chapter 6). With poor circulation, the foot will also feel colder. The foot is palpated in the non–weight-bearing and long leg sitting or supine positions. The following structures, including the joints between them, should be palpated.

Anteriorly and Anteromedially

Toes and Metatarsal, Cuneiform, and Navicular Bones. Starting on the medial side, the examiner can easily palpate the great toe and its two phalanges. Moving proximally, one will come to the first metatarsal bone (Fig. 12–78). The head of the first

metatarsal should be palpated carefully. On the lateral aspect, the examiner palpates for any evidence of a bunion (exostosis, callus, and inflamed bursa), which is often associated with hallux valgus. On the plantar aspect, the two sesamoid bones just proximal to the head of the first metatarsal may be palpated. The examiner then palpates the first metatarsal bone along its length to the first cuneiform bone and notes any tenderness, swelling, or signs of pathology. As the examiner moves proximally past the first cuneiform on its medial aspect, a bony prominence will be felt–the tubercle of the navicular bone. The examiner then returns to the first cuneiform bone and moves laterally on the dorsal and plantar surface, palpating the second and third cuneiforms (Fig. 12–79). Like the first cuneiform, the navicular and second and third cuneiform bones should be palpated on their dorsal and plantar aspects for signs of pathology (e.g., fracture, exostosis, or *Köhler's disease*–osteochondritis of the navicular bone).

Moving laterally, one palpates the three phalanges of each of the lateral four toes. Each of the lateral four metatarsals is palpated proximally to check for conditions such as Freiberg's disease (osteochondrosis of the second metatarsal head). Under the heads of the second and third metatarsals on the

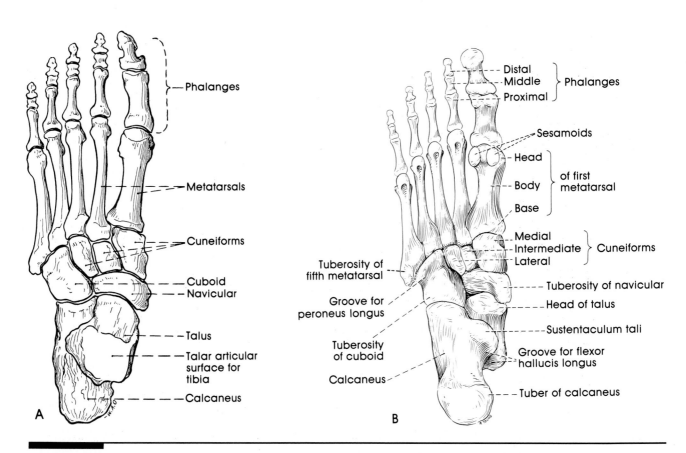

FIGURE 12–78. *Bones of the ankle and foot. (A) Dorsal view. (B) Plantar view. (Adapted from Hollinshead, W. H., and D. B. Jenkins: Functional Anatomy of the Limbs and Back. Philadelphia, W. B. Saunders Co., 1981, pp. 194,317.)*

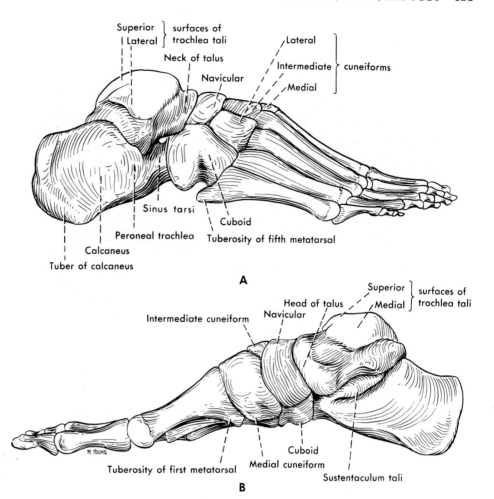

FIGURE 12–79. Bones of the foot from the lateral (A) and medial (B) sides. (From Hollinshead, W. H., and D. B. Jenkins: Functional Anatomy of the Limbs and Back. Philadelphia, W. B Saunders Co., 1991, p. 310.)

plantar aspect, one should feel for any evidence of a callus, which may indicate a fallen metatarsal arch. Care must be taken to palpate the base of the fifth metatarsal (styloid process) and adjacent cuboid bone for signs of pathology. Also, the lateral aspect of the head of the fifth metatarsal may demonstrate a bunion similar to that seen on the first toe; this is called a "tailor's bunion."

In addition to palpating the metatarsal bones, the examiner palpates between the bones for evidence of pathology (e.g., Morton's or interdigital neuroma) as well as the intrinsic muscles of the foot.

Medial Malleolus, Medial Tarsal Bones, and Posterior Tibial Artery. The examiner stabilizes the patient's heel by holding the calcaneus stable with one hand and palpates the distal edges of the medial malleolus for tenderness or swelling with the other hand. Palpating along the medial malleolus, one will come to its distal extent. Moving from that point along a line joining the navicular tubercle, the examiner moves along the talus until the head of the talus is reached. As the head of the talus is palpated, the examiner may evert and invert the foot, feeling the movement between the talar head and navicular bone. Eversion causes the head to become more prominent, as does the deformity pes

planus. At the same time, the tibialis posterior tendon may be palpated where it inserts into the navicular and cuneiform bones. Rupture (third-degree strain) of this tendon leads to a valgus foot. The four ligaments that make up the deltoid ligament (tibionavicular, tibiocalcanean, and anterior and posterior tibiotalar) may also be palpated for signs of pathology.

Returning to the medial malleolus at its distal extent, the examiner moves further distally (approximately one finger width) until another bony prominence—the sustentaculum tali of the calcaneus—is felt. This bony prominence is often small and difficult to palpate. Moving further posteriorly, one palpates the medial aspect of the calcaneus for signs of pathology (e.g., sprain, fracture, or tarsal tunnel syndrome). As the examiner moves to the plantar aspect of the calcaneus, the heel fat pad, intrinsic foot muscles, and plantar fascia are palpated for signs of pathology (e.g., heel bruise, plantar fasciitis, or bone spur).

The examiner then returns to the medial malleolus and palpates along its posterior surface, noting the movement of the tibialis posterior and long flexor tendons (and checking for tendinitis) during plantar flexion and dorsiflexion and noting any swelling or crepitus. At the same time, the posterior tibial artery, which supplies blood to 75 per cent of the foot, may be palpated as it runs posterior to the medial malleolus. This pulse is often difficult to palpate in individuals with "fat" ankles and in the presence of edema or synovial thickening.

Anterior Tibia, Neck of Talus, and Dorsalis Pedis Artery. The examiner moves to the anterior aspect of the medial malleolus following its course laterally onto the distal end of the tibia. As the examiner moves distally, the fingers will rest on the talus. If the foot is then plantar flexed and dorsiflexed, the anterior aspect of the articular surface of the talus can be palpated for signs of pathology (e.g., osteochondritis dissecans). As the examiner moves further distally, the fingers can follow the course of the neck of the talus to the talar head. Moving distally from the tibia, one should be able to palpate the long extensor tendons, tibialis anterior tendon, and, with care, the extensor retinaculum (Fig. 12–80). If the examiner moves further distally over the cuneiforms or between the first and second metatarsal bones, the dorsalis pedis pulse (branch of the anterior tibial artery) may be palpated. It may be found between the tendons of extensor digitorum longus and extensor hallucis longus over the junction of the first and second cuneiform bones. If one suspects an anterior compartment syndrome, this pulse should be palpated and compared with that of the opposite side. It should be remembered, however, that this pulse is normally absent in 10 per cent of the population.

Anteriorly and Anterolaterally

Lateral Malleolus, Calcaneus, Sinus Tarsi, and Cuboid Bone. The lateral malleolus is palpated at the distal extent of the fibula. One should note that the lateral malleolus extends further distally and lies more posterior than the medial malleolus. The examiner then stabilizes the calcaneus with one hand and palpates with the other hand as previously done. As the examiner moves distally from the lateral malleolus, the fingers lie along the lateral edge of the calcaneus, which is palpated with care. At the same time, the peroneal tendons can be palpated as they angle around the lateral malleolus to their insertion in the foot as well as to their origin in the peroneal muscles of the leg. The peroneal retinaculum, which holds the peroneal tendons in place as they angle around the lateral malleolus, is also palpated for tenderness (see Fig. 12–80). While palpating the retinaculum, the examiner should ask the patient to invert and evert the foot. If the peroneal retinaculum is torn, the peroneal tendons will often slip out of their groove or dislocate on eversion (see Fig. 12–44). While the lateral malleolus is being palpated, the lateral ligaments (calcaneofibular, pos-

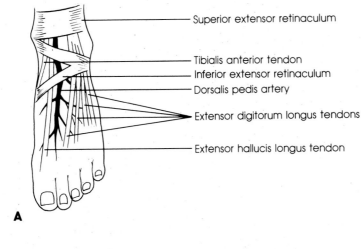

Superior extensor retinaculum

Tibialis anterior tendon
Inferior extensor retinaculum
Dorsalis pedis artery

Extensor digitorum longus tendons

Extensor hallucis longus tendon

A

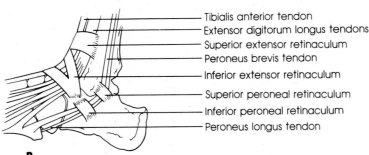

Tibialis anterior tendon
Extensor digitorum longus tendons
Superior extensor retinaculum
Peroneus brevis tendon
Inferior extensor retinaculum
Superior peroneal retinaculum
Inferior peroneal retinaculum
Peroneus longus tendon

B

FIGURE 12–80. Retinaculum of the ankle. (A) Anterior view. (B) Lateral view.

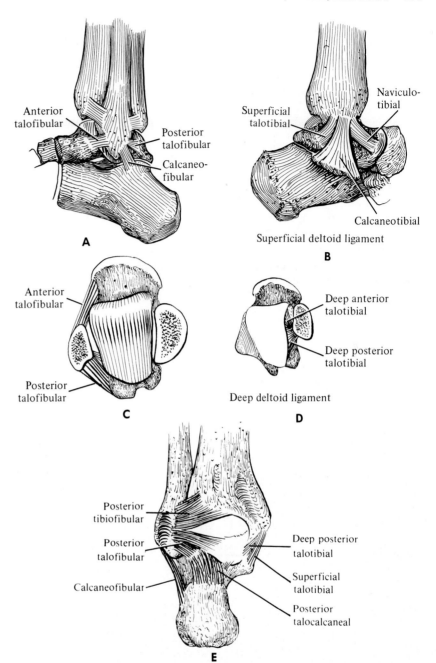

FIGURE 12–81. Ligaments of the ankle. (A) Ligaments of the lateral aspect. (B) Superior view of lateral ligaments. (C) Ligaments on the medial aspect (superficial deltoid ligaments). (D) Superior view of deep deltoid ligament on the medial aspect. (E) Posterior view of the ankle. (Adapted from Hamilton, W. C.: Anatomy: Traumatic Disorders of the Ankle. New York, Springer-Verlag, 1984, pp. 6–7.)

terior talofibular, and anterior talofibular) should be palpated for tenderness and swelling (Fig. 12–81).

Returning to the lateral malleolus, the examiner palpates its anterior surface and then moves anteriorly to the extensor digitorum muscle, the only muscle on the dorsum of the foot. If one palpates carefully and deeply through the muscle, a depression—the sinus tarsi—will be felt (Fig. 12–82). If the fingers are left in the depression and the foot is inverted, the neck of the talus will be felt and the fingers will be pushed deeper into the depression. Tenderness in this area may also be indicative of a sprain to the anterior talofibular ligament (see Fig. 12–82), the most frequently injured ligament in the lower leg, ankle, and foot.

The cuboid bone may be palpated in two ways. The examiner may move further distally from the sinus tarsi approximately one finger width and the fingers will lie over the cuboid bone, or the styloid process at the base of the fifth metatarsal bone may be palpated. As the examiner moves slightly proximally, the fingers will lie over the cuboid bone. In either case, the cuboid should be palpated on its dorsal, lateral, and plantar surfaces for signs of pathology.

Inferior Tibiofibular Joint, Tibia, and Muscles of the Leg. Starting at the lateral malleolus and following its anterior border, one should note any signs of pathology. The inferior tibiofibular joint is almost impossible to feel; however, it lies between

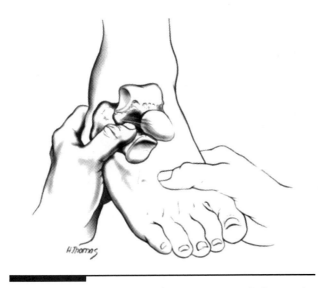

FIGURE 12–82. *Palpation of the sinus tarsi and the anterior talofibular ligament. (From Jahss, M. H.; Disorders of the Foot. Philadelphia, W. B. Saunders Co., 1991, p. 36.)*

the tibia and fibula and just superior to the talus. The examiner then follows the "shin" or crest of the tibia superiorly, looking for signs of pathology (e.g., shin splints, anterior tibial syndrome, or stress fracture). At the same time, the muscles of the lateral compartment (peronei) and anterior compartment (tibialis anterior and long extensors) should be carefully palpated for tenderness or swelling.

Posteriorly

The patient is then asked to lie in the prone position with the feet over the end of the examining table. The examiner palpates the following structures.

Calcaneus and Achilles Tendon. The examiner palpates the calcaneus and surrounding soft tissue for swelling (e.g., retrocalcaneal bursitis), exostosis (e.g., pump bump), or other signs of pathology. In

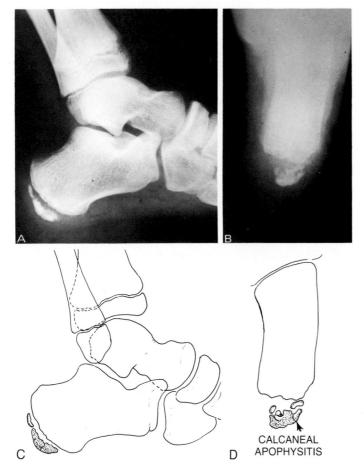

CALCANEAL
APOPHYSITIS

FIGURE 12–83. *Sever's disease (calcaneal apophysitis). Fragmentation of the posterior apophysis off the calcaneus, causing achillodynia. (A) Lateral roetgenogram of a 10-year-old boy with pain around the insertion of the Achilles tendon. (B) Axial view of the calcaneus. (C and D) Representations of the films above. (From Kelikian, H., and A. S. Kelikian: Disorders of the Ankle. Philadelphia, W. B. Saunders Co., 1985, p. 121.)*

children, one should take care palpating the calcaneal epiphysis for evidence of Sever's disease (calcaneal apophysitis) (Fig. 12–83). Moving proximally, one palpates the Achilles tendon, noting any swelling or thickening (e.g. tendinitis, retro-Achilles bursitis) or crepitation on movement. Any swelling from an intracapsular sprain of the ankle would also be evident posteriorly. Proximal to the Achilles tendon, the dome or superior surface of the calcaneus may also be palpated.

Posterior Compartment Muscles of the Leg. Moving further proximally, the examiner palpates the superficial (triceps surae) and deep (tibialis posterior and long flexors) posterior compartment muscles of the leg along their length for signs of pathology (e.g., strain or thrombosis).

Radiographic Examination

When viewing any radiograph, one should look for changes and differences between the right and left lower leg, ankle, and foot, such as osteoporosis or alterations in soft tissue, joint space, and alignment. Both weight-bearing and non–weight-bearing views should be taken. To be viewed properly, individual radiographs must be made of the ankle, lower leg, and foot (Fig. 12–84).[13, 32–34]

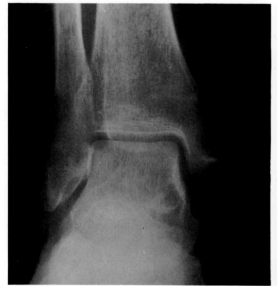

A

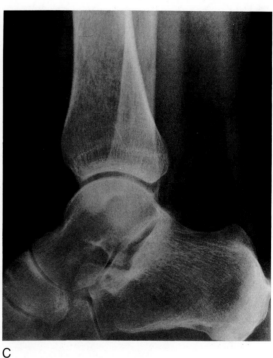

C

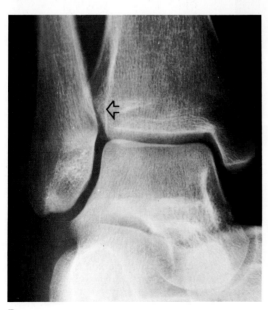

B

FIGURE 12–84. *Roentgenograms of normal ankle. (A) Anteroposterior view. (B) Internal oblique (mortise) view. Arrow demonstrates alignment of lateral talus with posterior cortex of tibia. (C) Lateral view. (From Weissman, B. N. W., and C. B. Sledge: Orthopedic Radiology. Philadelphia, W. B. Saunders Co., 1986, pp. 590–591.)*

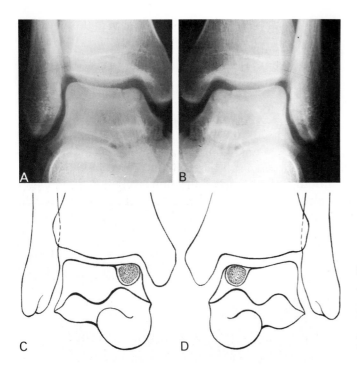

FIGURE 12–85. Bilateral osteochondritis dissecans of the talus. (A and B) Oblique anteroposterior films of the right and left ankles of a 29-year-old man without any antecedent trauma. (C and D) Illustrations of the roentgenograms above. (From Kelikian, H., and A. S. Kelikian: Disorders of the Ankle. Philadelphia, W. B. Saunders Co., 1985, p. 726.)

Anteroposterior View of the Ankle. The examiner notes the shape, position (whether the medial clear space is normal), and texture of the bones and determines whether there is any fractured or new subperiosteal bone. In addition, the configuration, congruity and inclination of the talar dome in relation to the tibial vault above it should be noted. If there are epiphyseal plates present, the examiner should note whether they appear normal. Any in-crease or decrease in joint space, greater reduction of the tibial overlap, widening of the interosseous space, and greater visibility of the digital fossa should also be noted.

One should also look for osteochondritis dissecans of the talus (medial side) (Fig. 12–85).[12]

Mortise View of Ankle. With this view, the ankle mortise and distal tibiofibular joint can be visualized. To obtain this view, which is a modification

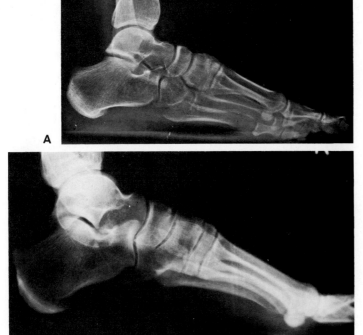

FIGURE 12–86. Lateral view of the foot. (A) Weight-bearing posture. Note the flattened soft-tissue pads beneath the heel and in the front part of the foot and that the first metatarsal head is elevated by the sesamoids beneath it. (B) Non–weight-bearing posture. The bony alignment and configuration are satisfactory, but the lack of resistance from the floor to the body weight permits variations, which make such views unsatisfactory for determining foot contours. (From Jahss, M. H.: Disorders of the Foot. Philadelphia, W. B. Saunders Co., 1991, pp. 68, 72.)

of the anteroposterior view, the foot and leg are medially rotated 15 to 30°.

Lateral View of Leg, Ankle, and Foot. With this view, the examiner notes the shape, position, and texture of bones, including the tibial tubercle (Fig. 12–86). Any fracture, new subperiosteal bone, or bone spurs should be noted (Fig. 12–87). One must note whether the epiphyseal lines are normal and whether there is any increase or decrease in joint space. Although this view clearly shows the talus and calcaneus, there is overlap of the midtarsal, metatarsal, and phalangeal structures. When view-

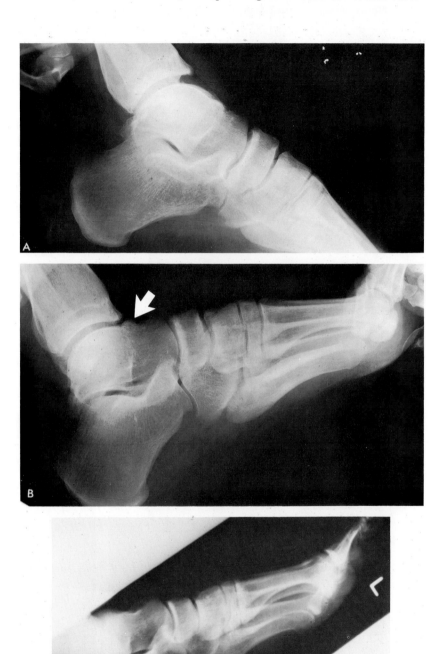

FIGURE 12–87. (A) Talotibial spurs. (B) Impingement occurs when the foot is dorsiflexed. (C) Heel spur. (A and B from O'Donoghue, D. H.; Treatment of Injuries to Athletes, 4th ed. Philadelphia, W. B. Saunders Co., 1984, p. 627.)

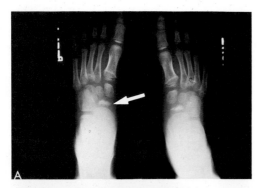

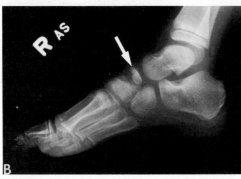

FIGURE 12–88. *Radiographs of the foot. (A) Bilateral involvement with condensation in the early stage of Köhler's disease. (B) The same foot 2 years later shows restoration of contour on the way to completion. (From Jahss, M. H.: Disorders of the Foot. Philadelphia, W. B. Saunders Co., 1991, p. 608.)*

ing lateral films, the examiner must also be aware of Sever's disease and Köhler's disease (Fig. 12–88).

Dorsoplanar View of the Foot. As with the previous view, the examiner should note the position, shape, and texture of the bones of the foot (Fig. 12–89). The presence of a metatarsus primus varus and conditions such as Köhler's disease should be noted. The dorsoplanar view is primarily used to project the forefoot.

Medial Oblique View of the Foot. This view is often taken because it gives the clearest picture of the tarsal bones and joints and the metatarsal shafts and bases (Fig. 12–90). The medial oblique view shows any pathology in the calcaneocuboid joint as well as the presence of a calcaneonavicular bar (Figs. 12–91 and 12–92).

Stress Oblique View. The examiner should note whether there is a calcaneonavicular bar or abnormality of the calcaneus or navicular bones.

Stress Film. The stress radiograph is used to compare the two ankles for integrity of the ligaments (Figs. 12–93 and 12–94).[17, 23, 35] With the application of an eversion or abduction stress, tilting of the talus more than 10° is considered pathological. An increase in the medial clear space (space between medial malleolus and talus) of more than 2 to 3 mm is considered pathological and usually indicates insufficiency of the deltoid ligament, especially the

Text continued on page 505

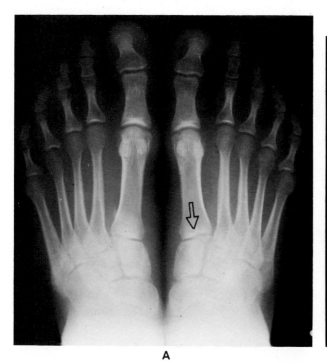

A

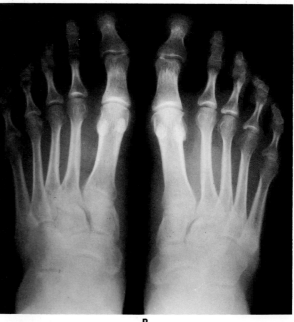

B

FIGURE 12–89. *Dorsoplanar view of the foot. (A) Weight-bearing posture. The cuneiform–first metatarsal joint is clearly seen (arrow), as are the transverse intertarsal joints, which is in contrast to the non–weight-bearing roentgenograms. (B) Non–weight-bearing posture. The joint between the medial and middle cuneiforms is clearly seen. The other midtarsal joints are obscure. (From Jahss, M. H.: Disorders of the Foot. Philadelphia, W. B. Saunders Co., 1991, pp. 69, 71.)*

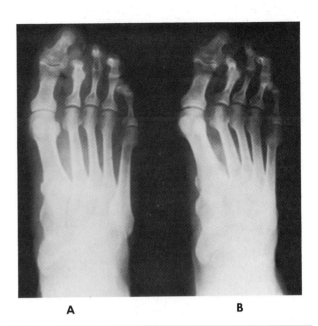

A   B

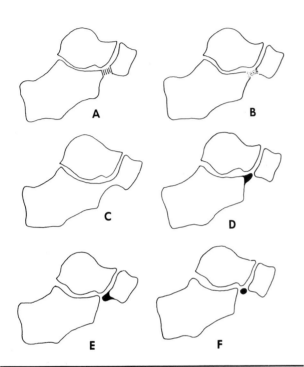

FIGURE 12–90. Metatarsals and phalanges. (A) With the beam centered directly over the foot, the metatarsal bases and adjacent tarsal bones are shown much more clearly than in B. (B) This is half of the examination of both feet with the tube centered between the feet. Marked overlap of metatarsal bases and adjacent tarsal bones is seen. The midtarsal joint can be seen as a continuous line or cyma. (From Klenerman, L.: The Foot and Its Disorders. Boston, Blackwell Scientific Publications, 1982, p. 306.)

FIGURE 12–91. Diagrammatic representation of the types of union. (A) Fibrous. (B) Cartilaginous. (C) Osseous. (D) Prominent process on the calcaneus. (E) Prominent process on the navicular. (F) Separate calcaneonavicular ossicle (calcaneum secondarium). (From Klenerman, L.: The Foot and Its Disorders. Boston, Blackwell Scientific Publications, 1982, p. 336.)

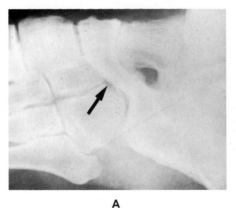
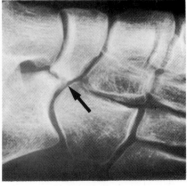

A   B

FIGURE 12–92. Calcaneonavicular coalition or bar. (A) Total bony union as well as bony breaks on the upper surfaces of the navicular and talus. The head of the talus may be small. (B) Fibrous or cartilaginous, rather than osseous, union between the bones is seen with osteoarthritic changes of the opposing bone surfaces and an enlarged navicular. (From Klenerman, L.: The Foot and Its Disorders. Boston, Blackwell Scientific Publications, 1982, p. 340.)

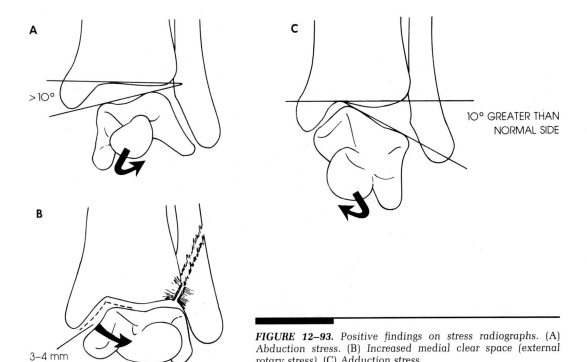

FIGURE 12–93. Positive findings on stress radiographs. (A) Abduction stress. (B) Increased medial clear space (external rotary stress). (C) Adduction stress.

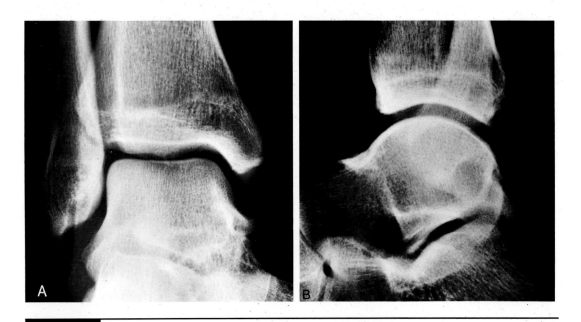

FIGURE 12–94. Abnormal stress views: anterior talofibular and calcaneofibular ligament tears. Anteroposterior (A) and lateral (B) views of the right ankle showing hypertrophic lipping from the anterior tibia and talus. The syndesmosis is slightly wide.

Illustration continued on opposite page

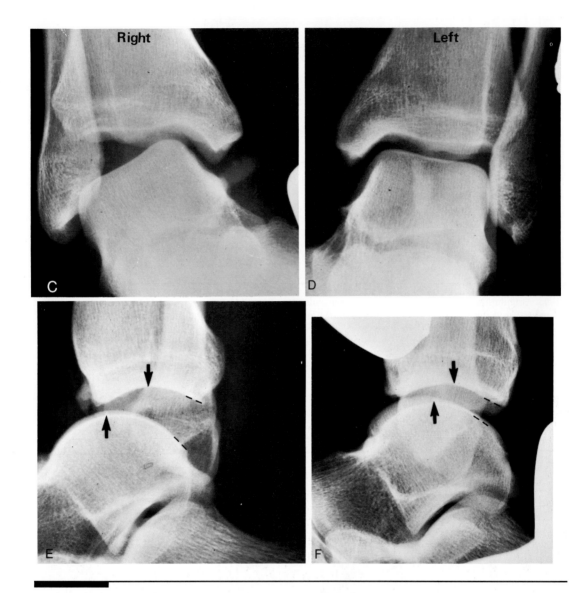

FIGURE 12–94 Continued Comparison varus stress views of the right (C) and left (D) ankles show abnormal talar tilt on the right, particularly compared with the normal left side. This is diagnostic of an anterior talofibular ligament tear on the right, with or without a calcaneofibular ligament tear. The anterior drawer test is abnormal on the right (E) compared with the left (F). Comparison can be made by noting the anterior shift of the midtalus in relation to the midtibia (arrows) on each side, the loss of parallelism of the subchondral cortices on the right, or the marked widening of the posterior joint space (lines) on the abnormal compared with the normal side. This is consistent with an anterior talofibular ligament tear on the right. (From Weissman, B. N. W., and C. B. Sledge: Orthopedic Radiology. Philadelphia, W. B. Saunders Co., 1986, p. 600.).

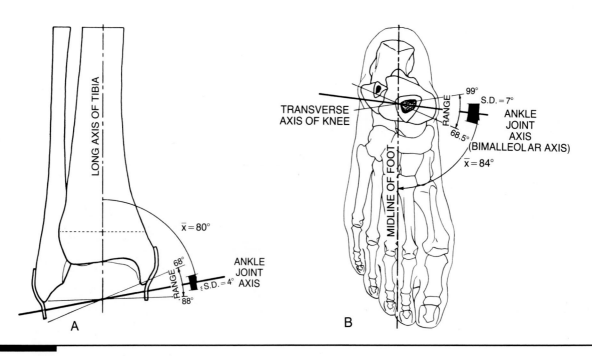

FIGURE 12–95. Orientation of the ankle joint axis. Mean values measure (A) 80° from a vertical reference and (B) 84° from the longitudinal reference of the foot. (Adapted from Novick, A.: Anatomy and biomechanics. In Hunt, G. C. (ed.): Physical Therapy of the Foot and Ankle. New York, Churchill Livingstone, 1988; and Isman, R. E., and V. T. Inman: Anthropometric Studies of the Human Foot and Ankle: Technical Report No. 58. University of California, San Francisco, 1968.)

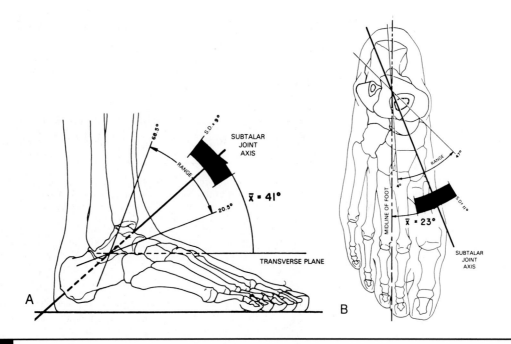

FIGURE 12–96. Orientation of the subtalar joint axis. Mean values measure (A) 41° from the transverse plane and (B) 23° medially from the longitudinal reference of the foot. (Adapted from Novick, A.: Anatomy and biomechanics. In Hunt, G. C. (ed.): Physical Therapy of the Foot and Ankle. New York, Churchill Livingstone, 1988; and Isman, R. E., and V. T. Inman: Anthropometric Studies of the Human Foot and Ankle: Technical Report No. 58. University of California, San Francisco, 1968.)

tibiotalar ligament. Instability may also be demonstrated by widening of the syndesmosis or the mortise. An inversion or adduction stress causing 8 to 10° more movement on one side than the other is considered pathological and is indicative of torn lateral ligaments. If the talus has not moved or it is fixed but its distal end is unduly prominent, subtalar instability is suggested.

Measurements on Plain Roentgenograms. Plain radiographs may be used to measure different angles and axes. For example, Figure 12–95 shows the ankle joint axis and Figure 12–96 shows the subtalar joint axis. Figures 12–97 and 12–98 show various angles measured in the ankle and foot.

Arthrograms. Arthrograms of the ankle are indicated when there is chronic ligament laxity or indications of loose body or osteochondritis dissecans (Figs. 12–99 and 12–100).[12] Leakage of the contrast medium indicates tearing of the joint capsule or capsular ligaments. Normally, the talocrural joint will admit only approximately 6 ml of contrast medium.

CT Scans. CT scans are useful for determining the relationships among the bones as well as for giving a view of the relation between bony and soft tissues (Figs. 12–101 and 12–102).

MRI. MRI is especially useful for delineating bony and soft tissues around the ankle and foot and is a technique that involves nonionization (Figs. 12–103 and 12–104).

Bone Scans. Bone scans are used in the lower limb, ankle, and foot to diagnose stress fractures, primarily those of the tibia (Fig. 12–105) and metatarsal bones.

Abnormal Ossicles or Accessory Bones. Because the foot often exhibits abnormal ossicles, this may lead to incorrect interpretation of films (Fig. 12–Text continued on page 510

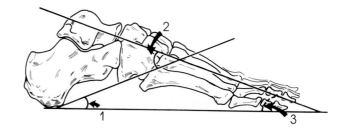
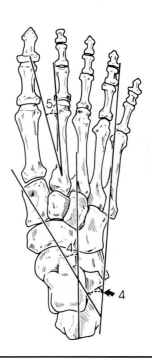

FIGURE 12–97. *Angles of the foot. (1) Lateral talocalcaneal angle. (2) Calcaneal inclination angle. (3) Talar declination angle. (4) Talocalcaneal angle (two methods). (5) Metatarsus adductus angle.*

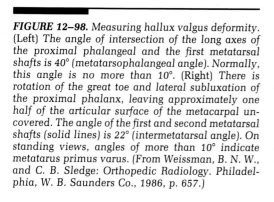

FIGURE 12–98. *Measuring hallux valgus deformity. (Left) The angle of intersection of the long axes of the proximal phalangeal and the first metatarsal shafts is 40° (metatarsophalangeal angle). Normally, this angle is no more than 10°. (Right) There is rotation of the great toe and lateral subluxation of the proximal phalanx, leaving approximately one half of the articular surface of the metacarpal uncovered. The angle of the first and second metatarsal shafts (solid lines) is 22° (intermetatarsal angle). On standing views, angles of more than 10° indicate metatarus primus varus. (From Weissman, B. N. W., and C. B. Sledge: Orthopedic Radiology. Philadelphia, W. B. Saunders Co., 1986, p. 657.)*

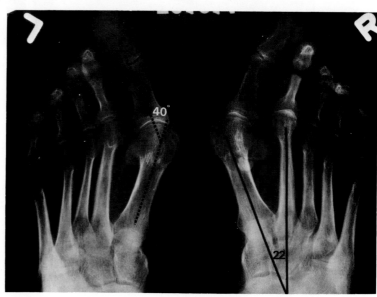

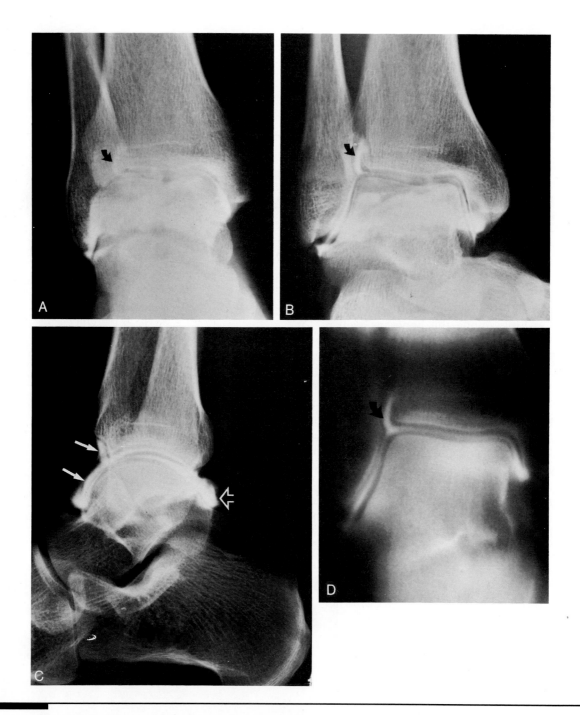

FIGURE 12–99. Normal positive-contrast ankle arthrogram. Anteroposterior (A), internal oblique (mortise; B), and lateral (C) views and a tomogram (D) in the internal oblique projection show contrast agent coating the articular surfaces and filling normally present anteriorly (white arrows), posteriorly (open arrow), and in syndesmotic (black arrows) recesses. There is no extension of contrast medium into the soft tissue medially or laterally. (From Weissman, B. N. W., and C. B. Sledge: Orthopedic Radiology. Philadelphia, W. B. Saunders Co., 1986, p. 596.)

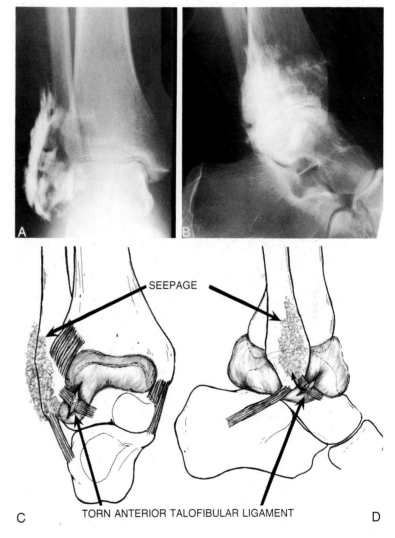

FIGURE 12–100. Contrast arthrography showing acute tear of the anterior tibiofibular ligament. (A) Anteroposterior arthrogram of the right ankle 14 hours after the injury showing extravasation of the contrast medium in front of and around the lateral aspect of the fibula. (B) Lateral view of the same. (C and D) Illustrations of the arthrograms above. (From Kelikian, H., and A. S. Kelikian: Disorders of the Ankle. Philadelphia, W. B. Saunders Co., 1985, p. 143.)

SEEPAGE

TORN ANTERIOR TALOFIBULAR LIGAMENT

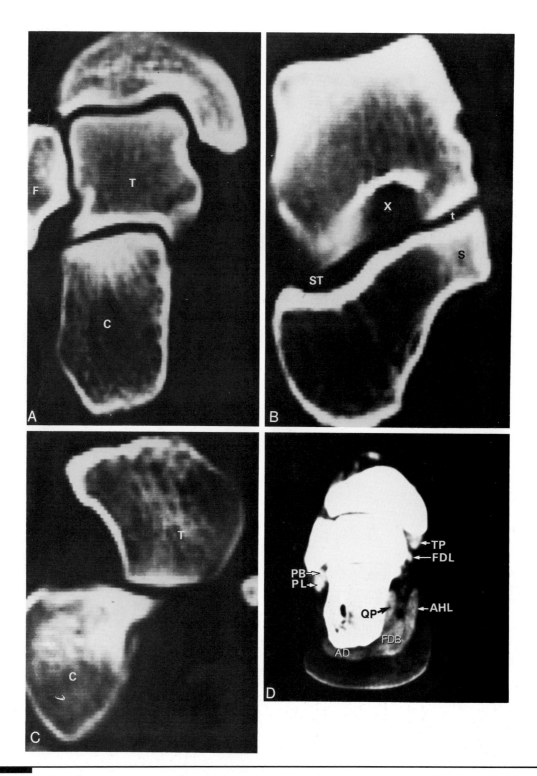

FIGURE 12–101. Normal CT anatomy. (A) Coronal section through the ankle and subtalar joint; T = talus, C = calcaneus, F = fibula. (B) Further anteriorly, the sustentaculum tali (S), the site of insertion of the talocalcaneal ligament (X), the subtalar joint (ST), and the midtalocalcaneonavicular joint (t) are seen. (C) Anterior to the sustentaculum tali, the talus (T) and the calcaneus (C) are seen. (D) The peroneus brevis (PB), peroneus longus (PL), posterior tibial (TP), and flexor digitorum longus (FDL) are seen. AHL = Abductor hallucis longus, FDB = flexor digitorum brevis, QP = quadratus plantae, AD = abductor digiti quinti pedis. This scan is at the level of the posterior aspect of the sustentaculum tali. (From Weissman, B. N. W., and C. B. Sledge: Orthopedic Radiology. Philadelphia, W. B. Saunders Co., 1986, p. 632.)

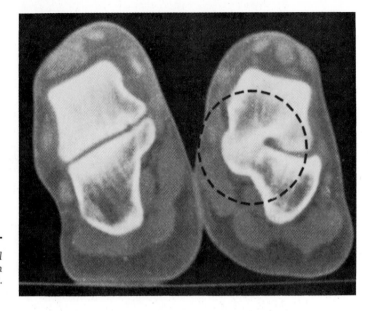

FIGURE 12–102. *Coronal CT view showing talocalcaneal coalition. (From Rettig, A. C., et al.: Radiographic evaluation of foot and ankle injuries in the athlete. Clin. Sports Med. 6:914, 1987.)*

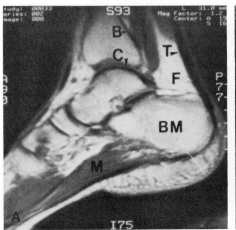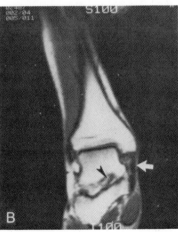

FIGURE 12–103. *MRI sagittal and coronal images of the ankle. (A) Sagittal projection— note the white bone marrow (BM), white subcutaneous fat (F), black tendons (T), black ligaments, gray muscles (M), gray articular cartilage (C), and black cortical bone (B). (B) Coronal projection—note the black appearance of the deltoid ligament (white arrow) and interosseous ligament (black arrowhead) between the talus and calcaneus. (From Kingston, S.: Magnetic resonance imaging of the ankle and foot. Clin. Sports Med. 7:19, 1988.)*

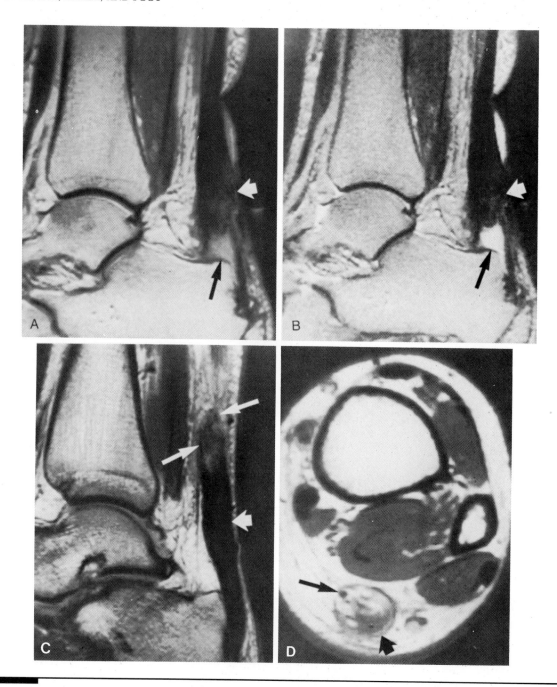

FIGURE 12–104. *MRI showing partial Achilles tendon tear. (A) Sagittal, proton-density and (B) T2-weighted MRI reveals a large tear at the Achilles insertion with intratendinous fluid (long arrow) and fraying and thickening of the distal tendon (short arrow). (C) Complete Achilles tendon tear. Sagittal, proton-density MRI reveals disruption of the Achilles tendon (long arrows) and thickening of its distal portion (short arrows). (D) On an axial, T1-weighted MRI, only gray granulation tissue is seen within the paratenon (short arrow). The intact plantaris tendon passes along the medial border of the paratenon (long arrow). (From Kerr, R., et al.: Magnetic resonance imaging of foot and ankle trauma. Orthop. Clin. North Am. 21:593, 1990.)*

106). These bones are parts of prominences of various tarsal bones that for some reason (e.g., fracture or a secondary ossification center) separated from the normal bone.[36] A sesamoid bone, on the other hand, is incorporated into the substance of a tendon, with one surface articulating with the adjacent

bones. A sesamoid bone moves with the tendon and is found over bony prominences or where the tendon makes a change in direction. In addition to the normal sesamoid bones under the big toe, sesamoid bones may also be found in the tendons of peroneus longus and tibialis posterior. Abnormal ossicles are

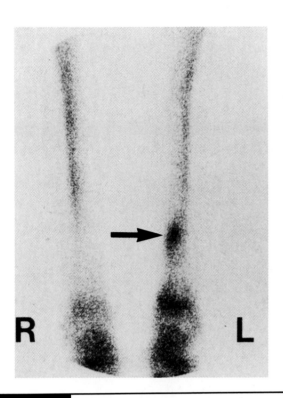

FIGURE 12–105. *Bone scan of lower tibia. Arrow indicates area of increased isotope uptake ("hot spot"), which is consistent with a stress-related lesion. Normal x-rays were negative. (From Williams, A., et al.: Imaging of Sports Injuries. London, Bailliere Tindall, 1989, pp. 135,137.)*

seen in club feet (Fig. 12–108). Although not all of the bones are present at birth, a series of films will show differences when compared with films of normal feet.

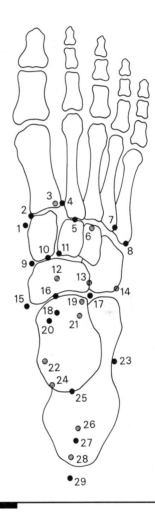

more likely to occur in the foot than anywhere else in the body. Some of the more common ossicles include the following:

1. Os trigonium (separate posterior talar tubercle).
2. Os tibiale externum (separate navicular tuberosity).
3. Bipartite medial cuneiform (into upper and lower halves).
4. Os vesalianum (separate tuberosity of the base of the fifth metatarsal).
5. Os sustentaculi (separate part of the sustentaculum tali).
6. Os supranaviculare (dorsum of the talonavicular joint).

Films Showing Bone Development. Like the bones of the hand, the bones of the foot form within a certain time period (Fig. 12–107). However, because the foot is subjected to greater forces and environmental effects than the hand, it is not usually used to determine skeletal age. X-rays of the foot will often show the developing bone deformities

FIGURE 12–106. *Accessory tarsal bones. (1) Os sesamoideum tibialis anterior, (2) Os cuneo-metatarsale I tibiale, (3) Os cuneo-metatarsale I plantare, (4) Os intermetatarsale I, (5) Os cuneo-metatarsale II dorsale, (6) Os unci, (7) Os intermetatarsale IV, (8) Os Vesalianum, (9) Os paracuneiforme, (10) Os naviculocuneiforme I dorsale, (11) Os intercuneiforme, (12) Os sesamoideum tibialis posterior (according to Trolle, this may be the same as No. 15), (13) Os cuboideum secundarium, (14) Os peroneum, (15) Os tibiale (externum), (16) Os talonaviculare dorsale, (17) Os calcaneus secundarius, (18) Os supertalare, (19) Os trochleae, (20) Os talotibiale dorsale, (21) Os in sinu tarsi, (22) Os sustentaculi proprium, (23) Calcaneus accessorius, (24) Os talocalcaneare posterior, (25) Os trigonum, (26) Os aponeurosis plantaris, (27) Os supracalcaneum, (28) Os subcalcaneum, (29) Os tendinis Achillis. (From Klenerman, L.: The Foot and Its Disorders. Boston, Blackwell Scientific Publications, 1982, p. 361.)*

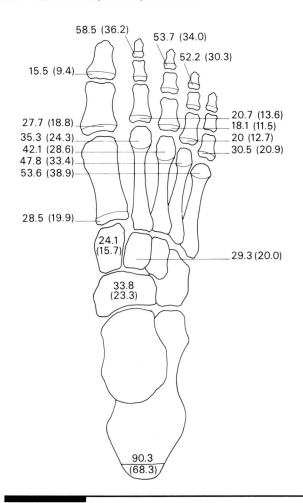

58.5 (36.2)
53.7 (34.0)
52.2 (30.3)
15.5 (9.4)
27.7 (18.8)
35.3 (24.3)
42.1 (28.6)
47.8 (33.4)
53.6 (38.9)
20.7 (13.6)
18.1 (11.5)
20 (12.7)
30.5 (20.9)
28.5 (19.9)
24.1 (15.7)
29.3 (20.0)
33.8 (23.3)
90.3 (68.3)

FIGURE 12–107. *Anteroposterior diagram of the foot showing the times of appearance (in months) of the centers of ossification for boys (girls in brackets). (From Hoerr, et al. (1962), with kind permission of Charles C Thomas, Springfield, IL.)*

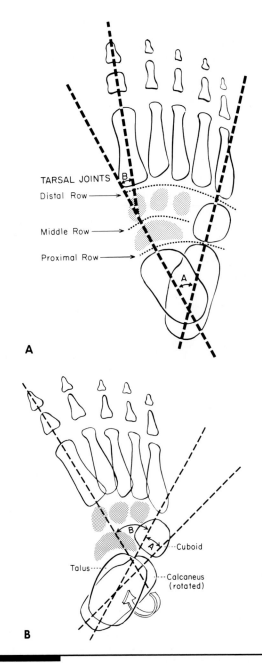

TARSAL JOINTS
Distal Row
Middle Row
Proximal Row
B
A

A

B
A
Cuboid
Talus
Calcaneus (rotated)

B

FIGURE 12–108. *X-ray illustrations of the foot. (A) Representation of the normal foot. The cuboid blocks medial movement of the foot at the midrow of tarsal joints because of its unique location. It alone occupies a position in both rows of tarsal joints. The talocalcaneal angle (angle A) is measured by drawing lines through the long axis of both of these bones. One should attempt to be as accurate as possible in making these measurements. The normal range for this measurement is 20 to 40° in the young child. The talo–first metatarsal angle (angle B) is measured by drawing lines through the long axis of the talus and along the long axis of the first metatarsal. The normal range is 0 to −20°; (B) Hindfoot varus, as manifest by a decreased talocalcaneal angle (angle A), and talonavicular subluxation, as manifest by a talocalcaneal angle of less than 15° and a talo–first metatarsal angle (angle B) of more than 15°. Talonavicular subluxation occurs through the medial movement of three bones, which move as a unit. The navicular, cuboid, and calcaneus move medially through the combined movements of medial translation and supination of the proximal tarsal bones, whereas the calcaneus inverts beneath the talus. (From Simons, G. W.: Orthop. Clin. North Am. 9:189, 1978.)*

PRÉCIS OF THE LOWER LEG, ANKLE, AND FOOT ASSESSMENT*

History
Observation
Examination
  Active movements (weight bearing—standing)
    Plantar flexion
    Dorsiflexion
    Supination
    Pronation
    Toe extension
    Toe flexion
  Active movements (non–weight bearing—sitting or supine lying)
    Plantar flexion
    Dorsiflexion
    Supination
    Pronation
    Toe extension
    Toe flexion
    Toe abduction
    Toe adduction
  Special tests (sitting)
  Passive movements (supine lying)
    Plantar flexion at the talocrural (ankle) joint
    Dorsiflexion at the talocrural joint
    Inversion at the subtalar joint
    Eversion at the subtalar joint
    Adduction at the midtarsal joints
    Abduction at the midtarsal joints
    Flexion of the toes
    Extension of the toes
    Adduction of the toes
    Abduction of the toes
  Resisted isometric movements (supine lying)
    Knee flexion
    Plantar flexion
    Dorsiflexion
    Supination
    Pronation
    Toe extension
    Toe flexion
  Special tests (supine lying)
  Reflexes and cutaneous distribution (supine lying)
  Joint play movements (supine and side lying)
    Long-axis extension
    Anteroposterior glide
    Talar rock
    Side tilt
    Rotation
    Side glide
    Tarsal bone mobility
  Palpation (supine lying and prone lying)
  Special tests (prone lying)
  Functional assessment (standing)
  Special tests (standing)
  Radiographic examination

After any examination, the patient should always be warned of the possibility of exacerbation of symptoms as a result of assessment.

*The précis is shown in an order that will limit the amount of moving that the patient has to do but ensure that all necessary structures are tested. It does not follow the order of the text.

CASE STUDIES

When doing these case studies, the examiner should list the appropriate questions to be asked and why they are being asked, what to look for and why, and what things should be tested and why. Depending on the patient's answers (and the examiner should consider different responses), several possible causes of the patient's problem may become evident (examples are given in parentheses). If so, a differential diagnosis chart should be made. The examiner can then decide how different diagnoses may affect the treatment plan.

1. A 38-year-old man ruptured his Achilles tendon 4 weeks earlier and had it surgically repaired. The cast has been removed. Describe your assessment plan for this patient.
2. A 24-year-old woman presents at your clinic with a painful left foot. There is no history of trauma; however, the pain has been present for approximately 6 years and has become worse in the last year. Describe your assessment plan for this patient (Morton's neuroma versus plantar fasciitis).
3. A 59-year-old man comes to you complaining of pain in his right calf and some numbness in his right foot. He also complains of some stiffness in his back. Describe your assessment plan for this patient (lumbar spondylosis versus tibial nerve palsy).
4. A 10-year-old boy recently had a triple arthrodesis for talipes equino varus. The cast has now been removed. Describe your assessment plan for this patient.
5. A 16-year-old female volleyball player come to you complaining of left ankle pain and difficulty walking after she stepped on another player's foot and went over on her ankle. The injury occurred 30 minutes ago and her ankle is swollen. Describe your assessment plan for this patient (malleolar fracture versus ligament sprain).
6. A 25-year-old woman presents telling you that she is training for a marathon but that every time she increases her mileage, her right foot hurts. Some time ago, someone told her she had a cavus foot. Describe your assessment plan for this patient.
7. Parents bring a 2-year-old boy to you expressing concern that the child appears to have flat feet and "pigeon toes." Describe your assessment plan for this patient.
8. A 32-year-old woman comes to you complaining of ankle pain. She states she sprained it 9 months earlier and thought it was better. However, she has now returned to training, and the ankle is bothering her. Describe your assessment plan for this patient (proprioceptive loss versus hypermobility).

REFERENCES

CITED REFERENCES

1. Kleiger, B.: Mechanisms of ankle injury. Orthop. Clin. North Am. 5:127, 1974.
2. Hunt, G. C., and R. S. Brocato: Gait and foot pathomechanics. *In* Hunt, G. C. (ed.): Physical Therapy of the Foot and Ankle. Clinics in Physical Therapy. Edinburgh, Churchill Livingstone, 1988.
3. Brown, L. P., and P. Yavorsky: Locomotor biomechanics and pathomechanics: A review. J. Orthop. Sports Phys. Ther. 9:3, 1987.

4. McPoil, T. G., and R. S. Brocato: The foot and ankle: Bio-mechanical evaluation and treatment. In Gould, J. A. (ed.): Orthopedic and Sports Physical Therapy. St. Louis, C. V. Mosby Co., 1990.
5. Root, M. L., W. P. Orien, and J. H. Weed: Normal and Abnormal Function of the Foot. Los Angeles, Clinical Bio-mechanics Corp., 1977.
6. McMaster, M. J.: The pathogenesis of hallux rigidus. J. Bone Joint Surg. 60B:82, 1978.
7. Durman, D. C.: Metatarsus primus varus and hallux valgus. Arch. Surg. 74:128, 1957.
8. Price, G. F. W.: Metatarsus primus varus—including various clinicoradiologic features of the female foot. Clin. Orthop. Relat. Res. 145:217, 1979.
9. Kapandji, I. A.: The Physiology of the Joints, vol. 2. Lower Limb. New York, Churchill Livingstone, 1970.
10. Lipscomb, A. B., and A. A. Ibrahim: Acute peroneal com-partment syndrome in the well conditioned athlete. Am. J. Sports Med. 5:154, 1977.
11. Williams, P. L., and R. Warwick (eds.): Gray's Anatomy, 36th British ed. Philadelphia, W. B. Saunders Co., 1980.
12. Kelikian, H., and A. S. Kelikian: Disorders of the Ankle. Philadelphia, W. B. Saunders Co., 1985.
13. Palmer, M. L., and M. Epler: Clinical Assessment Procedures in Physical Therapy. Philadelphia, J. B. Lippincott Co., 1990.
14. Jahss, M. H.: Disorders of the Foot. Philadelphia, W. B. Saunders Co., 1982.
15. Hamilton, J. J., and L. K. Ziemer: Functional Anatomy of the Human Ankle and Foot. American Association of Orthopedic Surgeons, Symposium on the Foot and Ankle. St. Louis, C. V. Mosby Co., 1983.
16. Hyslop, G. H.: Injuries of the deep and superficial peroneal nerves complicating ankle sprain. Am. J. Surg. 51:436, 1941.
17. Kaplan, P. E., and W. T. Kernahan: Tarsal tunnel syndrome: An electrodiagnostic and surgical correlation. J. Bone Joint Surg. 63A:96, 1981.
18. Mubarak, S., and A. Hargens: Exertional compartment syn-dromes. American Association of Orthopedic Surgeons, Sym-posium on the Foot and Leg in Running Sports. St. Louis, C. V. Mosby Co., 1982.
19. Reneman, R. S.: The anterior and the lateral compartmental syndrome of the leg due to the intensive use of muscles. Clin. Orthop. Relat. Res. 113:69, 1975.
20. Freeman, M. A. R., M. R. E. Dean, and I. W. F. Hanham: The etiology and prevention of functional instability of the foot. J. Bone Joint Surg. 47B:678, 1965.
21. Roy, S., and R. Irvin: Sports Medicine: Prevention, Evalua-tion, Management and Rehabilitation. Englewood Cliffs, N. J., Prentice-Hall, 1983.
22. Staheli, L. T.: Rotational problems of the lower extremities. Orthop. Clin. North Am. 18:503, 1987.
23. Colter, J. M.: Lateral ligamentous injuries of the ankle. In Hamilton, W. C. (ed.): Traumatic Disorders of the Ankle. New York, Springer-Verlag, 1984.
24. Hamilton, W. C.: Anatomy. In Hamilton, W. C. (ed.): Trau-matic Disorders of the Ankle. New York, Springer-Verlag, 1984.
25. Rasmussen, O., and I. Tovberg-Jansen: Anterolateral rota-tional instability in the ankle joint. Acta Orthop. Scand. 52:99, 1981.
26. Gungor, T.: A test for ankle instability: Brief report. J. Bone Joint Surg. 70B:487, 1988.
27. Mennell, J. M.: Foot Pain. Boston, Little, Brown & Co., 1969.
28. Wallace, L. A.: Limb length difference and back pain. In Grieve, G. P. (ed.): Modern Manual Therapy of the Vertebral Column. Edinburgh, Churchill Livingstone, 1986.
29. Thompson, T., and J. Doherty: Spontaneous rupture of the tendon of Achilles: A new clinical diagnostic test. Anat. Res. 158:126, 1967.
30. Blood, S. D.: Treatment of the sprained ankle. J. Am. Osteo-pathic Assoc. 79:680, 1980.
31. Kaltenborn, F. M.: Mobilization of the Extremity Joints. Oslo, Olaf Norlis Bokhandel, 1980.
32. Black, H.: Roentgenographic considerations. Am. J. Sports Med. 5:238, 1977.
33. Hoffman, J. D.: Radiography of the ankle. In Hamilton, W. C.

(ed.): Traumatic Disorders of the Ankle. New York, Springer-Verlag, 1984.
34. Renton, P., and W. J. Stripp: The radiology and radiography of the foot. In Klenerman, L. (ed): The Foot and Its Disorders, 2nd ed. Boston, Blackwell Scientific Publications, 1982.
35. Rubin, G., and M. Witten: The talar-tilt angle and the fibular collateral ligaments: A method for the determination of talar-tilt. J. Bone Joint Surg. 42:311, 1960.
36. Klenerman, L.: Examination of the foot. In Klenerman, L. (ed.): The Foot and Its Disorders, 2nd ed. Boston, Blackwell Scientific Publications, 1982.

GENERAL REFERENCES

American Academy of Orthopedic Surgeons: Athletic Training and Sports Medicine. Chicago, AAOS, 1984.
American Orthopaedic Association: Manual of Orthopaedic Sur-gery. Chicago, 1972.
Anderson, K. J., J. F. Lecocq, and E. A. Lecocq: Recurrent anterior subluxation of the ankle joint. J. Bone Joint Surg. 34A:853, 1952.
Basmajian, J. V., and G. Stecko: The role of muscles in arch support of the foot. J. Bone Joint Surg. 45A:1184, 1964.
Beetham, W. P., H. F. Polley, C. H. Slocumb, and W. F. Weaver: Physical Examination of the Joints. Philadelphia, W. B. Saun-ders Co., 1965.
Berridge, F. R., and J. G. Bonnin: The radiographic examination of the ankle joint including arthrography. J. Surg. Gynecol. Obstet. 79:383, 1944.
Bojsen-Moller, F.: Anatomy of the forefoot: Normal and patho-logic. Clin. Orthop. Relat. Res. 1422:10, 1979.
Cailliet, R.: Foot and Ankle Pain. Philadelphia, F. A. Davis Co., 1968.
Campbell, J. W., and V. T. Inman: Treatment of plantar fasciitis and calcaneal spurs with the UC-BL shoe insert. Clin. Orthop. Relat. Res. 103:57, 1974.
Carroll, N. C., R. McMurtry, and S. F. Leete: The pathoanatomy of congenital club-foot. Orthop. Clin. North Am. 9:225, 1978.
Case, W. S.: Ankle injuries. In Sanders, B. (ed.): Sports Physical Therapy. Norwalk, Conn., Appleton & Lange, 1990.
Catterall, A.: A method of assessment of the clubfoot deformity. Clin. Orthop. Relat. Res. 264:48–53, 1991.
Chen, S. C.: Ankle injuries. In Helal, B., J. B. King, and W. J. Grange (eds.): Sports Injuries: Their Treatment. London, Chap-man and Hall Medical, 1986
Clarkson, H. M., and G. B. Gilewich: Musculoskeletal Assess-ment—Joint Range of Motion and Manual Muscle Strength. Baltimore, Williams & Wilkins Co., 1989.
Close, J. R.: Some applications of the functional anatomy of the ankle joint. J. Bone Joint Surg. 38A:761, 1956.
Close, J. R., V. T. Inman, P. M. Poor, and F. N. Todd: The function of the subtalar joint. Clin. Orthop. Relat. Res. 50:159, 1967.
Cooper, D. L., and J. Fair: Managing the pronated foot. Phys. Sportsmed. 5:131, 1979.
Cox, J. S., and R. L. Brand: Evaluation and treatment of lateral ankle sprains. Phys. Sportsmed. 5:51, 1977.
Cyriax, J.: Textbook of Orthopaedic Medicine, vol. 1, 8th ed. Diagnosis of Soft Tissue Lesions. London, Bailliere Tindall, 1982.
Debrunner, H. U.: Orthopaedic Diagnosis. London, E & S Living-stone, 1970.
DeCarlo, M. S., and R. W. Talbot: Evaluation of ankle joint proprioception following injection of the anterior talofibular ligament. J. Orthop. Sports Phys. Ther. 8:70, 1986.
DeValentine, S.: Evaluation and treatment of ankle fractures. Clin. Podiatr. 2:325, 1985.
Donatelli, R.: Abnormal biomechanics of the foot and ankle. J. Orthop. Sports Phys. Ther. 9:11, 1987.
Ebbetts J.: Manipulation of the foot. Physiother. 57:194, 1971.
Edgar, M. A.: Hallux valgus and associated conditions. In Klenerman, L. (ed.): The Foot and Its Disorders, 2nd ed. Boston, Blackwell Scientific Publications, 1982.
Fixsen, J. A.: The foot in childhood. In Klenerman, L. (ed.): The Foot and Its Disorders, 2nd ed. Boston, Blackwell Scientific Publications, 1982.
Fromherz, W. A.: Examination. In Hunt, G. C. (ed.): Physical

Therapy of the Foot and Ankle. Clinics in Physical Therapy. Edinburgh, Churchill Livingstone, 1988.

Garbalosa, J. C., R. Donatelli, and M. J. Wooden: Dysfunction, evaluation and treatment of the foot and ankle. In Donatelli, R., and M. J. Wooden (eds.): Orthopedic Physical Therapy. Edinburgh, Churchill Livingstone, 1989.

Garrick, J. G.: The injured ankle: A sports medicine nemesis. Sports Med. Bull. 10:8, 1975.

Gartland, J. J.: Fundamentals of Orthopedics. Philadelphia, W. B. Saunders Co., 1979.

Gray, G. W.: Chain Reaction—Successful Strategies for Closed Chain Testing and Rehabilitation. Adrian, Mich., Wynn Marketing Inc., 1989.

Gutrecht, J. A., R. E. Espinosa, and P. J. Dyck: Early descriptions of common neurological signs. Mayo Clin. Proc. 43:807, 1968.

Ha' Eri, G. B., V. L. Fornasier, and J. Schatzker: Morton's neuroma: Pathogenesis and ultrastructure. Clin. Orthop. Relat. Res. 141:256, 1979.

Helfet, A. J., and D. M. Gruebel-Lee: Disorders of the Foot. Philadelphia, J. B. Lippincott Co., 1979.

Hlavac, H. F.: The Foot Book: Advice to Athletes. Mountain View, Calif., World Publications, 1977.

Hoerr, N. L., S. I. Pyle, and C. C. Francis: Radiographic Atlas of Skeletal Development of the Foot and Ankle. Springfield, Ill., Charles C Thomas, 1962.

Holden, C. E. A.: Compartment syndromes following trauma. Clini. Orthop. Relat. Res. 113:8, 1975.

Hollinshead, W. H., and D. B. Jenkins: Functional Anatomy of the Limbs and Back. Philadelphia, W. B. Saunders Co., 1981.

Hoppenfeld, S.: Physical Examination of the Spine and Extremities, New York, Appleton-Century-Crofts, 1976.

Hutton, W. C., J. R. R. Stott, and I. A. F. Stokes: The mechanics of the foot. In Klenerman, L. (ed.): The Foot and Its Disorders, 2nd ed. Boston, Blackwell Scientific Publications, 1982.

Inman, V. T.: The Joints of the Ankle, Baltimore, Williams & Wilkins Co., 1976.

Judge, R. D., G. D. Zuidema, and F. T. Fitzgerald: Clinical Diagnosis: A Physiological Approach. Boston, Little, Brown & Co., 1982.

Kaumeyer, G., and T. Malone: Ankle injuries: Anatomical and biomechanical considerations necessary for the development of an injury prevention program. J. Orthop. Sports Phys. Ther. 1:171, 1980.

Kerr, R., D. M. Forrester, and S. Kingston: Magnetic resonance imaging of foot and ankle trauma. Orthop. Clin. North Am. 21:591, 1990.

Kingston, S.: Magnetic resonance imaging of the ankle and foot. Clin. Sports Med. 7:15, 1988.

Kiruchi, S., M. Hasue, and M. Watanabe: Ischemic contracture in the lower limb. Clin. Orthop. Relat. Res. 134:185, 1978.

Kleiger, B.: The mechanism of ankle injuries. J. Bone Joint Surg. 38A:59, 1956.

Klenerman, L.: Functional anatomy. In Klenerman, L. (ed.): The Foot and Its Disorders, 2nd ed. Boston, Blackwell Scientific Publications, 1982.

Landeros, O., H. M. Frost, and C. C. Higgins: Post-traumatic anterior ankle instability. Clin. Orthop. Relat. Res. 56:169, 1968.

Lassiter, T. E., T. R. Malone, and W. E. Garrett: Injury to the lateral ligaments of the ankle. Orthop. Clin. North Am. 20:629, 1989.

Lattanga, L., G. W. Gray, and R. M. Kantner: Closed vs open kinetic chain measurements of subtalar joint eversion: Implications for clinical practice. J. Orthop. Sports Phys. Ther. 9:310, 1987.

Leach, R. E.: Achilles tendinitis. Am. J. Sports Med. 9:93, 1981.

MacConaill, M. A., and J. V. Basmajian: Muscles and Movements: A Basis for Human Kinesiology. Baltimore, Williams & Wilkins Co., 1969.

Maitland, G. D.: The Peripheral Joints: Examination and Recording Guide. Adelaide, Australia, Virgo Press, 1973.

Mann, R. A.: Surgical implications of biomechanics of the foot and ankle. Clin. Orthop. Relat. Res. 146:111, 1980.

Matsen, F. A.: Compartment syndrome: A unified concept. Clin. Orthop. Relat. Res. 113:8, 1975.

McRae, R.: Clinical Orthopaedic Examination. New York, Churchill Livingstone, 1976.

Milbauer, D. L., and S. Patel: Roentgenographic techniques. In Nicholas, J. A., and E. B. Hershman (eds.): The Lower Extremity and Spine in Sports Medicine, vol I. St. Louis, C. V. Mosby Co., 1986.

Morris, J. M.: Biomechanics of the foot and ankle. Clin. Orthop. Relat. Res. 122:10, 1977.

Morton, D. J.: The Human Foot: Its Evolution, Physiology and Functional Disorders. Cambridge, Cambridge University Press, 1935.

Mubarak, S. J., and A. R. Hargens: Compartment Syndrome and Volkmann's Contracture. Philadelphia, W. B. Saunders Co., 1981.

Nigg, B. M.: The assessment of loads acting on the locomotor system in running and other sports activities. Semin. Orthop. 3:197, 1988.

Norfray, J. F., L. Schlachter, W. T. Kernaham, et al.: Early confirmation of stress fractures in joggers. JAMA 243:1647, 1980.

O'Donoghue, D. H.: Treatment of Injuries to Athletes, 4th ed. Philadelphia, W. B. Saunders Co., 1984.

Post, M.: Physical Examination of the Musculoskeletal System. Chicago, Year Book Medical Pub., 1987.

Rettig, A. C., K. D. Shelbourne, H. F. Beltz, D. W. Robertson, and P. Arfken: Radiographic evaluation of foot and ankle injuries in the athlete. Clin. Sports Med. 6:905, 1987.

Root, M. L., W. P. Orien, and H. J. Weed: Normal and Abnormal Function of the Foot. Los Angeles, Clinical Biomechanics Corp., 1977.

Rorabeck, C. H., and I. Macnab: The pathophysiology of the anterior tibial compartment syndrome. Clin. Orthop. Relat. Res. 113:52, 1975.

Samuelson, K. M.: Functional anatomy. In Hamilton, W. C. (ed.): Traumatic Disorders of the Ankle, New York, Springer-Verlag, 1984.

Scheller, A. D., J. R. Kasser, and T. B. Quigley: Tendon injuries about the ankle, Orthop. Clin. North Am. 11:801, 1980.

Seligson, D., J. Gassman, and M. Pope: Ankle Instability: Evaluation of the lateral ligaments. Am. J. Sports Med. 8:39, 1980.

Sheehan, G.: Medical Advice for Runners. Mountain View, Calif., World Publications, 1978.

Sidey, J. D.: Weak ankles: A study of common peroneal entrapment neuropathy. Br. Med. J. 3:623, 1969.

Simons, G. W.: Analytical radiography and the progressive approach in talipes equinovarus. Orthop. Clin. North Am. 9:187, 1978.

Spring, J. M., and G. W. Hyatt: Treatment of sprained ankles. Gen. Pract. 36:78, 1967.

Staheli, L. T., D. E. Chew, and M. Corbett: The longitudinal arch. J. Bone Joint Surg. 69A:426, 1987.

Subotnick, S. I.: History and physical examination. In Subotnick, S. I. (ed.): Sports Medicine of the Lower Extremity. Edinburgh, Churchill Livingstone, 1989.

Subotnick, S. I.: Podiatric Sports Medicine. Mount Kisco, N. Y., Futura Publishing Co., 1975.

Subotnick, S. I.: The Running Foot Doctor, Mountain View, Calif., World Publications, 1977.

Sweetman, R.: Pes cavus. Physiother. 49:204, 1963.

Testa, V., G. Capasso, and N. Maffulli: Paresthesia of the anterior aspect of the ankle—An early sign of lumbar spinal disorders in sportsmen. Physiother. 75:205, 1989.

Vanderwilde, R., L. T. Staheli, D. E. Chew, and V. Malagon: Measurements on radiographs of the foot in normal infants and children. J. Bone Joint Surg. 70A:407, 1988.

Wadsworth, C. T.: Manual Examination and Treatment of the Spine and Extremities. Baltimore, Williams & Wilkins Co., 1988.

Walter, N. E., and M. D. Wolf: Stress fractures in young athletes. Am. J. Sports Med. 5:165, 1977.

Weissman, B. N. W., and C. B. Sledge: Orthopedic Radiology. Philadelphia, W. B. Saunders Co., 1986.

Williams, A., R. Evans, and P. D. Shirley: Imaging of Sports Injuries. London, Bailliere Tindall, 1989.

Yvars, M. F.: Osteochondral fractures of the dome of the talus. Clin. Orthop. Relat. Res. 114:185, 1976.

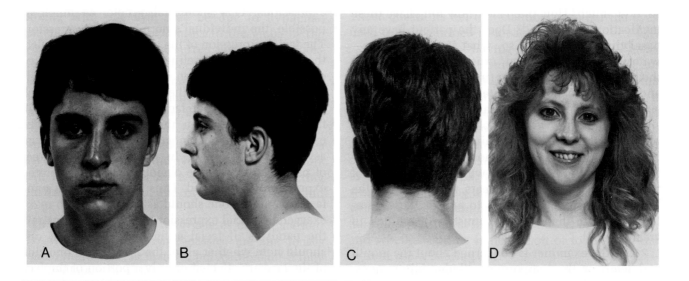

FIGURE 13–11. Views of the head and face. (A) Anterior. (B) Side. (C) Posterior. (D) Altered facial features with smile.

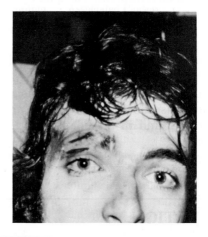

FIGURE 13–12. Laceration to the upper eyelid and eyebrow.

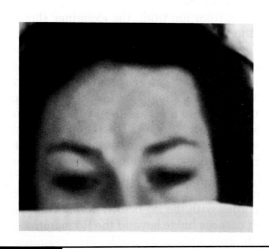

FIGURE 13–13. Contusion to the forehead due to racquetball.

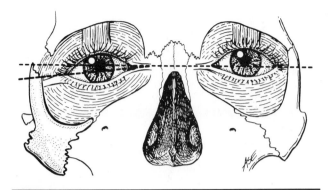

FIGURE 13–14. *Illustration demonstrating how inferior displacement of the zygoma results in depression of the lateral canthus and pupil because of depression of the suspensory ligaments that attach to the lateral orbital (Whitnall's) tubercle. (From Ellis, E.: Fractures of the zygomatic complex and arch. In Fonseca, R. J., and R. V. Walker [eds.]: Oral and Maxillofacial Trauma. Philadelphia, W. B. Saunders Co., 1991, p. 446.)*

Immediate referral for further examination by a specialist is required for an embedded corneal foreign body; haze or blood in the anterior chamber (hyphema); decreased or partial vision; irregular, asymmetric, or poor pupil action; diplopia or double vision; laceration of the eyelid or impaired lid function; perforation or laceration of the globe; broken contact lens or shattered eyeglass in the eye; unexplained eye pain that is stabbing or deep and throbbing; blurred vision that does not clear with blinking; loss of all or part of the visual field; protrusion

of one eye relative to the other; an injured eye that does not move as fully as the uninjured eye; or abnormal pupil size or shape. A teardrop pupil usually indicates iris entrapment in a corneal or scleral laceration. In addition, the eyes should be observed from the lateral aspect. The normal distance from the cornea to the angle of the eye is 16 mm or less. The distances between the upper and lower lids should be the same for both eyes. When the eyes open, the superior eyelid should cover a portion of the iris but not the pupil itself. If it does cover more of the iris than the other or extends over the iris or pupil, ptosis or drooping of that eyelid should be suspected. If the eyelid does not cover part of the iris, retraction of the eyelid should be suspected. One should also note if the eyelids are everted or inverted. Normally, they are neither. The examiner should also note whether the patient can close both eyes completely. If an eye injury is suspected, this action should be done very carefully because closing the eyes can increase intraocular pressure. The lids should be pressed together only enough to bring the eyelashes together. Any inflammation or masses, especially on the lid margin, should be noted. If present, a "black eye," or periorbital contusion, should also be noted (Fig. 13–16). The lashes should be viewed to see if there is

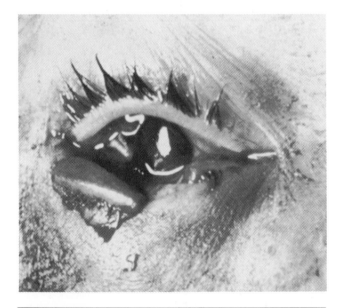

FIGURE 13–15. *A severe glancing or direct blow to this right eye has resulted in a ruptured globe. (From Pashby, T. J., and R. C. Pashby: Treatment of sports eye injuries. In Schneider, R. C., et al. [eds.]: Sports Injuries—Mechanisms, Prevention and Treatment. Baltimore, Williams & Wilkins, 1985, p. 589.)*

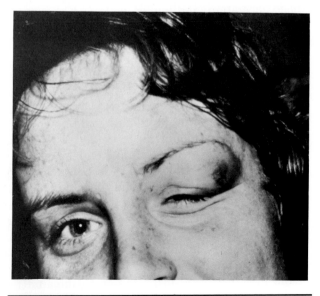

FIGURE 13–16. *Black eye (periorbital ecchymosis).*

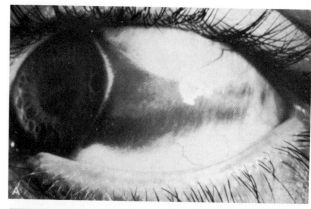
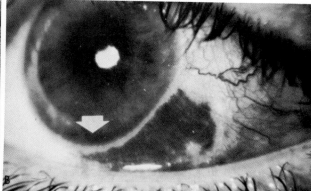
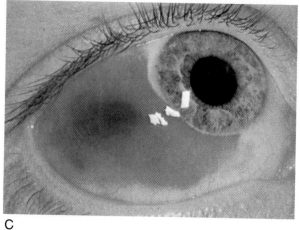

C

FIGURE 13–17. (A) Posttraumatic conjunctival hemorrhage without other ocular or orbital damage. (B) Posttraumatic conjunctival hemorrhage from blunt injury, with a small hyphema (arrow). In this case, the injury was significant because of the presence of blood in the anterior chamber. (From Paton, D., and M. F. Goldberg: Management of Ocular Injuries. Philadelphia, W. B. Saunders Co., 1976, p. 182.) (C) Subconjunctival ecchymosis with no lateral limit should instill in one a high index of suspicion of osseous orbital fractures. (From Lew, D., and D. P. Sinn: Diagnosis and treatment of midface fractures. In Fonseca, R. J., and R. V. Walker [eds.]: Oral and Maxillofacial Trauma. Philadelphia, W. B. Saunders Co., 1991, p. 520.)

even distribution along the lid margins. "Racoon eyes," which are purple discolorations of the eyelids and orbital regions, may indicate orbital fractures, basilar skull fractures, or a fracture of the base of the anterior cranial fossa.[4] However, this sign takes several hours to develop.

The conjunctiva should be inspected for hemorrhage, laceration, and foreign bodies.[8] If the patient complains of "something in the eye," eversion of the upper eyelid will usually reveal a foreign body that can often be easily brushed away. Displaced contact lenses are often found in this upper area of the eye. The conjunctival covering of the lower lid may be examined by having the patient look upward while the examiner draws the lower lid downward. The conjunctiva should be examined as being a continuous sheet of epithelium from the globe to the lids. The color of the sclera should also be noted. Posttraumatic conjunctival hemorrhage (Fig. 13–17) and possible scleral lacerations (Fig. 13–18) should be noted, if present. In dark-skinned patients, pigmented areas may show up as small dark spots or patches near the limbus. The shape and color of the cornea should be inspected. The anterior chambers of the eye should be inspected and compared for clarity and depth.[8] If present, hyphema in the form of haze or actual blood pooling (Fig. 13–19) in the

anterior eye chamber should be noted. If there is any potential for or evidence of bleeding in the anterior chamber of the eye, the patient's activity should be curtailed, as increased activity increases the chances of secondary hemorrhage during the first week after injury. Examination of the cornea

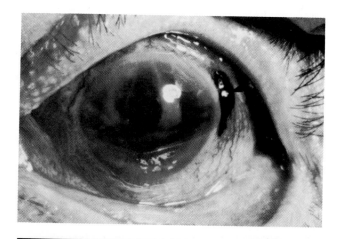

FIGURE 13–18. Scleral rupture (arrow) at the limbus after blunt trauma. Iris and ciliary body have prolapsed into the subconjunctival space. (From Paton, D., and M. F. Goldberg: Management of Ocular Injuries. Philadelphia, W. B. Saunders Co., 1976, p. 310.)

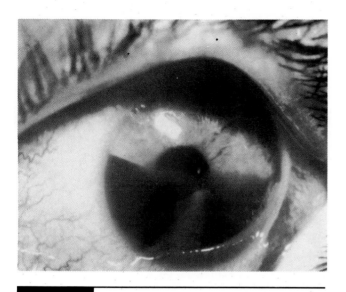

FIGURE 13–19. Hyphema in the anterior chamber of the eye. (From Easterbrook, M., and J. Cameron: Injuries in racquet sports. In Schneider, R. C., et al. [eds.]: Sports Injuries—Mechanisms, Prevention and Treatment. Baltimore, Williams & Wilkins, 1985, p. 556.)

with a pen light shone obliquely on the eye should be carried out to look for foreign bodies, abrasions, or lacerations. Corneal injuries can lead to lacrimation (tearing), photophobia (intolerance to light), or blepharospasm (spasm of the eyelid orbicular muscle) as well as extreme pain due to exposure of sensory nerve endings. Abrasions are readily outlined by a fluorescein strip dipped into tears that have been exposed as the lower lid is pulled downward.

The pupillary size (diameter range: 2–6 mm; $\bar{x}$:3.5 mm), shape (round), and symmetry should be compared with those of the other eye. Elliptical pupils often indicate a corneal laceration. The color of the irises of the eyes should be compared. When looking at the pupils, the examiner should note whether the pupils are equal. Are the pupils smaller or larger than normal? Are they round or irregularly shaped? The pupils are normally slightly unequal in 5 per cent of the population, but inequality of pupil size should initially be viewed with suspicion. Pupils tend to be smaller in infants, the elderly, and persons with hyperopia (farsightedness), whereas they tend to be slightly dilated in persons with myopia (nearsightedness) or light-colored irises.

The nose should be inspected for any deviations in shape, size, or color. The skin should be smooth without swelling and conform to the color of the face. The airways are usually oval and symmetrically proportioned. If a discharge is present, its character (i.e., color, smell, texture) should be noted and described. Bloody discharge occurs from epistaxis or trauma such as a nasal fracture, zygoma fracture, or skull fracture. Mucoid discharge is typical of rhinitis. Bilateral purulent discharge can occur with upper respiratory tract infection. Unilateral purulent, thick, greenish, and often malodorous discharge usually indicates the presence of a foreign body.

Depression of the nasal bridge can result from a fracture of the nasal bone. Nasal flaring is associated with respiratory distress, whereas narrowing of the airways on inspiration may be indicative of chronic nasal obstruction and be associated with mouth breathing. The nasal mucosa should be deep pink and glistening. A film of clear discharge is often apparent on the nasal septum. The nasal septum should be close to midline and fairly straight, appearing thicker anteriorly than posteriorly. If present, a hematoma in the septal area should be noted. Asymmetric posterior nasal cavities may indicate a deviation of the nasal septum.

With the patient's mouth closed, the lips should be observed for symmetry, color, edema, and surface abnormalities. Lipstick should be removed before the assessment. The lips should be pink and have vertical and horizontal symmetry, both at rest and with movement. Dry, cracked lips may be caused by dehydration due to wind or low humidity, whereas deep fissures at the corners of the mouth may indicate overclosure of the mouth or riboflavin deficiency.

Drooping of the mouth on one side, sagging of the lower eyelid, and flattening of the nasolabial fold suggest possible facial nerve (cranial nerve VII) involvement. The patient will also demonstrate an inability to pucker the lips to whistle.

The shape and position of the jaw and teeth should also be noted anteriorly and from the side. Asymmetry may indicate a fracture of the jaw (Fig. 13–20), whereas bleeding around the gums of the teeth may indicate fracture, avulsion, or loosening of the teeth (Fig. 13–21). If there are missing teeth, they must be accounted for. If they are not accounted for, an x-ray may be required to ensure that the teeth have not entered the abdominal or chest cavity (Fig. 13–22). If pain occurs on percussion of the teeth, it often indicates damage to the periodontal ligament.

From the side, the examiner should look for any asymmetry or depression, which may indicate pathology. The examiner should inspect the auricles of the ears for size, shape, symmetry, landmarks, color, and position on the head. To determine the position of the auricle, the examiner can draw an imaginary line between the outer canthus of the eye and occipital protuberance (Fig. 13–23). The top of the auricle should touch or be above this line.[4] The examiner can then draw another imaginary line perpendicular to the previous line and just anterior to the auricle. The auricle's position should be

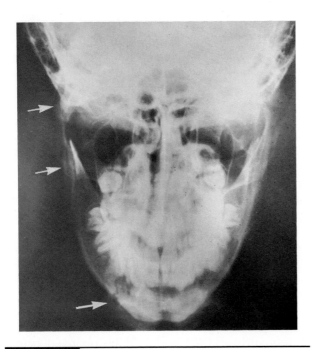

FIGURE 13–20. Fracture of the neck of the condyle on the right with fracture through the mandible on the same side. When one fracture is shown in the mandible, search carefully for the second. (From O'Donoghue, D. H.: Treatment of Injuries to Athletes. Philadelphia, W. B. Saunders Co., 1984, p. 115.)

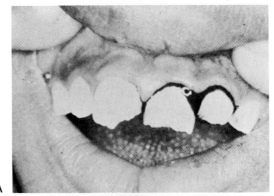

A

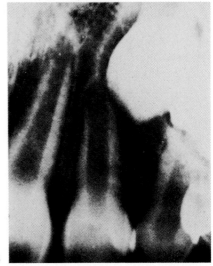

B

FIGURE 13–21. A 9-year-old boy was hit in the mouth with a ball while he was playing baseball. The right maxillary central and lateral incisors were chipped. (A) Avulsed teeth reimplanted with finger pressure. (B) Radiograph of root canal with wide-open apex. Reimplanted quickly, these teeth may not require root canal treatment. (From Torg, J. S.: Athletic Injuries to the Head, Neck and Face. Philadelphia, Lea & Febiger, 1982, p. 247.)

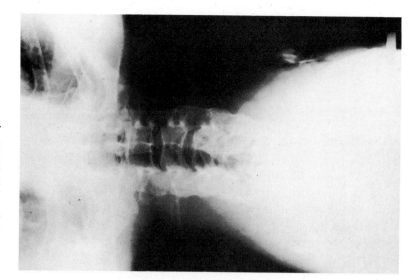

FIGURE 13–22. *The bicuspid was located on a chest radiograph in the right mainstem bronchus. Teeth are frequently aspirated during the traumatic episode and are usually located in this position. The tooth was removed by bronchoscopy before repair of the facial injury. (From Powers, M. P.: Diagnosis and management of dentoalveolar injuries. In Fonseca, R. J., and R. V. Walker [eds.]: Oral and Maxillofacial Trauma. Philadelphia, W. B. Saunders Co., 1991, p. 328. Courtesy of Mr. D. Patton, Swansea, Wales.)*

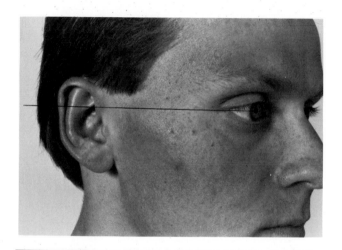

FIGURE 13–23. *Auricle alignment. Normal position shown.*

(height, protrusion) can be compared by observing from behind. A low hairline may indicate conditions such as Klippel-Feil syndrome. The examiner should also look for the presence of *Battle's sign.* This sign, which takes as long as 24 hours to show, is demonstrated by purple and blue discoloration of the skin in the mastoid area and may indicate a temporal bone or basilar skull fracture.

The examiner then views the patient from over-

almost vertical. If the angle is more than 10° posterior or anterior, it is considered abnormal. An auricle that is set low or is at an unusual angle may indicate chromosomal aberrations or renal disorders. In addition, the lateral and medial surfaces and surrounding tissues should be examined, noting any deformities, lesions, or nodules. The auricles should be the same color as the facial skin without moles, cysts, or other lesions or deformities. Athletes, especially wrestlers, may exhibit a cauliflower ear (hematoma auris), which is a keloid scar forming in the auricle due to friction to or twisting of the ear (Fig. 13–24). Blueness may indicate some degree of cyanosis. Pallor or excessive redness may be the result of vasomotor instability or increased temperature. Frostbite can cause extreme pallor or blistering (Fig. 13–25).

The examiner should look posteriorly for any asymmetry or depression. The positions of the ears

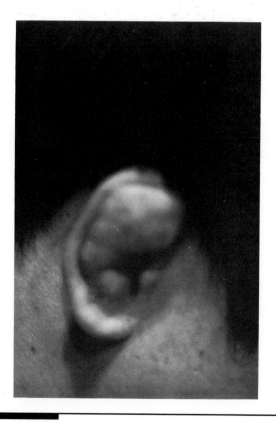

FIGURE 13–24. *Hematoma auris seen in a wrestler.*

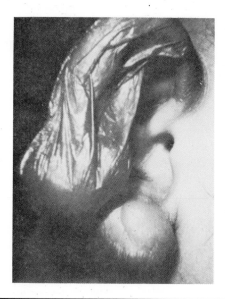

FIGURE 13–25. *Auricular frostbite with development of massive vesicles that are beginning to resolve spontaneously. (From Schuller, D. E., and R. A. Bruce: Ear, nose, throat and eye. In Strauss, R. H. [ed.] Sports Medicine, 2nd ed. Philadelphia, W. B. Saunders Co., 1991, p. 191.)*

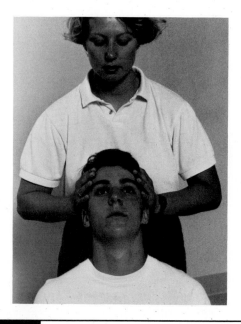

FIGURE 13–26. Viewing the patient from above.

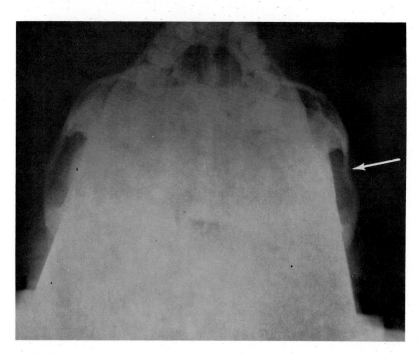

FIGURE 13–27. *Typical fracture of zygomatic arch on the right. Note normal arch on the left. (From O'Donoghue, D. H.: Treatment of Injuries to Athletes. Philadelphia, W. B. Saunders Co., 1984, p. 114.)*

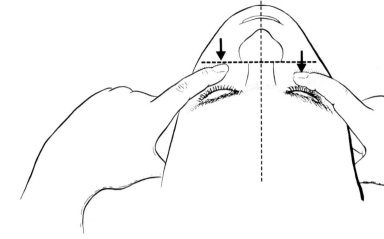

FIGURE 13–28. *Method of assessing posterior displacement of the zygomatic complex from behind the patient. The examiner should firmly but carefully depress the fingers into the edematous soft tissues while palpating along the infraorbital areas. (From Ellis, E.: Fractures of the zygomatic complex and arch. In Fonseca, R. J., and R. V. Walker [eds.]: Oral and Maxillofacial Trauma. Philadelphia, W. B. Saunders Co., 1991, p. 443.)*

head (superior view) to note any asymmetry from above (Fig. 13–26). This method is especially useful when looking for a possible fracture of the zygoma (Fig. 13–27). The deformity is easier to detect if the examiner places the index fingers below the infraorbital margins along the zygomatic bodies and then gently pushes into the edema to reduce the effect of the edema (Fig. 13–28).

EXAMINATION

The examination of the head and face differs from the orthopedic assessment of other areas of the body because the assessment does not involve articular joints. The only articular joints that could be included in the assessment are the temporomandibular joints, and these joints are discussed in Chapter 3.

Examination for a Head Injury

The examiner must remember that many problems in the head and face may be problems referred from the cervical spine, temporomandibular joint, or teeth. However, if one suspects a head injury, it is necessary to keep a close watch on the patient, noting any changes and when these changes occur. Thus, it is important that "*neural watch*" be implemented by the examiner so that any changes that occur over time can be easily determined (Table 13–5).

As the examination for a head injury is performed, the examiner should always be looking for the possibility of an expanding intracranial lesion primarily due to a leaking or torn blood vessel. Normally, the brain has a fixed volume that is enclosed in a nonexpansile structure, namely, the skull and dura mater. These lesions may be due to epidural hem-

TABLE 13–5. Neural Watch Chart*

Unit		Time 1 ( )	Time 2 ( )	Time 3 ( )
I Vital signs	Blood pressure Pulse Respiration Temperature			
II Conscious and	Oriented Disoriented Restless Combative			
III Speech	Clear Rambling Garbled None			
IV Will awaken to	Name Shaking Light pain Strong pain			
V Nonverbal reaction to pain	Appropriate Inappropriate "Decerebrate" None			
VI Pupils	Size on right Size on left Reacts on right Reacts on left			
VII Ability to move	Right arm Left arm Right leg Left leg			
VIII Sensation	Right side (normal/abnormal) Left side (normal/abnormal) Dermatome affected (specify) Peripheral nerve affected (specify)			

*Modified from American Academy of Orthopedic Surgeons: Athletic Training and Sports Medicine. Park Ridge, IL, AAOS, 1984, p. 399.

orrhage (usually tearing of one of the meningeal arteries as a result of high-speed impact), subarachnoid hemorrhage (usually as a result of an aneurysm), or subdural hemorrhage (usually as a result of tearing of bridging veins between the brain and cavernous sinus). These injuries are emergency conditions that must be looked after immediately because of their high mortality rate (as much as 50%). An expanding intracranial lesion is indicated by an altered lucid state (state of consciousness), development of inequality of the pupils, unusual slowing of the heart rate that primarily occurs after a lucid interval, irregular eye movements, and eyes that will no longer track properly. There is also a tendency for the patient to demonstrate increased body temperature and irregular respirations. Normal intracranial pressure measures from 4 to 15 mm Hg, and an intracranial pressure of more than 20 mm Hg is considered abnormal. Intracranial pressure of 40 mm Hg causes neurological dysfunction and impairment. Although the individual in the emergency care setting has no way of determining the intracranial pressure, the signs and symptoms previously mentioned indicate that the pressure is increasing. Most patients who experience an increase in intracranial pressure complain of severe headache, and this symptom is often followed by vomiting (sometimes projectile vomiting).

Signs and symptoms that indicate a good possibility of recovery from a head injury, especially after the patient experiences unconsciousness, include response to noxious stimuli, eye opening, pupil activity, spontaneous eye movement, intact oculovestibular reflexes, and appropriate motor function responses. Neurological signs that indicate a poor prognosis after a head injury include nonreactive pupils, absence of oculovestibular reflexes, severe extension patterns or no motor function response at all, and increased intracranial pressure.[3]

It is important when examining the unconscious patient for a possible head injury to determine the level of consciousness of the individual, which may be done with the *Glasgow Coma Scale* (Table 13–6). The first test relates to eye opening. Eye opening may be spontaneous, in response to speech, or in response to pain, or there may be no response at all. Each of these responses is given a value. For example, spontaneous eye opening is given a value of 4, response to speech is given a value of 3, response to pain is given a value of 2, and no response at all is given a value of 1. Spontaneous opening of the eyes indicates functioning of the ascending reticular activating system. This finding does not necessarily mean that the patient is aware of the surroundings or of what is happening, but it does imply that the patient is in a state of arousal. A patient who opens the eyes in response to the examiner's voice is probably responding to the stimulus of sound, not necessarily to the command to do something, such as opening the eyes. If unsure, the examiner may try different sound-making objects (e.g., bell, horn) to elicit an appropriate response.

The second test involves motor response; the patient is given a grade of 6 if there is a response to a verbal command. Otherwise, the patient is graded on a five-point scale depending on the motor response to a painful stimulus (see Table 13–6). When scoring motor responses, it is the ease with which

TABLE 13–6. Glasgow Coma Scale

			Time 1 ( )	Time 2 ( )
Eyes	Open	Spontaneously	4	
		To verbal command	3	
		To pain	2	
		No response	1	
Best motor response	To verbal command	Obeys	6	
	To painful stimulus*	Localizes pain	5	
		Flexion—withdrawal	4	
		Flexion—abnormal (decorticate rigidity)	3	
		Extension (decerebrate rigidity)	2	
		No response	1	
Best verbal response†		Oriented and converses	5	
		Disoriented and converses	4	
		Inappropriate words	3	
		Incomprehensible sounds	2	
		No response	1	
Total			3–15	

*Apply knuckles to sternum; observe arms.
†Arouse patient with painful stimulus if necessary.

The Glasgow Coma Scale, based on eye opening, verbal, and motor responses, is a practical means of monitoring changes in level of consciousness. If response on the scale is given a number, the responsiveness of the patient can be expressed by summation of the numbers. The lowest score is 3, and the highest is 15.

the motor responses are elicited that constitutes the criterion for the best response. Commands given to the patient should be simple, such as, "Move your arm." The patient should not be asked to squeeze the examiner's hand, nor should the examiner place something in the patient's hand and then ask the patient to grasp it. This action may cause a reflex grasp, not a response to a command.[3]

If the patient does not give a motor response to a verbal command, then the examiner should attempt to elicit a motor response to a painful stimulus. It is the type and quality of the patient's reaction to the painful stimulus that constitute the scoring criteria. The stimulus should not be applied to the face because painful stimulus in the facial area may cause the eyes to close tightly as a protective reaction. The painful stimulus may be applying a knuckle to the sternum, squeezing the trapezius muscle, or squeezing the soft tissue between the thumb and index finger (Fig. 13–29). If the patient moves a limb when the painful stimulus is applied to more than one point or tries to remove the examiner's hand that is applying the painful stimulus, the patient is localizing, and a value of 5 is given. If the patient withdraws from the painful stimulus rapidly, a normal reflex withdrawal is being shown, and a value of 4 is given. However, if application of a painful stimulus creates a decorticate or decerebrate posture (Fig. 13–30), an abnormal response is being demonstrated, and a value of 3 is given for the decorticate posture (injury above red nucleus) or a value of 2 is given for decerebrate posture (brain stem injury). Decorticate posturing results from lesions of the diencephalon area, whereas decerebrate posturing results from lesions of the midbrain. With decorticate posturing, the arms, wrists, and fingers are flexed, the upper limbs are adducted, and the legs are extended, medially rotated, and plantar flexed. Decerebrate posturing, which has a poorer prognosis, involves extension, adduction, and hyperpronation of the arms, whereas the lower limbs are the same as for decorticate posturing.[9] Decerebrate rigidity is usually bilateral. If the patient exhibits no reaction to the painful stimulus, a value of 1 is given. It is important to be sure the "no" response is due to a head injury and not due to a spinal cord injury and, thus, lack of feeling or sensation. Any difference in reaction between limbs should be carefully noted, as this finding may be indicative of a specific focal injury.[3]

In the third test, verbal response is graded on a five-point scale and measures the person's speech in response to simple questions such as "Where are you?" or "Are you winning the game?" For verbal responses, the patient who converses appropriately will show proper orientation, being aware of oneself and the environment, and is given a grade of 5. The patient who is confused will be disoriented and unable to completely interface with the environment; this patient will be able to converse using the appropriate words and is given a grade of 4. The patient exhibiting inappropriate speech will be unable to sustain a conversation with the examiner; this individual would be given a grade of 3. A vocalizing patient will only groan or make incomprehensible sounds. This finding leads to a grade of 2. Again, the examiner should make note of any possible mechanical reason for the inability to verbalize. If the patient makes no sounds and thus has no verbal response, a grade of 1 is assigned.

It is vital that the initial score on the Glasgow Coma Scale be obtained as soon as possible after the onset of the injury at the scene of the injury. With the Glasgow Coma Scale, the initial score is used as a basis for determining the severity of the patient's head injury. Patients who maintain a score of 8 or less on the Glasgow Coma Scale for 6 hours or longer are considered to have a serious head injury. A patient who scores between 9 and 11 is considered moderately head injured, and one who scores 12 or higher is considered to have a mild head injury.[3]

The Rancho Los Amigos Scale of Cognitive Function may also be used to assess the patient's cognitive abilities. This scale is an eight-level progression from level 1, where the patient is nonresponsive, to level 8, where the patient's behavior is purposeful and appropriate (Table 13–7). The Rancho Los Amigos scale provides an assessment of cognitive function and behavior only, not of physical functioning.[3]

If an individual receives a head injury such as a mild concussion and is not referred to the hospital, the examiner should ensure that someone accompanies the individual home and that someone at home knows what has happened so he or she can monitor the patient in case the patient's condition worsens. Appropriate written instructions should be sent home concerning the individual. The Head Injury Card (Table 13–8) is such an example.

The examiner may also wish to determine if the patient has suffered an upper motor neuron lesion. Testing the deep tendon reflexes (see Table 1–11) or the pathological reflexes (see Table 1–13) or having the patient perform various balance and coordination tests may help to determine if this type of lesion has occurred. It must be remembered, however, that the pathological reflexes may not be elicited owing to shock. Deep tendon reflexes will be accentuated on the side of the body opposite to which the brain injury has occurred. Balance can play an important role in the assessment of a head-injured patient. Balance involves the integration of several inputs (e.g., visual, proprioceptive, and vestibular systems) by the brain that are analyzed to allow a proper action. For example, in standing, the body is inher-

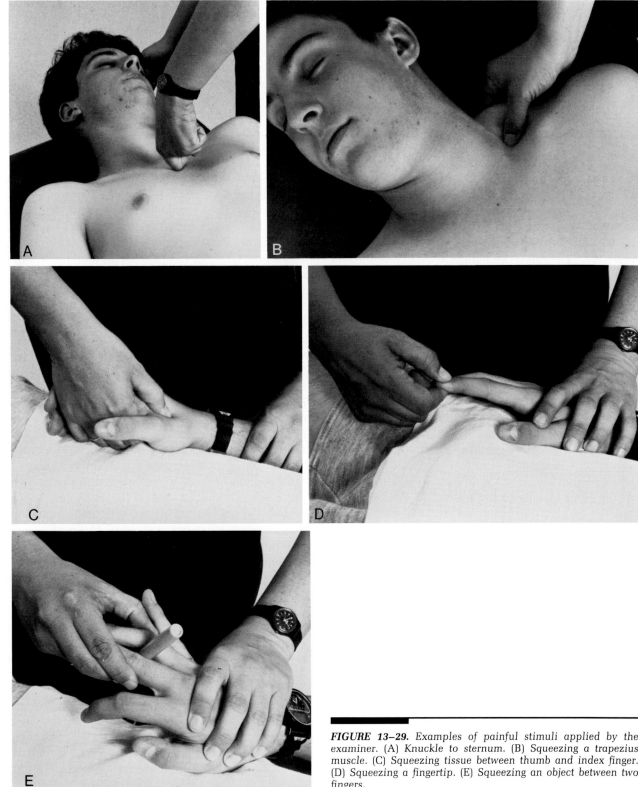

FIGURE 13–29. Examples of painful stimuli applied by the examiner. (A) Knuckle to sternum. (B) Squeezing a trapezius muscle. (C) Squeezing tissue between thumb and index finger. (D) Squeezing a fingertip. (E) Squeezing an object between two fingers.

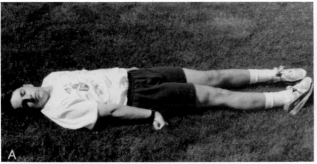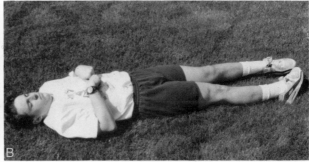

FIGURE 13–30. (A) *Decorticate rigidity.* (B) *Decerebrate rigidity.*

TABLE 13–7. Rancho Los Amigos Scale of Cognitive Function*

Level I	No response
Level II	Generalized response
Level III	Localized response
Level IV	Confused, agitated
Level V	Confused, inappropriate
Level VI	Confused, appropriate
Level VII	Automatic, appropriate
Level VIII	Purposeful, appropriate

*From Hagen, C., Malkmus, D., and Durham, P.: Levels of cognitive functioning. *In* Rehabilitation of the Brain Injured Adult—Comprehensive Management. Professional Staff Association of Rancho Los Amigos, Downey, California, 1980.

TABLE 13–8. Head Injury Card

HEAD INJURY CARD

Please Read Carefully

(Give one to an accompanying person, and one to the player)

NAME _____ AGE _____

SUSTAINED A HEAD INJURY AT _____
                                        (time)

ON _____
       (date)

IMPORTANT WARNING:
(S)He is to be taken to a hospital or a doctor immediately if (s)he:

- VOMITS
- DEVELOPS A HEADACHE
- BECOMES RESTLESS OR IRRITABLE
- BECOMES DIZZY, DROWSY OR CANNOT BE ROUSED
- HAS A FIT (CONVULSION)
- ANYTHING ELSE UNUSUAL OCCURS

For the **rest of today** (s)he should:

- REST QUIETLY
- NOT CONSUME ALCOHOL
- NOT DRIVE A VEHICLE

AND

(S)He should not train or play again without medical clearance by **a doctor.**

_____ PHONE _____
       (Doctor)

DATE _____

Queensland Health Department ● Division of Health Promotion

pected. The muscles of the face are different from most muscles in that they move the skin and soft tissues rather than the joints, if one excludes the temporomandibular joint. For example, the frontalis muscle may be weak if the eyebrows do not raise symmetrically. The corrugator muscle draws the eyebrows medially and downward (frowning). The orbicularis oris muscle approximates and compresses the lips, whereas the zygomaticus muscles raise the lateral angle of the mouth (smiling).

Examination for an Eye Injury[5-7]

If the eyelids are swollen shut, the examiner should assume that the globe has been ruptured. A penetrating wound of the eyelid should be assessed carefully, as it may be associated with a globe injury. Therefore, the examiner should not force the eyelid open, as intraocular pressure can force extrusion of the ocular contents if the globe has been ruptured. The patient should also be instructed not to squeeze the eyelids tight, as this action increases the intraocular pressure from a normal value of 15 mm Hg up to approximately 70 mm Hg.

To examine the normal functioning of the eye muscles, the examiner asks the patient to move through the six cardinal positions of gaze (Fig. 13–37). The examiner holds the patient's chin steady with one hand and asks the patient to follow the examiner's other hand while the examiner traces a large "H" in the air. The examiner should hold the index finger or pencil approximately 25 cm from the patient's nose. From the midline, the finger or pencil is moved approximately 30 cm to the patient's right and held. It is then moved up approximately 20 cm and held, moved down 40 cm (20 cm relative to midline) and held, and moved slowly back to midline. The same movement is repeated on the other side. The examiner should observe movement

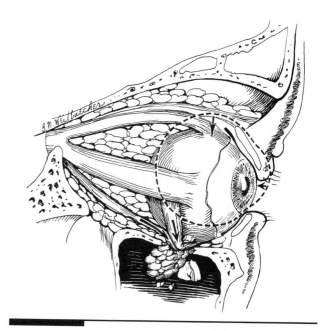

FIGURE 13–38. *Blow-out fracture of the orbital floor. The dotted line indicates normal position of the globe. The inferior oblique and inferior rectus muscles are restrained by the incarcerated orbital tissues. (From Paton, D., and M. F. Goldberg: Management of Ocular Injuries. Philadelphia, W. B. Saunders Co., 1976, p. 63.)*

of both eyes, noting whether the eyes follow the finger or pencil smoothly. The examiner should also observe any parallel movement of the eyes in all directions. If the eyes do not move in unison or only one eye moves, there is something affecting the action of the muscles. One of the most common causes of one eye not moving after trauma to the eye is a "blow-out" fracture of the orbital floor (Fig. 13–38). Because the inferior muscles become "caught" in the fracture site, the affected eye will demonstrate limited movement (Fig. 13–39), especially upward. The patient with this type of fracture may also demonstrate depression of the eye globe, blurred vision, double vision, and conjunctival hemorrhage.

Occasionally, when looking to the extreme side, the eyes will develop a rhythmic motion called *end point nystagmus*. Nystagmus is a rhythmic movement of the eyes with an abnormal slow drifting away from fixation and rapid return. With end point nystagmus, there is a quick motion in the direction of the gaze followed by a slow return. This test differentiates end point nystagmus from *pathological nystagmus*, in which there is a quick movement of the eyes in the same direction regardless of gaze. Pathological nystagmus exists when it is seen in the region of full binocular vision, not just at the periphery. It produces a rapid component (rapid shift of the eye) in the same direction regardless of the direction in which the eyes are looking. Cerebellar

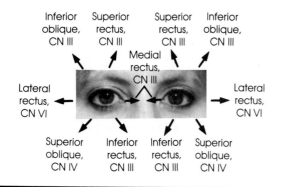

FIGURE 13–37. *The eye's six cardinal fields of gaze showing muscles and cranial nerves involved in the movement.*

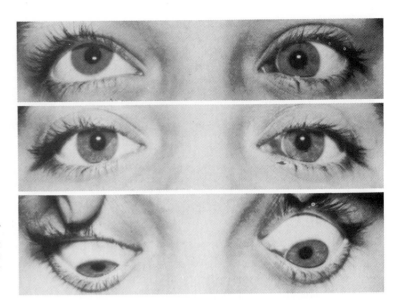

FIGURE 13–39. Fresh blow-out fracture of left orbit with limitation of upward and downward movements of the left eye. (From Paton, D., and M. F. Goldberg: Management of Ocular Injuries. Philadelphia, W. B. Saunders Co., 1976, p. 65.)

nystagmus is greater when the eyes are deviated toward the side of the lesion.

While testing the cardinal positions, the examiner should also watch for lid lag. Normally, the upper lid covers the top of the iris, rising when the patient looks up and quickly lowering as the eye lowers. With lid lag, the upper lid will delay lowering as the eye lowers.

Peripheral vision or the visual field (peripheral limits of vision) can be tested with the confrontation test (Fig. 13–40). The patient is asked to cover the right eye while the examiner covers the left eye, so the open eyes of the examiner and of the patient are directly opposite each other. Both the examiner and the patient should look into each other's eye. While this is occurring, the examiner fully extends the arm on the same side midway between the patient and the examiner and then moves it toward them with the fingers waving. The patient tells the examiner when the moving fingers are first seen. The examiner then compares the patient's response with the time or distance that the examiner first noted the fingers. The nasal, temporal, superior, and inferior fields should all be tested in a similar fashion. The visual field should describe angles of 60° nasally, 90° temporally, 50° superiorly, and 70° inferiorly. Double simultaneous testing may also be performed. This method uses two stimuli (e.g., moving fingers) that are simultaneously presented in the right and left visual fields, and the patient is asked which finger is moving. Normally, the patient should say "both" without hesitation. Any loss of vision field demands referral, which means if the patient is unable to see in the same visual fields as before, the patient should be referred.

The eyelids should be everted to look at the underside of the eyelid and to give a clearer view of the globe, especially if the patient complains of a foreign body. The upper eyelid may be everted using a special lid retractor or a cotton swab (Fig. 13–41). The patient is asked to look down and to the right and then down and to the left while the superior aspect of the eye is examined. The examiner can check the inferior aspect of the eye and its conjunctival lining by carefully pulling the lower eyelid downward and gently holding it against the bony orbit. Next, the patient is asked to look up and to the right and then up and to the left while the inferior aspect of the eye is examined. These two techniques may also be used to look for a contact lens that has migrated away from the cornea.

Both eyelids should be checked for laceration. Lacerations in the area of the lacrimal gland are especially important to detect (Fig. 13–42).

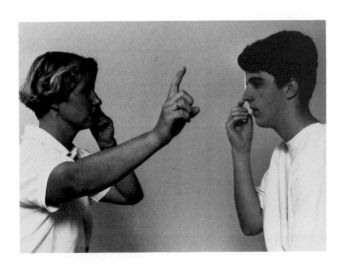

FIGURE 13–40. Confrontation eye test.

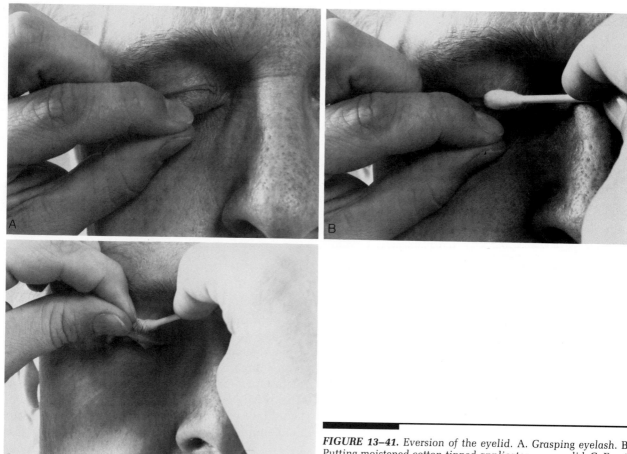

FIGURE 13–41. Eversion of the eyelid. A. Grasping eyelash. B. Putting moistened cotton-tipped applicator over eyelid. C. Everting eyelid over cotton-tipped applicator.

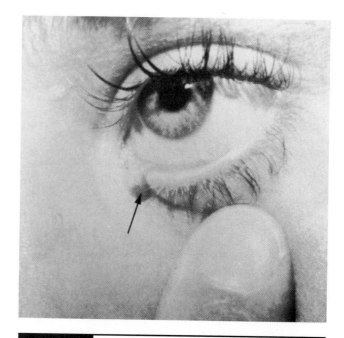

FIGURE 13–42. A lower lid laceration (arrow). (From Pashby, T, J., and R. C. Pashby: Treatment of sports eye injuries. In Schneider, R. C., et al. [eds.]: Sports Injuries—Mechanisms, Prevention and Treatment. Baltimore, Williams & Wilkins, 1985, p. 576.)

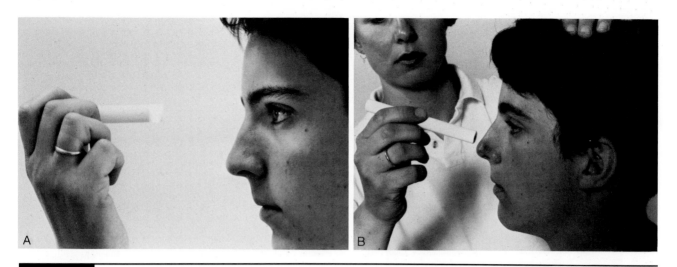

FIGURE 13–43. Testing the pupils for reaction to light. A. Light shining in eye. B. Light away from eye.

The reaction of the pupils to light should then be tested. First, the light in a room is dimmed. The examiner should remember that the pupils dilate in a dark environment or with a long focal distance, and constrict in a light environment or with a short focal distance. The examiner shines a pen light directly into one of the patient's eyes for approximately 5 seconds (Fig. 13–43). Normally, the examiner will observe constriction of the pupil, followed by slight dilation. The pupillary reaction is classified as brisk (normal), sluggish, nonreactive, or fixed. An oval or slightly oval pupil or one fixed and dilated pupil indicates increased intracranial pressure. The fixation and dilation of both pupils are terminal signs of anoxia and ischemia to the brain. If the redilation is significant, an injury to the optic nerve may be suspected. If both pupils are midsize, midposition, and nonreactive, midbrain damage is usually indicated. In a fully conscious, alert individual who has sustained a blow near the eye, a dilated fixed pupil usually implies injury to the ciliary nerves of the eye rather than brain injury. The other eye is tested similarly, and the results are compared. Normally, both pupils constrict when a light is shined in one eye. The reaction of the eye being tested is called the *direct light reflex*. The reaction of the other pupil is called the *consensual light reflex*. This reaction is brisker in the young and people with blue eyes.[8] If the optic nerve is damaged, the affected pupil constricts in response to light in the opposite eye (consensual) and dilates in response to light shone into it (direct). If the oculomotor nerve is affected, the affected pupil will be fixed and dilated and will not respond to light (directly or consensually). If the pupils do not react, it is an indication of injury to the oculomotor nerve and its connections or of injury to the head. The eye will also appear laterally displaced owing to paresis

of the medial rectus muscle. The pupil is then tested for "constriction to accommodation." The patient is asked to look at a distant object and then at a test object—a pencil or the examiner's finger held 10 cm from the bridge of the nose. The pupils will dilate when the patient looks at a far object and constrict when the patient focuses on the near object. The eyes will also adduct (going "cross-eyed") when the patient looks at the close object. These actions are called the *accommodation-convergence reflex*.[8] When looking at distant objects, the eyes should be parallel. Deviation or lack of parallelism is called *strabismus* and indicates weakness of one of the extraocular muscles or lack of neural coordination.[12]

When inspected under normal overhead light, the lens of the eye should be transparent. Shining a light on the lens may cause it to appear gray or yellow. The cornea should be smooth and clear. If the patient has extreme pain in the corneal area, a corneal abrasion should be suspected (Fig. 13–44). An appropriate specialist may test for corneal abrasion by using a fluorescein strip and a slit lamp. The cornea should be crystal clear when it is viewed, and the iris details should match those of the other eye.

To check for depth of the anterior chamber of the eye or a narrow corneal angle, the examiner shines a light obliquely across each eye. Normally, it illuminates the entire iris. When the corneal angle is narrow because of a shallow anterior chamber, the examiner will be able to see a crescent-shaped shadow on the side of the iris away from the light (Fig. 13–45). This finding indicates an anatomic predisposition to narrow-angled glaucoma.

To test for symmetry of gaze, the examiner aims a light source approximately 60 cm from the patient while standing directly in front of the patient and holding the light distant enough to prevent conver-

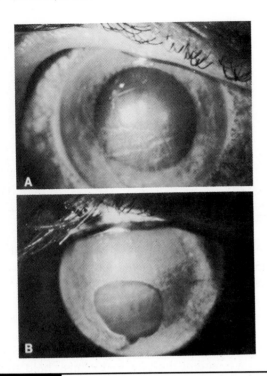

FIGURE 13-44. Corneal abrasion. (A) Without fluorescein. (B) With fluorescein. (From Torg, J. S.: Athletic Injuries to the Head, Neck and Face. Philadelphia, Lea & Febiger, 1982, p. 262.)

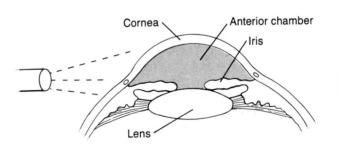

NORMAL ANGLE

FIGURE 13-45. Normal and narrow corneal angle (depth of anterior chamber). (From Swartz, M. H.: Textbook of Physical Diagnosis. Philadelphia, W. B. Saunders Co., 1989, p. 144.)

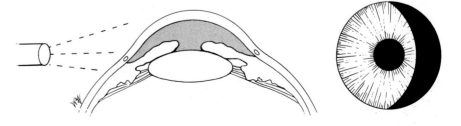

NARROW ANGLE

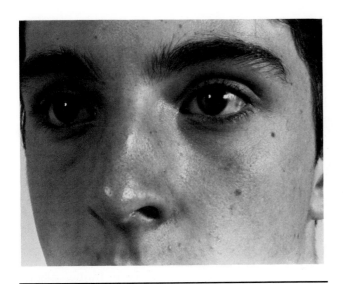

FIGURE 13–46. *Symmetry of gaze. Note white "dots" of light on pupil.*

gence of the patient's gaze. The patient is asked to stare at the light. The dots of reflected light on the two corneas should be in the same location (Fig. 13–46). When one eye does not look directly at the light, the reflected dot of light moves to the side opposite the deviation. For example, if the eye deviates medially, the reflection appears more laterally placed than in the other eye. The examiner can approximate the angle of deviation by noting the position of the reflection. Each millimeter of displacement reflection represents approximately 7°

of ocular deviation. To bring out a mild deviation, a cover-uncover test may be used (Fig. 13–47). The patient looks at a specific point, such as the bridge of the examiner's nose. One of the patient's eyes is then covered with a card. Normally, the uncovered eye will not move. If it moves, it was not straight before the other eye was covered. The other eye is then tested in a similar fashion.

Visual acuity is tested using a vision chart. Visual acuity is the ability of the eye to perceive fine detail, for example, when reading. If a standard eye wall chart is not available, a pocket visual acuity card may be used (Fig. 13–48). This pocket card is usually viewed at a distance of approximately 35 to 36 cm. As with the wall chart, the patient is asked to examine the smallest line possible. If neither eye chart is available, any printed material may be used. If glasses or contact lenses are worn, the patient should be tested both without and with the corrective lenses. The test is done quickly so the patient cannot memorize the chart. Visual acuity is recorded as a fraction in which the numerator indicates the distance of the patient from the chart (e.g., 20 ft) and the denominator indicates the distance at which the normal eye can read the line. Thus, 20/100 means the patient can read at 20 ft what the average person can read at 100 ft. The smaller the fraction, the worse the myopia (nearsightedness). Corrected vision of less than 20/40 should be referred to the appropriate specialist.[8]

Intraocular examination with an ophthalmoscope, if available, may reveal lens, vitreous, or retinal damage.

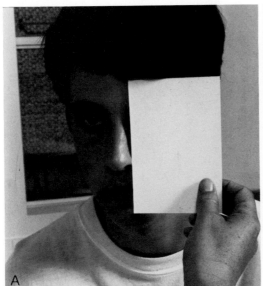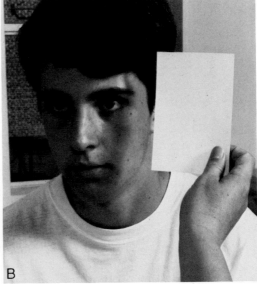

A B

FIGURE 13–47. *Cover-uncover test.*

CLARK'S CHARTS
EYE EXAM

To test visual acuity: hold chart 14 inches from eyes in good light. Test each eye separately and then jointly, with and without corrective lenses. If bifocals are present have patient read with them.

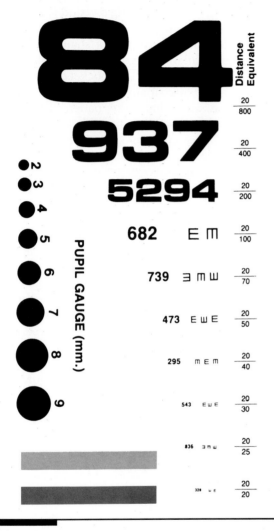

FIGURE 13–48. *Hand-held vision chart. (Top solid bar is red, and bottom solid bar is green.)*

Examination of the Nose[5–7]

Patency of the nasal passages can be determined by occluding one nostril by pushing a finger against the side of it. The patient is then asked to breathe in and out of the opposite nostril with the mouth closed. The process is repeated on the other side. Normally, no sound should be heard, and the patient can breathe easily through the open nostril.

If available, a nasal speculum and light may be used to inspect the nasal cavity. The nasal mucosa and turbinates can be inspected for color, foreign bodies, and abnormal masses (e.g., polyp). The nasal septum should be in midline and straight and is normally thicker anteriorly than posteriorly. If the nasal cavities are asymmetric, it may indicate a deviated septum. If the patient demonstrates a septal hematoma, it must be treated fairly quickly, as the hematoma may cause excessive pressure on the septum, making it avascular. This avascularity may result in a "saddle nose" deformity owing to necrosis and absorption of the underlying cartilage (Fig. 13–49).

Illumination of the frontal and maxillary sinuses may be performed if sinus tenderness is present or infection is suspected. The examination must be performed in a completely darkened room. To illuminate the maxillary sinuses, the examiner places the light source lateral on the nose just beneath the medial aspect of the eye. The examiner then looks through the patient's open mouth for illumination of the hard palate. To illuminate the frontal sinuses, the examiner places the light source against the medial aspect of each supraorbital rim. The examiner looks for a dim red glow as light is transmitted

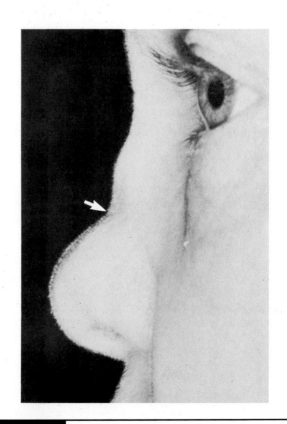

FIGURE 13–49. *"Saddle nose" deformity (arrow) that occurred as a result of loss of septal cartilage support secondary to septal hematoma and abscess. (From Handler, S. D.: Diagnosis and management of maxillofacial injuries. In Torg, J. S. (ed.): Athletic Injuries to the Head, Neck and Face. Philadelphia, Lea & Febiger, 1982, p. 232.)*

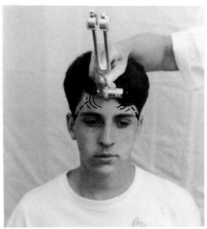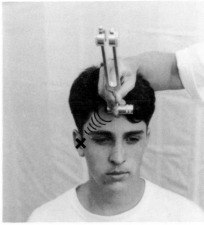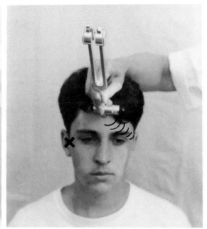

FIGURE 13–50. The Weber test. When a vibrating tuning fork is placed on the center of the forehead, the sound will be heard in the center without lateralization to either side (normal response). (A) In the presence of a conductive hearing loss, the sound will be heard on the side of the conductive loss. (B) In the presence of the sensorineural loss, the sound will be better heard on the opposite (unaffected) side.

just below the eyebrow. The sinuses will usually show differing degrees of illumination. The absence of a glow indicates either that the sinus is filled with secretions or that it has never developed.

Internal examination of the nose may be performed using a nasal illuminator or a light and nasal speculum, if available. In this case, the examiner notes the septum, nasal membrane, and turbinates for signs of pathology.

Examination of the Teeth[5–7]

The examiner should observe the teeth to see if they are in normal position and whether any teeth are missing or depressed (see Figure 13–21). Using the index finger, the examiner can apply mild pressure to each tooth, pressing inward toward the tongue and outward toward the lips. Normally, a small amount of movement will be seen. If a tooth is loose, a positive test is indicated by excessive movement or increased pain or numbness relative to other teeth. A tooth that has been avulsed may be cleansed with warm water and reinserted into the socket. The patient is then referred to the appropriate specialist.

Examination of the Ear[5–7]

Examination of the ear deals primarily with whether the patient is able to hear. There are several tests that may be used to test hearing.

Whispered Voice Test. The patient's response to the examiner's whispered voice can be used to determine hearing ability. The examiner masks the hearing in one of the patient's ears by placing the examiner's finger gently in the patient's ear canal. Standing approximately 30 to 60 cm away from the patient, the examiner whispers one- or two-syllable words very softly and asks the patient to repeat the words heard. If the patient has difficulty, the examiner gradually increases the loudness of the whisper until the patient responds appropriately. The procedure is repeated in the other ear. The patient should be able to hear softly whispered words in each ear at a distance of 30 to 60 cm and respond correctly at least 50 per cent of the time.[4, 5]

Ticking Watch Test. The ticking watch test uses a nonelectric ticking watch to test high-frequency hearing. The examiner positions the watch approximately 15 cm from each ear, slowly moving it toward the ear. The patient is asked to tell the examiner when the ticking is heard. The distance can be measured and will give some idea of the patient's ability to hear high-frequency sound.[4, 5]

Weber Test. The examiner places the base of a vibrating tuning fork on the midline vertex of the patient's head. The patient is asked if the sound is heard equally well in both ears or is heard better in one ear (lateralization of sound) (Fig. 13–50). The patient should hear the sound equally well in both ears. If the sound is lateralized, the patient is asked to identify through which ear the sound is heard better. To test the reliability of the patient's response, the examiner repeats the procedure while occluding one ear with a finger and asks the patient through which ear the sound is heard better. It should be heard better in the occluded ear.[4, 5]

Rinne Test. The Rinne test is performed by placing the base of the vibrating tuning fork against the patient's mastoid bone. The examiner counts or times the interval with a watch. The patient is asked

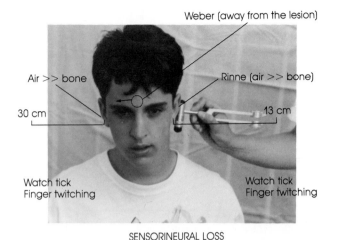

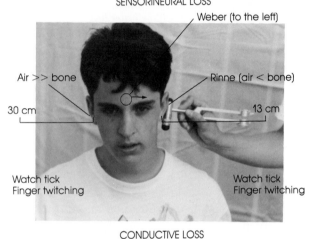

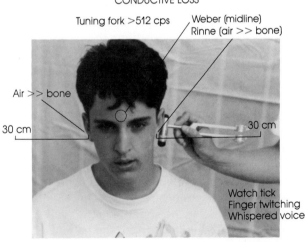

FIGURE 13–51. *Bedside hearing tests. (Reproduced with permission from Branch, W. T., and H. H. Funkenstein: Vertigo. In Branch, W. T. [ed.]: Office Practice of Medicine. Philadelphia, W. B. Saunders Co., 1982, p. 341.) (From Reilly, B. M.: Practical Strategies in Outpatient Medicine. Philadelphia, W. B. Saunders Co., 1984.)*

to tell the examiner when the sound is no longer heard, and the examiner notes the number of seconds. The examiner then quickly positions a still-vibrating tine 1 to 2 cm from the auditory canal, and the patient is asked to tell the examiner when the sound is no longer heard. The examiner then compares the number of seconds the sound was heard by bone conduction versus by air conduction. The counting or timing of the interval between the two sounds determines the length of time that sound is heard by air conduction. Air-conducted sound should be heard twice as long as bone-conducted sound. For example, if bone conduction is heard for 15 seconds, the air conduction should be heard for an additional 30 seconds.[4–6]

Schwabach Test. This test is a comparison of the patient's and examiner's hearing by bone conduction. The examiner alternately places the vibrating tuning fork against the patient's mastoid process and against the examiner's mastoid bone until one of them no longer hears a sound. The examiner and patient should hear the sound for equal amounts of time.[4, 5]

Conductive hearing loss implies the patient experiences reduction of all sounds rather than difficulty in interpreting sounds. Sensorineural or perceptual hearing loss indicates there is a defect in that the patient has difficulty interpreting the sounds heard (Fig. 13–51).

Internal examination of the ear may be accomplished using an otoscope, if available. In this case, the examiner would note the canal as well as the eardrum (tympanic membrane), noting any blockage, excessive wax, swelling, redness, transparency (usually pearly gray), bulging, retraction, or perforation of the eardrum.

Special Tests

Tests for Expanding Intracranial Lesions

For each of these tests, the patient must be able to stand normally when the eyes are open.

Neurological Control Test—Upper Limb. The patient is asked to stand with the arms forward flexed 90° and the eyes closed. The patient is asked to hold this position for approximately 30 seconds. If the examiner notes that one arm tends to move or "drift" outward and downward, the test is considered positive for an expanding intracranial lesion on the side opposite the side with the drift.

Neurological Control Test—Lower Limb. The patient is asked to sit on the edge of a table or in a chair with the legs extended in front and not touching the ground. The patient is then asked to close the eyes for approximately 20 to 30 seconds. If the examiner notes that one leg tends to move or drift, the test is considered positive for an expanding intracranial lesion on the side opposite that with the drift.

Romberg Test. The patient is asked to stand with the feet together and arms by the side with the eyes open. The examiner notes whether the patient has any problem with balance. The patient is then asked to close the eyes, and the examiner notes any differences. A positive Romberg test is elicited when the patient sways or falls to one side when the eyes are closed and is indicative of an expanding intracranial lesion.

Walk or Stand in Tandem. Patients with expanding intracranial lesions will demonstrate increasing difficulty in walking in tandem ("walking the white line") or standing in tandem. (Standing in tandem is more difficult to perform than walking in tandem.)

Tests for Coordination

Heel to Knee Test. The patient, who is lying supine with the eyes open, is asked to take the heel of one foot and touch the opposite knee with the heel and then slide the heel down the shin. The test is repeated with the eyes closed, and both legs are tested. The test can be repeated several times with increasing speed, with examiner noting any differences in coordination or the presence of tremor. Normally, the tests should be accomplished easily, smoothly, and quickly with the eyes open and closed.

Finger to Nose Test. The patient stands or sits with the eyes open and is asked to bring the index finger to the nose. The test is repeated with the eyes closed. Both arms are tested several times with increasing speed. Normally, the tests should be accomplished easily, smoothly, and quickly with the eyes open and closed.

Finger-Thumb Test. The patient is asked to touch each finger with the thumb of the same hand. The normal or uninjured side is tested first, followed by the injured side. The examiner compares both sides for coordination and timing.

Hand Flip Test. The patient is asked to touch the back of the opposite hand with the anterior aspect of the fingers, "flip" the hand over, and touch the opposite hand with the posterior aspect of the fingers. The movement is repeated several times, with both sides being tested. The examiner compares the two sides for coordination and speed.

Finger Drumming Test. The patient is asked to "drum" the index and middle finger of one hand up and down as quickly as possible on the back of the other hand. The test is repeated with the other hand.

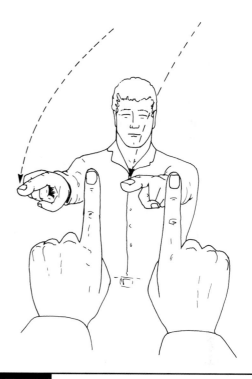

FIGURE 13–52. *Past pointing. The patient is asked to raise the hands over the head and then, with the eyes closed, touch the examiner's fingers. This figure illustrates abnormal past pointing to the right—past pointing often points toward the side of the vestibular lesion. (From Reilly, B. M.: Practical Strategies in Outpatient Medicine. Philadelphia, W. B. Saunders Co., 1991, p. 195.)*

The examiner compares the two sides for coordination and speed.

Hand-Thigh Test. The patient is asked to pat the thigh with the hand as quickly as possible. The uninjured side is tested first. While doing the test, the patient may be asked to supinate and pronate the hand between each hand-thigh contact to make the test more complex. The examiner watches for speed and coordination and compares the two sides.

Past Pointing Test. The patient and examiner face each other. The examiner holds up both index fingers approximately 15 cm apart. The patient is asked to lift the arms over the head and then bring the arms down to touch the patient's index fingers to the examiner's index fingers (Fig. 13–52). The test is repeated with the patient's eyes closed. Normally, the test can be performed without difficulty. Patients with vestibular disease have problems with past pointing. The test may also be used to test proprioception.

Tests for Proprioception

Proprioceptive Finger-Nose Test. The patient keeps the eyes closed. The examiner lightly touches one of the patient's fingers and asks the patient to touch the patient's nose with that finger. The examiner then touches another finger on the other hand, and the patient again touches the nose. Patients with proprioceptive loss have difficulty doing the test without visual input.

Proprioceptive Movement Test. The patient keeps the eyes closed. The examiner moves the patient's finger or toe up or down by grasping it on the sides to lessen clues given by pressure. The patient then tells the examiner which way the digit moved.

Proprioceptive Space Test. The patient keeps the eyes closed. The examiner places one of the patient's hands or feet in a selected position in space. The patient is then asked to imitate that position with the other limb or to find the hand or foot with the other limb. True proprioceptive loss will cause the patient to be unable to properly position or to find the normal limb with the limb that has proprioceptive loss.

Past Pointing Test. The test is performed as described above.

Reflexes and Cutaneous Distribution

With a head injury patient, deep tendon reflexes (see Table 1–11) should be performed. Accentuation of one or more of the reflexes may indicate trauma to the brain on the opposite side. Pathological reflexes (see Table 1–13) may also be altered with a head injury.

The corneal reflex (trigeminal nerve, cranial nerve V) is used to test for damage or dysfunction to the pons. The patient looks to one side to avoid involuntary blinking. The examiner touches the cornea (not the eyelashes or conjunctiva) with a small, fine point of cotton (Fig. 13–53). The normal response is a bilateral blink because the reflex arc connects both facial nerve nuclei. If the reflex is absent, the test is considered positive.

The gag reflex may be tested using a tongue depressor that is inserted into the posterior pharynx and depressed toward the hypopharynx. The reflex tests cranial nerves IX and X, and its absence in a trauma setting may indicate caudal brain stem dysfunction.

Consensual light reflex may be tested by shining a light into one eye. This action will cause the "lighted" pupil to constrict. If there is normal communication between the two oculomotor nerves, the "nonlighted" pupil will also constrict.

The jaw reflex is usually tested only if the temporomandibular joint or cervical spine is being examined. The examiner should check the sensation

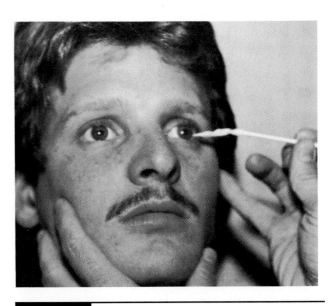

FIGURE 13–53. *Testing corneal sensitivity. (From Seidel, H. M., et al.: Mosby's Guide to Physical Examination. St. Louis, C. V. Mosby Co., 1987, p. 178.)*

of the head and face, keeping in mind the difference in dermatome and sensory nerve distributions (Fig. 13–54). Lip anesthesia or paresthesia is often seen in patients with mandibular fracture.

Joint Play Movements

Because no articular joints are involved in the assessment of the head and face, there are no joint play movements to test.

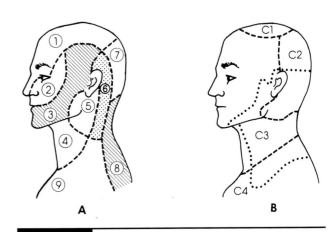

FIGURE 13–54. *(A) Sensory nerve distribution of the head, neck, and face. (1) Ophthalmic nerve. (2) Maxillary nerve. (3) Mandibular nerve. (4) Transverse cutaneous nerve of neck (C2–C3). (5) Greater auricular nerve (C2–C3). (6) Lesser auricular nerve (C2). (7) Greater occipital nerve (C2–C3). (8) Cervical dorsal rami (C3–C5). (9) Suprascapular nerve (C5–C6). (B) Dermatome pattern of the head, neck, and face. C3 is shown in dotted lines because of overlap.*

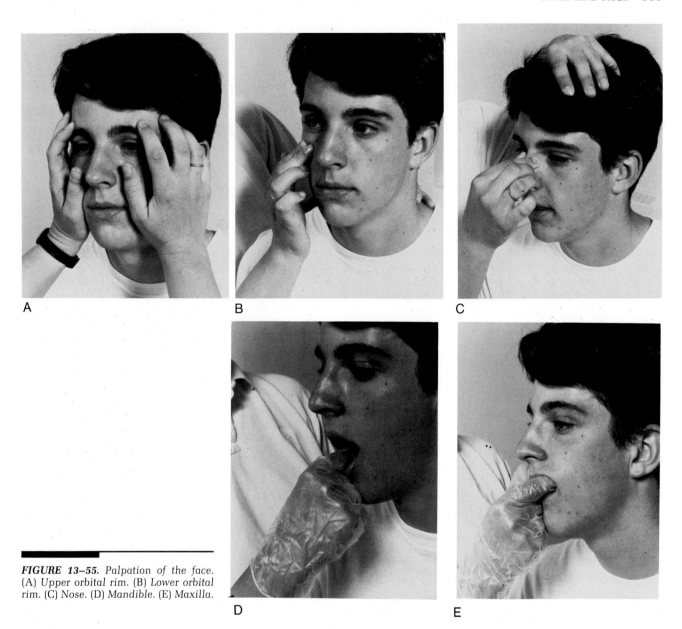

FIGURE 13–55. *Palpation of the face. (A) Upper orbital rim. (B) Lower orbital rim. (C) Nose. (D) Mandible. (E) Maxilla.*

Palpation

During palpation of the head and face, the examiner should note any tenderness, deformity, crepitus, or other signs and symptoms that may indicate the source of pathology. The examiner should note the texture of the skin and surrounding bony and soft tissues. Normally, the patient is palpated in the sitting or supine position, beginning with the skull and moving from anterior to posterior, to the face, and finally to the lateral and posterior structures of the head.

The skull is palpated by a gentle rotary movement of the fingers progressing systematically from front to back. Normally, the skin of the skull moves freely and has no tenderness, swelling, or depressions.

The temporal area and temporalis muscle should be laterally palpated for tenderness and deformity. The external ear or auricle and the periauricular area should also be palpated for tenderness or lacerations.

The occiput should be posteriorly palpated for tenderness. The presence of Battle's sign should be noted, if observed, as this sign is indicative of a basilar skull fracture.

The face is palpated beginning superiorly and working inferiorly in a systematic manner. Like the skull, the forehead is palpated by gentle rotary movements of the fingers feeling the movement of the skin and the occipitofrontalis muscle underneath. Normally, the skin of the forehead moves freely and is smooth and even with no tender areas. The examiner then palpates around the eye socket or orbital rim, moving over the eyebrow and supraorbital rims around the lateral side of the eye and along the zygomatic arch to the infraorbital rims, looking for deformity, crepitus, tenderness, and lacerations (Fig. 13–55A and B). The orbicularis oculi

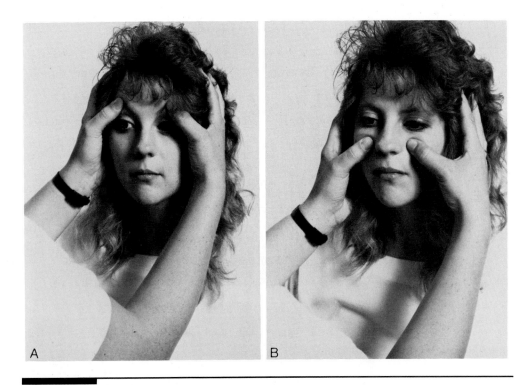

FIGURE 13–56. (A) *Palpation of frontal sinuses.* (B) *Palpation of maxillary sinuses.*

muscles surround the orbit. The medial side of the orbital rim and nose are then palpated for tenderness, deformity, and fracture. The nasal bones, including the lateral and alar cartilage, are palpated for any crepitus or deviation (Fig. 13–55C). The septum should be inspected to see if it has widened, which may indicate a septal hematoma, which often occurs with a fracture. It should also be determined whether the patient can breathe through the nose or smell.

The frontal and maxillary sinuses should be inspected for swelling. To palpate the frontal sinuses, the examiner uses the thumbs to press up under the bony brow on each side of the nose (Fig. 13–56A). The examiner then presses under the zygomatic processes using either the thumbs or index and middle fingers to palpate the maxillary sinuses (Fig. 13–56B). No tenderness or swelling over the soft tissue should be present. The sinus areas may also be percussed to detect tenderness. A light tap directly over each sinus with the index finger can be used to detect tenderness.

The examiner then moves inferiorly to palpate the jaw. The examiner palpates the mandible along its entire length, noting any tenderness, crepitus, or deformity. The examiner, using a rubber glove, may also palpate along the mandible interiorly, noting any tenderness or pain (Fig. 13–55D). The "outside" hand may be used to stabilize the jaw during this procedure. The mandible may also be tapped with a finger along its length to see if tenderness is

elicited. The muscles of the cheek (buccinator) and mouth (orbicularis oris) should be palpated at the same time.

The maxilla may be palpated in a similar fashion, both internally and externally, noting position of the teeth, tenderness, and any deformity (Fig. 13–55E). The examiner may grasp the teeth anteriorly to see if the teeth and mandible move in relation to

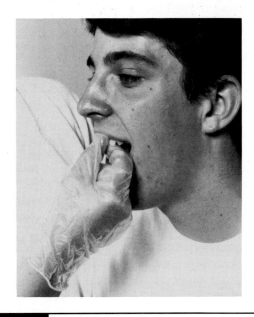

FIGURE 13–57. *Palpation for maxillary fracture with anteroposterior "rocking" motion.*

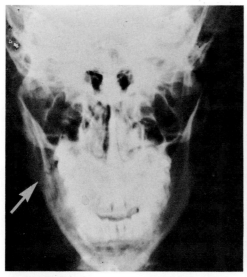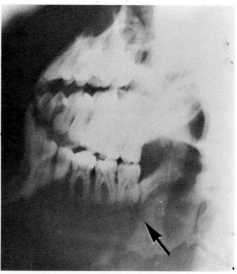

FIGURE 13–58. *Incomplete fracture of angle of mandible on the left. (From O'Donoghue, D. H.: Treatment of Injuries to Athletes. Philadelphia, W. B. Saunders Co., 1984, p. 114.)*

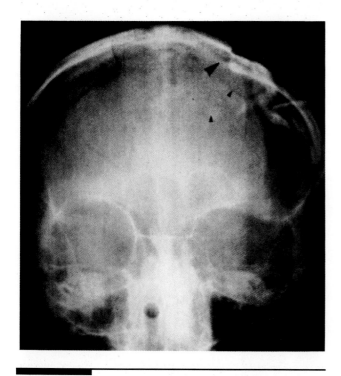

FIGURE 13–59. *Anteroposterior skull roentgenogram to illustrate a depressed parietal skull fracture (large arrow) with multiple bony fragments into the brain (small arrows). (From Albright, J. P., et al.: Head and neck injuries in sports. In Scott, W. N., et al. [eds.]: Principles of Sports Medicine. Baltimore, Williams & Wilkins, 1984, p. 53.)*

the rest of the face, which may indicate a Le Fort fracture (Fig. 13–57).

The trachea should be palpated for midline position. The examiner places a thumb along each side of the trachea, comparing the spaces between the trachea and the sternocleidomastoid muscle, which should be symmetric. The hyoid bone and the thyroid and cricoid cartilages should be identified. Normally, they are smooth and nontender and move when the patient swallows.

Radiographic Examination

Anteroposterior View. The examiner should note the normal bone contours, looking for fractures of the various bones (Figs. 13–58, 13–59, and 13–60).

Lateral View. The examiner should again note bony contours, looking for the possibility of fractures (Figs. 13–58 and 13–61).

CT Scans. CT scans help to differentiate between bone and soft tissue and give a more precise view of fractures (Figs. 13–62 and 13–63).

MRI. MRI is especially useful for demonstrating lesions of the soft tissues of the head and face and for differentiating between bone and soft tissue (Figs. 13–64 and 13–65).

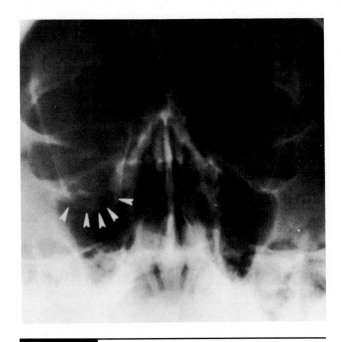

FIGURE 13–60. Plain posteroanterior view showing blow-out fracture of the orbit (arrows). (From Paton, D., and M. F. Goldberg: Management of Ocular Injuries. Philadelphia, W. B. Saunders Co., 1976, p. 70.)

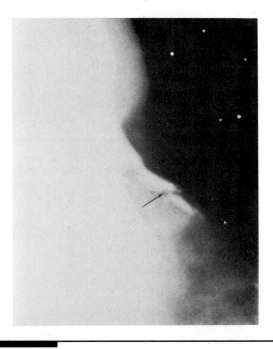

FIGURE 13–61. Lateral radiograph of the nasal bones demonstrating a nasal fracture (arrow). (From Torg, J. S.: Athletic Injuries to the Head, Neck and Face. Philadelphia, Lea & Febiger, 1982, p. 229.)

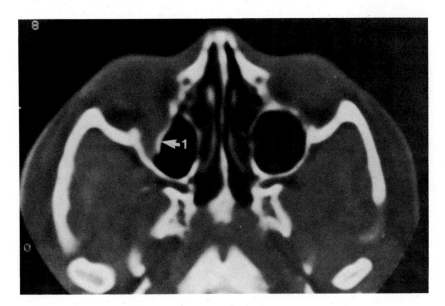

FIGURE 13–62. Axial CT of orbital blow-out fracture showing fracture of the orbit (1) with orbital contents herniated into the maxillary sinus. (From Sinn, D. P., and N. D. Karas: Radiographic evaluation of facial injuries. In Fonseca, R. J., and R. V. Walker [eds.]: Oral and Maxillofacial Trauma. Philadelphia, W. B. Saunders Co., 1991.)

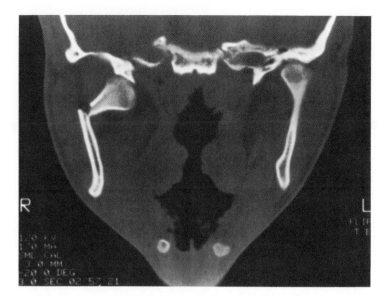

FIGURE 13–63. CT scan is ideal for condylar fractures. (From Bruce, R., and R. J. Fonseca: Mandibular fractures. In Fonseca, R. J., and R. V. Walker [eds.]: Oral and Maxillofacial Trauma. Philadelphia, W. B. Saunders Co., 1991, p. 389.)

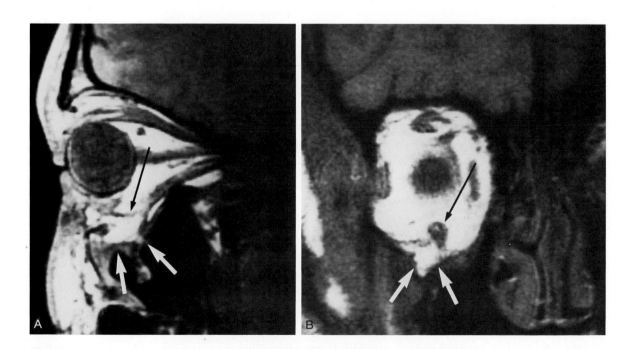

FIGURE 13–64. MRI showing blow-out fracture. Sagittal (A) and coronal (B) T1-weighted scans demonstrate a blow-out fracture of the right orbit with depression of the orbital floor (arrows) into the superior maxillary sinus. The inferior rectus muscle (long arrow) is clearly identified and is not entrapped by the floor fracture. (From Harms, S. E.: The orbit. In Edelman, R. R., and J. R. Hesselink [eds.]: Clinical Magnetic Resonance Imaging. Philadelphia, W. B. Saunders Co., 1990, p. 619.)

T₁ AXIAL

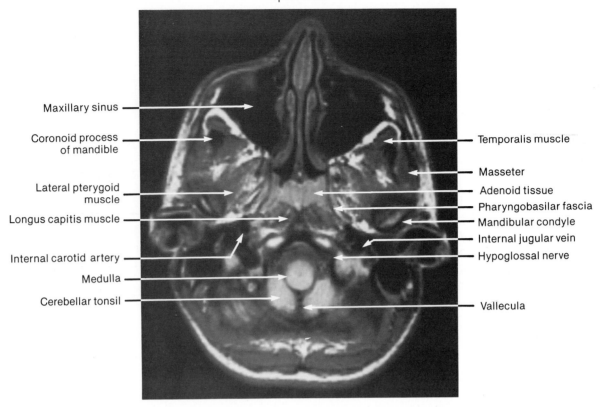

Maxillary sinus

Coronoid process of mandible

Lateral pterygoid muscle

Longus capitis muscle

Internal carotid artery

Medulla

Cerebellar tonsil

Temporalis muscle

Masseter

Adenoid tissue

Pharyngobasilar fascia

Mandibular condyle

Internal jugular vein

Hypoglossal nerve

Vallecula

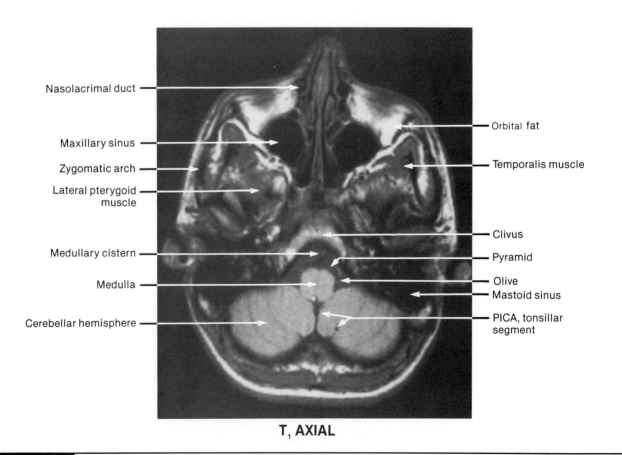

Nasolacrimal duct

Maxillary sinus

Zygomatic arch

Lateral pterygoid muscle

Medullary cistern

Medulla

Cerebellar hemisphere

Orbital fat

Temporalis muscle

Clivus

Pyramid

Olive

Mastoid sinus

PICA, tonsillar segment

T₁ AXIAL

FIGURE 13–65. MRI of the head and brain at two levels. (From Greenberg, J. J., et al.: Brain: Indications technique atlas. In Edelman, R. R., and J. R. Hesselink [eds.]: Clinical Magnetic Resonance Imaging. Philadelphia, W. B. Saunders Co., 1990, p. 384.)

PRÉCIS OF THE HEAD AND FACE ASSESSMENT*

History (sitting)
Observation (sitting)
Examination* (sitting)
  Head injury
    Neural watch
    Glasgow Coma Scale
  Facial injury
  Eye injury
  Nasal injury
  Tooth injury
  Ear injury
  Special tests
  Reflexes and cutaneous distribution
  Palpation
  Radiographic examination

---

*When examining the head and face, if only one area has been injured (e.g., the nose), then only that area needs to be examined provided the examiner is certain that adjacent structures have not also been injured.

After any examination, the patient should always be warned of the possibility of exacerbation of symptoms as a result of the assessment.

CASE STUDIES

When doing these case studies, the examiner should list the appropriate questions to be asked and why they are being asked, what to look for and why, and what things should be tested and why. Depending on the answers of the patient (and the examiner should consider different responses), several possible causes of the patient's problem may become evident (examples given in parentheses). If so, a differential diagnosis chart should be made up. The examiner can then decide how different diagnoses may affect the treatment plan.

1. A 13-year-old boy received "an elbow" in the nose and cheek while play-wrestling. The nose is crooked and painful and bled after the injury, and the cheek is sore. Describe your assessment plan for this patient (nasal fracture versus zygomal fracture).

2. A 23-year-old woman was in an automobile accident. She was a passenger in the front seat and was not wearing a seat belt. The car in which she was riding hit another car, which had run a red light. The woman's face hit the dashboard of the car, and she received a severe facial injury. Describe your assessment plan for this patient (Le Fort fracture versus mandibular fracture).

3. An 83-year-old man tripped in the bathroom and hit his chin against the bathtub, knocking himself unconscious. Describe your assessment plan for this patient, (cervical spine lesion versus mandibular fracture).

4. An 18-year-old woman was playing squash. She was not wearing eye protectors and was hit in the eye with the ball. Describe your assessment plan for this patient (ruptured globe versus "blow-out" fracture).

5. A 27-year-old man was playing football. He received "a knee to the head," rendering him unconscious for approximately 3 minutes. Describe your assessment plan

for this patient (concussion versus expanding intracranial lesion).

6. A 15-year-old boy was playing field hockey. He was not wearing a mouth guard and was hit in the mouth and jaw by the ball. There was a large amount of blood. Describe your assessment plan for this patient (tooth fracture versus mandible fracture).

7. A 16-year-old male wrestler comes to you complaining of ear pain. He has just finished a match, which he lost. Describe your assessment plan for this patient (cauliflower ear versus external otitis).

8. A 17-year-old female basketball player comes to you complaining of eye pain. She says she received a "finger in the eye" when she went up to get the ball. Describe your assessment plan for this patient (hyphema versus corneal abrasion).

REFERENCES

CITED REFERENCES

1. Albright, J. P., J. Van Gilder, G. El Khoury, E. Crowley, and D. Foster: Head and neck injuries in sports. In Scott, W. N., B. Nisonson, and J. A. Nicholas (eds.): Principles of Sports Medicine. Baltimore, Williams & Wilkins, 1984.
2. Torg, J. S.: Athletic Injuries to the Head, Neck and Face. Philadelphia, Lea & Febiger, 1982.
3. Manzi, D. B., and P. A. Weaver: Head Injury: The Acute Care Phase. Thorofare, New Jersey, Slack Inc., 1987.
4. Seidel, H. M., J. W. Ball, J. E. Dains, and G. W. Benedict: Mosby's Guide to Physical Examination. St. Louis, C.V. Mosby Co., 1987.
5. Swartz, M. H.: Textbook of Physical Diagnosis: History and Examination. Philadelphia, W. B. Saunders Co., 1989.
6. Reilly, B. M.: Practical Strategies in Outpatient Medicine. Philadelphia, W. B. Saunders Co., 1984.
7. Novey, D. W.: Rapid Access Guide to the Physical Examination. Chicago, Year Book Medical Pub., 1988.
8. Pashby, T. J, and R. C. Pashby: Treatment of sports eye injuries. In Schneider, R. C., J. C. Kennedy, and M. L. Plant (eds.): Sports Injuries—Mechanisms, Prevention and Treatment. Baltimore, Williams & Wilkins, 1985.
9. Topel, J. L.: Examination of the comatose patient. In Weiner, W. J., and C. G. Goetz (eds.): Neurology for the Non-Neurologist. Philadelphia, J. B. Lippincott, 1989.
10. Fonseca, R. J., and R. V. Walker: Oral and Maxillofacial Trauma. Philadelphia, W. B. Saunders Co., 1991.
11. Pollock, R. A., and R. O. Dingman: Management and reconstruction of athletic injuries of the face, anterior neck, and upper respiratory tract. In Schneider, R. C., J. C. Kennedy, and M. L. Plant (eds.): Sports Injuries—Mechanisms, Prevention and Treatment. Baltimore, Williams & Wilkins, 1985.
12. Simpson, J. F., and K. R. Magee: Clinical Evaluation of the Nervous System. Boston, Little, Brown and Co., 1973.

GENERAL REFERENCES

American Academy of Orthopedic Surgeons: Athletic Training and Sports Medicine. Chicago, AAOOS, 1984.
Booher, J. M., and G. A. Thibodeau: Athletic Injury Assessment. St. Louis, C. V. Mosby Co., 1989.
Boyd-Monk, H.: Examining the external eye. Nursing 80:58–63, 1980.
Bruce, R., and R. J. Fonseca: Mandibular fractures. In Fonseca R. J., and R. V. Walker (eds.): Oral and Maxillofacial Trauma. Philadelphia, W. B. Saunders Co., 1991.
Bruno, L. A., T. A. Gennarelli, and J. S. Torg: Head injuries in athletics. In Welsh R. P., and R. J. Shephard (eds.): Current Therapy in Sports Medicine 1985–1986. St. Louis, C. V. Mosby Co., 1985.

Bruno, L. A., T. A. Gennarelli, and J. S. Torg: Management guidelines for head injuries in athletics. Clin. Sports Med. 6:17–29, 1987.

Burde, R. M.: Eye movements and vestibular system. *In* Pearlman, A. L., and R. C. Collins (eds.): Neurological Pathophysiology. New York, Oxford University Press, 1984.

Canter, R. C.: Guidelines for return to contact sports after a cerebral concussion. Phys. Sportsmed. 14:75–83, 1986.

Cox, M. S., C. L. Schepens, and H. M. MacKenzie Freeman: Retinal detachment due to ocular contusion. Arch. Ophthal. 76:678–685, 1966.

Diamond, G. R., G. E. Quinn, T. J. Pashby, and M. Easterbrook: Ophthalmologic injuries. Clin . Sports Med. 1:469–482, 1982.

Easterbrook, M., and J. Cameron: Injuries in racquet sports. *In* Schneider, R. C., J. C. Kennedy, and M. L. Plant (eds.): Sports Injuries—Mechanisms, Prevention and Treatment. Baltimore, Williams & Wilkins, 1985.

Edelman, R. R., and J. R. Hesselink: Clinical Magnetic Resonance Imaging. Philadelphia, W. B. Saunders Co., 1990.

Ellis, E.: Fractures of the zygomatic complex and arch. *In* Fonseca, R. J., and R. V. Walker (eds.): Oral and Maxillofacial Trauma. Philadelphia, W. B. Saunders Co., 1991.

Fahey, T. D.: Athletic Training–Principles and Practice. Palo Alto, Calif., Mayfield Pub. Co., 1986.

Foreman, S. M., and A. C. Croft: Whiplash Injuries–The Cervical Acceleration/Deceleration Syndrome. Baltimore, Williams & Wilkins, 1988.

Frost, D. E., and B. D. Kendall: Applied surgical anatomy of the head and neck. *In* Fonseca, R. J., and R. V. Walker (eds.): Oral and Maxillofacial Trauma. Philadelphia, W. B. Saunders Co., 1991.

Garrison, D. W.: Cranial Nerves–A Systems Approach. Springfield, Ill., Charles C Thomas Pub., 1986.

Gorman, B. D.: Ophthalmology and sports medicine. *In* Scott, W. N., B. Nisonson, and J. A. Nicholas (eds.): Principles of Sports Medicine. Baltimore, Williams & Wilkins, 1984.

Halling, A. H.: The importance of clinical signs and symptoms in the evaluation of facial fractures. Athletic Training 17:102–103, 1982.

Havener, W. H., and T. A. Makley: Emergency management of ocular injuries. Ohio State Med. J. 71: 776–779, 1975.

Hildebrandt, J. R.: Dental and maxillofacial injuries. Clin. Sports Med. 1:449–468, 1982.

Jenkins, D. B.: Hollinshead's Functional Anatomy of the Limbs and Back. Philadelphia, W. B. Saunders Co., 1991.

Jordan, B. D.: Head injury in sports. *In* Jordan, B. D., P. Tsairis, and R. F. Warren (eds.): Sports Neurology. Rockville, Maryland. Aspen Publishers Inc., 1989.

Kulund, D. N.: The Injured Athlete. Philadelphia, J. B. Lippincott Co., 1988.

Lampert, P. W., and J. M. Hardman: Morphological changes in brains of boxers. J. A. M. A. 251:2676-2679, 1984.

Lew, D., and D. P. Sinn: Diagnosis and treatment of midface fractures. *In* Fonseca, R. J., and R. V. Walker (eds.): Oral and Maxillofacial Trauma. Philadelphia, W. B. Saunders Co., 1991.

Liebgott, B.: The Anatomical Basis of Dentistry. Philadelphia, W. B. Saunders Co., 1988.

Mueller, F. D.: Catastrophic head and neck injuries. Phys. Sportsmed. 7:710–714, 1979.

Nasher, L. M.: A Systems Approach to Understanding and Assessing Orientation and Balance Disorders. NeuroCom International Inc., Clackamas, Oregon: 1987.

O'Donoghue, D. H.: Treatment of Injuries to Athletes. Philadelphia, W. B. Saunders Co., 1984.

Pashby, R. C., and T. J. Pashby: Ocular injuries in sports. *In* Welsh R. P., and R. J. Shephard (eds.): Current Therapy in Sports Medicine 1985—1986. St. Louis, C. V. Mosby Co., 1985.

Paton, D., and M. F. Goldberg: Management of Ocular Injuries. Philadelphia, W. B. Saunders Co., 1976.

Powers, M. P.: Diagnosis and management of dentoalveolar injuries. *In* Fonseca, R. J., and R. V. Walker (eds.): Oral and Maxillofacial Trauma. Philadelphia, W. B. Saunders Co., 1991.

Rimel, R. W., B. Giordani, J. T. Barth, T. J. Boll, and J. J. Jane: Disability caused by minor head injury. Neurosurg. 9:2212–228, 1981.

Ross, R. J., I. R. Casson, O. Siegel, and M. Cole: Boxing injuries: Neurologic, radiologic and neuropsychologic evaluation. Clin. Sports Med. 6:41–51, 1987.

Rousseau, A. P.: Ocular trauma in sports. *In* MacKenzie Freeman H. M. (ed.): Ocular Trauma in Sports. New York, Appleton-Century-Crofts, 1979.

Roy, S., and R. Irvin: Sports Medicine–Prevention, Evaluation, Management and Rehabilitation. Englewood Cliffs, N. J. Prentice-Hall Inc., 1983.

Sandusky, J. C.: Field evaluation of eye injuries. Athletic Training 16:254–258, 1981.

Schneider, R. C.: Head and Neck Injuries in Football—Mechanisms, Treatment and Prevention. Baltimore, Williams & Wilkins, 1973.

Schneider, R. C., T. R. Peterson, and R. E. Anderson: Football. *In* Schneider, R. C., J. C. Kennedy, and M. L. Plant (eds.): Sports Injuries—Mechanisms, Prevention and Treatment. Baltimore, Williams & Wilkins, 1985.

Schuller, D. E., and R. A. Bruce: Ear, nose, throat, and eye. In Strauss R. H. (ed.): Sports Medicine. Philadelphia, W. B. Saunders Co., 1984.

Schultz, R. C., and D. L. de Camara: Athletic facial injuries. J. A. M. A. 252:3395–3398, 1984.

Scott, W. N., B. Nisonson, and J. A. Nicholas: Principles of Sports Medicine. Baltimore, Williams & Wilkins, 1984.

Sinn, D. P., and N. D. Karras: Radiographic evaluation of facial injuries. *In* Fonseca, R. J., and V. Walker (eds.): Oral and Maxillofacial Trauma. Philadelphia, W. B. Saunders Co., 1991.

Sitler, M.: Nasal septal injuries. Athletic Training 21:10–12, 1986.

Solon, R. C.: Maxillofacial trauma. *In* Scott, W. N., B. Nisonson, and J. A. Nicholas (eds.): Principles of Sports Medicine. Baltimore, Williams & Wilkins, 1984.

Untevharnscheidt, F.: Boxing injuries. *In* Schneider, R. C., J. C. Kennedy, and M. L. Plant (eds.): Sports Injuries—Mechanisms, Prevention and Treatment. Baltimore, Williams & Wilkins, 1985.

Vegso, J. J., and R. C. Lehman: Field evaluation and management of head and neck injuries. Clin. Sports Med. 6:1–15, 1987.

Vinger, P. F.: How I manage corneal abrasions and lacerations. Phys. Sportsmed. 14:170–179, 1986.

Gait Assessment

Walking is the simple act of falling forward and catching oneself. One foot is always in contact with the ground, and within a cycle there are two periods of single-leg support and two periods of double-leg support. When one runs, there is a period of time during which one foot is not always in contact with the ground, and there is a period called "double float."

The locomotion pattern tends to be variable and irregular until about the age of 7 years. There are several functional tasks involved in gait, including forward progression, which is executed in a stepping movement in a wide range of rapid and comfortable walking speeds. Second, one must alternately balance the body on one limb and then the other; this is accompanied by repeated adjustments of limb length. Finally, there is support of the upright body.

This chapter gives a basic overview of normal gait but does not go into a detailed description; this task is left to other authors.[1-4] The various terms commonly used to describe gait, the normal pattern of gait, the assessment of gait, and common abnormal gaits are reviewed.

DEFINITIONS[1-4]

Gait Cycle

The gait cycle is the time interval or sequence of motions occurring between two consecutive initial contacts for the same foot (Fig. 14–1). For example, if heel strike is the initial contact, the gait cycle for the right leg is from one heel strike to the next heel strike on the same foot. The gait cycle consists of two phases for each foot: *stance phase* and *swing phase*. In addition, there are two periods of *double support* and one period of *single-leg stance* during the gait cycle.

Stance Phase

The stance phase of gait occurs when the foot is on the ground and bearing weight (Fig. 14–2). It allows the lower leg to support the weight of the body and allows for the advancement of the body over the supporting limb. Normally, this makes up 60 per cent of the gait cycle and consists of five subphases, or *instants*:

1. Initial contact (heel strike).
2. Load response (foot flat).
3. Midstance (single-leg stance).
4. Terminal stance (heel-off).
5. Preswing (toe-off).

The initial contact instant is the *weight-loading* or *weight acceptance* period of the stance leg, which accounts for the first 10 per cent of the gait cycle. During this period, one foot is coming off the floor while the other foot is accepting body weight and absorbing the shock of initial contact so that both feet are in contact with the floor; it is thus a period of *double-leg support* or *double-leg stance*.

The load response and midstance instants compose the *single-leg support* or *single-leg stance*, which accounts for the next 40 per cent of the gait cycle. During this period, one leg alone carries the body weight while the other leg goes through its swing phase. The stance leg must be able to hold the weight of the body, and the body must be able to balance on the one stance leg. In addition, lateral hip stability must be exhibited to maintain the balance, and the tibia of the stance leg must advance over the stationary foot.

The terminal stance and preswing instants make up the *weight-unloading period*, which accounts for the next 10 per cent of the gait cycle. During this period, the stance leg is unloading the body weight to the contralateral limb and prepares the leg for the swing phase. As with the first two instants, both

the normal gait cycle and takes up approximately 30 per cent of the cycle.

NORMAL PARAMETERS OF GAIT[2-5]

Base Width

The normal base width, which is the distance between the two feet, is 5 to 10 cm (Fig. 14–5). If the base is wider than this amount, one may suspect some pathology, such as cerebellar or inner ear problems, which results in the balance being poor, or diabetes or peripheral neuropathy, which may indicate a loss of sensation. In either case, the patient tends to have a wider base to maintain balance.

Gait (Step) Length

Gait length is the distance between successive contact points on opposite feet. Normally, this distance is 35 to 41 cm and should be equal for both legs. It varies with age and sex, with children taking smaller steps than adults and females taking smaller steps than males. Height also has an effect as a taller person takes larger steps. Step length tends to de-

crease with age, fatigue, pain, and disease. If gait length is normal for both legs, the rhythm of walking will be smooth. If there is pain in one limb, the patient will attempt to take weight off that limb as quickly as possible, altering the rhythm.

Stride Length

Stride length is the linear distance in the plane of progression between successive points of foot-to-floor contact of the same foot. The stride length is normally about 70 to 82 cm in length and in reality is one gait cycle.

Lateral Pelvic Shift (Pelvic List)

Lateral pelvic shift is the side-to-side movement of the pelvis during walking and is necessary to center the weight of the body over the stance leg for balance (Fig. 14–6). The lateral pelvic shift is normally 2.5 to 5 cm. It increases if the feet are farther apart.

Vertical Pelvic Shift (Pelvic Tilt)

Vertical pelvic shift keeps the center of gravity from moving up and down more than 5 cm during normal gait. By means of a vertical pelvic tilt, the high point

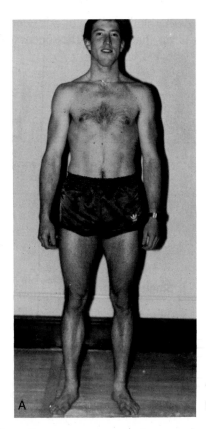
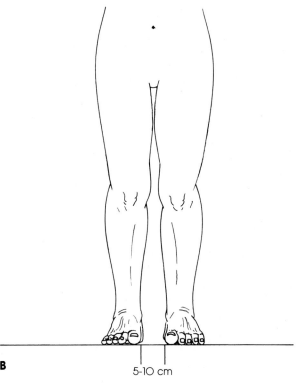

5-10 cm

FIGURE 14–5. (A) Photograph shows individual standing with wider-than-normal base width. (B) Normal base width.

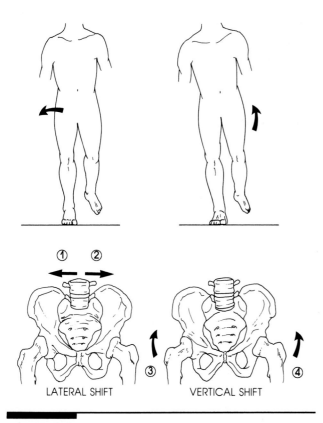

FIGURE 14–6. *Pelvic shift. Numbers indicate that one lateral or vertical shift occurs, and then the other; they do not occur at the same time. 1, Right lateral shift. 2, Left lateral shift. 3, Right vertical shift. 4, Left vertical shift.*

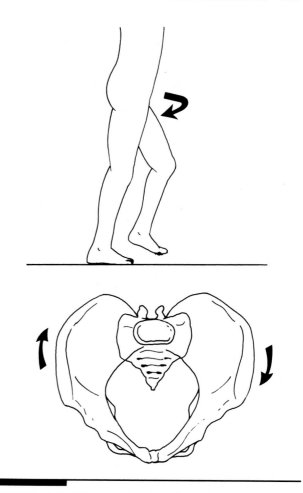

FIGURE 14–7. *Pelvic rotation. Left forward pelvic rotation is illustrated.*

occurs during midstance and the low point occurs during initial contact, although the height of these points may increase during the swing phase if the knee is fused. On the swing phase, the hip is lower on the swing side, and the patient must flex the knee and dorsiflex the foot to clear the toe. This action shortens the extremity length at midstance and decreases the center of gravity rise.

Pelvic Rotation

Pelvic rotation is necessary to lessen the angle of the femur with the floor, and in so doing it lengthens the femur (Fig. 14–7). It decreases the center-of-gravity path amplitude of displacement and thus decreases the center-of-gravity dip. There is a total of 8° pelvic rotation, with 4° forward on the swing leg and 4° posteriorly on the stance leg. For balance to be maintained, the thorax rotates in the opposite direction of the pelvis. Thus, when the pelvis rotates clockwise, the thorax rotates counterclockwise, and vice versa. These concurrent rotations provide counterrotation forces and help regulate the individual's speed of walking.

Center of Gravity

Normally, in the standing position, the center of gravity is 5 cm anterior to the second sacral vertebra; it tends to be slightly higher in males than in females because males tend to have a greater body mass in the shoulder area. The vertical and horizontal displacements of the center of gravity describe a "figure-eight" occupying a 5-cm square within the pelvis during walking. The vertical displacement can be observed from the side. The patient's head will descend during weight-loading and weight-unloading periods and will rise during single-leg stance.

Normal Cadence

The normal cadence is between 90 and 120 steps per minute. With age, the cadence decreases. Figure 14–8 illustrates the cadence of normal gait from heel strike to toe-off. With pathology or deformity (e.g., a cavus foot), this pattern may be altered. As the pace of walking increases, the stride width increases, and the toeing-out angle decreases.

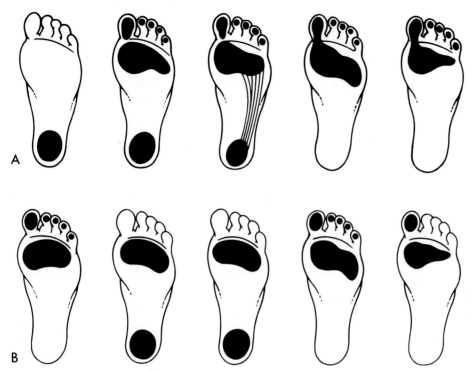

FIGURE 14–8. The cadence of gait. (A) Normal foot. (B) Cavus foot. (From Viladot, A.: Patología del Antepié. Barcelona, Ediciones Toray, S.A., 1975.)

NORMAL PATTERN OF GAIT[1–4, 6]

Stance Phase

As previously mentioned, there are five instants involved during the stance phase of gait. These are now described in order of occurrence. This phase is the closed kinetic chain phase of gait. The action occurring at the various joints causes a "chain reaction" due to the stresses put on the joints and supporting structures with weight bearing. The foot now becomes the fixed stable segment, and alterations occur from the foot up, with the joints of the foot adapting first, followed by the ankle, knee, hip, pelvis, and spine. Thus, the relationship between the joints changes. During the swing phase, the alterations occur from the spine, pelvis, and hip down.

INITIAL CONTACT

During the initial contact, the hip is flexed 30 to 49° and is medially rotated; the knee is slightly flexed, or extended; the ankle is at 90° with the foot supinated; and the hindfoot is everted. The pelvis is level and medially rotated on the initial contact side while the trunk is aligned between the two lower limbs. At this instant, there is little force going through the limb. If pain occurs in the heel at this time, it may be due to a heel spur, bone bruise, heel fat pad bruise, or bursitis. If the knee is weak, the patient may extend the knee by using the hand or may hit the heel hard on the ground to "whip" the knee into extension. A patient may do this because of weakness of the muscles (e.g., a reflex inhibition, poliomyelitis, or other condition), an internal derangement of the knee, a nerve root lesion (L2, L3, or L4), or femoral neuropathy. In the past, this instant was referred to as "heel strike"; however, with some pathological gaits, heel strike may not be the first instant. Instead, the toes, the forefoot, or the entire foot may initially contact the ground. If the dorsiflexor muscles are weak, instead of heel contact, the foot "slaps" or "flops" down. The weakness may be due to a peroneal neuropathy or nerve root lesion (L4).

LOAD RESPONSE

Load response is a critical event in that the person subconsciously decides whether the limb will be able to bear the weight of the body. The forefoot is pronated to enable it to absorb the shock more effectively, and the plantar aspect is in contact with the floor. The ankle is plantar flexed, and the hindfoot is inverted. The foot is pronated, since this position unlocks the foot and enables it to adapt to different terrains and postures. The flexed and laterally rotated hip begins going into extension while the knee flexes 15 to 25°. The pelvis drops slightly on the swing leg side and medially rotates on the same side. The trunk is aligned with the stance leg. The tibia will begin to move forward over the fixed foot, and the body swings over the foot.

MIDSTANCE

The midstance instant is a period of stationary foot support. Normally, the weight of the foot is evenly distributed over the entire foot. The trunk is aligned over the stance leg, while the pelvis shows a slight drop to the swing leg side.

During this stage, there is maximum extension of the hip (10 to 15°) with lateral rotation, and the greatest force is on the hip. The knee begins to flex, and the ankle is locked at 5 to 8° of dorsiflexion, rolling forward on the forefoot (roll-off). The foot is in contact with the floor with the forefoot pronated and the hindfoot inverted. This instant is another critical event for the ankle. If the pain is elicited during this period, it may be due to conditions such as arthritis, rigid pes planus, fallen metatarsal or longitudinal arches, plantar fasciitis, or Morton's metatarsalgia. If the gluteus medius (L5 nerve root) is weak, the Trendelenburg sign will be positive.

TERMINAL STANCE AND PRESWING

In the final stages, the hip begins to flex and moves from lateral rotation to medial rotation, while the knee is flexed to 50 to 60°. At the ankle, there is plantar flexion. This action helps to smooth the center-of-gravity pathway. The forefoot is initially in contact with the floor, and the foot progresses so that only the big toe is in contact with the floor. The forefoot begins to move from inversion to eversion.

The pelvis is initially level and laterally rotated and then dips to the swing leg side, remaining laterally rotated. The trunk is initially aligned over the lower limbs and moves toward the stance leg. If pain is elicited during these instants, it may be due to a hallux rigidus. With hallux rigidus, the patient is unable to push off on the medial aspect of the foot; instead, the patient pushes off on the lateral aspect of the foot to compensate for the painful metatarsal arch resulting from increased pressure on the metatarsal heads. If the plantar flexors are weak (e.g., S1–S2 nerve root), push-off may be absent. The foot pronates so that there is a rigid lever for better push-off.

Swing Phase

The swing phase of gait involves the lower limb in an open kinetic chain; the foot is not fixed on the ground, and the stresses on the limb are therefore less and easier to dissipate. During this phase, alterations occur from the pelvis and hip down as these structures provide the most stability in the lower limb during non–weight bearing. As previously mentioned, there are three instants involved during the swing phase of gait. These are now described in order of occurrence.

INITIAL SWING

During the first subphase of acceleration (Fig. 14–9), flexion and medial rotation of the hip and flexion of the knee occur. The pelvis medially rotates and

dips the swing leg side. The trunk is aligned with the stance leg. In addition, the ankle continues to plantar flex. The foot is not in contact with the floor. The forefoot continues supinating while the hindfoot continues everting. The dorsiflexor muscles contract to allow the foot to clear the ground, and the knee exhibits its maximum flexion of about 60°. If the quadriceps muscles are weak, the pelvis is thrust forward to provide forward momentum to the leg.

MIDSWING

During the midswing instant, the hip continues to flex and medially rotate, and the knee continues to flex. The ankle is in the anatomic position for the first 25 per cent of the stance phase to permit the foot and midtarsal joints to unlock for the foot to adapt to uneven terrain while weight bearing. The forefoot is supinated, and the hindfoot is everted. The pelvis and trunk are in the same position as during the previous stage. If the dorsiflexor muscles are weak, the patient will demonstrate a high steppage gait. In such a gait, the hip flexes excessively so that the toes can clear the ground.

TERMINAL SWING

During the final subphase, also called deceleration, the hip continues to flex and medially rotate, while the knee reaches its maximum extension. At the ankle, dorsiflexion has occurred. The forefoot is supinated, and the hindfoot is everted. The trunk and pelvis maintain the same position as before. The hamstring muscles are contracting during the terminal phase to slow the swing; if the hamstrings are weak (e.g., S1–S2 nerve root lesion), heel strike may be excessively harsh.

Other Patterns in Gait

Hip. The function of the hip is to extend the leg during the stance phase and flex the leg during the swing phase. The ligaments of the hip help to stabilize it in extension. If there is loss of movement of the hip, the compensatory mechanisms are increased mobility of the knee on the same side and increased mobility of the contralateral hip. In addition, the lumbar spine shows increased mobility. The hip extensors help to initiate movement, as do the hip flexors; therefore, both groups of muscles work phasically. The hip flexors (primarily, the iliopsoas muscle) fire to slow extension; the hip extensors (primarily, hamstring muscles) fire to slow flexion. In this way, they work eccentrically. The abductor muscles provide stability during single-leg support, another critical event for the hip.

Knee. When the knee is in flexion during the first three instants of the stance phase of gait, it acts as a shock absorber. Painful knees are not able to do this.

NORMAL GAIT

	SWING 40%			STANCE 60%				
	INITIAL SWING	MID-SWING	TERMINAL SWING	INITIAL CONTACT	LOADING RESPONSE	MID-STANCE	TERMINAL STANCE	PRE-SWING
TRUNK	ERECT NEUTRAL	ERECT NEUTRAL	ERECT NEUTRAL	ERECT NEUTRAL	ERECT NEUTRAL	ERECT NEUTRAL	ERECT NEUTRAL	ERECT NEUTRAL
PELVIS	LEVEL; BACKWARD ROTATION 5°	LEVEL; NEUTRAL ROTATION	LEVEL; FORWARD ROTATION 5°	LEVEL; MAINTAINS FORWARD ROTATION	LEVEL; LESS FORWARD ROTATION	LEVEL; NEUTRAL ROTATION	LEVEL; BACKWARD ROTATION 5°	LEVEL; BACKWARD ROTATION 5°
HIP	FLEXION 20° NEUTRAL ROTATION ABDUCTION ADDUCTION	FLEXION 20°→30° NEUTRAL ROTATION ABDUCTION ADDUCTION	FLEXION 30° NEUTRAL ROTATION ABDUCTION ADDUCTION	FLEXION 30° NEUTRAL ROTATION ABDUCTION ADDUCTION	FLEXION 30° NEUTRAL ROTATION ABDUCTION ADDUCTION	EXTENDING TO NEUTRAL NEUTRAL ROTATION ABDUCTION ADDUCTION	APPARENT HYPEREXT 10° NEUTRAL ROTATION ABDUCTION ADDUCTION	NEUTRAL EXTENSION NEUTRAL ROTATION ABDUCTION ADDUCTION
KNEE	FLEXION 60°	FROM 60° TO 30° FLEXION	EXTENSION TO 0°	FULL EXTENSION	FLEXION 15°	EXTENDING TO NEUTRAL	FULL EXTENSION	FLEXION 35°
ANKLE	PLANTAR FLEXION 10°	NEUTRAL	NEUTRAL	NEUTRAL HEEL FIRST	PLANTAR FLEXION 15°	FROM PLANTAR FLEXION TO 10° DORSIFLEXION	NEUTRAL WITH TIBIA STABLE AND HEEL OFF PRIOR TO INITIAL CONTACT OPPOSITE FOOT	PLANTAR FLEXION 20°
TOES	NEUTRAL	NEUTRAL	NEUTRAL	NEUTRAL	NEUTRAL	NEUTRAL	NEUTRAL IP EXTENDED MP	NEUTRAL IP EXTENDED MP

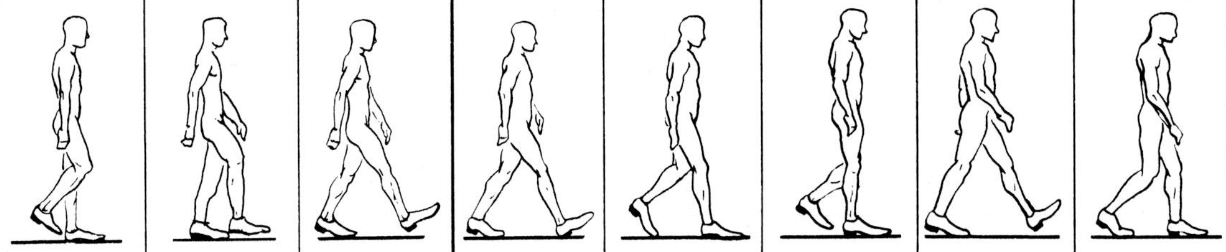

FIGURE 14–9. Normal gait cycle. Pathokinesiology Service and Physical Therapy Department: *Normal and Pathological Gait Syllabus,* p. 11. (Courtesy of Ranchos Los Amigos Hospital, Downey, Calif.)

One of the critical events of the knee is extension. The functions of the knee during gait are to bear weight, absorb shock, extend the stride length, and allow the foot to move through its swing. The quadriceps muscles use only 4 to 5 per cent of their maximum voluntary contraction to extend the knee, but in so doing they help to control weight acceptance. The hamstring muscles flex the knee and slow the leg down in the swing phase, working eccentrically. If the knee has a flexion deformity, the hip is flexed and therefore loses its extension power, which is a critical event for the hip. By observing the knee anteriorly, the examiner can usually see the rotation occurring.

Gastrocnemius and Soleus. The gastrocnemius and soleus muscles are important in gait. They use 85 per cent of their maximum voluntary contraction during normal walking. These muscles help to restrain the body's own forward momentum during gait.

Foot and Ankle. The ankle and foot play major roles in gait in that the various joints allow the foot to accommodate to the ground. The joints in the foot and ankle work interdependently during normal gait. When the heel contacts with the ground, the lower limb becomes a closed kinetic chain, and movements and stresses must be absorbed by the structures of the lower limb.

OBSERVATION AND EXAMINATION

Overview and Patient History

The observation of an individual's gait should be included in any assessment of the lower limb. One must keep in mind that the posture of the head, neck, thorax, and lumbar spine can affect gait when no pathology is evident in the lower limb. The examiner must be able to identify the action of each body segment and note any deviation from normal during the individual phases of gait. For this reason, it is important to understand the normal parameters of gait and the mechanism of gait as it occurs. If one understands these normal events and how, when, and why they occur, how the gait is altered under pathological conditions can be better understood.

The examiner should first perform a general overview of the patient's gait, looking at stride length, step frequency, time of swing, speed of walking, and duration of the complete walking cycle. Once this overview is completed, the examiner can look at specific parts of gait in terms of phases and what happens at each joint during these phases.

Because gait constantly changes as one stops and starts, hurries, dawdles, and walks with others, it is important to remember whether the movements the patient is capable of are normal and whether the speeds, phases, strides, and duration of the cycles occur in normal combinations. Thus, in addition to the patient walking at a normal speed, slow and fast gait speed should be examined to see if these changes affect the gait. The examiner must be able to see the lumbar spine, pelvis, hips, knees, feet, and ankles. Female patients should be in a bra and briefs, and male patients should be in shorts. The patient should walk barefoot. In this way, the motions of the toes, feet, legs, pelvis, and trunk can be properly observed.

It is important that one read the patient's charts and take a history from the patient regarding any disease or injury, past or present, that may be causing gait problems. The examiner should ask the patient to walk in the usual manner, using any aids necessary, for example, parallel bars, crutches, walker, or canes. While the patient is doing this, an initial general observation of any obvious limp or deformity should be made.

Sequential Observation

The examiner should observe the gait from the front, behind, and the side, in each instance observing from proximal to distal and watching the pelvis and lumbar spine down to the ankle and foot. This method will provide a sequential, thorough manner to the assessment.

ANTERIOR VIEW

When observing from the front as the patient walks, one should note whether any lateral tilt to the pelvis occurs, whether there is any sideway swaying of the trunk, whether the pelvis rotates on a horizontal plane, and whether the trunk and upper extremity rotate in the opposite direction to the pelvis. Usually, the trunk and upper extremity rotation is approximately 180° out of phase with the pelvis, (i.e., as the pelvis and lower limb rotate one way, the trunk and upper limb rotate in the opposite direction). This action helps provide a balancing effect and smoothes the forward progression of the body. One should note any bowing of the femur or the tibia, any medial or lateral rotation of the hips, and the position of the feet as the patient goes through the gait cycle (Fig. 14–10). This view is best used to examine the weight-loading period of the gait cycle. It should also be noted whether there is any abduction or circumduction of the swing leg, atrophy of the musculature of the anterior thigh and leg, and a normal base width.

LATERAL VIEW

During the gait cycle, the examiner should observe from the side any lumbar lordosis, hip movement, or limitation of flexion or extension of the hip. This view enables one to examine the interactions be-

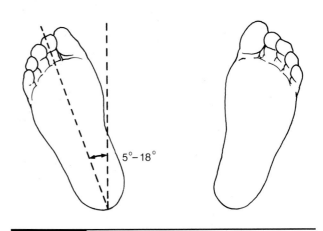

FIGURE 14–10. *During stance and gait, the toes angle out 5 to 18° (Fick angle).*

tween the walking surface and the various body parts.

As the patient moves from initial contact to loading response, the foot flexes immediately while the knee flexes until the foot is flat on the floor. During this period, the hip is also flexed.

During midstance, the ankle dorsiflexes as the body pivots in an arc over the stationary foot. At the same time, the hip and knee extend, lengthening the leg.

As the patient moves from terminal stance to preswing, the ankle plantar flexes to raise the heel, and the hip and knee flex as the weight is transferred to the opposite leg.

During the initial swing, the ankle is plantar flexed, and the hip and knee are maximally flexed. As the leg progresses to midswing, the ankle dorsiflexes while the hip and knee begin to extend. As the patient moves from midswing to terminal swing, the ankle remains in the neutral position while the hip and knee continue extending. As the leg moves from terminal swing to initial contact, the knee reaches maximum extension while the ankle remains in neutral. No further hip extension occurs at this stage.

One must remember that there may be some compensation by the lumbar spine for limitation of movement of the hip. The patient should be observed to determine whether there is (1) sufficient knee extension at initial contact, followed almost immediately by slight flexion until the foot makes contact with the floor; (2) control of the slightly flexed knee during load response and midstance; and (3) sufficient flexion during preswing and initial swing. Also, any hyperextension of the knee during the gait cycle should be noted.

When looking at the ankle, the examiner should observe immediate plantar flexion at initial contact. The foot then dorsiflexes through midstance or single-leg stance, with maximum dorsiflexion being reached just before heel-off. It should be noted whether there is sufficient plantar flexion during push-off.

Finally, the examiner should note whether there

TABLE 14–1. Detailed and Total Locomotion Score in Chronic Arthritis*

UPPER EXTREMITIES

A. Subjective score (max. 100 points)

1. **Pain (max. 33 points)**
    33 None at ordinary activity ____
    25 Mild, inconstant, unilaterally, not interfering with normal activity
    17 Mild bilateral or moderate unilateral, constant use of analgetics
    10 Severe pain despite large doses of analgetics, affecting activity
    5 Severe pain despite large doses of analgetics, affecting activity
    0 Severe bilateral, unable to work and use walking supports, prevents physical activity

2–4. **Pain score reduction** ____
    –10% Unilateral hand pain
    –25% Bilateral hand pain
    –25% Severe pain from both lower extremities or neck
                                                        Sum: ____

ABILITY (max. 67 points)

Degree of disability

General (max. 20 points)	None	Mild	Moderate	Severe or unable	
5–6. Manage work, household routines, shopping, children care (min. 3 of 4)	8 ☐	6 ☐	3 ☐	0 ☐ R 5 ☐ L 6	
7–8. ADL (home and kitchen chore, personal care, dressing, etc.)	7 ☐	5 ☐	2 ☐	0 ☐ R 7 ☐ L 8	
9–10. Drive a car or use public transportation	5 ☐		2 ☐	0 ☐ R 9 ☐ L 10	

Special (max. 47 points)

	None	Mild	Moderate	Severe or unable
11–12. Feeding (hold knife, cup, open milk pack)	10 ☐	7 ☐	4 ☐	0 ☐ R 11 ☐ L 12
13–14. Carry 3 kg burden	5 ☐		2 ☐	0 ☐ R 13 ☐ L 14
15–18. Use telephone	5 ☐		2 ☐	0 ☐ R 15 ☐ L 16
17–18. Comb hair, brush teeth, shave	5 ☐		2 ☐	0 ☐ R 17 ☐ L 18
19–20. Wash the axillas	5 ☐		2 ☐	0 ☐ R 19 ☐ L 20
21–22. Reach things over shoulder level	5 ☐		2 ☐	0 ☐ R 21 ☐ L 22
23–24. Use of walking support(s)	12 ☐	7 ☐	4 ☐	0 ☐ R 23 ☐ L 24

Sum: right ____ left ____ Both (R/2 + L/2) ____

SUBJECTIVE SCORE: (pain: ____, ability: ____)   _____

B. Objective score—physical signs (max. 100 points)

		Right	Left
Shoulder (max. 35 points)			
25–26. Flexion:	>90° = 10p, 45-90° = 5 p, <45° = 0p	☐25	☐26
27–28. Extension:	>20° = 5p, 0-20° = 3p, 0° = 0p	☐27	☐28
29–30. Abduction:	>90° = 10p, 45-90° = 5p, <45° = 0p	☐29	☐30
31–32. Internal rot.:	>15° = 5p, <15° = 0p	☐31	☐32
33–34. External rot.:	>10° = 5p, <10° = 0p	☐33	☐34
Elbow (max. 35 points)			
35–36. Flexion (from 90°):	>120° = 10p, 100-120° = 7p, 90-100° = 4p, 0° = 0p	☐35	☐36
37–38. Extension defect:	0-30° = 10p, 30-60° = 7p, 60-90° = 4p, 90° = 0p	☐37	☐38
39–40. Deformity: none + stable = 5p, rigid deformity = 2p, laxid = 0p		☐39	☐40
41–42. Varus-valgus: <5° = 10p, 5-10° = 7p stressed varus-valgus >15° = 3p, >25° = 0p		☐41	☐42
Wrist (max. 15 points)			
43–44. Deformity (rigid, laxid): none = 15p, mild = 10p, moderate = 5p, severe = 0p		☐43	☐44
Hand (max. 15 points)			
45–46. Deformity (rigid, laxid): none = 15p, mild = 10p, moderate = 5p, severe = 0p		☐45	☐46

Sum: right ____ left ____ Both (R/2 + L/2) ____

OBJECTIVE SCORE: ____   SUBJ. + OBJ. SCORE: ☐ (a)
                                              (upper extremities)

is (1) coordination of movement among the hip, knee, and ankle; (2) even or uneven gait length; and (3) equal or uneven duration of steps.

POSTERIOR VIEW

When observing the gait cycle from behind, one should notice the same structures that were viewed from the front. Any abnormal abduction or adduction movements as well as lateral displacement of the different body segments should be noted. This view is best to examine the weight-unloading period of the gait cycle. The examiner can note whether heel rise is equal for both feet and whether the heels turn in or out. The observation should also include lateral movement of the spine and the musculature of the back, buttocks, posterior thigh, and calf.

Footwear

The patient should be asked to walk in normal footwear as well as in bare feet. The examiner should take time to observe the patient's footwear and observe any wearing down of the heels and/or socks, the condition of the shoe uppers, creases, and so on. The feet should also be examined for callus formations, blisters, corns, and bunions.

Compensatory Mechanisms

The examiner must try to determine the primary cause of gait faults and the compensatory factors used to maintain an energy-saving gait. An individual tries to use the most energy-saving gait possible. By assessing this way, one will be able to set appropriate goals and plan a logical approach to treatment.

Locomotion Score.[7] In addition to the detailed assessment of gait, a locomotion scale or grading system has been developed that includes subjective and objective scores, which are combined for a total score. Table 14–1 is a locomotion scoring scale that was developed for rheumatoid arthritis. In addition to including all aspects of locomotion, it gives an overall estimation of functional disability for patients with rheumatoid arthritis.

TABLE 14–1. Detailed and Total Locomotion Score in Chronic Arthritis* *Continued*

LOWER EXTREMITIES

C. Subjective score (max. 100 points)

47. **Pain (max. 44 points)** ——
   44 None at ordinary activity
   40 Slight, occasional ache or awareness of pain, not influencing activity
   30 Mild bilateral or moderate unilateral, may take analgesics
   20 Moderate, affecting ordinary activities and work, consistent use of analgesics.
   10 Severe pain in spite of optimal medication
   0 Severe, preventing most of activity or patient bedridden

48–50. **Pain score reduction** ——
   −25% Moderate or severe pain from more than one ipsilateral joint
   −50% Moderate or severe pain from more than one contralateral joint
   −10% Severe pain from upper extremities or neck

Sum: ——

ABILITY (max. 56 points)

Walk (max. 36 points)

51.	Limp:	none = 12p, slight = 8p, moderate = 5p, severe = 0p	☐
		none = 12p, cane for long walks = 8p, cane most of time = 5p	
52.	Support:	one crutch or can't use = 3p, two canes = 2p	☐
		two crutches or can't walk = 0p	
53.	Distance:	unlimited = 12p, >400m = 8p, <400m = 5p	☐
		indoors only = 2p, bed or chair = 0p	

Special (max. 20 points)

54.	Climb stairs:	without difficulty = 6p	☐
		with difficulty or by using banister = 3p	
		with great difficulty or unable = 0p	
55.	Shoes and socks:	without difficulty = 6p, with difficulty = 3p, unable = 0p	☐
56.	Sitting:	without difficulty = 6p, only short time or on high chair = 3p, unable to use any chair = 0p	☐

| 57. | Transportation: | can use public transportation = 2p, unable = 0p | ☐ |

Sum: pain: ——, ability: —— (walk: ——, special: ——)

SUBJECTIVE SCORE: ——

D. Objective score—physical signs (max. 100 points)

			Right	Left
Hip (max. 35 points)				
58–59.	Flexion:	>90° = 10p, 60–90° = 5p, <60° = 0p	☐58	☐59
60–61.	Extension defect:	0-10° = 10p, 10–30° = 5p, >30° = 0p	☐60	☐61
62–63.	Abduction/adduction:	>10° = 10p, −10–10° = 5p, <−10° = 0p	☐62	☐63
64–65.	Rotation:	>0° = 5p, 0° = 0p	☐64	☐65
Knee (max. 35 points)				
66–67.	Flexion:	>100° = 10p, 80–100° = 8p, 60–80° = 5p	☐66	☐67
68–69.	Extension defect:	0° = 10p, 0–10° = 8p, 10–20° = 5p		
		20-30° = 2p, >30° = 0p	☐68	☐69
70–71.	Varus-valgus:	<7° = 10p, 7–15° = 8p		
		stressed v/v 15–30° = 5p, >30° = 0p	☐70	☐71
72–73.	Deformity:	none + stable = 5p, rigid = 2p, laxid = 0p	☐72	☐73
Ankle (max. 15 points)				
74–75.	Deformity (rigid, laxid): none = 15p, mild = 10p, moderate = 5p, severe = 0p		☐74	☐75
Feet (max. 15 points)				
76–77.	Deformity (rigid, laxid): None = 15p, mild = 10p, moderate = 5p, severe = 0p		☐76	☐77

SUM: right: —— left: ——   Both (R/2 + L/2): ——

OBJECTIVE SCORE: ——   **SUBJ. + OBJ. SCORE:** ☐ (b)
                                          (lower extremities)

TOTAL LOCOMOTION SCORE: (a + b) ——

---

*Modified from Larsson, S. E., and B. Jonsson: Locomotion score in rheumatoid arthritis. Acta Orthop. Scand. 60:272, 1989 © Munksgaard International Publishers Ltd., Copenhagen, Denmark.

ABNORMAL GAIT

Discussed next are some of the more common gait abnormalities; this list is by no means all-inclusive.

Antalgic Gait

The antalgic gait is self-protective and is the result of pain caused by injury to the hip, knee, ankle, or foot. The stance phase on the affected leg is shorter than that on the nonaffected leg as the patient attempts to remove weight from the affected leg as quickly as possible. In addition, the painful region is often supported by one hand, if it is within reach, whereas the other arm, acting as a counterbalance, is outstretched. If a painful hip is causing the problem, the patient will also shift the body weight over the painful hip because this shift decreases the pull of the abductor muscles. This action decreases the pressure on the femoral head from more than twofold body weight to approximately body weight as the load is now vertically over the hip instead of at an angle.

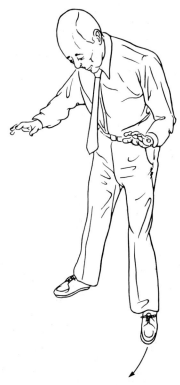

FIGURE 14–11. Ataxic gait. In cerebellar ataxia, the patient has poor balance and a broad base and, therefore lurches, staggers, and exaggerates all movements. In sensory ataxia, the patient has a broad-based gait. Because the patient cannot feel the feet, the patient slaps them against the ground and looks down at them while walking. In both types of ataxias, the gait is irregular, jerky, and weaving. (From Judge, R. D., G. D. Zuidema, and F. T. Fitzgerald: Clinical Diagnosis: A Physiological Approach. Boston, Little, Brown & Co., 1982, p. 438.)

Arthrogenic Gait

The arthrogenic gait results from stiffness, laxity, or deformity, and it may be painful or pain free. If the knee or hip is fused or the knee has recently been removed from a cylinder cast, the pelvis must be elevated by exaggerated plantar flexion of the opposite ankle and circumduction of the stiff leg to provide toe clearance. This movement compensates for the lack of flexion in the hip or knee.

Ataxic Gait

If the patient has poor sensation or lacks muscle coordination, there is a tendency toward poor balance and a broad base (Fig. 14–11). The gait of an individual with cerebellar ataxia includes a lurch or stagger, and all movements are exaggerated. The feet of an individual with sensory ataxia slap the ground because they cannot be felt. The patient also watches the feet while walking. The resulting gait is irregular, jerky, and weaving.

Gluteus Maximus Gait

If the gluteus maximus muscle is weak, the patient will thrust the thorax posteriorly at initial contact to maintain hip extension of the stance leg. The resulting gait has a characteristic lurch (Fig. 14–12).

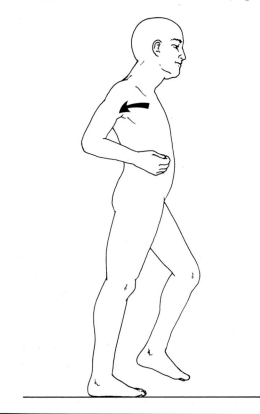

FIGURE 14–12. Gluteus maximus gait.

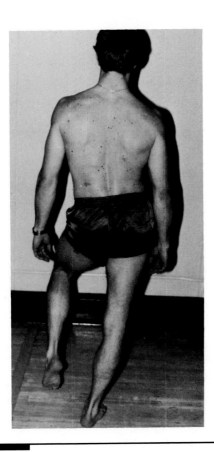

FIGURE 14–13. Gluteus medius (Trendelenburg) gait.

Gluteus Medius (Trendelenburg) Gait

If the gluteus medius muscle is weak, the patient will exhibit an excessive lateral list in which the thorax is thrusted laterally to keep the center of gravity over the stance leg (Fig. 14–13). A positive Trendelenburg sign will also be exhibited. If there is bilateral weakness of the gluteus medius muscles, the gait will show accentuated side-to-side movement, resulting in a "wobbling" gait or "chorus girl swing." This gait may also be seen in patients with congenital dislocation of the hip and coxa vara.

Hemiplegic or Hemiparetic Gait

The patient with hemiplegic or hemiparetic gait swings the paraplegic leg outward and ahead in a circle (circumduction) or pushes it ahead (Fig. 14–14). In addition, the affected upper limb is carried across the trunk for balance. This is sometimes referred to as a neurogenic or flaccid gait.

Parkinsonian Gait

The neck, trunk, and knees of a patient with parkinsonian gait are flexed. The gait is characterized by shuffling or short rapid steps (marche à petits pas) at times. The arms are held stiffly and do not have their normal associative movement (Fig. 14–15).

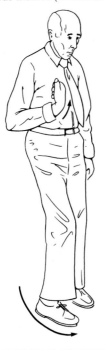

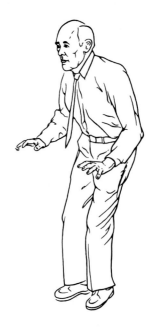

FIGURE 14–14. Hemiplegic (hemiparetic) gait. The arm is carried across the trunk, adducted at the shoulder. The forearm is rotated, the arm is flexed at the elbow and wrist, and the hand is flexed at the metacarpophalangeal joints. The leg is extended at the hip and knee. The patient either swings the affected leg outward in a circle (circumduction) or pushes it ahead. (From Judge, R. D., G. D. Zuidema, and F. T. Fitzgerald: Clinical Diagnosis: A Physiological Approach. Boston, Little, Brown & Co., 1982, p. 438.)

FIGURE 14–15. Parkinsonism. The head, trunk, and knees are flexed, and the arms are held rather stiffly with poor associative movement. The gait is shuffling or characterized at times by short, rapid steps (marche à petits pas). The patient may lean forward and walk progressively faster, seemingly unable to stop (festination). (From Judge, R. D., G. D. Zuidema, and F. T. Fitzgerald: Clinical Diagnosis: A Physiological Approach. Boston, Little, Brown & Co., 1989, p. 496.)

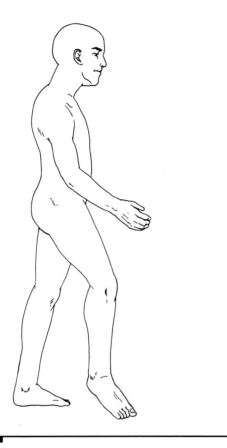

FIGURE 14–16. Psoatic limp. Note external rotation, flexion, and abduction of affected hip.

During the gait, the patient may lean forward and walk progressively faster as though unable to stop (festination).

Psoatic Limp

The psoatic limp is seen in patients with conditions affecting the hip, such as Legg-Calvé-Perthes disease. The limp may be due to weakness or reflex inhibition of the psoas major muscle. Classic manifestations of this limp are lateral rotation, flexion, and adduction of the hip (Fig. 14–16). The patient will exaggerate movement of the pelvis and trunk to help move the thigh into flexion.

Scissors Gait

This gait is the result of spastic paralysis of the hip adductor muscles and causes the knees to be drawn together so that the legs can be swung forward only with great effort (Fig. 14–17). This is seen in spastic paraplegics and may be referred to as a neurogenic or spastic gait.

Short Leg Gait

If one leg is shorter than the other or there is a deformity in one of the bones of the leg, the patient

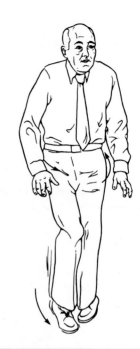

FIGURE 14–17. Scissors gait. Spasticity of thigh adduction, seen in spastic paraplegics, draws the knees together. The legs are advanced (with great effort) by swinging the hips. (From Judge, R. D., G. D. Zuidema, and F. T. Fitzgerald: Clinical Diagnosis: A Physiological Approach. Boston, Little, Brown & Co., 1982, p. 439.)

will demonstrate a lateral shift to the affected side and the pelvis will tilt down on the affected side, creating a limp (Fig. 14–18). The weight-bearing period may be the same for the two legs. With proper

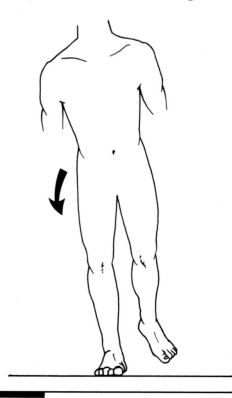

FIGURE 14–18. Short leg gait.

footwear, the gait may appear normal. This may also be termed painless osteogenic gait.

Steppage or Foot Drop Gait

The patient with this gait has weak or paralyzed dorsiflexor muscles, resulting in a foot drop. To compensate and avoid dragging the toes against the ground, the patient lifts the knee higher than normal; this results in a high steppage gait (Fig. 14–19). At initial contact, the foot slaps on the ground because of loss of control of the dorsiflexor muscles.

Stiff Knee or Hip Gait

The patient with this gait lifts the entire leg higher than normal to clear the ground because of a stiff hip or knee. To do this, excessive plantar flexing of the other foot occurs, and the affected leg swings through an arc, moving the leg anteriorly (Fig. 14–20). The arc of movements helps to decrease the elevation needed to "clear" the affected leg. Because of the loss of flexibility in the hip, knee, or both, the gait lengths will be different for the two legs. When the stiff limb is weight bearing, the gait length will usually be smaller.

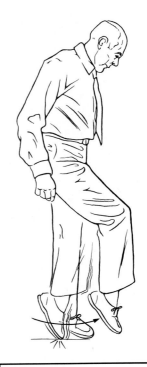

FIGURE 14–19. Steppage or foot drop gait. To avoid dragging the toes against the ground (because the patient dorsiflexes the foot), the patient lifts the knee high and slaps the foot to the ground on advancing. (From Judge, R. D., G. D. Zuidema, and F. T. Fitzgerald: Clinical Diagnosis: A Physiological Approach. Boston, Little, Brown & Co., 1982, p. 438.)

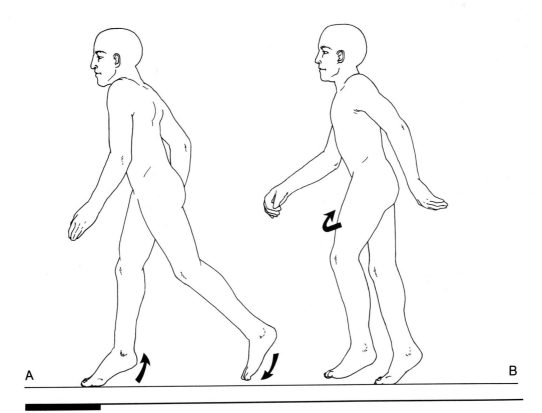

FIGURE 14–20. Stiff knee or hip gait. (A) Excessive plantar flexion. (B) Circumduction.

REFERENCES

CITED REFERENCES

1. Bowker, J. H., and C. B. Hall: Normal human gait. *In* Atlas of Orthotics: Biomechanical Principles and Applications. St. Louis, C.V. Mosby Co., 1975.
2. Inman, V. T., H. J. Ralston, and F. Todd: Human Walking. Baltimore, Williams & Wilkins, 1981.
3. Koerner, I. B.: Normal Human Locomotion and the Gait of the Amputee. Edmonton, University of Alberta Bookstore, 1979.
4. Koerner, L: Observation of Human Gait. Videotapes produced by the Health Sciences Audiovisual Education, University of Alberta, 1984.
5. Hoppenfeld, S.: Physical Examination of the Spine and Extremities. New York, Appleton-Century-Crofts, 1976.
6. Perry, J., and H. J. Hislop: The mechanics of walking: A clinical interpretation. *In* Perry J and H. J. Hislop (eds.): Principles of Lower-Extremity Bracing. New York, American Physical Therapy Association, 1970.
7. Larsson, S. E., and B. Jonsson: Locomotion score in rheumatoid arthritis. Acta Orthop. Scand. 60:272, 1989.

GENERAL REFERENCES

Brown, L. P., and P. Yavorsky: Locomotor biomechanics and pathomechanics: A review. J. Orthop. Sports Phys. Ther. 9:3, 1987.
Chondera, J. D.: Analysis of gait from footprints. Physiother. 60:179, 1974.
Eberhart, H. D., V. T. Inman, and B. Bresler: Principal elements in human locomotion. *In* Klopsteg, P. E. and P. D. Wilson (eds.): Human Limbs and Their Substitutes. New York, McGraw-Hill Co., 1954.
Finley, F. R., K. A. Cody, and R. V. Finizie: Locomotion patterns in elderly women. Arch. Phys. Med. Rehabil. 50:140, 1969.
Garbalosa, J. C., R. Donatelli, and M. J. Wooden: Dysfunction, evaluation and treatment of the foot and ankle. *In* Donatelli, R., and M. J. Wooden (eds.): Orthopedic Physical Therapy. Edinburgh, Churchill Livingstone, 1989.
Gray, G. W.: Chain Reaction—Successful Strategies for Closed Chain Testing and Rehabilitation. Adrian, Michigan, Wynn Marketing, 1989.
Grieve, D. W.: The assessment of gait. Physiother. 55:452, 1969.

Gruebel-Lee, D. M.: Disorders of Hip. Philadelphia, J. B. Lippincott Co., 1983.
Inman, V. T.: The Joints of the Ankle. Baltimore, Williams & Wilkins, 1976.
Inman, V. T.: Functional aspects of the abductor muscles of the hip. J. Bone Joint Surg. 29:607, 1947.
Judge, R. D., G. D. Zuidema, and F. T. Fitzgerald: Clinical Diagnosis: A Physiological Approach. Boston, Little, Brown and Co., 1982.
Kotok, Y., E. Y. Chao, R. K. Laughman, E. Schneider, and B. F. Morrey: Biomechanical analysis of foot function during gait and clinical applications. Clin. Orthop. Relat. Res. 177:23, 1983.
Macleod, J.: Clinical Examination. New York, Churchill Livingstone, 1976.
Murray, M. P., A. B. Brought, and R. C. Kory: Walking patterns of normal men. J. Bone Joint Surg. 46A:335, 1964.
Murray, M. P.: Gait as a total pattern of movement. Am. J. Phys. Med. 46:290, 1967.
Murray, M. P., D. R. Gore, and B. H. Clarkson: Walking patterns of patients with unilateral pain due to osteoarthritis and avascular necrosis. J. Bone Joint Surg. 53A:259, 1971.
Normal Gait Chart. Rancho Los Amigos Hospital, Downey, Calif., 1981.
Perry, J.: Anatomy and biomechanics of the hindfoot. Clin. Orthop. Relat. Res. 177:9, 1983.
Perry, J.: Pathologic gait. *In* Atlas of Orthotics: Biomechanical Principles and Applications. St. Louis, C. V. Mosby Co., 1975.
Root, M. L., W. P. Orien, and J. H. Weed: Normal and Abnormal Function of the Foot. Los Angeles, Clinical Biomechanics Corp. 1977.
Saunders, J. B. M., V. T. Inman, and H. O. Eberhart: The major determinants in normal and pathological gait. J. Bone Joint Surg. 35A:543, 1953.
Simon, S. R., R. A. Mann, J. L. Hogy, and L. J. Larsen: Role of the posterior calf muscles in a normal gait. J. Bone Joint Surg. 60A:465, 1978.
Thurston, A. J., and J. D. Harris: Normal kinematics of the lumbar spine and pelvis. Spine 8:199, 1983.
Tiberio, D., and G. W. Gray: Kinematics and kinetics during gait. *In* Donatelli, R., and M. J. Wooden (eds.): Orthopedic Physical Therapy. Edinburgh, Churchill Livingstone, 1989.
Wadsworth, C. T.: Manual Examination and Treatment of the Spine and Extremities. Baltimore, Williams & Wilkins, 1988.
Wright, D. G., S. M. Desai, and W. H. Henderson: Action of the subtalar and ankle joint complex during the stance phase of walking. J. Bone Joint Surg. 46A:361, 1964.

CHAPTER 15
Assessment of Posture

POSTURE DEVELOPMENT

Posture, which is the relative disposition of the body at any one moment, is a composite of the positions of the different joints of the body at that time. Thus, the position of one joint has an effect on the position of the other joints. Correct posture is the position in which minimum stress will be applied to each joint. Any position that increases the stress to the joints may be called *faulty* posture. If the individual has strong and flexible muscles, faulty postures may not affect the joints because the individual has the ability to change position readily so the stresses do not become excessive. If the joints are stiff or too mobile and the muscles are weak, however, the posture cannot be easily altered to the correct alignment, and the result can be some form of pathology. The pathology may be the result of the cumulative effect of repeated small stresses over a long period of time or of constant abnormal stresses over a short period of time. These chronic stresses can result in the same problems that are seen when a sudden (acute) severe stress is applied to the body. The abnormal stresses cause excessive wearing of the articular surfaces of joints and produce osteophytes and traction spurs, which are the result of the attempt of the body to alter its structure to accommodate these repeated stresses. The soft tissue (e.g., muscles and ligaments) may become weakened, stretched, or traumatized by increased stress. The application of an acute stress on the chronic stress may exacerbate the problem and produce the signs and symptoms that initially prompt the patient to seek aid.

At birth, the entire spine is *concave* forward, or flexed (Fig. 15–1). Curves of the spine found at birth are called *primary curves*. The curves that maintain this position—those of the thoracic spine and sacrum—are thus classified as primary curves of the spine. As the child grows (Fig. 15–2), *secondary curves* appear and are *convex* forward, or extended. At about the age of 3 months, when the child begins to be able to lift the head, the cervical spine becomes convex forward, producing the cervical lordosis. In the lumbar spine, the secondary curve develops slightly later (6 to 8 months), when the child begins to sit up and walk. In old age, the secondary curves again begin to disappear as the spine starts to return to a flexed position as the result of disc degeneration, ligamentous calcification, osteoporosis, and vertebral wedging.

In the child, the center of gravity is at the level of the T12 vertebra. As the child grows older, the center of gravity drops, eventually reaching the level of the second sacral vertebra in adults (slightly higher in males). The child will stand with a wide base to maintain balance, and the knees will be flexed. Initially, the knees will be slightly bowed (genu varum) until about 18 months of age. The child then becomes slightly knock-kneed (genu valgum) until the age of 3 years. By the age of 6 years, the legs should naturally straighten out (see Fig. 15–24). The lumbar spine in children has an exaggerated lumbar curve, or excessive lordosis. This accentuated curve is due to the presence of large abdominal contents, weakness of the abdominal musculature, and the small pelvis characteristic of children this age.

Initially, a child is flatfooted, or appears to be, as the result of the minimal development of the medial

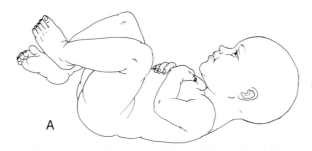

FIGURE 15–1. Postural development. (A) Flexed posture in a newborn. (B) Development of secondary cervical curve. (C) Development of secondary lumbar curve.

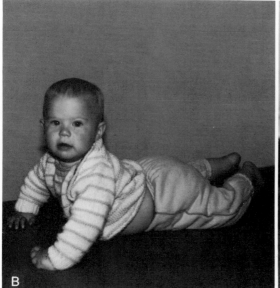

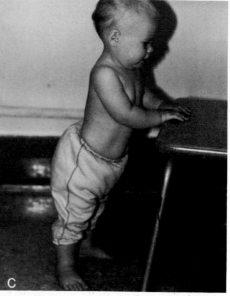

FIGURE 15–2. Postural changes with age. Apparent kyphosis at ages 6 and 8 is due to scapular winging. (From McMorris, R. O.: Faulty posture. Pediatr. Clin. North Am. 8:214, 1961.)

No. 1	No. 2	No. 3	No. 4	No. 5	No. 6
2 yrs.	4 yrs.	6 yrs.	8 yrs.	10 yrs.	18 yrs.

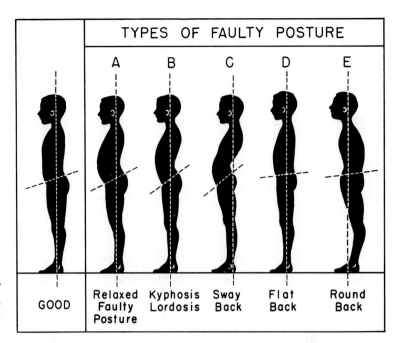

FIGURE 15–3. *Types of faulty posture. (From Mc-Morris, R. O.: Faulty posture. Pediatr. Clin. North Am. 8:217, 1961.)*

longitudinal arch and a fat pad that is found in the arch. As the child grows, the fat pad slowly decreases in size, making the medial arch more evident. In addition, as the foot develops and the muscles strengthen, the arches of the feet develop normally and become more evident.

The advantage of an erect posture, as seen in human beings, is that it enables the hands to be free and the eyes to be farther from the ground so that the individual can see farther ahead. The disadvantages include an increased strain on the spine and lower limbs and comparative difficulties in respiration and transport of the blood to the brain.

Factors Affecting Posture

Several anatomic factors may affect correct posture, including the following:

1. Bony contours (e.g., hemivertebra).
2. Laxity of ligamentous structures.
3. Fascial and musculotendinous tightness (e.g., hamstrings, tensor fasciae latae, pectorals, hip flexors).
4. Muscle tonus (e.g., gluteus maximus, abdominals, erector spinae).
5. Pelvic angle (normal is 30°).
6. Joint position and mobility.
7. Neurogenic outflow and inflow.

These factors may be further enhanced or cause additional problems when combined with pathological or congenital states, such as Klippel-Feil syndrome, Scheuermann's disease (juvenile kyphosis), scoliosis, or disc disease.

Causes of Poor Posture

There are many causes of poor posture (Fig. 15–3). Some of these causes are *postural* (positional), and some are *structural*.

Postural Factors

The most common postural problem is poor postural habit (i.e., for whatever reason, the individual does not maintain a correct posture). This type of posture is often seen in the individual who stands or sits for long periods of time and begins to slouch. Maintaining a correct posture requires muscles that are strong, flexible, and easily adaptable to environmental change. These muscles must continually work against gravity and in harmony with one another to maintain an upright posture.

Another cause of poor postural habits, especially in children, is not wanting to appear taller than one's peers. If a child has an early, rapid growth spurt, for example, there will be a tendency to slouch to not appear different. Such a spurt may also result in the unequal growth of the various structures, and this may lead to altered posture; for example, the growth of muscle may not keep up with the growth of bone. This process is sometimes evident in adolescents with tight hamstrings.

Another cause of poor posture is muscle imbalance or muscle contracture. For example, a tight iliopsoas muscle increases the lumbar lordosis in the lumbar spine.

Pain may also cause poor posture. Pressure on a nerve root in the lumbar spine can lead to pain in the back and result in a scoliosis as the body unconsciously adopts a posture that decreases the pain.

Respiratory conditions (e.g., emphysema), general weakness, excess weight, loss of proprioception, or muscle spasm (as seen in cerebral palsy) may also lead to poor posture.

Structural Factors

Structural deformities may cause an alteration of posture. For example, a significant difference in leg length or anomalies of the spine, such as a hemivertebra, may alter the posture.

COMMON SPINAL DEFORMITIES

Lordosis

Lordosis is an excessive anterior curvature of the spine (Fig. 15–4).[1–5] Pathologically, it is an exaggeration of the normal curves found in the cervical and lumbar spines. Causes of increased lordosis include (1) postural deformity; (2) lax muscles, especially the abdominal muscles; (3) a heavy abdomen due to excess weight or pregnancy; (4) compensatory mechanisms that result from another deformity, such as

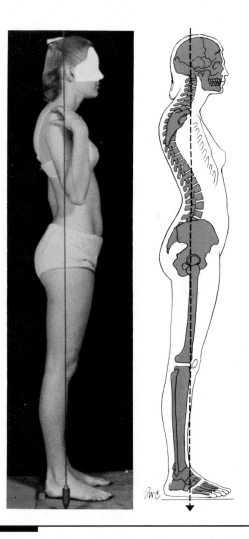

FIGURE 15–5. *Faulty posture illustrating exaggerated lordosis and kyphosis. (From Kendall, F. P., and E. K. McCreary: Muscles: Testing and Function. Baltimore, Williams & Wilkins, 1983, p. 281.)*

kyphosis (Fig. 15–5); (5) hip flexion contracture; (6) spondylolisthesis; (7) congenital problems, such as congenital dislocation of the hip; (8) failure of segmentation of the neural arch of a facet joint segment; or (9) fashion. For example, wearing high heels will increase the lordotic curve.

In the patient with lordosis, one may often observe sagging shoulders, medial rotation of the legs, and poking forward of the head so that it is in front of the center of gravity. This posture is adopted by the individual in an attempt to keep the center of gravity where it should be. Deviation in one part of the body often leads to deviation in another part of the body in an attempt to maintain the correct center of gravity and the correct visual plane.

The pelvic angle, normally approximately 30°, is increased with lordosis. With excessive lordosis, there is an increase in the pelvic angle to approximately 40°, accompanied by a mobile spine and an

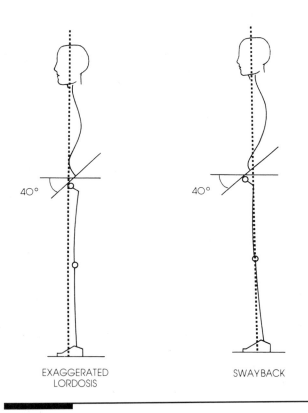

EXAGGERATED LORDOSIS

SWAYBACK

FIGURE 15–4. *Examples of lordosis.*

anterior pelvic tilt. With a *swayback* deformity, there is increased pelvic inclination to approximately 40°, and the thoracolumbar spine exhibits a kyphosis (Fig. 15–6). A swayback deformity results in the spine bending back rather sharply at the lumbosacral angle.

Kyphosis

Kyphosis is excessive posterior curvature of the spine (Figs. 15–7 and 15–8).[3, 5–10] Pathologically, it is an exaggeration of the normal curve found in the thoracic spine. There are several causes of kyphosis, including tuberculosis, vertebral compression fractures, Scheuermann's disease, ankylosing spondylitis, senile osteoporosis, tumors, compensation in conjunction with lordosis, and congenital anomalies.[6] Some of these congenital anomalies include a partial segmental defect, as seen in osseous metaplasia, or centrum hypoplasia and aplasia.[9, 11, 12] In addition, paralysis may lead to a kyphosis because of the loss of muscle action needed to maintain the correct posture combined with the forces of gravity.

There are four types of kyphoses:

Round Back. The individual with a round back has a long, rounded curve with decreased pelvic inclination (less than 30°) and thoracolumbar kyphosis. The patient will often present with the trunk flexed forward and a decreased lumbar curve.

Humpback or Gibbus. With humpback, there is a localized sharp posterior angulation in the thoracic spine (Fig. 15–9).

Flat Back. An individual with flat back has decreased pelvic inclination to 20° and a mobile lumbar spine (Fig. 15–10).

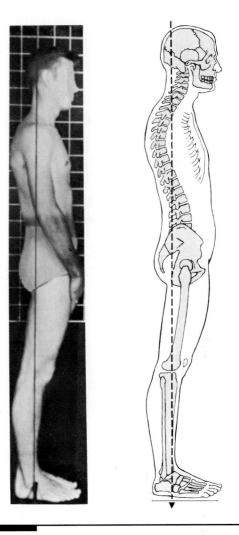

FIGURE 15–6. Faulty posture illustrating a swayback. (From Kendall, F. P., and E. K. McCreary: Muscles: Testing and Function. Baltimore, Williams & Wilkins, 1983, p. 284.)

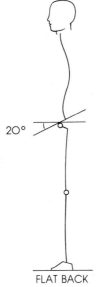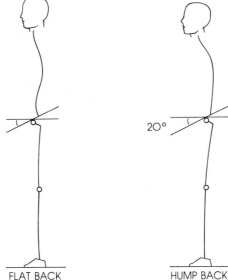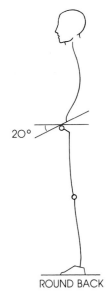

FIGURE 15–7. Examples of kyphosis.

FLAT BACK   HUMP BACK   ROUND BACK

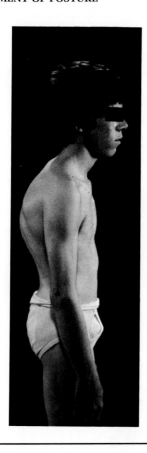

FIGURE 15–8. *Faulty posture illustrating thoracic kyphosis. (From Moe, J. H., D. S. Bradford, R. B. Winter, and J. E. Lonstein: Scoliosis and Other Spinal Deformities. Philadelphia, W. B. Saunders Co., 1978, p. 152.)*

Dowager's Hump. This is often seen in older individuals, especially women. The deformity is due to osteoporosis, in which the thoracic vertebral bodies begin to degenerate and wedge in an anterior direction and result in a kyphosis (Fig. 15–11).

Pathological conditions such as Scheuermann's vertebral osteochondritis may also result in a structural kyphosis (Fig. 15–12). In this condition, inflammation of the bone and cartilage occurs around the ring epiphysis of the vertebral body. The condition often leads to an anterior wedging of the vertebra. It is a growth disorder that affects approximately 10 per cent of the population, and several vertebrae are usually affected. The most common area for the disease to occur is between T10 and L2.

Scoliosis

Scoliosis is a lateral curvature of the spine.[6, 8, 13–19] In the cervical spine, a scoliosis is called a *torticollis* (Fig. 15–13). There are several types of scoliosis, some of which are nonstructural (see Fig. 15–13) and some which are structural. *Nonstructural scoliosis* may be due to postural problems, hysteria, nerve root irritation, inflammation, or compensation caused by leg length discrepancy or contracture (in the lumbar spine).[18] *Structural scoliosis* may be congenital and due to wedge vertebra, hemivertebra

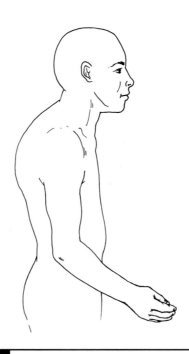

FIGURE 15–9. *Humpback or gibbus deformity.*

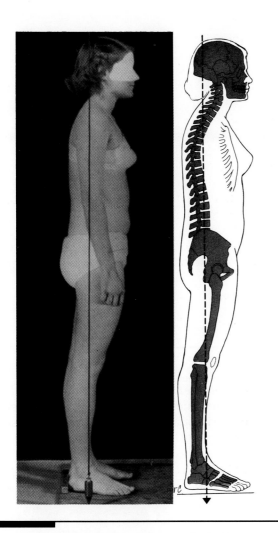

FIGURE 15–10. Faulty posture illustrating flat back. (From Kendall, F. P., and E. K. McCreary: Muscles: Testing and Function. Baltimore, Williams & Wilkins, 1983, p. 285.)

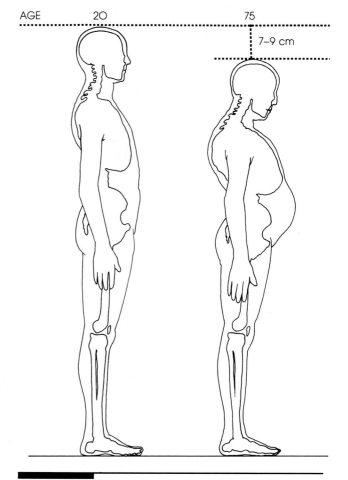

FIGURE 15–11. Loss of height resulting from osteoporosis and leading to "dowager's hump." Note the flexed head and protruding abdomen, which occur in part to maintain the center of gravity in its normal position.

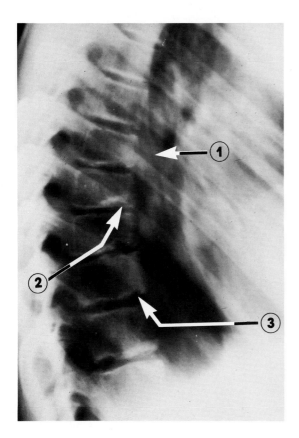

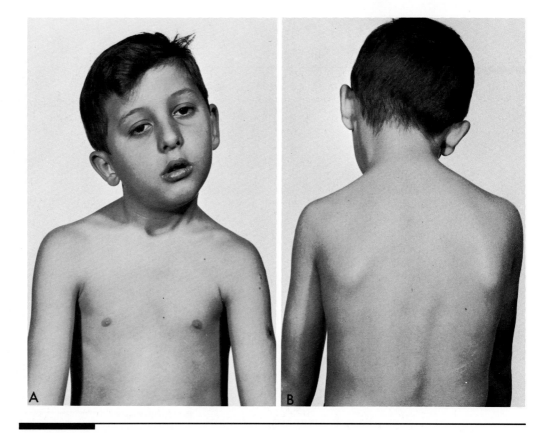

FIGURE 15–12. A classic radiographic appearance of the spine in a patient with Scheuermann's disease. Note the wedged vertebra (1), Schmorl's nodules (2), and marked irregularity of the vertebral end plates (3). (From Moe, J. H., D. S. Bradford, R. B. Winter, and J. E. Lonstein: Scoliosis and Other Spinal Deformities. Philadelphia, W. B. Saunders Co., 1978, p. 332.)

FIGURE 15–13. Congenital muscular torticollis on the right in a 10-year-old boy. Note the contracted sternocleidomastoid muscle. (From Tachdjian, M. O.: Pediatric Orthopedics. Philadelphia, W. B. Saunders Co., 1990, p. 118.)

(Fig. 15–14), or failure of segmentation; idiopathic (genetic) (Fig. 15–15) or neuromuscular and the result of upper or lower motor neuron lesion; myopathic and the result of muscular dystrophy; or arthrogryposis and the result of persistent joint flexure or contracture.[12] In addition, scoliosis may result from conditions such as neurofibromatosis, mesenchymal disorders, or trauma. It is also seen in infection, tumors, and inflammatory conditions and in conjunction with malocclusion and ear problems.

With regard to nonstructural scoliosis, there is no bony deformity, and it is not progressive. The spine will show segmental limitation, and side bending is usually symmetric. The scoliotic curve will disappear on forward flexion. This type of scoliosis is usually found in the cervical, lumbar, or thoracolumbar area.

In structural scoliosis, the patient lacks normal flexibility, and side bending becomes asymmetric. This type of scoliosis may be progressive, and the curve will not disappear on forward flexion.

Idiopathic scoliosis accounts for 75 to 85 per cent of all cases of (structural) scoliosis. The vertebral

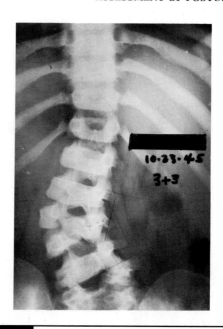

FIGURE 15–14. *Scoliosis caused by hemivertebra. (From Moe, J. H., D. S. Bradford, R. B. Winter, and J. E. Lonstein: Scoliosis and Other Spinal Deformities. Philadelphia, W. B. Saunders Co., 1978, p. 134.)*

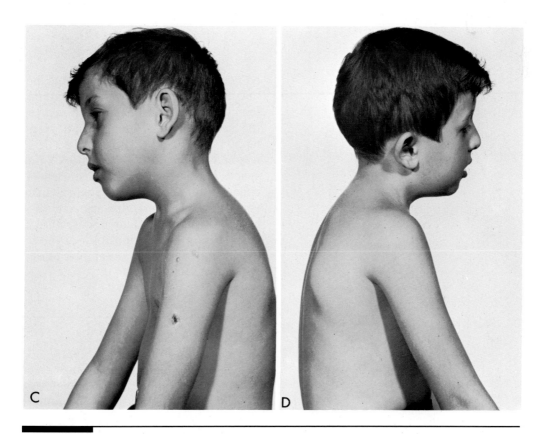

FIGURE 15–13 Continued See legend on opposite page

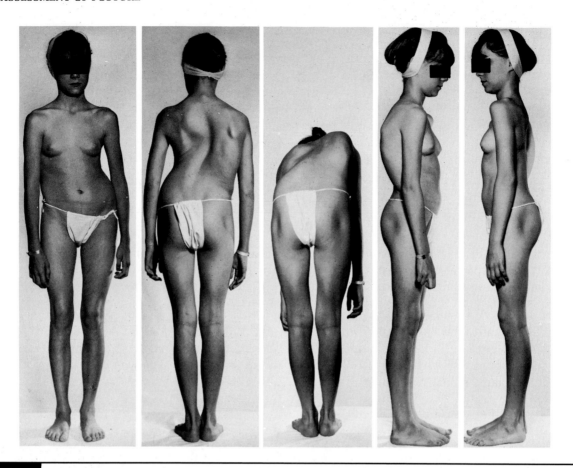

FIGURE 15–15. Idiopathic structural right thoracic scoliosis. (From Tachdjian, M. O.: Pediatric Orthopedics. Philadelphia, W. B. Saunders Co., 1990, p. 2274.)

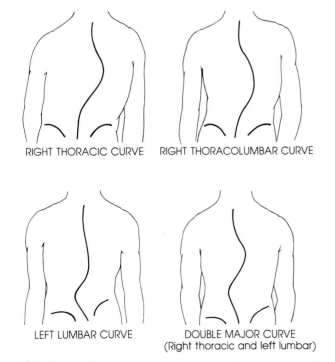

RIGHT THORACIC CURVE RIGHT THORACOLUMBAR CURVE

LEFT LUMBAR CURVE DOUBLE MAJOR CURVE
(Right thoracic and left lumbar)

FIGURE 15–16. Examples of scoliosis curve patterns.

bodies rotate into the convexity of the curve, with the spinous processes going toward the concavity of the curve. There is a fixed rotational prominence on the convex side, which is best seen on forward flexion from the "skyline" view. This prominence is sometimes called a "razorback spine." The disc spaces are narrowed on the concave side and widened on the convex side. There is distortion of the vertebral body, and vital capacity is considerably lowered when the lateral curvature exceeds 60°; compression and malposition of the organs within the rib cage also occur. Examples of scoliotic curves are shown in Figure 15–16.

POSTURAL HISTORY

As with any history, one must ensure that the information obtained is as complete as possible. By listening to the patient, the examiner will often be able to comprehend the problem. The information should include a history of the problem, the patient's general condition and health, and family history. If a child is being examined, the examiner must also obtain prenatal and postnatal histories including the health of the mother during pregnancy, any complications during pregnancy or delivery, and drugs taken by the mother during that period, especially the first trimester.

It should be remembered that it is unusual for an individual to present with just a postural problem. It is the symptoms produced by pathology caused by or causing the postural abnormality that initiate the consultation. Thus, the examiner must be cognizant of various underlying pathological conditions when assessing posture. The following questions should be asked:

1. Does the family have any history of back problems or other special problems? Conditions such as hemivertebra, scoliosis, and Klippel-Feil syndrome may be congenital.

2. Has the patient had any previous illnesses, surgery, or severe injuries?

3. Is there a history of any other conditions, such as connective tissue diseases, that have a high incidence of associated spinal problems?

4. Has there been any previous treatment? If so, what was it?

5. How old is the patient? Many spinal problems begin in childhood or are the result of degeneration.

6. In the child, has there been a growth spurt? If so, when did it begin?

7. For females, when did menarche begin? Does back pain appear to be associated with menses? Menarche indicates the point at which approximately two thirds of adolescent growth spurt has been completed.

8. For males, has there been a voice change? If so, when?

9. For children, is there difficulty in fitting clothes? For example, with scoliosis, the hem of a dress is usually uneven because of the spinal curvature.

10. If a deformity is present, is it progressive or stationary?

11. Does the patient have any difficulty breathing?

12. Which hand is the dominant one? Often, the dominant side will show a lower shoulder with the hip slightly deviated to that side (Fig. 15–17). The spine may deviate slightly to the opposite side, and

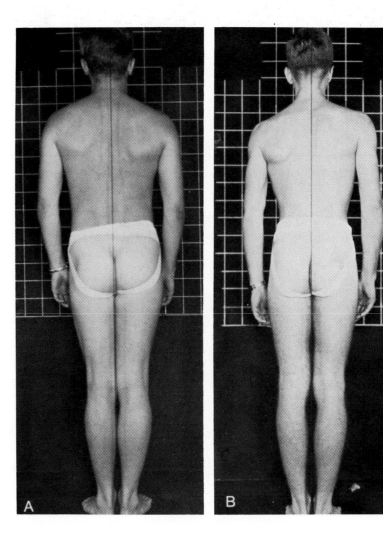

FIGURE 15–17. Effect of handedness on posture. (A) Right hand dominant. (B) Left hand dominant. (From Kendall, F. P., and E. K. McCreary: Muscles: Testing and Function. Baltimore, Williams & Wilkins, 1983, p. 294.)

the opposite foot will be slightly more pronated.[3] The gluteus medius on the dominant side may also be weaker.

13. Does the patient experience any neurological symptoms (e.g., "pins and needles" or numbness)?

14. What is the nature, extent, type, and duration of the pain?

15. What positions or activities increase the pain or discomfort?

16. What positions or activities decrease the pain or discomfort?

OBSERVATION

To assess posture correctly, the patient must be adequately undressed. Male patients should be in shorts, and female patients should be in a bra and shorts. Ideally, the patient should not wear shoes or stockings. However, if the patient uses walking aids, braces, collars, or orthotics, they should be noted and may be used after the patient has been assessed in the "natural" state to determine the effect of the appliances.

The patient should be examined in the habitual, relaxed posture that is usually adopted. Often, it may take some time for the patient to adopt the usual posture because of tenseness or uncertainty.

In the standing and sitting positions, the assessment is the same as the observation for the upper and lower limb scanning examinations of the cervical and lumbar spines. Assessment of posture should be carried out with the patient in the standing, sitting, and lying (supine and prone) positions. Once the patient has been examined in these positions, the examiner may decide to include other habitual postures assumed by the patient to see whether these postures increase or alter symptoms. The patient may also be assessed wearing different footwear to determine the effects on the posture and symptoms.

Standing

The examiner should first determine body type (Fig. 15–18).[19] There are three body types: ectomorphic, mesomorphic, and endomorphic. The *ectomorph* is

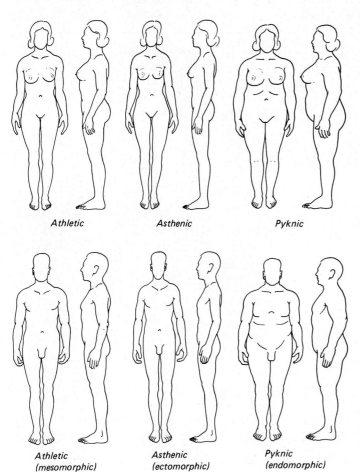

Athletic   Asthenic   Pyknic

Athletic
(mesomorphic)   Asthenic
(ectomorphic)   Pyknic
(endomorphic)

FIGURE 15–18. Male and female body types. (From Debrunner, H. U.: Orthopaedic Diagnosis. London, E & S Livingstone, 1970, p. 86.)

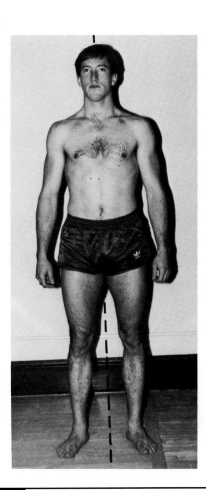

FIGURE 15–19. *Normal posture in the standing position (anterior view).*

Anterior View

When observing the patient from the front (Fig. 15–19), the examiner should ensure that the following conditions hold true:

1. The head is straight on the shoulders (in midline). The examiner should note whether the head is tilted to one side or rotated habitually (Fig. 15–20). The cause of altered head position must be established. For example, it may be the result of weak muscles, trauma, a hearing loss, temporomandibular joint problems, or the wearing of bifocal glasses.

2. The posture of the jaw is normal. In the resting position, normal jaw posture is when the lips are gently pressed together, the teeth are slightly apart (freeway space), and the tip of the tongue is behind the upper teeth in the roof of the mouth. This position maintains the mandible in a good posture (i.e., slight negative pressure in the mouth reduces the work of the muscles). It also enables respiration through the nose and diaphragmatic breathing.

3. The tip of the nose is in line with the manubrium sternum, xiphisternum, and umbilicus. This line is the anterior line of reference used to divide the body into right and left halves. If the umbilicus is used as a reference point, the examiner should remember that the umbilicus is almost always slightly off center.

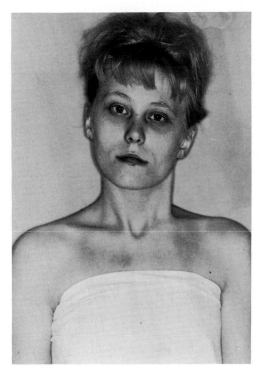

FIGURE 15–20. *Congenital torticollis in 18-year-old girl. Note the asymmetry of the face. (From Tachdjian, M. O.: Pediatric Orthopedics. Philadelphia, W. B. Saunders Co., 1990, p. 114.)*

a person who has a thin body build characterized by a relative prominence of structures developed from the embryonic ectoderm. The *mesomorph* has a muscular or sturdy body build characterized by relative prominence of structures developed by the embryonic mesoderm. The *endomorph* has a heavy or fat body build characterized by relative prominence of structures developed from the embryonic endoderm.

In addition to body type, one should note the emotional attitude of the patient. Is the patient tense, bored, or lethargic? What is the appearance? Does the patient appear to be healthy, emaciated, or overweight? Answers to these questions can help the examiner determine how much will have to be done to correct any problems. For example, if the patient is lethargic, it may take longer to correct the problem than if the individual appears truly interested in correcting the problem. The examiner must remember that posture is an expression of one's personality, sense of well-being, and self-esteem.

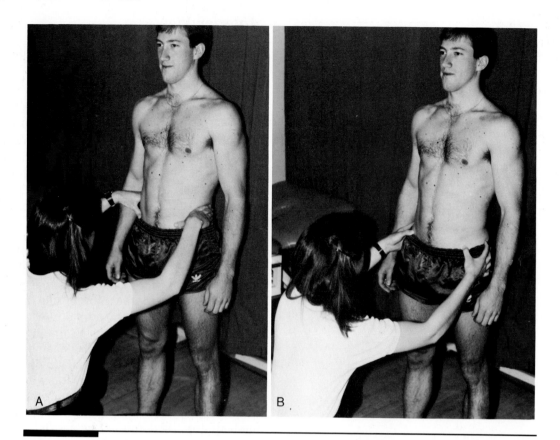

FIGURE 15–21. *Viewing height equality. (A) Iliac crests. (B) Anterior superior iliac spines (ASIS).*

4. The trapezius neck line is equal on both sides. The muscle bulk of the trapezius muscles should be equal, and the slope of the muscles should be close to equal. Because the dominant arm usually shows greater laxity by being slightly lower, the slope on the dominant side may be slightly greater.

5. The shoulders are level. In most cases, the dominant side will be slightly lower.

6. The clavicles and acromioclavicular joints are level and equal. They should be symmetric. Any deviation should be noted. Deviations may be due to subluxations or dislocations of the acromioclavicular or sternoclavicular joints, fractures, or clavicular rotation.

7. There is no protrusion, depression, or lateralization of the sternum, ribs, or costocartilage. If there are changes, they should be noted.

8. The waist angles are equal, and the arms are equidistant from the waist. If a scoliosis is present, one arm will hang closer to the body than the other arm. The examiner should also note whether the arms are equally rotated medially or laterally.

9. The carrying angle at each elbow is equal. Any deviation should be noted. The normal carrying angle varies from 5 to 15°.

10. The palms of both hands face the body in the relaxed standing position. Any differences should be noted and may give an indication of rotation in the upper limb.

11. The high points of the iliac crest are the same height on each side (Fig. 15–21). With a scoliosis, the patient may feel that one hip is "higher" than the other. This apparent high pelvis is due to the lateral shift of the trunk. The pelvis will usually be level. The same condition can cause the patient to feel that one leg is shorter than the other.

12. The anterior superior iliac spines (ASIS) are level. If one ASIS is higher than the other, there is a possibility that one leg will be shorter than the other or that the pelvis may be rotated more or shifted up or down more on one side relative to the other side.

13. The pubic bones are level at the symphysis pubis. Any deviation should be noted.

14. The patellae of the knees point straight ahead. Sometimes the patellae face outward ("frog eyes" patella) or inward ("squinting" patella). The position of the patella may be altered by torsion of the femur or tibia.

15. The knees are straight. The knees may be in genu varum or genu valgum. The examiner should note whether the deformity results from the femur, tibia, or both bones. In children, the knees go through a progression of being straight, going into

genu varum (Fig. 15–22), being straight, going into genu valgum (Fig. 15–23), and finally being straight again during the first 6 years of life (Fig. 15–24).[8]

16. The heads of the fibulae are level.

17. The medial and lateral malleoli of the ankles are level. Normally, the medial malleoli are slightly anterior to the lateral malleoli, but the lateral malleoli extend farther distally.

18. The arches are present in the feet and equal on the two sides. In this position, only the medial longitudinal arch will be visible. The examiner should note any pes planus (flatfoot), pes cavus ("hollow" foot), or other deformities.

19. The feet angle out equally (usually 10°) (Fig. 15–25). This finding means that the tibias are normally slightly laterally rotated. The presence of "pigeon toes" usually indicates medial rotation of the tibias.

20. There is no bowing of bone. Any bowing may indicate diseases such as osteomalacia or osteoporosis.

21. The bony and soft-tissue contours are equal on the two halves of the body.

The patient's skin is observed for abnormalities such as hairy patches (e.g., from diastematomyelia), pigmented lesions (e.g., from café-au-lait spots or neurofibromatosis), subcutaneous tumors, and scars (e.g., Ehlers-Danlos syndrome), all of which may lead to or contribute to postural problems (Fig. 15–26).

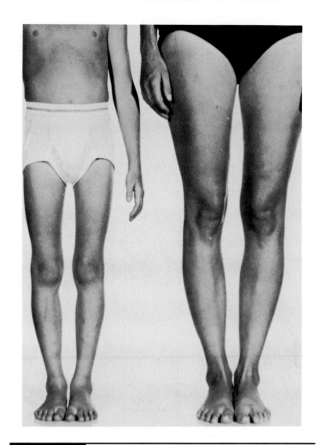

FIGURE 15–22. *Bilateral genu varum in mother and son. Note the associated internal tibial torsion. (From Tachdjian, M. O.: Pediatric Orthopedics. Philadelphia, W. B. Saunders Co., 1990, p. 2823.)*

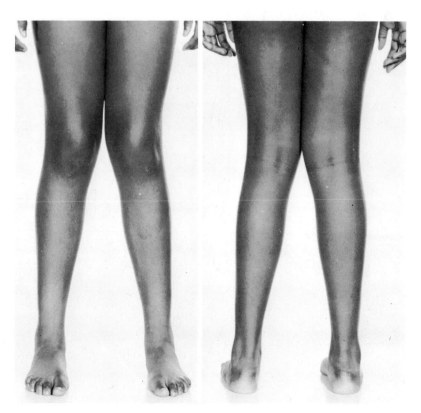

FIGURE 15–23. *Bilateral genu valgum in an adolescent. (From Tachdjian, M. O.: Pediatric Orthopedics. Philadelphia, W. B. Saunders Co., 1990, p. 2827.)*

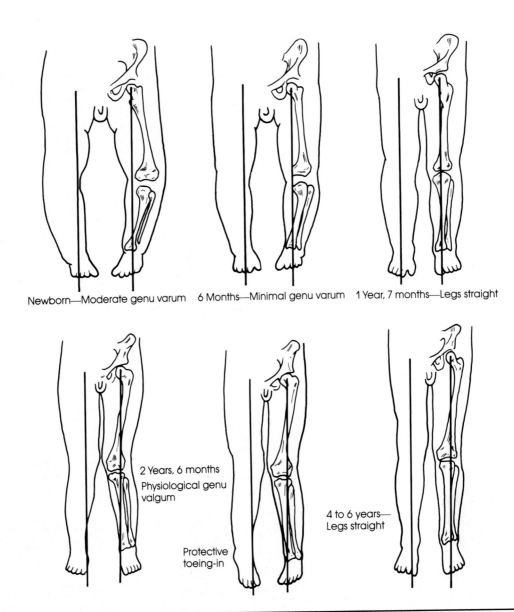

Newborn—Moderate genu varum   6 Months—Minimal genu varum   1 Year, 7 months—Legs straight

2 Years, 6 months
Physiological genu valgum

Protective toeing-in

4 to 6 years—Legs straight

FIGURE 15–24. Physiological evolution of lower limb alignment at various ages in infancy and childhood. (Redrawn from Tachdjian, M. O.: Pediatric Orthopedics. Philadelphia, W. B. Saunders Co., 1972, p. 1463.)

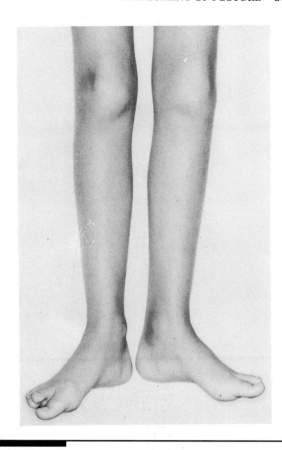

FIGURE 15–25. Exaggerated tibial torsion. In stance, with the patellae facing straight forward, the feet point outward. (From Tachdjian, M. O.: Pediatric Orthopedics. Philadelphia, W. B. Saunders Co., 1990, p. 2816.)

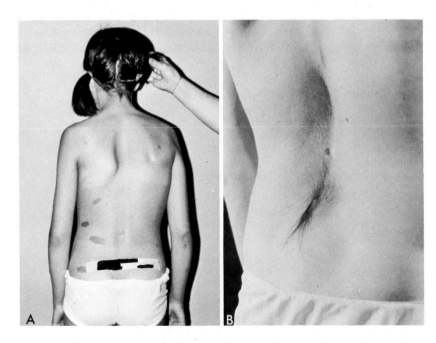

FIGURE 15–26. Abnormal skin markings. (A) Café-au-lait areas of pigmentation seen in neurofibromatosis. (B) Lumbar hair patch seen in diastematomyelia. (From Moe, J. H., D. S. Bradford, R. B. Winter, and J. E. Lonstein: Scoliosis and Other Spinal Deformities. Philadelphia, W. B. Saunders Co., 1978, p. 20.)

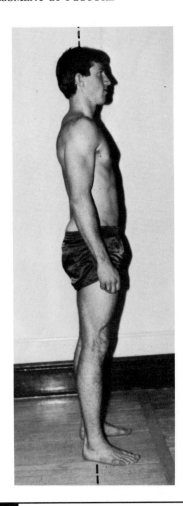

FIGURE 15–27. *Posture in the standing position (side view).*

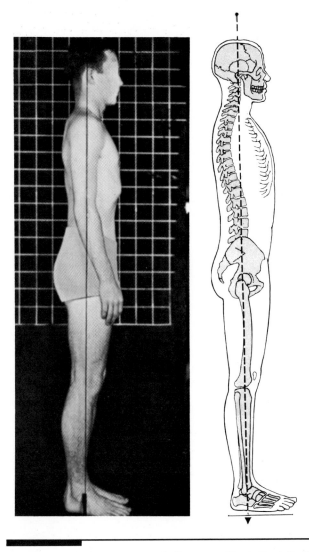

FIGURE 15–28. *Correct postural alignment. (From Kendall, F. P., and E. K. McCreary: Muscles: Testing and Function. Baltimore, Williams & Wilkins, 1983, p. 280.)*

Lateral View

From the side, the examiner should look to ensure the following:

1. The ear lobe is in line with the tip of the shoulder (acromion process) and the high point of the iliac crest. This line is the lateral line of reference dividing the body into front and back halves (Fig. 15–27). If the chin pokes forward, an excessive lumbar lordosis may also be present. This compensatory change is due to the body's attempt to maintain the center of gravity in the normal position.

2. Each spinal segment has a normal curve (Fig. 15–28). Large gluteus maximus muscles or excessive fat may give the appearance of an exaggerated lordosis. One should look at the spine in relation to the sacrum. Likewise, the scapulae may give the optical illusion of an increased kyphosis in the thoracic spine.

3. The shoulders are in proper alignment. If the shoulders droop forward, "rounded shoulders" are indicated. This improper alignment may be due to habit or tight pectoral muscles.

4. The chest, abdominal, and back muscles have proper tone. Weakness or spasm of any of these muscles can lead to postural alterations.

5. There are no chest deformities, such as pectus carinatum (undue prominence of the sternum) or pectus excavatum (undue depression of the sternum).

6. The pelvic angle is normal (30°) (Fig. 15–29).

7. The knees are straight, flexed, or in recurvatum (hyperextended). Usually, in the normal standing position, the knees are slightly flexed (0 to 5°). Hyperextension of the knees may cause an increase in lordosis in the lumbar spine. Tight hamstrings can also cause knee flexion.

Figure 15–30 illustrates the normal posture and some of the abnormal deviations seen when viewing the patient from the side.

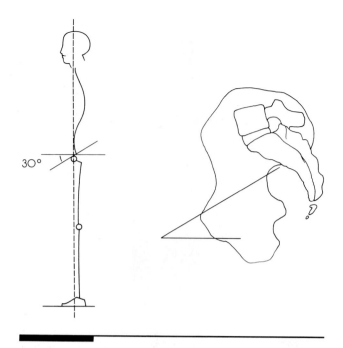

30°

FIGURE 15-29. *Normal pelvic angle.*

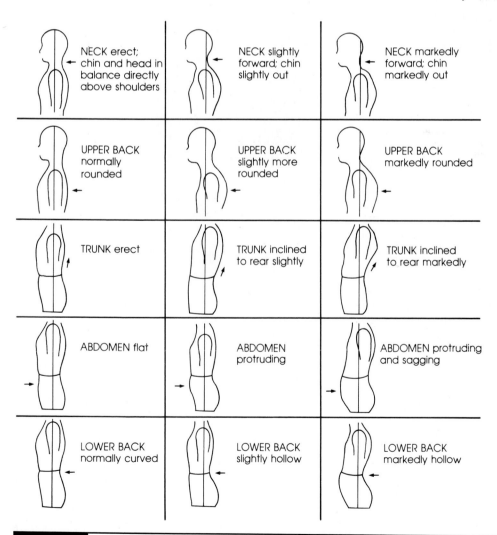

NECK erect; chin and head in balance directly above shoulders

NECK slightly forward; chin slightly out

NECK markedly forward; chin markedly out

UPPER BACK normally rounded

UPPER BACK slightly more rounded

UPPER BACK markedly rounded

TRUNK erect

TRUNK inclined to rear slightly

TRUNK inclined to rear markedly

ABDOMEN flat

ABDOMEN protruding

ABDOMEN protruding and sagging

LOWER BACK normally curved

LOWER BACK slightly hollow

LOWER BACK markedly hollow

FIGURE 15-30. *Postural deviations obvious from the side view. (Redrawn from Reedco Research, Auburn, N.Y.)*

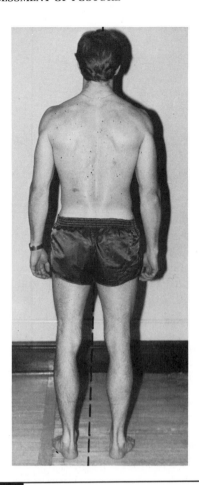

FIGURE 15–31. Posture in the standing position (posterior view).

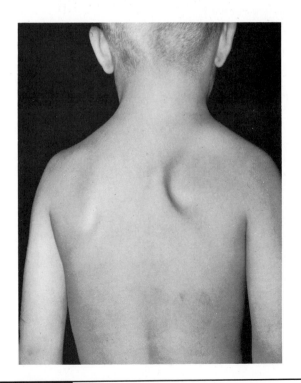

FIGURE 15–33. Sprengel's deformity. Note the small, high scapula on the right. (From Tachdjian, M. O.: Pediatric Orthopedics. Philadelphia, W. B. Saunders Co., 1990, p. 139.)

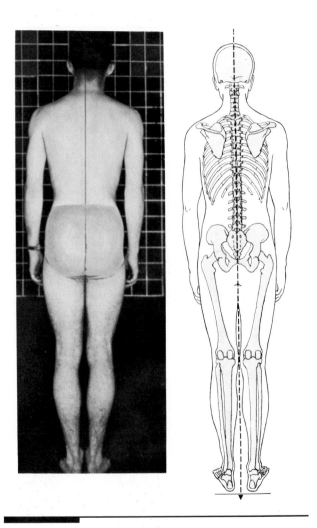

FIGURE 15–32. Correct postural alignment. (From Kendall, F. P., and E. K. McCreary: Muscles: Testing and Function. Baltimore, Williams & Wilkins, 1983, p. 290.)

Posterior View

When viewing from behind (Fig. 15–31), the examiner should note whether:

1. The shoulders are level, and the head is in midline. These findings should be compared with those from the anterior view.

2. The spines of the scapula and inferior angles of the scapula are level (Fig. 15–32). Defects such as Sprengel's deformity should be noted (Fig. 15–33).

3. The spine is straight or curved laterally, indicating scoliosis. A plumb line may be dropped from the spinous process of the seventh cervical vertebra (Fig. 15–34). The distance from the vertical string to the gluteal cleft can be measured. This distance is sometimes used as a measurement of spinal imbalance, and it is noted whether the devia-

tion is to the left or right. If a torticollis or cervicothoracic scoliosis is present, the plumb line should be dropped from the occipital protuberance.[6]

4. The ribs protrude.

5. The waist angles are level.

6. The arms are equidistant from the body and equally rotated.

7. The posterior superior iliac spines (PSIS) are level (Fig. 15–35). If one is higher than the other, one leg may become shorter or it may be due to rotation of the pelvis. The examiner should note how the posterior superior iliac spines relate to the anterior superior iliac spines (ASIS). If the ASIS on one side is higher and the PSIS on the same side is lower than the ASIS and the PSIS on the other side, there is a torsion deformity at the sacroiliac joint. If the ASIS and PSIS on one side are higher than the ASIS and PSIS on the other side, there may be an upslip at the sacroiliac joint on the high side.

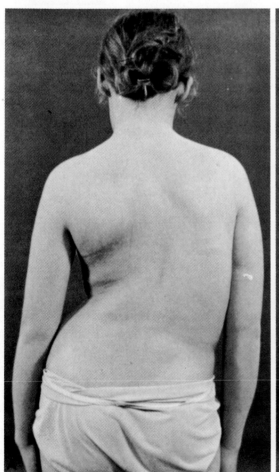
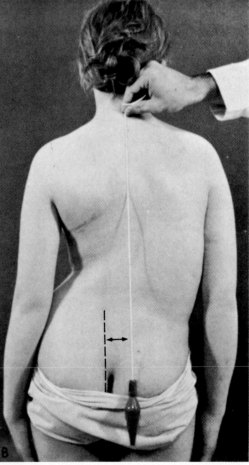

FIGURE 15–34. *The patient is viewed from the back to evaluate the spine deformity. (A) A typical right thoracic curve is shown. The left shoulder is lower, and the right scapula is more prominent. Note the decreased distance between the right arm and the thorax, with the shift of the thorax to the right. The left iliac crest appears higher, but this is due to the shift of the thorax with fullness on the right and elimination of the waistline. Thus the "high" hip is only apparent, not real. (B) Plumb line dropped from the prominent vertebra of C7 (vertebra prominens) measures the decompensation of the upper thorax over the pelvis. The distance from the vertical plumb line to the gluteal cleft is measured in centimeters and is recorded noting the direction of fall from the occipital protuberance (inion). (From Moe, J. H., D. S. Bradford, R. B. Winter, and J. E. Lonstein: Scoliosis and Other Spinal Deformities. Philadelphia, W. B. Saunders Co., 1978, p. 14.)*

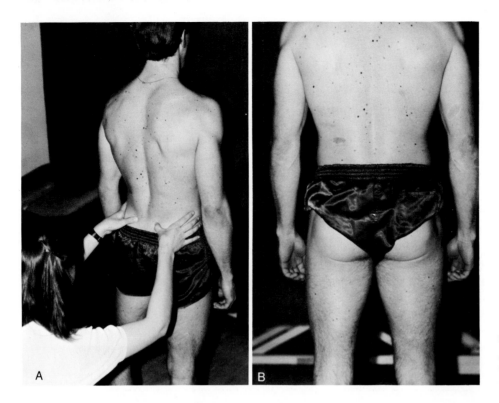

FIGURE 15–35. Viewing height of equality. (A) Posterior superior iliac spines. (B) Gluteal folds.

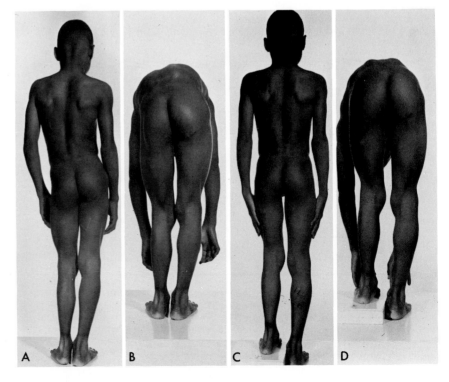

FIGURE 15–36. (A and B) Functional scoliosis resulting from short leg. (C and D) The spinal position with short leg is corrected. (From Tachdjian, M. O.: Pediatric Orthopedics. Philadelphia, W. B. Saunders Co., 1972, p. 1192.)

8. The gluteal folds are level. Muscle weakness, nerve root problems, or nerve palsy may lead to asymmetry.

9. The knee joints are level. If they are not, it may indicate that one leg is shorter than the other (Fig. 15–36).

10. Both of the Achilles tendons descend straight to the floor. If the tendons angle out, it may indicate flatfeet (pes planus).

11. The heels are straight or angled in (varus) or out (valgus).

12. Bowing of bones is present.

Figure 15–37 illustrates the normal posture and some of the abnormal deviations seen when viewing from behind.

When viewing posture, the examiner should remember that the pelvis is usually the key to proper back posture. The normal pelvic angle is 30° and is held or balanced in this position by muscles. For the pelvis to "sit properly" on the femur, the following muscles must be strong, supple, and balanced: abdominals, hip flexors, hip extensors, back extensors, hip rotators, and hip abductors and adductors.

If the height of the patient is measured, especially

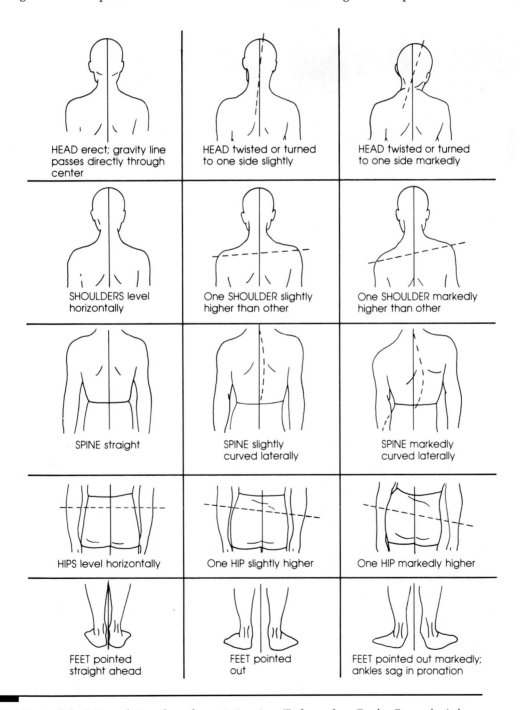

FIGURE 15–37. *Postural deviations obvious from the posterior view. (Redrawn from Reedco Research, Auburn, N.Y.)*

TABLE 15–1. Percentage of Mature Height Attained at Different Ages*

Chronological Age (Years)	Percentage of Eventual Height	
	Boys	*Girls*
1	42.2	44.7
2	49.5	52.8
3	53.8	57.0
4	58.0	61.8
5	61.8	66.2
6	65.2	70.3
7	69.0	74.0
8	72.0	77.5
9	75.0	80.7
10	78.0	84.4
11	81.1	88.4
12	84.2	92.9
13	87.3	96.5
14	91.5	98.3
15	96.1	99.1
16	98.3	99.6
17	99.3	100.0
18	99.8	100.0

*From Bayley, N.: The accurate prediction of growth and adult height. Mod. Probl. Pediatr. 7:234–255, 1954.

in a child, one could estimate the focal height of the child by using a chart such as the one shown in Table 15–1.[20]

Forward Flexion

Having completed the assessment of normal standing, the examiner asks the patient to flex forward at the hips with the fingertips of both hands together so that the arms drop vertically (Fig. 15–38). The feet should be together, and both knees should be

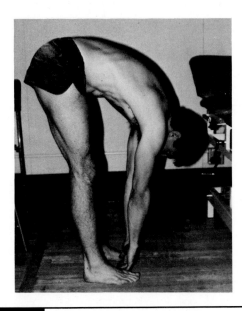

FIGURE 15–38. Posture in forward flexion. Note flattening or "rounding" of lumbar curve.

straight. Any alteration from this posture will cause the spine to rotate, giving a false view.

From this position, using the anterior and posterior skyline view, the examiner can note the following:

1. Whether there is any asymmetry of the rib cage (e.g., rib hump). If a hump is present, a level and tape measure may be used to obtain the perpendicular distance between the hump and hollow (Fig. 15–39).[6]

2. Whether there is any asymmetry in the spinal musculature.

3. Whether a kyphosis is present.

4. Whether the lumbar spine straightens or flexes.

5. Whether there is any restriction to forward bending such as spondylolisthesis or tight hamstrings (Figs. 15–40 and 15–41).

Sitting

With the patient seated on a stool so that the feet are on the ground and the back is unsupported, the examiner looks at the individual's posture (Fig. 15–42). This observation is carried out, as in the standing position, from the front, back, and side. If any anteroposterior or lateral deviations of the spine are observed, one should remember whether they were present when the patient was examined while standing. It should be noted whether the spinal curves increase or decrease when the patient is in the sitting position. From the front, it can be noted whether the knees are the same distance from the floor. If they are not, this may indicate a shortened tibia. From the side, it can be noted whether one knee protrudes farther than the other. If it does, this may indicate a shortened femur.

Supine Lying

With the patient in the supine lying position, the examiner notes the position of the head and cervical spine as well as the shoulder girdle. The chest area is observed for any protrusion, such as pectus carinatum, or sunken areas, such as pectus excavatum.

The abdominal musculature should be observed to see whether it is strong or flabby, and the waist angles should be noted to see whether they are equal. As in the standing position, the anterior superior iliac spines should be viewed to see if they are level. Any extension in the lumbar spine should be noted. In addition, it should be noted whether bending the knees helps to decrease the lumbar curve. If it does, it may indicate tight hip flexors. The lower limbs should descend parallel from the

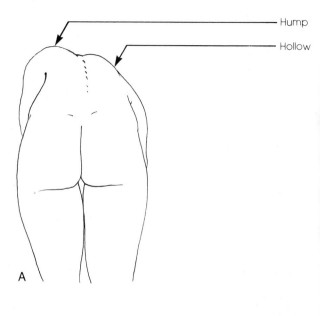

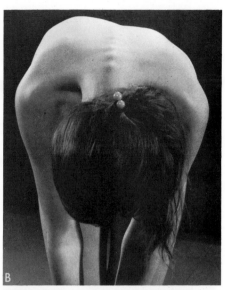

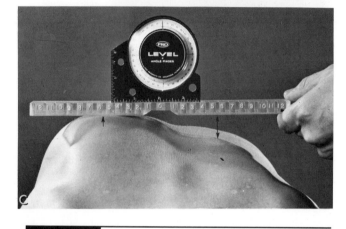

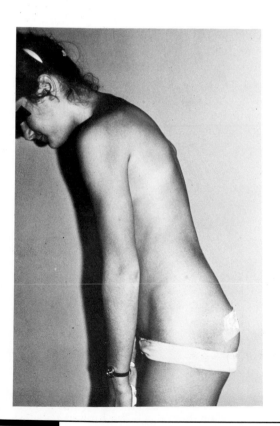

FIGURE 15–39. Rib hump in forward bending test. (A) Posterior view. (B) Anterior view. The two sides are compared. Note the presence of a right thoracic prominence. (C) Measurement of the prominence. The spirit level is positioned with the zero mark over the palpable spinous process in the area of maximal prominence. The level is made horizontal, and the distance to the apex of the deformity (5 to 6 cm) is noted. The perpendicular distance from the level to the valley is measured at the same distance from the midline. A 2.4-cm right thoracic prominence is shown. (From Moe, J. H., D. S. Bradford, R. B. Winter, and J. E. Lonstein: Scoliosis and Other Spinal Deformities. Philadelphia, W. B. Saunders Co., 1978, p. 17.)

FIGURE 15–40. Abnormal forward bending resulting from tight hamstrings, as seen in this patient with spondylolisthesis. (From Moe, J. H., D. S. Bradford, R. B. Winter, and J. E. Lonstein: Scoliosis and Other Spinal Deformities. Philadelphia, W. B. Saunders Co., 1978, p. 19.)

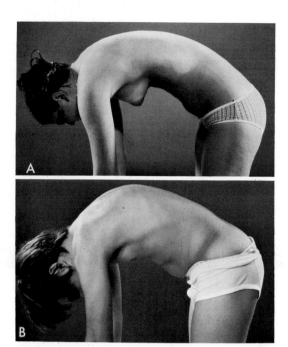

FIGURE 15–41. Forward bending position for viewing kyphosis (lateral view). (A) Normal thoracic roundness is demonstrated with a gentle curve to the entire spine. (B) An area of increased bending is seen in the thoracic spine, indicating structural changes—Scheuermann's disease, in this example. (From Moe, J. H., D. S. Bradford, R. B. Winter, and J. E. Lonstein: Scoliosis and Other Spinal Deformities. Philadelphia, W. B. Saunders Co., 1978, p. 18.)

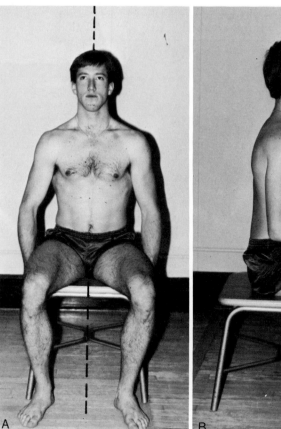

FIGURE 15–42. Posture in sitting positions (A and B).

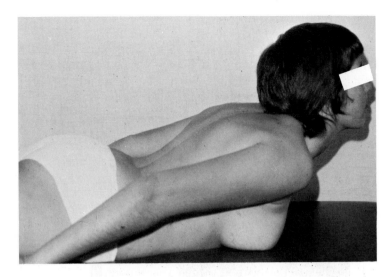

FIGURE 15–43. Structural kyphosis does not disappear on extension. (From Moe, J. H., D. S. Bradford, R. B. Winter, and J. E. Lonstein: Scoliosis and Other Spinal Deformities. Philadelphia, W. B. Saunders Co., 1978, p. 339.)

pelvis. If they do not or if they cannot be aligned parallel and at right angles to a line joining the anterior superior iliac spines, it may indicate an abduction or adduction contracture at the hip.

Prone Lying

With the patient lying prone, the examiner notes the position of the head, neck, and shoulder girdle as previously. The head should be positioned so that it is not rotated, side flexed, or extended. Any condition such as Sprengel's deformity or rib hump should be noted, as should any spinal deviations. The examiner should determine whether the posterior superior iliac spines are level and should ensure that the musculature of the buttocks, posterior thigh, and calves is normal (Fig. 15–43).

EXAMINATION

Assessment of posture, as previously mentioned, primarily involves history and observation. If on completing the history and observation the examiner feels that an examination is necessary, other chapters of this text should be referred to, and the procedure outlined for that area of the body should be followed.

With every postural assessment, however, the examiner should always perform two tests—the leg length measurement[21–24] and the straight leg raising test.

Leg Length Measurement. The patient lies supine with the pelvis set square or "balanced" on the legs (i.e., the legs at an angle of 90° to a line joining the ASISs). The legs should be 15 to 20 cm apart and parallel to each other (Fig. 15–44).

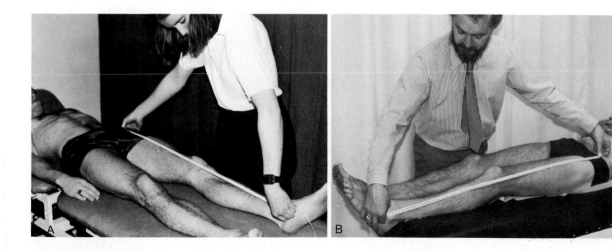

FIGURE 15–44. Measuring leg length to medial malleolus (A) and to lateral malleolus (B).

The examiner then places one end of the tape measure against the distal aspect of the ASIS, holding it firmly against the bone. The index finger of the other hand is placed immediately distal to the medial or lateral malleolus and pushed against it. The thumbnail is brought down against the tip of the index fingers so that the tape measure is pinched between them. A reading is taken where the thumb and finger pinch together. A slight difference, up to 1.0 to 1.5 cm, is considered normal but can still be relevant.

Further information on measuring true leg length may be found in Chapter 10.

Straight Leg Raising Test. The patient lies in the supine position with the knees extended and hips medially rotated (Fig. 15–45). The examiner passively flexes the patient's hip, keeping the knee extended and the hip medially rotated until the patient complains of pain or tightness in the back of the leg. The hip is then extended slightly until no pain or tightness is felt. The patient is asked to flex the head so that the chin rests on the chest. If the pain returns, it is an indication of a nerve root injury. If the pain does not return, it may be an indication of tight hamstrings. The other leg should be tested in a similar fashion, and any differences should be noted.

Further information on the straight leg raising test may be found in Chapter 8.

Additional Tests. Other tests may also be performed based on what the examiner has observed.

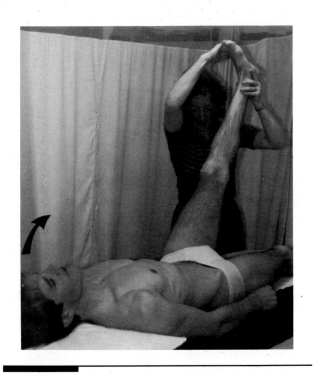

FIGURE 15–45. *Straight leg raising test.*

For example, if the hip flexors appear tight, the Thomas test should be performed (see Chapter 10).

Refer to Table 15–2 for a detailed presentation of postural problems.

TABLE 15–2. Good and Faulty Posture: Summary Chart*

Good Posture	Part	Faulty Posture
Head is held erect in a position of good balance.	Head	Chin up too high. Head protruding forward. Head tilted or rotated to one side.
Arms hang relaxed at the sides with palms of the hands facing toward the body. Elbows are slightly bent, so forearms hang slightly forward. Shoulders are level, and neither one is more forward or backward than the other when seen from the side. Scapulae lie flat against the rib cage. They are neither too close together nor too wide apart. In adults, a separation of approximately 4 in. is average.	Arms and shoulders	Holding the arms stiffly in any position forward, backward, or out from the body. Arms turned so that palms of hands face backward. One shoulder higher than the other. Both shoulders hiked up. One or both shoulders drooping forward or sloping. Shoulders rotated either clockwise or counterclockwise. Scapulae pulled back too hard. Scapulae too far apart. Scapulae too prominent, standing out from the rib cage ("winged scapulae").
A good position of the chest is one in which it is slightly up and slightly forward (while the back remains in good alignment). The chest appears to be in a position about halfway between that of a full inspiration and a forced expiration.	Chest	Depressed, or "hollow-chest" position. Lifted and held up too high, brought about by arching the back. Ribs more prominent on one side than on the other. Lower ribs flaring out or protruding.
In young children up to about the age of 10, the abdomen normally protrudes somewhat. In older children and adults, it should be flat.	Abdomen	Entire abdomen protrudes. Lower part of the abdomen protrudes while the upper part is pulled in.

TABLE 15–2. Good and Faulty Posture: Summary Chart* *Continued*

Good Posture	Part	Faulty Posture
The front of the pelvis and the thighs are in a straight line. The buttocks are not prominent in back but instead slope slightly downward. The spine has four natural curves. In the neck and lower back, the curve is forward, and in the upper back and lowest part of the spine (sacral region), it is backward. The sacral curve is a fixed curve, whereas the other three are flexible.	Spine and pelvis (side view)	The low back arches forward too much (lordosis). The pelvis tilts forward too much. The front of the thigh forms an angle with the pelvis when this tilt is present. The normal forward curve in the low back has straightened out. The pelvis tips backward and there is a slightly backward slant to the line of the pelvis in relation to the front of the hips (flat back). Increased backward curve in the upper back (kyphosis or round upper back). Increased forward curve in the neck. Almost always accompanied by round upper back and seen as a forward head. Lateral curve of the spine (scoliosis); toward one side (C-curve), toward both sides (S-curve).
Ideally, the body weight is borne evenly on both feet, and the hips are level. One side is not more prominent than the other as seen from front or back, nor is one hip more forward or backward than the other as seen from the side. The spine does not curve to the left or the right side. (A *slight* deviation to the left in right-handed individuals and to the right in left-handed individuals should not be considered abnormal. Also, because a tendency toward a *slightly* low right shoulder and *slightly* high right hip is frequently found in right-handed people, and vice versa for left-handed, such deviations should not be considered abnormal.)	Hips, pelvis, and spine (back view)	One hip is higher than the other (lateral pelvic tilt). Sometimes it is not really much higher but appears so because a sideways sway of the body has made it more prominent. (Tailors and dressmakers often notice a lateral tilt because the hemline of skirts or length of trousers must be adjusted to the difference.) The hips are rotated so that one is farther forward than the other (clockwise or counter-clockwise rotation).
Legs are straight up and down. Patellae face straight ahead when feet are in good position. Looking at the knees from the side, the knees are straight (i.e., neither bent forward nor "locked" backward).	Knees and legs	Knees touch when feet are apart (genu valgum). Knees are apart when feet touch (genu varum). Knee curves slightly backward (hyperextended knee) (genu recurvatum). Knee bends slightly forward, that is, it is not as straight as it should be (flexed knee). Patellae face slightly toward each other (medially rotated femurs). Patellae face slightly outward (laterally rotated femurs).
Toes should be straight, that is, neither curled downward nor bent upward. They should extend forward in line with the foot and not be squeezed together or overlap.	Toes	Toes bend up at the first joint and down at middle and end joints so that the weight rests on the tips of the toes (hammer toes). This fault is often associated with wearing shoes that are too short. Big toe slants inward toward the midline of the foot (hallus valgus). This fault is often associated with wearing shoes that are too narrow and pointed at the toes.
In standing, the longitudinal arch has the shape of a half dome. Barefoot or in shoes without heels, the feet toe-out slightly. In shoes with heels, the feet are parallel. In walking with or without heels, the feet are parallel, and the weight is transferred from the heel along the outer border to the ball of the foot. In running, the feet are parallel or toe-in slightly. The weight is on the balls of the feet and toes because the heels do not come in contact with the ground.	Foot	Low longitudinal arch or flatfoot. Low metatarsal arch, usually indicated by calluses under the ball of the foot. Weight borne on the inner side of the foot (pronation). "Ankle rolls in." Weight borne on the outer border of the foot (supination). "Ankle rolls out." Toeing-out while walking or while standing in shoes with heels ("outflared" or "slue-footed"). Toeing-in while walking or standing ("pigeon-toed").

*Modified from Kendall, F. P., and E. K. McCreary: Muscles: Testing and Function. Baltimore, Williams & Wilkins, 1983.

PRÉCIS OF POSTURAL ASSESSMENT

History
Observation
    Standing (front, side, and behind)
    Forward flexion (front, side, and behind)
    Sitting (front, side, and behind)
    Supine lying
    Prone lying
Examination
    Leg length measurement
    Straight leg raising test
Examination of specific joints (see appropriate chapter)

As with any assessment, the patient must be warned that there may be some discomfort after the examination and that this discomfort is normal. Discomfort after any assessment should decrease within 24 hours. The examiner must always keep in mind that several joints may be affected at the same time, either as the result of or as the cause of faulty posture. Thus, the examination of posture may be an extensive one, with observation of the posture in general but also several specific joints in detail.

REFERENCES

CITED REFERENCES

1. Fahrni, W. H.: Backache: Assessment and Treatment. Vancouver, Musquean Publishers, Ltd., 1976.
2. Finneson, B. E.: Low Back Pain. Philadelphia, J. B. Lippincott Co., 1981.
3. Kendall, F. P., and E. K. McCreary: Muscles: Testing and Function. Baltimore, Williams & Wilkins, 1983.
4. McKenzie, R. A.: The Lumbar Spine: Mechanical Diagnosis and Therapy. Waikanae, New Zealand, Spinal Publications, 1981.
5. Wiles, P., and R. Sweetnam: Essentials of Orthopaedics. London, J & A Churchill Co., 1965.
6. Moe, J. H., D. S. Bradford, R. B. Winter, and J. E. Lonstein: Scoliosis and Other Spinal Deformities. Philadelphia, W. B. Saunders Co., 1978.
7. McMorris, R. O.: Faulty posture. Pediatr. Clin. North Am. 8:213, 1961.
8. Tachdjian, M. O.: Pediatric Orthopedics. Philadelphia, W. B. Saunders Co., 1972.
9. Tsou, P. M.: Embryology and congenital kyphosis. Clin. Orthop. Relat. Res. 128:18, 1977.
10. White, A. A., M. M. Panjabi, and C. C. Thomas: The clinical biomechanics of kyphotic deformities. Clin. Orthop. Relat. Res. 128:8, 1977.
11. Hensinger, R. N.: Kyphosis secondary to skeletal dysplasias and metabolic disease. Clin. Orthop. Relat. Res. 128:113, 1977.
12. Tsou, P. M., A. Yau, and A. R. Hodgson: Embryogenesis and prenatal development of congenital vertebral anomalies and their classification. Clin. Orthop. Relat. Res. 152:211, 1980.
13. Cailliet, R.: Scoliosis: Diagnosis and Management. Philadelphia, F. A. Davis Co., 1975.
14. Figueiredo, U. M., and J. I. P. Mames: Juvenile idiopathic scoliosis. J. Bone Joint Surg. 63B:61, 1981.
15. Goldstein, L. A., and T. R. Waugh: Classification and terminology of scoliosis. Clin. Orthop. Relat. Res. 93:10, 1973.
16. James, J. I. P. : The etiology of scoliosis. J. Bone Joint Surg. 52B:410, 1970.
17. White, A. A.: Kinematics of the normal spine as related to scoliosis. J. Biomech. 4:405, 1971.
18. Papaioannou, T., I. Stokes, and J. Kenwright: Scoliosis associated with limb length inequality. J. Bone Joint Surg. 64A:59, 1982.
19. Debrunner, H. U.: Orthopaedic Diagnosis. London, E & S Livingstone, 1970.
20. Bayley, N.: The accurate prediction of growth and adult height. Mod. Probl. Pediatr. 7:234, 1954.
21. Clarke, G. R.: Unequal leg length: An accurate method of detection and some clinical results. Rheumat. Phys. Med. 11:385, 1972.
22. Fisk, J. W., and M. L. Baigent: Clinical and radiological assessment of leg length. N. Z. Med. J. 81:477, 1975.
23. Nichols, P. J. R., and N. T. J. Bailey: The accuracy of measuring leg-length differences. Br. Med. J. 2:1247, 1955.
24. Woerman, A. L., and S. A. Binder-Macleod: Leg-length discrepancy assessment: Accuracy and precision in five clinical methods of evaluation. J. Orthop. Sports Phys. Ther. 5:230, 1984.

GENERAL REFERENCES

Anderson, B. J. G., R. Ortengon, A. I. Nachemson, et al.: The sitting posture: An electromyographic and discometric study. Orthop. Clin. North Am. 6:105, 1975.
Cailliet, R.: Nerve and Arm Pain. Philadelphia, F. A. Davis Co., 1964.
Cyriax, J.: Textbook of Orthopaedic Medicine, vol. 1: Diagnosis of Soft Tissue Lesions. London, Bailliere Tindall, 1982.
During, J., H. Goudfrooij, W. Keessen, T. W. Beeker, and A. Crowe: Towards standards for posture-postural characteristics of the lower back system in normal and pathological conditions. Spine 10:83, 1985.
Kapandji, I. A.: The Physiology of the Joints, vol. 2: The Trunk and Vertebral Column. New York, Churchill Livingstone, 1974.
Kappler, R.: Postural balance and motion patterns. J. Am. Osteopath. Assoc. 81:598, 1982.
Littler, W. A.: Cardiorespiratory failure and scoliosis. Physiother. 60:69, 1974.
MacDougall, J. D., H. A. Wenger, and H. J. Green: Physiological Testing of the Elite Athlete. Ottawa, Canadian Association of Sports Sciences, 1982.
Matthews, D. K.: Measurement in Physical Education. Philadelphia, W. B. Saunders Co., 1973.
Mennell, J.: Back Pain: Diagnosis and Treatment Using Manipulative Techniques. Boston, Little, Brown and Co., 1960.
Murray, M. P., A. Seireg, and R. C. Scholz: Centre of gravity, centre of pressure and supportive forces during human activities. J. Appl. Physiol. 23:831, 1967.
Opila, K. A.: Gender and somatotype differences in postural alignment: Response to high-heeled shoes and simulated weight gain. Clin. Biomech. 3:145, 1988.
Opila, K. A., S. S. Wagner, S. Schiowitz, and J. Chen: Postural alignment in barefoot and high-heeled stance. Spine 13:542, 1988.
Portnoy, H., and F. Morin: Electromyographic study of postural muscles in various positions and movements. Am. J. Physiol. 186:122, 1956.
Rothman, R. H., and F. A. Simeone: The Spine. Philadelphia, W. B. Saunders Co., 1982.
Torcell, G., A. Nordwall, and A. Nachemson: The changing pattern of scoliosis treatment due to effective screening. J. Bone Joint Surg. 63A:337, 1981.
Wolfson, L. I., R. Whipple, P. Amerman, and A. Kleinberg: Stressing the postural response—A quantitative method for testing balance. J. Am. Geriatr. Soc. 34:845, 1986.

Emergency Sports Assessment

This chapter is provided to enable the health care professional to immediately assess a patient before application of first aid or transportation to the hospital. Such an assessment should be divided into two parts. The first part concerns the primary evaluation or survey, which is usually done at the location in which the patient is found to ensure that life-threatening situations are handled immediately. The secondary evaluation is performed when the examiner has more time and the patient is not under immediate threat of death or permanent disability.

PRE-EVENT PREPARATION

Before any sporting event, the examiner should establish and practice emergency protocols. This preparation includes designating personnel for specific tasks and establishing emergency vehicle routes and entrances. The examiner and the assistants should know the location of additional medical assistance, emergency equipment (e.g., spinal board, neck supports, sandbags, stretchers, blankets, and emergency first-aid kit), and a telephone. Near the telephone, the examiner should post emergency telephone numbers (e.g., ambulance, physician, and dentist), name and address of the sports facility, entrance to be used, and any obvious landmarks, because the person making the emergency call may forget information or give inappropriate information when under stress.

The examiner should take the time to give the facility a safety check by looking for potential hazards. Visiting teams should also be informed of emergency protocols. In addition, emergency situations and protocols must be practiced repeatedly to ensure proper care will be given in an emergency.

PRIMARY ASSESSMENT

After an injury occurs, the examiner must first take control of the situation and ensure that minimal additional harm comes to the patient. The examiner is designated as the *charge person*, or person in control. The examiner takes control by not allowing the patient to be moved until some type of assessment is made, the spine is supported as much as possible, and, if required, assistance is obtained.

While performing the initial assessment, the examiner must keep in mind that six situations can immediately threaten the life of a patient: airway obstruction, respiratory failure, cardiac arrest, severe heat injury, head (craniocerebral) injury, and cervical spine injury.[1]

Initially, the examiner stabilizes and immobilizes the patient's head and cervical spine in case the patient has suffered a cervical spine injury (Fig. 16–1). Simultaneously, the examiner talks to the patient, explains what the examiner is going to do, and reassures the patient. The patient should be left in the original position until the nature and severity of the injury have been determined, except in cases of respiratory or cardiac distress. A spinal cord injury should be suspected, at least initially, if the patient has neck pain; the patient's head position is asymmetric or abnormal; the patient is having respiratory difficulty, especially if the chest is not moving (absence of abdominal or diaphragmatic breathing); the patient is demonstrating priapism (erection of the penis); or the patient is unconscious after a fall or other contact activity. Other indications of neurological injuries in the conscious patient include numbness, tingling, or burning, especially below the clavicles; muscle weakness; twitching; or paralysis

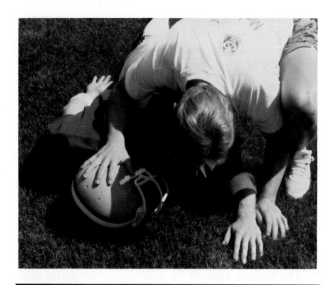

FIGURE 16–1. Stabilization of the patient's head and neck before initial assessment.

of the arms and/or legs, especially bilaterally (flaccid paralysis).[2]

The examiner must quickly determine whether the patient is conscious. At this early stage, the examiner simply determines whether the patient is alert (fully conscious), confused (drowsy), in delirium, in obtundation (dulled sensations, especially pain and touch), in a stupor, or in a coma. A patient is classified as alert if able to carry on an appropriate conversation with no delays and is aware of time, place, and identity. A classification of confused implies that the patient is disoriented to time, place, and/or identity, has a short attention span, is easily bewildered, and has difficulty following commands. A patient in a delirious state is disoriented, restless, and irritable and may have hallucinations. A patient in obtundation appears drowsy and lethargic but readily replies to verbal stimulation if the questions are simple. A patient is classified as stuporous if responses are elicited only from loud noises or painful stimulation. This type of patient is lethargic and does not respond to normal verbal communication. In a comatose state, the patient appears to be asleep and does not respond to verbal or painful stimuli, except in a rudimentary way (e.g., pulling away from a painful stimulus).

The level of consciousness or arousal should be determined by talking to the patient, not by moving the patient. Some individuals refer to this as the "shake and shout" stage, in which the examiner tries to arouse the unconscious individual by gently shaking the patient (without allowing movement of the head and neck) and by shouting into each ear. If the patient does not respond to this verbal stimulus, the examiner can, at least initially, assume that the patient is unconscious or not fully conscious and proceed under that assumption. Further neurological assessment is left until the examiner is sure that the patient has a patent airway, is breathing normally, and has a heartbeat. If the patient is conscious, the examiner should reassure the patient that help has arrived. The patient should be informed of what the examiner is doing and proposes to do in terms of examining and moving the patient. Regardless of the patient's state of consciousness, the patient should not move or be moved until the examiner has had an opportunity to examine the patient.

The primary assessment should take no more than 30 seconds to 2 minutes, with the maximum on-scene time being 10 minutes.[3] If the injury is severe, the longer the assessment takes, the higher the mortality rate is likely to be.

For the primary emergency assessment, the examiner should call at least one individual to provide immediate assistance, relay messages, and obtain additional help, if necessary. This person is designated the *call person* and should know the location of the closest telephone and what telephone numbers to call in specific emergencies. When telephoning, the call person should state the caller's name, the number of the telephone being used, the exact emergency (type of injury), the degree of urgency, and the exact location of the facility; ask for an estimated time of arrival; and explain what the best entrance is to the facility for the responding emergency personnel. Other individuals (as many as six or seven) may be called as necessary to act as transporters or help move the patient.

Establishing the Airway

While waiting for assistance, the examiner can immediately begin to check for abnormal or arrested breathing, abnormal or arrested pulse, internal and external bleeding, and shock. This initial assessment is called the *ABCs* (Airway, Breathing, and Circulation) of cardiopulmonary resuscitation (CPR). The first priority is to maintain an adequate airway, normal ventilation, and hemodynamic stability (Table 16–1).[4, 5] Also, obvious bleeding should be controlled by compression.

While the cervical spine is protected and immobilized, the airway is quickly assessed for patency.[3] Respirations can be determined by watching for movement of the chest, feeling the breath on the cheek, or hearing the air move in and out (Fig. 16–2). The normal resting ranges of respirations are 10 to 25 breaths per minute for adults and 20 to 25 breaths per minute for children. If a patient is not breathing and has no heartbeat, clinical death will

TABLE 16–1. Priorities in the Management of Injuries: Beware of Injury to the Cervical Spine!

Highest priority
1. Respiratory and cardiovascular impairment: Facial, neck, and chest injuries
2. Hemorrhage: External, severe

High priority
3. Retroperitoneal injuries: Shock, hemorrhage
4. Intraperitoneal injuries: Shock, hemorrhage
5. Craniocerebral spinal cord injuries: Open or closed, observation
6. Severe burns: Extensive soft-tissue wounds

Low priority
7. Lower genitourinary tract: Hemorrhage, extravasation
8. Peripheral vascular, nerve, locomotor injuries: Open or closed
9. Facial and neck injuries: Except priorities 1 and 2
10. Cold exposure

Special
11. Fractures, dislocations: Splinting
12. Tetanus prophylaxis

From Steichen, F. M.: The emergency management of the severely injured. J. Trauma 12:787, 1972.

occur between 0 and 4 minutes (Fig. 16–3). If breathing and heartbeat are not restored within 4 to 6 minutes, brain damage is probable. If there is no breathing and no heartbeat for 6 to 10 minutes, biological death occurs, and brain damage is very likely.[6]

If the conscious patient exhibits abnormal or arrested breathing (asphyxia), the examiner should look for possible causes. Causes include compression of the trachea; falling back of the tongue, blocking the airway; foreign bodies; swelling of the tissues, for example, owing to a bee sting that results in anaphylactic shock; fluid in the air passages; presence of harmful gases or fumes; and suffocation. Falling back of the tongue is the most common cause of airway obstruction after a sport injury, especially

in the unconscious patient. Normally, the tone of the muscles of the tongue ensures airway patency. However, in the unconscious individual, especially those in the supine position, muscle tone is lost and the tongue falls back, potentially leading to an obstruction. If the tongue is the cause of obstruction, the examiner can simply pull the chin forward in a *chin-lift* (Fig. 16–4A) or *jaw-thrust maneuver* (Fig. 16–4B) to restore the airway, being careful that movement of the cervical spine is kept to a minimum; the chin-lift maneuver is less likely to compromise the cervical spine.[7] Either maneuver pulls the retropharyngeal musculature forward, thus opening the airway. If the examiner can see an object obstructing the airway, an oral screw and tongue forceps can be used to remove the object (Fig. 16–5). The mouth should be held open with the oral screw or something similar, and the examiner can use a finger to sweep the mouth clear of debris (e.g., broken teeth, dentures, mouth guard, chewing gum, or tobacco). If the jaw is not held open and blocked from closing, the examiner should put fingers in the patient's mouth only with caution. If the examiner is concerned about maintaining a patent airway, an oropharyngeal airway may be used (Fig. 16–6). As a last resort, a wide-bore needle (18-gauge or larger) may be inserted into the trachea to ensure an airway.

If the patient is not breathing, artificial ventilation (mouth-to-mouth resuscitation) must be initiated immediately using the breathing portion of the CPR techniques (Fig. 16–7) or by "bagging" the patient (Fig. 16–8).

If the patient is conscious but obviously in respiratory and/or cardiac distress, the examiner must immediately deal with the presenting situation (Table 16–2). If the patient does not have a patent airway, an airway must be established as described above.

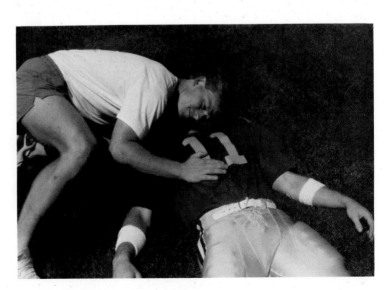

FIGURE 16–2. Examiner positioning to determine respiration of the patient. The examiner can feel the breath on the cheek, hear the breath, and watch the chest move.

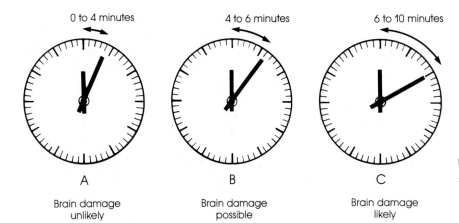

0 to 4 minutes

4 to 6 minutes

6 to 10 minutes

A

Brain damage
unlikely

B

Brain damage
possible

C

Brain damage
likely

FIGURE 16–3. *If the brain is deprived of oxygen for 4 to 6 minutes, brain damage is possible. After 6 minutes, brain damage is extremely likely.*

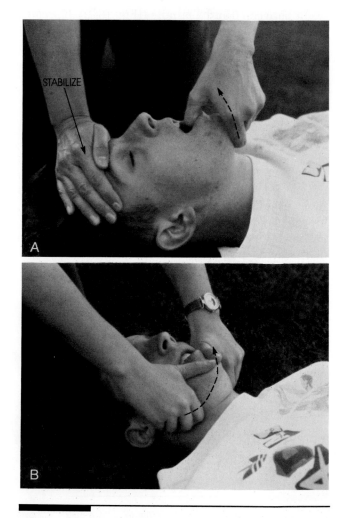

FIGURE 16–4. *Chin lift (A) and jaw thrust (B) maneuvers. In both cases, the head should not be tilted if a cervical injury is suspected.*

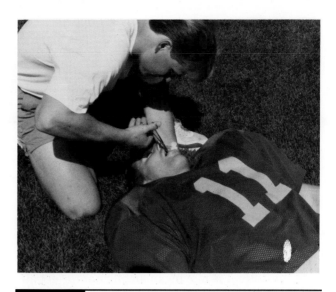

FIGURE 16–5. Use of tongue forceps and oral screw to maintain patent airway.

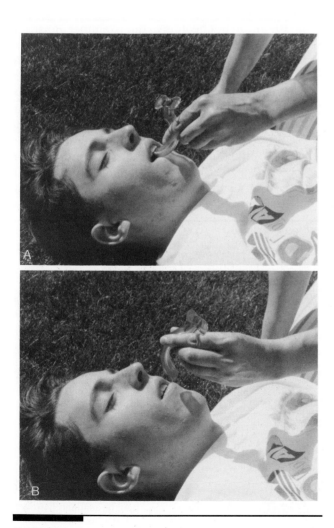

FIGURE 16–6. Insertion of an oropharyngeal airway to establish a patent airway. (A) Inserting the oral airway; insert the airway wrong way up and gently rotate once in the mouth. (B) The airway in its final position in the mouth.

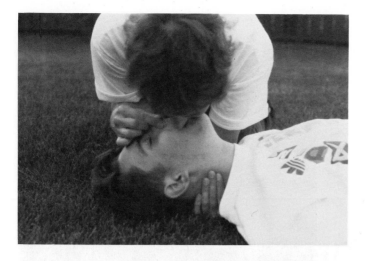

FIGURE 16–7. *Mouth-to-mouth resuscitation.*

If the patient is moving in an attempt to "get air," the examiner may assume that a severe cervical injury is less likely to have occurred. However, movement of the head in relation to the cervical spine should be kept to a minimum. A rapid assessment of the brain and spinal cord can be accomplished by asking the patient to "stick out the tongue," "wiggle the toes" or "move the feet," and "squeeze the [examiner's] fingers."[8] Keeping in mind the possibility of a cervical injury, the examiner should position the patient so that airway clearance and resuscitation can be easily accomplished. This change in position must be performed very carefully to ensure that movement of the cervical spine is kept to a minimum.

If the patient is reasonably comfortable in the side-lying or prone position and there is no problem with cardiac function or breathing, it is not necessary to move the patient to the supine position.

Once the airway has been established, whether by the use of an airway (see Fig. 16–6), proper head or jaw positioning (see Fig. 16–4), tongue forceps (see Fig. 16–5), or tracheotomy, the examiner must ensure that the airway is maintained and that the patient continues breathing. Endotracheal intubation is necessary when nasopharyngeal bleeding, secretions, or aspirations prevent maintenance of an adequate airway or end-ventilation.[4] Transtracheal ventilation is the treatment of choice for patients with breathing problems caused by brain, cervical spine, or maxillofacial injuries. An endotracheal tube may cause straining and venous hypertension and lead to increased brain edema, and extension of the head and neck to open upper airways may

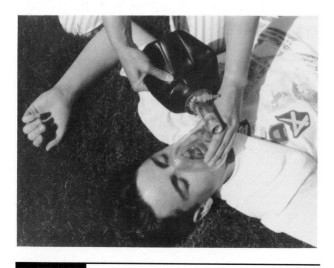

FIGURE 16–8. *Use of a "bagger" to maintain air supply to a patient.*

TABLE 16–2. Airway Obstruction*

Conscious Athlete	Unconscious Athlete
1. If patient is breathing or coughing, leave alone but continue to watch	1. Head tilt if no cervical spine injury is suspected
2. If no air is going in and out of lungs, administer: Four abdominal thrusts (Heimlich maneuver); some people also administer four back blows	2. No response—try to ventilate
	3. No success—reposition head and try to ventilate again
3. Repeat until: Patient can breathe independently Patient becomes unconscious	4. If unsuccessful, follow with four abdominal thrusts (Heimlich maneuver); some people also administer four back blows
	5. Quick sweep of the mouth
	6. If unsuccessful, repeat steps 1 through 5 until: There is no longer obstruction, or qualified help arrives; a tracheotomy may follow if obstruction continues

*Adapted from American Academy of Orthopedic Surgeons: Athletic Training and Sports Medicine. Park Ridge, IL, AAOS, 1984, p. 454.

aggravate cervical spine injuries. Also, hemorrhage in maxillofacial injuries prevents the effective use of a breathing mask and does not allow adequate visualization.[5]

Positioning the Patient

If the conscious patient is prone and in respiratory difficulty, the examiner, with assistance, should log-roll the patient (Fig. 16–9) onto a spinal board so that an attempt can be made to restore the airway. During any movement of the patient, traction must be applied to the cervical spine by the examiner to maintain stability. The patient should be reassured that others are going to carefully move the patient while the patient remains still. Before any movement is attempted, the patient as well as those who are going to assist the examiner should know what the examiner plans to do and what their jobs will be.

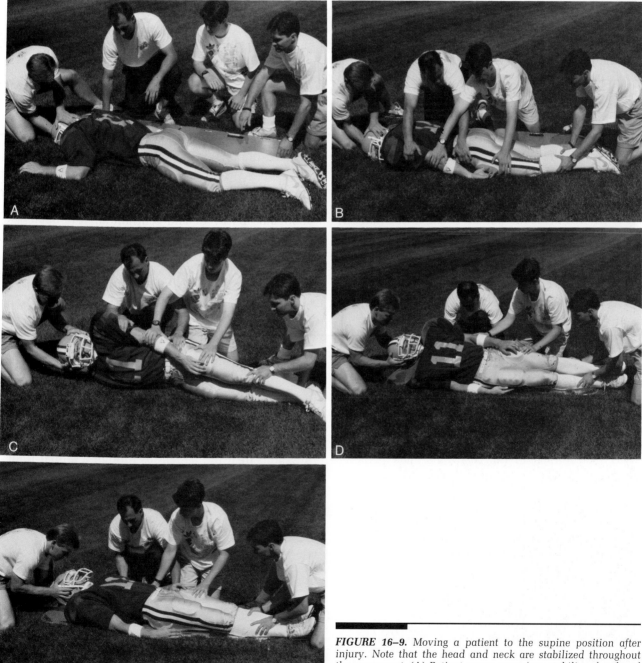

FIGURE 16–9. Moving a patient to the supine position after injury. Note that the head and neck are stabilized throughout the movement. (A) Patient prone, examiner stabilizes head and gives instruction to helpers. (B) through (E) Patient is log-rolled onto spinal board.

The sequence of movement and positioning of the extremities and the body of the patient should be thought out beforehand so that everyone is aware of what is going to happen. The proper procedure for moving the patient should be practiced often to ensure competency.

To roll the patient, at least three assistants are needed. There should also be two-way communication between the examiner and the patient at all times to continually evaluate the patient's comfort level and neurological signs. The assistants should place the spinal board beside the patient and then kneel beside the spinal board and patient (see Fig. 16–9A). They should reach over the patient and hold the shoulder, hip, and knees (Fig. 16–9B). On command from the examiner, the assistants should roll the patient toward them while the examiner stabilizes the head (see Fig. 16–9C and D) until the patient is lying supine on the spinal board (see Fig. 16–9E). Only rolling—not lifting—should occur. With the patient in the supine position, proper CPR techniques may be applied or the patient may be transported. The patient may also be covered with a blanket to provide warmth.

If a spinal injury is suspected and the conscious patient is in the prone position but having no difficulty in breathing, the patient is log-rolled halfway toward the assistants while another assistant slides the spinal board as close as possible to the patient's side. The patient is then rolled directly onto the spinal board in the prone position. Similarly, if a spinal injury is suspected and the patient is in the supine position and breathing normally, the patient is rolled toward the assistants while another assistant slides the spinal board under the patient as far as possible. The patient is then rolled back onto the spinal board in the supine position. If a spinal injury is suspected and the patient is in side lying, the patient is log-rolled directly onto the spinal board into the supine position. In each of these cases, the examiner controls the head, applies traction, and gives instructions to the assistants. The patient's head is then stabilized and immobilized with sand-bags, a head immobilizer, or triangular bandages, and the patient is strapped to the spinal board with restraining belts. It must be remembered that any major injury such as a head injury, a spinal injury, or a fracture requires appropriate handling, slow and deliberate management, and proper transportation to provide a satisfactory outcome. Thus, these techniques must be practiced repeatedly.

If possible and time permits, especially if the individuals are not used to working together, a simulated roll and transport using an uninjured person should be attempted before moving the patient to ensure that all involved know what they are doing in terms of patient positioning, movement sequence, and specific handling (e.g., head, hands, and feet) so that any transfer or movement of the patient is effective and organized.

During the emergency assessment, if the patient is nauseated, is vomiting, or has fluid draining from the mouth and breathing and circulation are normal, the patient should be placed in the recovery position (Fig. 16–10) provided that there is no suspicion of a spinal injury. This side-lying position will enable the patient to be continually monitored and will allow any change in condition to be easily observed while waiting for emergency personnel. The head should be positioned to keep the airway open and allow drainage from the throat and mouth. If the blood flow to the heart and brain has diminished, circulation can be improved by elevating the lower limbs, provided that the position change can be accomplished without causing further pain or breathing problems. If the patient has breathing difficulties or a chest injury or has experienced a heart attack or stroke, it may be desirable to lower blood pressure in the injured parts by elevating the upper part of the body slightly, if the position change can be accomplished without causing further pain or breathing problems.

If the patient is unconscious (Table 16–3), the examiner should reassess the level of unconsciousness and treat the patient as though a spinal injury has occurred. In the unconscious patient, the ex-

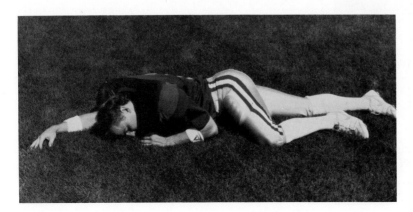

FIGURE 16–10. Recovery position.

aminer should watch for spontaneous limb movement, especially after the application of a painful stimulus, because movement indicates that the patient is less likely to have suffered a severe cervical injury.[2] In addition, the examiner should look for posturing, which indicates a severe head injury. Decerebrate rigidity is evidenced by all four extremities in extension. With decorticate rigidity, the lower limbs are in extension and the upper limbs are in flexion (see Fig. 13–30).

If cardiac or circulatory function is not compromised, the patient should be left in the original position until consciousness is regained. However, if the patient is unconscious and lying supine, the examiner should always watch for the possibility that the patient may "swallow" the tongue and

TABLE 16–3. Some Common Causes of Unconsciousness in Patients*

Category	Problem	Cause	Pathophysiology	Management
General	Loss of consciousness	Injury or disease	Shock, head injury, other injuries, diabetes, arteriosclerosis	Need for CPR, triage
Disease	Diabetic coma	Hyperglycemia and acidosis	Inadequate use of sugar, acidosis	Complex treatment for acidosis
	Insulin shock	Hypoglycemia	Excess insulin	Sugar
	Myocardial infarct	Damaged myocardium	Insufficient cardiac output	Oxygen, CPR, transport
	Stroke	Damaged brain	Loss of arterial supply to brain or hemorrhage within brain	Support, gentle transport
Injury	Hemorrhagic shock	Bleeding	Hypovolemia	Control external bleeding, recognize internal bleeding, CPR, transport
	Respiratory shock	Insufficient oxygen	Paralysis, chest damage, airway obstruction	Clear airway, supplemental oxygen, CPR, transport
	Anaphylactic shock	Acute contact with agent to which patient is sensitive	Allergic reaction	Intramuscular epinephrine, support, CPR, transport
	Cerebral contusion, concussion, or hematoma	Blunt head injury	Bleeding into or around brain, concussive effect	Airway, supplemental oxygen, CPR, careful monitoring, transport
Emotions	Psychogenic shock	Emotional reaction	Sudden drop in cerebral blood flow	Place supine, make comfortable, observe for injuries
Environment	Heatstroke	Excessive heat, inability to sweat	Brain damage from heat	Immediate cooling, support, CPR, transport
	Electric shock	Contact with electric current	Cardiac abnormalities, fibrillation	CPR, transport; do not treat until current controlled
	Systemic hypothermia	Prolonged exposure to cold	Diminished cerebral function, cardiac arrhythmias	CPR, rapid transport, warming at hospital
	Drowning	Oxygen, carbon dioxide, breath holding, water	Cerebral damage	CPR, transport
	Air embolism	Intravascular air	Obstruction to arterial blood flow by nitrogen bubbles	CPR, recompression
	Decompression sickness ("bends")	Intravascular nitrogen	Obstruction to arterial blood flow by nitrogen bubbles	CPR, recompression
Injected or ingested agents	Alcohol	Excess intake	Cerebral depression	Support, CPR, transport
	Drugs	Excess intake	Cerebral depression	Support, CPR, transport (bring drug)
	Plant poisons	Contact, ingestion	Direct cerebral or other toxic effect	Support, recognition, CPR, identify plant, local wound care, transport
	Animal poisons	Contact, ingestion, injection	Direct cerebral or other toxic effect	Recognition, support, CPR, identify agent, local wound care, transport
Neurological	Epilepsy	Brain injury, scar, genetic predisposition, disease	Excitable focus of motor activity in brain	Support, protect patient, transport in status epilepticus

*From the American Academy of Orthopedic Surgeons: Athletic Training and Sports Medicine, 2nd ed. Park Ridge, IL, AAOS, 1991, pp 618–619.

obstruct the airway. Also, an unconscious patient loses the cough reflex, and if vomiting or bleeding occurs, vomitus, mucus, or blood may enter and obstruct the airway. Thus, the examiner may elect to put the patient in the recovery position.

If the patient is unconscious and in respiratory or cardiac distress, the examiner must quickly assess the patient and attempt to restore respiratory and/or cardiac function. This patient is treated the same as the conscious patient.

If the patient's spine is twisted or flexed and the patient is reasonably comfortable, the patient should be stabilized in that position until a spinal injury is ruled out. If there has been a loss of breathing or cardiac function, the examiner must carefully correct the deformity, place the patient in the supine lying position, and perform the appropriate measures to deal with the problem.

If the patient is in the water and unconscious, the patient must be reached as quickly as possible. The rescuer should not jump into the water because this action will create waves that may rock the victim's head and could cause severe consequences if a neck injury has occurred. The examiner should approach the patient head-on and place an extended arm down the middle of the patient's back with the patient's head in the examiner's axilla. The examiner then grasps the patient's biceps with the forearm around the patient's forehead, slowly lifts the arm, and turns the patient face-up. The examiner's forearm locks the patient's head in the examiner's axilla during the turn. Once the patient is supine, both of the examiner's arms support the patient's head and spine in the water. An assistant then slides the spinal board under the patient in the water and blocks the patient's head with towels. The patient is next strapped to the spinal board with restraining straps and is lifted out of the water.[9] If a spinal board is not available and a cervical injury is suspected, the patient should be supported in the water until emergency personnel arrive.

If the patient is unconscious after playing a sport such as football in which a helmet is worn, the helmet should not be removed unless the examiner is absolutely certain that there has not been a neck injury. If the patient is in respiratory distress, facemasks can be easily removed using bolt cutters or an Exacto knife to cut the restraining straps while holding the mask in place (Figs. 16–11 and 16–12). If for whatever reason the decision is made to remove the head gear, the neck and head must be held as rigid as possible. To remove the helmet, in-line traction is first applied *to the helmet* by one individual, usually the assistant, to ensure initial stability. A second individual, usually the examiner, then stands at the side of the patient and applies in-

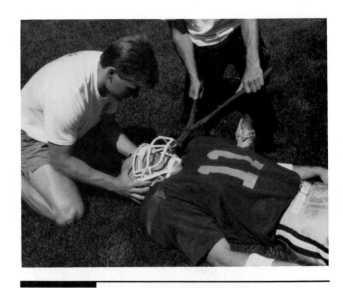

FIGURE 16–11. *Use of bolt cutters to remove mask.*

line traction by applying a traction force through the patient's chin and occiput (Fig. 16–13). The first individual stops applying traction and applies bilateral expansion to the helmet so the ears are cleared as the helmet is removed. Once the helmet is removed, the first individual reapplies in-line traction from the head, and the second individual releases the traction and continues the primary examination.[10] If desired, the examiner may apply a cervical collar such as the Stifneck collar but should do so only with caution because cervical collars do not completely eliminate movement in the cervical spine.[11]

If the patient is breathing with no difficulty, the rate and rhythm of the respirations and their characteristics should be noted. Cheyne-Stokes and

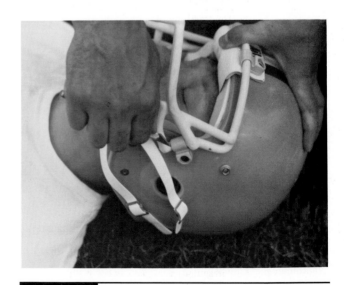

FIGURE 16–12. *Use of Exacto knife to cut mask restraining straps.*

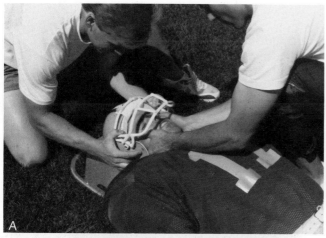

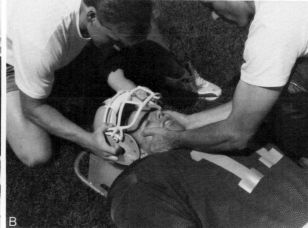

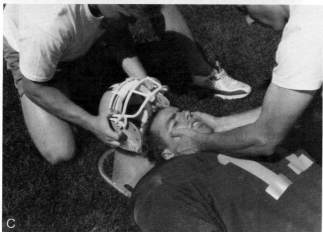

FIGURE 16–13. Removal of helmet. (A) Stabilize neck. (B) and (C) Remove helmet.

TABLE 16–4. Abnormal Breathing Patterns*

Term	Description	Location of Possible Neurological Lesions
Hyperpnea	Abnormal increase in the depth and rate of the respiratory movements	
Apnea	Periods of nonbreathing	Pons
Ataxic breathing (Biot's respiration)	Irregular breathing pattern, with deep and shallow breaths occurring randomly	Medulla
Hyperventilation	Prolonged, rapid hyperpnea, resulting in decreased carbon dioxide blood levels	Midbrain, pons
Cheyne-Stokes respirations	Periods of hyperpnea regularly alternating with periods of apnea, characterized by regular acceleration and deceleration in depth	Cerebrum, cerebellum, midbrain, pons
Cluster breathing	Breaths follow each other in disorderly sequence, with irregular pauses between them	Pons, medulla

*Adapted from Hickey, J. V.: The Clinical Practice of Neurological and Neurosurgical Nursing. Philadelphia, J. B. Lippincott Co., 1986, p. 138.

ataxic respirations are often associated with head injuries.[2] Table 16–4 indicates some of the abnormal breathing patterns that may be seen in a patient in an emergency situation.

Establishing Circulation

While the examiner is determining whether breathing is normal, the circulation should be checked (Table 16–5) for 10 or 15 seconds using the carotid (preferred), brachial, radial, or femoral pulse (Fig. 16–14). For a sedentary adult, the normal heart rate is 60 to 90 beats/min. For children, it is 80 to 100 beats/min. In the highly trained athlete of either sex, the rate may be as low as 40 beats/min. The examiner should note whether the pulse is absent, rapid and rebounding, or weak and diminishing.

The pulse is most often checked at the carotid artery because this artery is large and easy to locate. Therefore, the examiner has less chance of missing the pulse and does not have to move from the area of the patient's head to perform palpation. If a pulse cannot be detected, it is assumed that the patient

TABLE 16–5. Rapid Assessment Criteria for Circulation*

1. Skin color
2. Carotid pulse palpable (systolic blood pressure, $\geq$ 60 mm Hg)
   Femoral pulse palpable (systolic blood pressure, $\geq$ 70 mm Hg)
   Radial pulse palpable (systolic blood pressure, $\geq$ 80 mm Hg)

*Modified from Driscoll, P., and D. Skinner: Initial assessment and management—I: Primary survey. Br. Med. J. 300:1266, 1990.

does not have a heartbeat, and CPR should be initiated. When the pulse is assessed, the examiner should estimate its rate, strength, and rhythm to obtain an indication of the cardiac output. Circulatory sufficiency may also be determined by squeezing the nail bed or hypothenar eminence. Capillary refill is delayed if the pink color does not return to

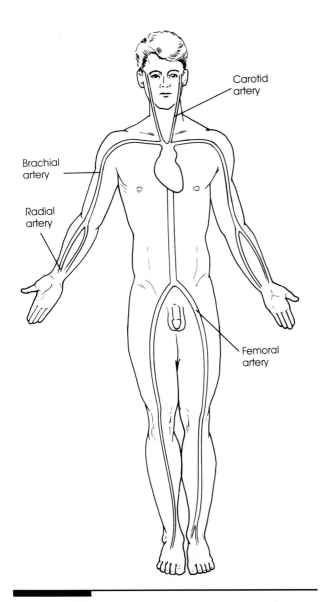

FIGURE 16–14. Location of commonly used pulses: carotid, brachial, radial, femoral.

Carotid artery
Brachial artery
Radial artery
Femoral artery

the nail bed or the hypothenar eminence within 2 seconds of the pressure's being released.[12] (Squeezing the hypothenar eminence is a better indicator when the patient is hypothermic.)

The pulse may also be used to determine the patient's blood pressure. If a carotid pulse can be palpated (Table 16–5), systolic blood pressure is 60 mm Hg or higher. If the femoral pulse can be palpated, systolic blood pressure is 70 mm Hg or higher. If the radial pulse can be palpated, systolic blood pressure is 80 mm Hg or higher.[2, 8, 12]

A weak or rapid pulse usually indicates shock, heat exhaustion, hypoglycemia, fainting, or hyperventilation. A slowing pulse is sometimes seen when there is a large increase in intracranial pressure, which usually indicates a severe lower brain stem compression.[13] A pulse that is rebounding and rapid is often the result of hypertension, fright, heat stroke, or hyperglycemia.

If the pulse rate is beginning to weaken, the patient may be going into *shock* (Fig. 16–15). Shock is characterized by signs and symptoms that occur when the cardiac output is insufficient to fill the arterial tree and the blood is under insufficient pressure to provide organs and tissues with adequate blood flow. Common types of shock and their causes are listed in Table 16–6. A patient becoming "shocky" becomes restless and anxious. The pulse will slowly become weak and rapid, and the skin will become cold and wet, often "clammy." Sweating may be profuse, and the face will initially be pale and later become cyanotic (blue) around the mouth. Respirations may be shallow, labored, rapid, or possibly irregular and gasping, especially if a chest injury has occurred. The eyes usually become dull and lusterless, and the pupils become increasingly dilated. The patient may complain of thirst and feel nauseated or vomit. If shock develops quickly, the patient may lose consciousness. To prevent or delay the onset of shock, the examiner may cover the patient, elevate the patient's legs, or attempt to eliminate the cause of the problem.

Circulatory collapse in trauma patients is primarily due to blood loss or hypovolemic shock, but the

TABLE 16–6. Types of Shock and Their Causes

Type	Cause
Hemorrhagic (hypovolemic)	Blood loss
Respiratory	Inadequate blood supply
Neurogenic	Loss of vascular control by nervous system
Psychogenic	Common fainting
Cardiogenic	Insufficient pumping of blood by the heart
Septic	Severe infection and blood vessel damage
Anaphylactic	Allergic reaction
Metabolic	Loss of body fluid

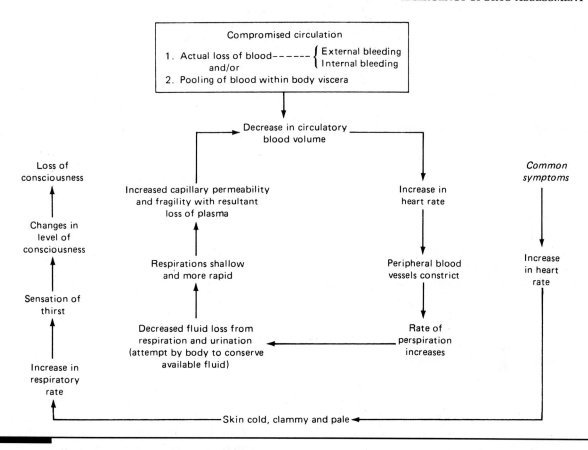

FIGURE 16–15. The shock cycle. (From Roy, S., and R. Irvin: Sports Medicine—Prevention, Evaluation, Management and Rehabilitation. © 1983, p. 84. Reprinted by permission of Prentice-Hall, Inc., Englewood Cliffs, N. J.)

examiner must remember that shock in trauma may also be due to tension pneumothorax, central nervous system injury, or pericardial tamponade (heart compression due to blood in the pericardium). The normal ranges of blood pressure are 100 to 120 mm Hg for systolic pressure and 60 to 80 mm Hg for diastolic pressure. With shock, the blood pressure will gradually decrease. If one is able to measure the blood pressure, it is best to assume that shock is developing in any injured adult whose systolic blood pressure is 100 mm Hg or less.

If the examiner is caring for a dark-skinned individual, it is often difficult to determine from observation whether the patient is going into shock. A healthy person with dark skin will usually have a red undertone and show a healthy pink color in the nail beds, lips, and mucous membranes of the mouth and tongue. A dark-skinned individual in shock, however, will have a gray cast to the skin around the nose and mouth (Fig. 16–16), especially if respiratory shock is being experienced. The mucous membranes of the mouth and tongue, lips, and nail

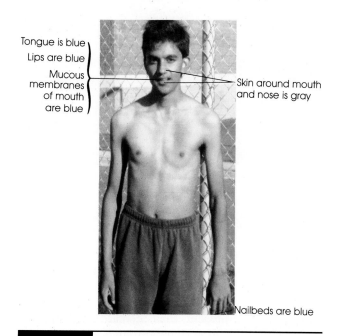

FIGURE 16–16. Determining shock in a dark-skinned victim.

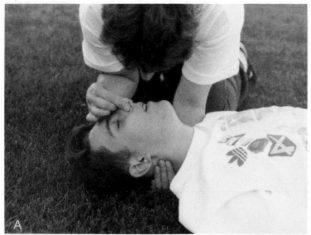

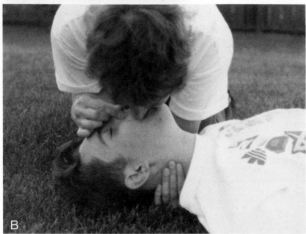

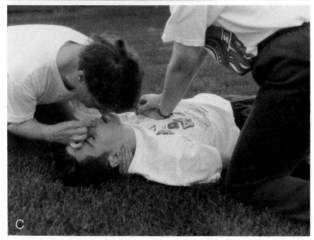

FIGURE 16–17. *The ABCs of cardiopulmonary resuscitation. (A) Checking airway. (B) Applying breath to patient. (C) Cardiac compressions for circulation.*

beds will have a blue tinge. If the shock is due to hypovolemia, the mucous membranes of the mouth and tongue will not be blue but rather will have a pale, graying, waxy pallor.[14]

If no pulse is present, then the cardiac portion of CPR techniques should be initiated (Fig. 16–17). Equipment such as shoulder or rib pads should be

removed, at least anteriorly, to give the examiner clear access to the anterior chest wall. It should be remembered that CPR provides only approximately 25% of normal cardiac output, so it is imperative that it is performed properly by knowledgeable individuals.[15] CPR is maintained until the patient recovers or emergency personnel arrive. If the patient might have a cervical spine injury, CPR must be done with care, because compression to the heart can cause repeated flexion/extension of the cervical spine.[5]

The examiner should look for any signs of external bleeding or hemorrhage. The types of wounds in which external bleeding or hemorrhage may be seen are incisions, which involve clean cuts, or lacerations, which have jagged edges. A contusion may produce internal bleeding, whereas a puncture or abrasion may also show bleeding or oozing on the surface. Of the five types of wounds, the puncture wound is probably the most difficult to treat because it has the highest probability of infection. The examiner should watch for bleeding from the lungs, which is indicated by bright, red, frothy blood appearing in the mouth. If there is bleeding from the stomach, it usually appears with vomitus and looks like coffee grounds. Bleeding from the upper bowel will produce tarry-black stools. If the bleeding is from the lower bowel, the blood appears normal when it accompanies the stools. If the bleeding is from the kidneys, it will cause the urine to have a smoky, red appearance. If the bleeding occurs in the bladder, the urine will have a redder appearance, and the patient may have difficulty urinating. If the liver, spleen, or kidney is injured, serious internal bleeding may result, and the blood will not be visible but will be contained within the abdominal cavity. In this case, the patient may experience abdominal rigidity, pain, and difficulty in breathing.

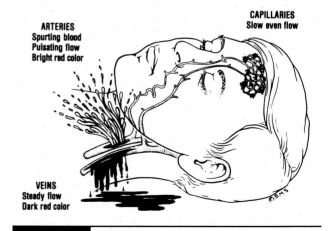

FIGURE 16–18. *Bleeding characteristics. (From Hafen, B. Q., and K. J. Karren: First Aid and Emergency Care Skills Manual. Englewood, NJ, Morton Pub. Co., 1982, p. 70.)*

When inspecting a bleeding structure, the examiner should note the type of vessel affected. For example, an artery will spurt blood, whereas a vein will provide an even flow. Capillaries tend to ooze bright blood (Fig. 16–18).[6] Because arterial bleeding is of greatest concern, the examiner must be aware of the pressure points in the body (Fig. 16–19) to apply proper treatment. The examiner chooses the pressure point closest to the area of bleeding and applies pressure to the artery to slow or stop the bleeding. Tourniquets should be used only with extreme caution and in selected instances (e.g., accidental amputation of a limb, very severe bleeding from a major artery, or the need to apply CPR with no assistance available). If a tourniquet is used, the time of tourniquet application should be carefully noted. Hemodynamic stability is best maintained by applying direct pressure to an open wound, keeping the patient in a recumbent position, and minimizing the number of times the patient is moved.[4]

If signs and symptoms of shock are present but visible bleeding is minimal, the examiner should suspect hidden bleeding within the abdomen, chest, or extremities.[2, 16] If bleeding is suspected in the abdomen, the examiner should check the abdominal wall for shape and distention. To check for bleeding in the chest or extremities, the examiner should look for deformities (e.g., fractures). Using the fingers to percuss the chest area and noting any loss of hollow sounds may help locate the presence of fluid or blood. Hyporesonance may indicate a solid organ or the presence of fluid or blood. Hyperresonance usually indicates air- or gas-filled spaces.[2]

Once the airway and the pulmonary and circulatory systems have been assessed and controlled, the examiner can proceed to the remainder of the primary assessment. The examiner should check the ears and nose for the presence of cerebrospinal fluid. If blood or cerebrospinal fluid leaks from the ear, it may be indicative of a skull fracture. The examiner should incline the head toward the affected side to facilitate drainage, unless a cervical injury is suspected. The examiner can place a gauze pad over the ear or nose where the bleeding is occurring to collect the fluid on the gauze (Fig. 16–20). The examiner should look for an "orange halo" forming on the pad (see Fig. 13–36). The halo is cerebrospinal fluid, the presence of which is a good indication of a skull fracture.[17]

Pupil Check

The examiner checks the pupils for shape and for response to light by using a pen light or covering the eye with one hand and then taking it away. Pupil reactions are normally the result of the intensity of light or focal distance. The pupils dilate in a dark environment or with a long focal distance, and they constrict in a light environment or with a short

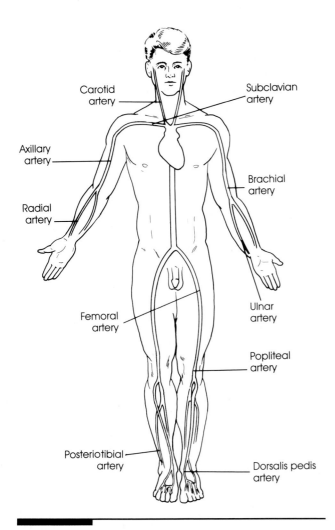

FIGURE 16–19. Pressure points in the body.

Carotid artery
Subclavian artery
Axillary artery
Radial artery
Brachial artery
Femoral artery
Ulnar artery
Popliteal artery
Posteriotibial artery
Dorsalis pedis artery

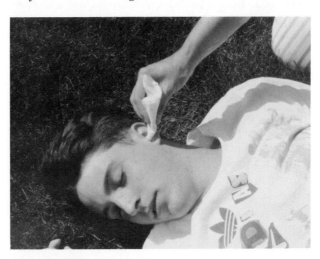

FIGURE 16–20. Checking the ear for possible bleeding and/or cerebrospinal fluid.

focal distance. Normally, the pupils are equally or almost equally dilated (diameter range of 2 to 6 mm and mean of 3.5 mm), but injury to the central nervous system (e.g., head injury) may cause the pupils to dilate unevenly. In a fully conscious, alert individual who has sustained a blow near the eye, a dilated fixed pupil is most likely the result of trauma to the short ciliary nerves of that eye rather than the result of third cranial nerve compression due to brain herniation.[4] Drugs may also affect the pupillary size. For example, opiate drugs cause pinpoint pupils, whereas amphetamines may cause dilated pupils.[2]

To test pupil reaction, the examiner holds one hand over one eye, moves the hand away quickly, or shines the light from a pen light into the eye, and then observes the pupil's reaction. The examiner tests the other eye in a similar fashion and compares the results. The pupillary reaction is classified as brisk (normal), sluggish, nonreactive, or fixed. An ovoid, or slightly oval, pupil or one fixed and dilated pupil indicates increasing intracranial pressure.[2] If both pupils are midsize, midposition, and nonreactive, midbrain damage is usually indicated. The fixation and dilation of both pupils are terminal signs of anoxia and ischemia to the brain.[2, 18]

Neural Watch

The patient's level of consciousness is then reassessed. The examiner should institute a *neural watch* (Table 16–7) or a similar observation scheme to note changes, if present, in the patient over time. The neural watch should be performed continuously every 5 to 15 minutes, as it also facilitates monitoring the patient's vital signs.[2] Once the patient has stabilized, neural watch recordings may be made every 15 to 30 minutes.[13] If possible, reassessment by the same examiner allows the detection of subtle changes.

The examination should include evaluation of the patient's facial expression; determination of the patient's orientation to time, place, and person; and presence of both posttraumatic amnesia and retrograde amnesia. Signs and symptoms that demand emergency action in an individual who has sustained a blow to the head are increased headache, nausea and vomiting, inequality of pupils, disorientation, progressive or sudden impairment of consciousness, gradual increase in blood pressure, and diminution of pulse rate.

Reaction to pain and level of consciousness can be determined by using physical and verbal stimuli. Verbal stimuli may include calling the patient's name and shaking and shouting at the patient if there is no cervical injury. Physical stimuli include

TABLE 16–7. Neural Watch Chart*

Unit		Time 1 ( )	Time 2 ( )	Time 3 ( )
I. Vital signs	Blood pressure Pulse Respirations Temperature			
II. Conscious and	Oriented Disoriented Restless Combative			
	Unconscious			
III. Speech	Clear Rambling Garbled None			
IV. Will awaken to	Name Shaking Light pain Strong pain			
V. Nonverbal reaction to pain	Appropriate Inappropriate "Decerebrate" None			
VI. Pupils	Size on right Size on left Reacts on right Reacts on left			
VII. Ability to move	Right arm Left arm Right leg Left leg			
VIII. Sensation	Right side (normal/abnormal) Left side (normal/abnormal) Dermatome affected (specify) Peripheral nerve affected (specify)			

*Modified from American Academy of Orthopedic Surgeons: Athletic Training and Sports Medicine. Park Ridge, IL, AAOS, 1984, p. 399.

squeezing the Achilles tendon, squeezing the trapezius muscle, squeezing the soft tissue between the patient's thumb and index finger, squeezing an object (pen or pencil) between the patient's fingers, squeezing a fingertip, or applying a knuckle to the sternum (this must be done with caution as it may cause bruising) (Fig. 16–21). In comatose patients, a motor response to a painful stimulus to an extremity may indicate intact pain appreciation from that site, especially if it is accompanied by a more remote response such as a grimace or a change in respirations or pulse.[4]

The level of consciousness can be best determined with the *Glasgow Coma Scale* (GCS)[19] (Table 16–8).

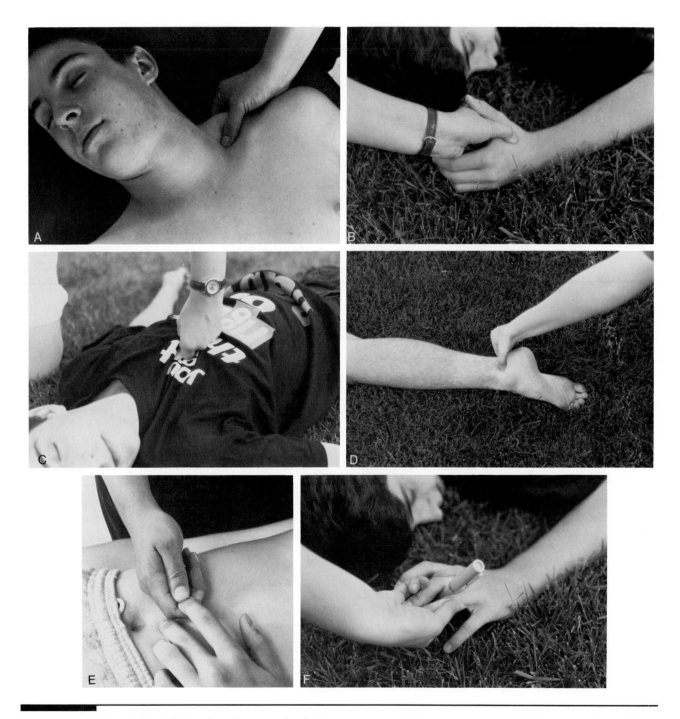

FIGURE 16–21. Use of physical stimuli to determine level of consciousness. (A) Squeezing trapezius. (B) Squeezing the soft tissue between thumb and index finger. (C) Knuckle to sternum. (D) Squeezing the Achilles tendon. (E) Squeezing a fingertip. (F) Squeezing a pen with the fingers.

TABLE 16–8. Glasgow Coma Scale

				Time 1 (___)	Time 2 (___)
Eyes	Open	Spontaneously	4		
		To verbal command	3		
		To pain	2		
		No response	1	_____	_____
Best motor response	To verbal command	Obeys	6		
	To painful stimulus*	Localizes pain	5		
		Flexion-withdrawal	4		
		Flexion-abnormal (decorticate rigidity)	3		
		Extension (decerebrate rigidity)	2		
		No response	1	_____	_____
Best verbal response†		Oriented and converses	5		
		Disoriented and converses	4		
		Inappropriate words	3		
		Incomprehensible sounds	2		
		No response	1	_____	_____
Total			3–15	_____	_____

*Apply knuckles to sternum; observe arms.
†Arouse patient with painful stimulus if necessary.
The Glasgow Coma Scale, which is based on eye opening, verbal, and motor responses, is a practical means of monitoring changes in level of consciousness. If responses on the scale are given grades, the overall responsiveness of the patient can be expressed in a score that is the summation of the grades. The lowest score is 3, and the highest is 15.

The sooner the patient is tested using this scale, the better, as the initial assessment can be used as a baseline for improvement or deterioration in the patient. The GCS is often performed in conjunction with the neural watch.

The first test of the GCS relates to eye opening. Eye opening may be spontaneous, in response to speech or in response to pain, or there may be no response at all. Each of these responses is given a score. For example, spontaneous eye opening is given a value of 4, response to speech is given a value of 3, response to pain is given a value of 2, and no response at all is given a value of 1. Spontaneous opening of the eyes indicates functioning of the ascending reticular activating system. This finding does not necessarily mean that the patient is aware of the surroundings or what is happening but does imply that the patient is in a state of arousal. A patient who opens the eyes in response to the examiner's voice is probably responding to the stimulus of sound, not necessarily to the command to do something, such as opening the eyes. If unsure, the examiner may try different sound-making objects (e.g., bell, horn, whistle) to elicit an appropriate response.

Motor response is given a value of 6 if the patient responds to a verbal command. Otherwise, the patient is scored on a five-point scale depending on the motor response to a painful stimulus. When scoring motor responses, it is the ease with which the motor responses are elicited that constitutes the criteria on for the best response. Commands given to the patient should be simple, such as "Move your arm." The patient should not be asked to squeeze the examiner's hand, nor should the examiner place something in the patient's hand and then ask the patient to grasp it. This action may cause a reflex grasp rather than a response to a command.[20]

If the patient does not give a motor response to a verbal command, the examiner should attempt to elicit a motor response to a painful stimulus. The type and quality of the patient's reaction to the painful stimulus constitute the scoring criteria. The stimulus should not be applied to the face because painful stimuli in the facial area may cause the eyes to close tightly as a protective reaction. Examples of applying a painful stimulus are shown in Figure 16–21. The painful stimulus should be applied to an area in which no injury has occurred and only in an amount sufficient to evoke a response. If the patient moves a limb when the painful stimulus is applied to more than one point or the patient tries to remove the hand of the examiner that is applying the painful stimulus, the patient is localizing, and a value of 5 should be given. If the patient withdraws rapidly from the painful stimulus, a normal reflex withdrawal is being shown, and a value of 4 should be assigned. However, if application of a painful stimulus creates a decorticate or decerebrate posture (see Fig. 13–30), an abnormal response is being demonstrated, and a value of 3 for the decorticate posture or a value of 2 for the decerebrate posture is given. With decorticate posturing, the arms, wrists, and fingers are flexed, the upper limbs are adducted, and the legs are extended, medially rotated, and plantar flexed. Decerebrate posturing, which has a poorer prognosis, involves extension, adduction, and hyperpronation of the arms, whereas the lower limbs are the same as for decorticate posturing.[21] Decerebrate rigidity is usually bilateral.

If the patient exhibits no reaction to the painful stimulus, a value of 1 is assigned. It is important to be sure that the "no" response is due to a head injury and not due to a spinal cord injury (flaccid paralysis) and thus lack of feeling or sensation. Any difference in reaction between limbs should be carefully noted, as this finding may be indicative of a specific focal injury.[22]

Verbal response is graded on a five-point scale and measures the person's speech in response to simple questions such as "Where are you?" or "Are you winning the game?"[21] For verbal responses, the patient who converses appropriately will show proper orientation and be aware of self as well as of the environment and is given a grade of 5. The patient who is confused will be disoriented and unable to completely interface with the environment. The patient will be able to converse with the appropriate words and will be given a grade of 4. The patient exhibiting inappropriate speech will be unable to sustain a conversation with the examiner. This individual will be given a grade of 3. The term "vocalizing patient" implies that the patient will only groan or make incomprehensible sounds. This finding is assigned a grade of 2. Again, the examiner should make note of any possible mechanical reason for the inability to verbalize. If the patient makes no sounds and thus has no verbal response, a grade of 1 is assigned.

It is vital that the initial scores on the GCS and the neural watch be obtained as soon as possible after the onset of the injury because amnesia may occur 10 to 20 minutes after a blow to the head or there may be an expanding intracranial lesion.[20] With the GCS, the initial score is used as a basis for determining the severity of the patient's head injury. Patients who maintain a score of 8 or less on the GCS for 6 hours or longer are considered to have a serious head injury. A patient who scores from 9 to 11 is considered to have a moderate head injury, and one who scores 12 or more is considered to have a mild head injury.[22]

Deterioration of consciousness may be due to many conditions, such as increased intracranial pressure caused by an expanding intracranial lesion, hypoxia (which can aggravate cerebral edema and increase intracranial pressure), epilepsy, meningitis, or fat embolism. The examiner should always look for signs of expanding intracranial lesions, especially if the patient is conscious. These lesions are emergency conditions that must be attended to immediately because of their potentially high mortality rate (up to 50%). An expanding intracranial lesion is indicated by an altered lucid state (state of consciousness), developing of inequality of the pupils, unusual slowing of the heart rate (which primarily occurs after a lucid interval), irregular eye movements, and eyes that no longer track properly. There is also a tendency for the patient to demonstrate increased body temperature and irregular respiration. Normal intracranial pressure ranges from 4 to 15 mm Hg, and intracranial pressure of more than 20 mm Hg is considered abnormal. Intracranial pressure of 40 mm Hg causes neurological dysfunction and impairment. Although the examiner in the emergency care setting has no way of determining the intracranial pressure, the signs and symptoms previously mentioned will provide an indication that the pressure is increasing. Most patients who experience an increase in intracranial pressure complain of severe headache followed by vomiting that may be projectile.

Signs and symptoms that indicate a good possibility of recovery for a head-injured patient, especially after unconsciousness, include response to noxious stimuli, eye opening, pupil activity, spontaneous eye movement, intact oculovestibular reflexes, and appropriate motor function responses. Neurological signs indicating a poor prognosis after a head injury include nonreactive pupils, absence of oculovestibular reflexes, severe extension patterns or no motor response at all, and increased intracranial pressure.[22]

If the patient experiences loss of consciousness or appears to have disturbed senses, is seeing stars or colors, is dizzy, or has auditory hallucinations, or a severe headache, the patient should not be left alone or allowed to return to activity (Table 16–9). In addition, nausea, vomiting, lethargy, increasing blood pressure, disturbed sensation of smell, or diminished pulse would lead the examiner to the same conclusion. Amnesia, hyperirritability, an open wound, unequal pupils, or leaking of cerebrospinal fluid or blood from the ears or nose also indicates an emergency condition. Numbness on one side of the body or a large contusion in the head area would likewise lead the examiner to handle the patient with care. If the frontal area of the brain is affected, the patient may experience lapses of memory, personality changes, or impairment of judgment. If the temporal lobe has been affected, the patient may experience feelings of unreality, déja vu, and hallucinations involving odors, sounds or visual disturbances such as macropsia (seeing objects as larger than they really are) and micropsia. The literature indicates that head injury is dependent not only on the magnitude and direction of impact and the structural features and physical reactions of the skull but also on the state of the head at the moment of impact.[1, 10, 21]

Assessment for Movement

The examiner asks the patient to move the limbs to reassess for a cervical spine injury and look for

mation should be clarified in an attempt to find out what happened and what injury or injuries the patient feels have occurred. (See the different chapters in this book for appropriate questions related to specific joints or areas of the body.) The patient can often provide the examiner with the diagnosis if the examiner listens carefully. Once the patient has been thoroughly questioned, others who witnessed the accident or injury may also be questioned to complete the history. Informed conversation with other individuals sometimes helps to detect abnormal behavior that might not be initially noticed. If the patient has a previous medical file, it may also prove beneficial to review the contents for information regarding preexisting conditions, previous trauma, and medications.

As the patient history is obtained, the examiner continues to observe the patient and notes levels of consciousness, developing symptoms, pain patterns, and altered functional abilities. In addition, the examiner should carefully watch for developing signs and symptoms such as expanding intracranial lesions by noting changes in facial expression, the pupils, and the level of consciousness by performing the neural watch and GCS several times. The basic observation stage is the same as the observation demonstrated during joint assessment by noting bony and soft-tissue contours, scars, deformities, the ability to move, and body alignment.

The next part of the secondary assessment is the scanning examination, in which the examiner quickly scans the entire body through observation, by asking the patient to make particular movements (depending on where the suspected injury has occurred), and by testing myotomes, dermatomes, and reflexes. During this phase, the examiner should explain what is being done and why, not only to reassure the patient but also to ensure cooperation and relaxation. This part of the examination may be done without removing the patient's clothes, although it is better to do so because clothing may obstruct the view of the injured area. However, if the examination is being performed in the presence of other people, clothing removal, especially if the patient will be embarrassed, should be left to a later time, or the patient should be moved to a more appropriate location. If the clothes must be removed, the patient should be warned, especially if in a public place, and every effort should be made to maintain the patient's dignity.

Once the specific area or areas of injury have been narrowed down through the scanning examination, the examiner can perform a detailed assessment of the different parts of the body, as specified previously in other chapters. Failure to perform a proper examination may lead to a missed assessment and more problems than originally anticipated.

TABLE 16–13. Emergency Care Levels of Decision*

1. Is the injury life threatening?
2. What care (first-aid) must be given on-site or "on the field"?
3. Can and should the patient be moved?
4. If the patient is to be moved, what is the best way to do it?
5. What steps are to be taken before the patient is moved? Spinal board? Splinting? Instruction?
6. If the patient is to be moved, where to? Side lines? Locker room? Training room? Hospital?
7. How is the patient to be transported? Ambulance? Parent's vehicle?
8. If the injury is not severe enough to require transportation to the hospital, what protocols are to be followed for return to activity?
9. If the patient is not allowed to return to activity, what protocols are to be followed?

*Adapted from Haines, A.: Principles of emergency care. Athletic J. 26:66–67, 1984.

The patient must be immediately sent to a hospital or trauma center if at any time during the primary or secondary evaluation the following signs are exhibited: pupillary or extraocular movement abnormality, facial or extremity weakness, amnesia, confusion or lethargy, sensory or cranial nerve abnormality, Babinski sign, deep tendon reflex asymmetry, or posttraumatic seizures.[18, 34] Proper care for the patient must always be uppermost in the mind of the examiner. Table 16–13 outlines the levels of decision making required of the examiner in the emergency sports assessment.

PRÉCIS OF THE EMERGENCY SPORTS ASSESSMENT (Fig. 16–22)

CASE STUDIES

When reviewing or practicing these case studies, the examiner should outline the necessary protocol for dealing with the described situations. The examiner can develop different scenarios depending on the degree of severity of the injury. These scenarios, including assessment and movement of the patient, should be practiced often so that the examiner is fully aware of how to handle emergency situations.

1. A diver misjudges his take-off from the 10-m board, hits his head on the concrete platform, and falls unconscious into the pool, displaying decorticate rigidity as he falls. Describe your emergency protocol for this patient.
2. A squash player is playing a game and is struck near the eye by her opponent's squash racquet. Describe your emergency protocol for this patient.

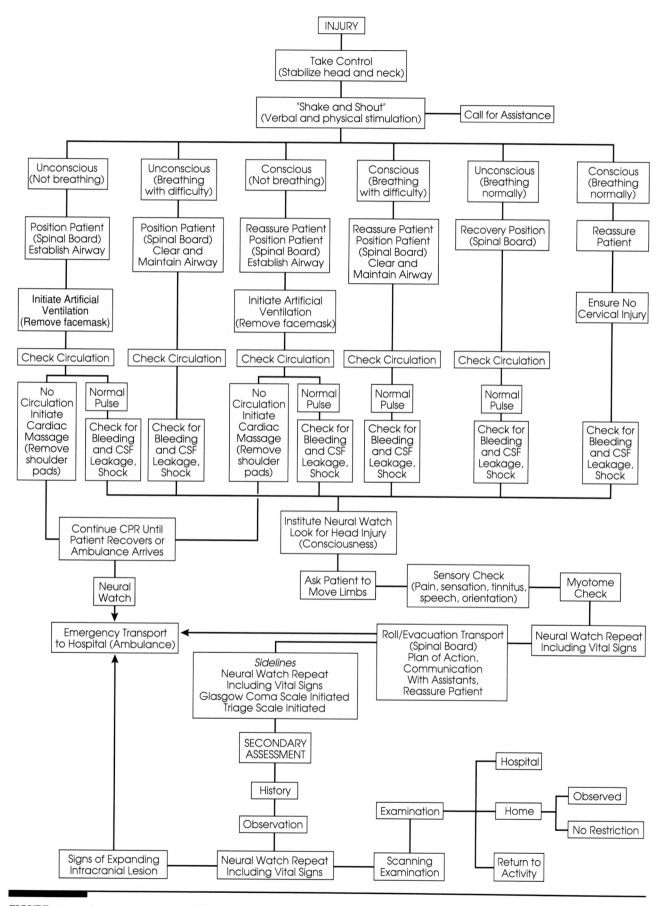

FIGURE 16–22. *Assessment sequence following acute injury.*

3. A 22-year-old professional basketball player is playing in a game. He is under his own net and suddenly collapses and lapses into unconsciousness. Describe your emergency protocol for this patient.

4. During a race on a hot, humid day, a 10,000-m runner collapses on the track during the event and lies motionless. Describe your emergency protocol for this patient.

5. During a baseball game, a batter is hit on the chest by a pitched ball and collapses at home plate. Describe your emergency protocol for this patient.

6. A defensive back tackles a runner and makes the tackle but does not move when the other players get up, even though he is conscious. He is having difficulty breathing. Describe your emergency protocol for this patient.

7. A rugby player hits his head during a collapsing scrum. He is knocked unconscious, is not breathing, and has no pulse. Describe your emergency protocol for this patient.

8. A hockey player receives a deep cut to the neck when another player's skate accidentally cuts him. He is bleeding profusely. Describe your emergency protocol for this patient.

9. A gymnast on the balance beam misses her dismount and lands on her head, neck, and shoulder and is knocked unconscious. Describe your emergency protocol for this patient.

10. A wrestler is thrown to the mat near the end of the first round. He lands quite hard on the side of his face with his neck twisted. He is lying prone and unconscious. Describe your emergency protocol for this patient.

11. While playing soccer, an athlete is stung by a bee and develops anaphylactic shock. Describe your emergency protocol for this patient.

12. A hockey player is "boarded" into the boards from behind. He falls to the ice and has difficulty breathing; he had been chewing gum. Describe your emergency protocol for this patient.

REFERENCES

CITED REFERENCES

1. Torg, J. S., T. C. Quedenfeld, and W. Newell: When the athlete's life is threatened. Phys. Sportsmed. 3:54–60, 1975.
2. Ward, R.: Emergency nursing priorities of the head injured patient. AXON 11:9–12, 1989.
3. Beaver, B. M.: Care of the multiple trauma victim—The first hour. Nurs. Clin. North Am. 25:11–21, 1990.
4. Hugenholtz, H., and M. T. Richard: The on-site management of athletes with head injuries. Phys. Sportsmed. 11:71–78, 1983.
5. Steichen, F. M.: The emergency management of the severely injured. J. Trauma 12:786–790, 1972.
6. American Academy of Orthopedic Surgeons: Emergency Care and Transportation of the Sick and Injured. Chicago, A. A. O. S., 1981.
7. Hochbaum, S. R.: Emergency airway management. Emerg. Med. Clin. North Am. 4:411–425, 1986.
8. Driscoll, P., and D. Skinner: Initial assessment and management—I: Primary survey. Br. Med. J. 300:1265–1266, 1990.
9. Richards, R. N.: Rescuing the spine-injured diver. Phys. Sportsmed. 3:67–71, 1975.
10. Vegso, J. J., M. H. Bryant, and J. S. Torg: Field evaluation of head and neck injuries. In Torg, J. S. (ed.): Athletic Injuries to the Head, Neck and Face. Philadelphia, Lea & Febiger, 1982.
11. Aprahamian, C., B. M. Thompson, W. A. Finger, and J. C. Darin: Experimental cervical spine injury model: Evaluation of airway management and splinting techniques. Ann. Emerg. Med. 13:584–587, 1984.
12. Keitz, J. E.: Emergent assessment of the multiple trauma patient. Ortho. Nurs. 8:29–32, 1989.
13. Hayward, R.: Management of Acute Head Injuries. Oxford, Blackwell Scientific Pub., 1980.
14. Hafen, B. Q., and K. J. Karren: First Aid and Emergency Care Skills Manual. Englewood, Colorado. Morton Pub. Co., 1982.
15. Jackson, R. E., and S. B. Freeman: Hemodynamics of cardiac massage. Emerg. Med. Clin. North Am. 1:501–513, 1983.
16. Rose, C. C.: Radiologic triage of the multiply-injured patient. Emerg. Med. Clin. North Am. 3:425–436, 1985.
17. Booher, J. M., and G. A. Thibodeau: Athletic Injury Assessment. St. Louis, C. V. Mosby Co., 1989.
18. Mahoney, B. D., and E. Ruiz: Acute resuscitation of the patient with head and spinal cord injuries. Emerg. Med. Clin. North Am. 1:583–594, 1983.
19. Teasdale, G., and B. Jennett: Assessment of coma and impaired consciousness—A practical scale. Lancet 2:81–83, 1974.
20. Topel, J. L.: Examination of the comatose patient. In Weiner, W. J., and C. G. Goetz (eds.): Neurology for the Non-Neurologist. Philadelphia, J. B. Lippincott, 1989.
21. Gerberich, S. G., J. D. Priest, J. Grafft, and R. C. Siebert: Injuries to the brain and spinal cord—Assessment, emergency care and prevention. Minn. Med. Nov:691–696, 1982.
22. Manzi, D. B., and P. A. Weaver: Head Injury: The Acute Care Phase. Thorofare, New Jersey, Slack Inc., 1987.
23. Davidoff, G., M. Jakubowski, D. Thomas, and M. Alpert: The spectrum of closed-head injuries in facial trauma victims: Incidence and impact. Ann. Emerg. Med. 17:27–30, 1988.
24. Baker, S. P., B. O'Neill, W. Haddon, and W. B. Long: The Injury Severity Score: A method for describing patients with multiple injuries and evaluating emergency care. J. Trauma 14:187–196, 1974.
25. Baker, S. P., and B. O'Neill: The Injury Severity Score: An update. J. Trauma 16:882–885, 1976.
26. Greenspan, L., B. A. McLellan, and H. Greig: Abbreviated Injury Scale and Injury Severity Score: A scoring chart. J. Trauma 25:60–64, 1985.
27. Champion, H. R., W. J. Sacco, A. J. Carnazzo, W. Copes, and W. J. Fouty: Trauma Score. Crit. Care Med. 9:672–676, 1981.
28. Champion, H. R., W. J. Sacco, D. S. Hannon, R. L. Lepper, E. S. Atzinger, W. S. Copes, and R. H. Prall: Assessment of injury severity: The triage index. Crit. Care Med. 8:201–208, 1980.
29. Lindsey, D.: Teaching the initial management of major multiple system trauma. J. Trauma 20:160–162, 1980.
30. Hawkins, M. L., R. C. Treat, and A. R. Masberger: Trauma victims: Field triage guidelines. South. Med. J. 80:562–565, 1987.
31. Clemmer, T. P., J. F. Orme, F. Thomas, and K. A. Brooks: Prospective evaluation of the CRAMS scale for triaging major trauma. J. Trauma 25:188–191, 1985.
32. Kirkpatrick, J. R., and R. L. Youmans: Trauma index—An aid in the evaluation of injury victims. J. Trauma 11:711–714, 1971.
33. Hugenholtz, H., and M. T. Richard: Return to athletic competition following concussion. C. M. A. J. 127:827–829, 1982.
34. Jones, R. K.: Assessment of minimal head injuries: Indications for in-hospital care. Surg. Neurol. 2:101–104, 1974.

GENERAL REFERENCES

American Academy of Orthopedic Surgeons: Athletic Training and Sports Medicine. Chicago, A. A. O. S., 1984.
Andrews, J.: Difficult diagnoses in blunt thoracoabdominal trauma. J. Emerg. Nurs. 15:399–404, 1989.
Arnheim, D. D.: Modern Principles of Athletic Training. St. Louis, C. V. Mosby Co., 1985.
Axe, M. J.: Limb-threatening injuries in sport. Clin. Sports Med 8:101–109, 1989.

Bailes, J. E., and J. C. Maroon: Management of cervical spine injuries in athletes. Clin. Sports Med. 8:43–58, 1989.

Dailey, R. H.: Acute upper airway obstruction. Emerg. Med. Clin. North Am. 1:261–277, 1983.

Davies, G. J., and C. Y. Anast: The fractured femur: Acute emergency care treatment. J. Orthop. Sports Phys. Ther. 1:53–58, 1979.

De Podesta, M.: A practical and effective approach in dealing with emergency situations. C. A. T. A. J. 9:5–8, 1982.

Diamond, D. L.: Sports-related abdominal trauma. Clin. Sports Med. 8:91–99, 1989.

Fahey, T. D.: Athletic Training—Principles and Practice. Palo Alto, Calif., Mayfield Pub. Co., 1986.

Gansche, M., D. P. Henderson, and J. S. Seidel: Vital signs as part of the prehospital assessment of the pediatric patient: A survey of paramedics. Ann. Emerg. Med. 19:173–178, 1990.

Greensher, J., H. C. Mofenson, and N. J. Merlis: First aid for school athletic emergencies. N. Y. State J. Med. 79:1058–1062, 1979.

Haines, A.: Principles of emergency care. Athletic J. 26:8–10+, 1984.

Halpern, J. S.: Clinical notebook—Upper extremity peripheral nerve assessment. J. Emerg. Nurs. 15:261–265, 1989.

Halpern, J. S.: Clinical notebook—Lower extremity peripheral nerve assessment. J. Emerg. Nurs. 15:333–337, 1989.

Hawkins, M. L., R. C. Treat, and A. R. Mansberger: The Trauma Score: A simple method to evaluate quality of care. Am. Surg. 54:204–206, 1988.

Hickey, J. V.: The Clinical Practice of Neurological and Neurosurgical Nursing. Philadelphia, J. B. Lippincott, 1986.

Jacobs, L. M., A. Sinclair, A. Beisner, and R. B. D'Agostino: Prehospital advanced life support: Benefits in trauma. J. Trauma 24:8–13, 1984.

Kane, G., R. Engelhardt, J. Celentino, W. Koenig, J. Yamanka, P. McKinney, M. Brewer, and D. Fife: Empirical development and evaluation of prehospital trauma triage instruments. J. Trauma 25:482–489, 1985.

Levin, H. S., V. M. O'Donnell, and R. G. Grossman: The Galveston orientation and amnesia test (G. O. A. T.)—A practical scale to assess cognition after head injury. J. Nerv. Ment. Dis. 167:675–684, 1979.

Long, S. E., S. E. Reid, H. J. Sweeney, and W. W. Johnson: Removing football helmets safely. Phys. Sportsmed. 8(10):119, 1980.

McKnight, W.: Understanding the patient in emergency. Can. Nurse July:20–23, 1976.

Meislen, H. W., K. V. Iserson, K. R. Kaback, M. Kobernick, A. B. Sanders, and S. Seifert: Airway trauma. Emerg. Med. Clin. North Am. 1:295-312, 1983.

Moore, S.: Airway maintenance—A primary consideration in the unconscious athlete. Athletic Training Spring:48–49, 1981.

Round Table: Guidelines to help you in giving on-field care. Phys. Sportsmed. 3:51–63, 1975.

Roy, S., and R. Irvin: Sports Medicine—Prevention, Evaluation, Management, and Rehabilitation. Englewood Cliffs, N. J. Prentice Hall, 1983.

Ryan, A. J.: On-field diagnosis of head injuries. Phys. Sportsmed. 4:82-84, 1976.

San Diego Sports Medicine Center: Athletic Injury Disaster Plan. San Diego, Valhalla High School, 1987.

Schneider, R. C., and F. C. Kiss. First aid and diagnosis—The treatment of head injuries. In Schneider, R. C. (ed.): Head and Neck Injuries in Football. Baltimore, Williams & Wilkins, 1973.

Schneider, R. C.: The treatment of the athlete with neck, cervical spine and cervical cord trauma. In Schneider, R. C., J. C. Kennedy, and M. L. Plant (eds.): Sports Injuries—Mechanisms, Prevention and Treatment. Baltimore, Williams & Wilkins, 1985.

Shatney, C. H.: Initial resuscitation and assessment of patients with multisystem blunt trauma. South. Med. J. 81:501–506, 1988.

Shires, G. T.: Initial management of the severely injured patient. J. A. M. A. 213:1872–1878, 1970.

Teasdale, G., and B. Jennett: Assessment of coma and impaired consciousness—A practical scale. Lancet 2 (July):81–83, 1974.

Walters, B. C., and I. McNeill: Improving the record of patient assessment in the trauma room. J. Trauma 30:398–409, 1990.

Weigelt, J. A.: Initial management of the trauma patient. Crit. Care Clin. 2:705–716, 1986.

Werman, H. A., R. N. Nelson, J. E. Campbell, R. L. Fowler, and P. Gandy: Basic trauma life support. Ann. Emerg. Med. 16:1240–1243, 1987.

West, J. G., M. A. Murdock, L. C. Baldwin, and E. Whalen: A method for evaluating field triage criteria. J. Trauma 26:655–659, 1986.

Wilberger, J. E., and J. C. Maroon: Head injuries in athletes. Clin. Sports Med. 8:1–9, 1989.

Yarnell, P. R., and S. Lynch: The "ding": Amnesic states in football trauma. Neurology 23:196–197, 1973.

Index